Medical Office Procedures

7TH Edition

Nenna L. Bayes, BBA, M.Ed.
Professor, Program Coordinator of Office Systems
Administration, Ashland Community and Technical College

Bonnie J. Crist, M.Ed., CMA (AAMA)
Medical Program Director, Harrison College

Karonne J. Becklin, M.Ed., CMA
Anoka Technical College

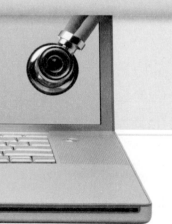

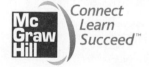

Connect
Learn
Succeed™

The McGraw-Hill Companies

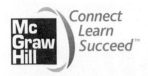

MEDICAL OFFICE PROCEDURES, SEVENTH EDITION

Published by McGraw-Hill, a business unit of The McGraw-Hill Companies, Inc., 1221 Avenue of the Americas, New York, NY, 10020. Copyright © 2012 by The McGraw-Hill Companies, Inc. All rights reserved. Previous editions © 1996, 1999, 2003, and 2006. No part of this publication may be reproduced or distributed in any form or by any means, or stored in a database or retrieval system, without the prior written consent of The McGraw-Hill Companies, Inc., including, but not limited to, in any network or other electronic storage or transmission, or broadcast for distance learning.

Some ancillaries, including electronic and print components, may not be available to customers outside the United States.

This book is printed on acid-free paper.

3 4 5 6 7 8 9 0 DOW/DOW 1 0 9 8 7 6 5 4 3

ISBN 978-0-07-340198-0
MHID 0-07-340198-6

Vice president/Editor in chief: *Elizabeth Haefele*
Vice president/Director of marketing: *John E. Biernat*
Publisher: *Kenneth S. Kasee Jr.*
Senior sponsoring editor: *Natalie J. Ruffatto*
Director of development: *Sarah Wood*
Managing developmental editor: *Michelle L. Flomenhoft*
Executive marketing manager: *Roxan Kinsey*
Lead digital product manager: *Damian Moshak*
Director, Editing/Design/Production: *Jess Ann Kosic*
Lead project manager: *Rick Hecker*
Senior buyer: *Michael R. McCormick*
Senior designer: *Srdjan Savanovic*
Lead photo research coordinator: *Carrie K. Burger*

Digital production coordinator: *Brent dela Cruz*
Media project manager: *Cathy L. Tepper*
Cover design: *Alexa Viscius*
Interior design: *Jesi Lazar*
Typeface: *10.5/13 Adobe Jenson Pro*
Compositor: *Aptara®, Inc.*
Printer: *RR Donnelley*
Cover credit: Phone: ©Fuse, Getty Images; Computer: ©Ryan McVay/Getty Images; Tablet: ©Commstock/PunchStock; Mouse: ©Nicholas Eveleigh/Getty Images; Arrow: ©Devon Ford and Michael Glascott; Screenshot + Medisoft logo: ©McKesson
Credits: The credits section for this book begins on page B-1 and is considered an extension of the copyright page.

Library of Congress Cataloging-in-Publication Data

Bayes, Nenna L., author.
    Medical office procedures / Nenna L. Bayes, BBA, MEd, Professor, Program Coordinator of Office Systems Administration, Ashland Community and Technical College, Bonnie J. Crist, MEd, CMA, (AAMA), Medical Program, Harrison College, Karonne J. Becklin, MEd, CMA, Anoka Technical College, Anoka, MN. — Seventh Edition.
        p. ; cm.
    Includes index.
    ISBN-13: 978-0-07-340198-0 (alk. paper)
    ISBN-10: 0-07-340198-6 (alk. paper)
    1. Medical assistants. 2. Medical offices—Management.   I. Crist, Bonnie J., author.   II. Becklin, Karonne J., author.
III. Becklin, Karonne J. Medical office procedures. revision of (work)   IV. Title.
    [DNLM: 1. Office Management. 2. Practice Management, Medical. W 80]
R728.8.B44 2012
610.68—dc22   2010047117

The Internet addresses listed in the text were accurate at the time of publication. The inclusion of a Web site does not indicate an endorsement by the authors or McGraw-Hill, and McGraw-Hill does not guarantee the accuracy of the information presented at these sites.

Medisoft® is a Registered Trademark of McKesson Corporation. Screenshots and Material pertaining to Medisoft® Software used with permission of MCKESSON Corporation. © 2010 MCKESSON Corporation. All Rights Reserved.

The Medidata (student data file), illustrations, instructions, and exercises in MEDICAL OFFICE PROCEDURES are compatible with the Medisoft® Advanced Version 16 Patient Accounting software available at the time of publication. Note that Medisoft® Advanced Version 16 Patient Accounting software must be available to access the Medidata. It can be obtained by contacting your McGraw-Hill sales representative.

Practice Partner® is a Registered Trademark of McKesson Corporation. Screenshots and Material pertaining to Practice Partner® Software used with permission of MCKESSON Corporation. © 2010 MCKESSON Corporation. All Rights Reserved.

The ABHES standards included appear with permission of The Accrediting Bureau of Health Education Schools.

2008 Standards and Guidelines for the Accreditation of Educational Programs in Medical Assisting, Appendix B, Core Curriculum for Medical Assistants, Medical Assisting Education Review Board (MAERB), 2008.
Inclusion of this Core Curriculum does not constitute any form of endorsement of this textbook by the Medical Assisting Education Review Board (MAERB) or the Commission on Accreditation of Allied Health Education Programs (CAAHEP).

All brand or product names are trademarks or registered trademarks of their respective companies.
CPT five-digit codes, nomenclature, and other data are © 2010 American Medical Association. All rights reserved. No fee schedules, basic unit, relative values, or related listings are included in the CPT. The AMA assumes no liability for the data contained herein.
CPT codes are based on CPT 2011.
ICD-9-CM codes are based on ICD-9-CM 2011.
All names, situations, and anecdotes are fictitious. They do not represent any person, event, or medical record.

www.mhhe.com

Table of Contents

About the Authors v

Preface vi

To the Student xiv

Guided Tour xvi

Acknowledgments xix

Part 1 THE ADMINISTRATIVE MEDICAL ASSISTANT'S CAREER 1

Chapter 1 The Administrative Medical Assistant 2

1.1 Tasks and Skills 4

1.2 Administrative Medical Assisting Personal Attributes 7

1.3 Employment Opportunities 9

1.4 Work Ethics and Professionalism 11

1.5 Professional Growth and Certification 17

1.6 Interpersonal Relationships 19

Chapter 2 Medical Ethics, Law, and Compliance 34

2.1 Medical Ethics 36

2.2 Medical Law 39

2.3 HIPAA 50

2.4 Medical Compliance Plans and Safeguards Against Litigation 57

Part 2 ADMINISTRATIVE RESPONSIBILITIES 69

Chapter 3 Office Communications 70

3.1 The Communication Cycle 72

3.2 Nonverbal Communication 74

3.3 Written Communication 75

3.4 Telephone Skills 89

3.5 Scheduling 102

3.6 Processing Incoming Mail and Preparing Outgoing Mail 112

Chapter 4 Managing Health Information 126

4.1 Computer Usage 128

4.2 The Medical Record 139

4.3 Documentation Formats 142

4.4 Ownership, Quality Assurance, and Record Retention 147

4.5 Filing Systems 151

4.6 Electronic Health Records (EHRs) 164

4.7 Medical Terminology and Abbreviations 166
4.8 Technologies for Data Input 166
Simulation 1 182

Chapter 5 Office Management 186
5.1 Physical Environment 188
5.2 Types of Management 190
5.3 The Office Manager's Role 194
5.4 Editorial Research Projects 196
5.5 Travel and Meeting Arrangements 197
5.6 Patient and Employee Education 205

Part 3 PRACTICE FINANCIALS 219

Chapter 6 Insurance and Coding 220
6.1 Insurance Terminology 222
6.2 Insurance Plans: Identifying Plans and Payers 224
6.3 Participation and Payment Methods 229
6.4 Procedural and Diagnostic Coding and Compliance 234
6.5 ICD-10-CM 244

Chapter 7 Billing, Reimbursement, and Collections 254
7.1 Recording Transactions 256
7.2 Insurance Claims 260
7.3 Payments from Patients 271
7.4 Delinquent Accounts 274
Simulation 2 288

Chapter 8 Practice Finances 290
8.1 Essential Financial Records 292
8.2 Identity Theft and Red Flag Requirements 297
8.3 Banking 298
8.4 Payroll 304
Simulation 3 315

Part 4 PREPARING FOR EMPLOYMENT 317

Chapter 9 Preparing for Employment in the Medical Office 318
9.1 Searching Sources of Employment Opportunities 320
9.2 Completing an Online and a Traditional Application 322
9.3 Preparing a Cover/Application Letter 324
9.4 Preparing Résumés 326
9.5 The Interview 336
9.6 The Follow-up Contact Letter 342

Appendix A Introduction to Medisoft® A-1
Appendix B Transcription .... available online at www.mhhe.com/bayes7e
Glossary G-1
Bibliography B-1
Index I-1
Working Papers WP-1

About the Authors

Nenna L. Bayes, BBA, M.Ed., has coauthored and reviewed various titles within the medical administrative fields. She earned an associate of applied business degree, a bachelor of business administration degree, and a masters of arts in education from Morehead State University. During her tenure, she has taught numerous courses within the administrative and medical administrative curriculum. She is a professor in and the program coordinator for the Office Systems Technology program at Ashland Community and Technology College in Ashland, Kentucky, and has received many teaching excellence awards. Prior to teaching, she worked in various medical office environments. Additionally, she is a member of the American Academy of Professional Coders (AAPC).

She lives in Flatwoods, Kentucky, with her husband and is blessed to have two children, their spouses, and one granddaughter. She is actively involved in music and enjoys camping in her leisure time.

Bonnie J. Crist, M.Ed., CMA (AAMA), is a healthcare professional focused on educating adult learners. She is currently the medical program director at Harrison College in Indianapolis, Indiana, where she manages both the Medical Assisting Associate's Degree Program and the Medical Office Assisting Diploma Program. Bonnie also teaches online for Harrison College. Bonnie began her career as a certified medical assistant, and she quickly moved into management and training. Since her initial experience of training medical externship students, Bonnie has focused on the importance of soft skills or professionalism in healthcare, as well as the importance of understanding how the adult learner learns best.

She earned her associate's of applied science degree in medical assisting from Indiana Business College, her undergraduate degree in healthcare management from National American University, and her master's degree in healthcare education from A. T. Still University.

Bonnie currently lives in Indianapolis, Indiana, with her family. Her interests include spending time with her family, reading, writing, and volunteering.

Karonne J. Becklin, M.Ed., CMA This book owes much to its previous editions, written by Karonne J. Becklin of Anoka Technical College.

Preface

The medical profession is complex and demanding. The typical physician rarely has time to attend to the administrative responsibilities of the office. Successfully performing the work of an administrative medical assistant requires a foundation of procedural knowledge as well as continuing education to keep up to date with technology, including computer skills and new computer software. This seventh edition of *Medical Office Procedures (MOP)*, the long-awaited revision of this widely used textbook, provides the required background for the responsibilities of the administrative medical assistant. To prepare students for the ever-increasing use of technology in the medical office, this revision places continued importance on the computerization of routine tasks and of communications.

Job opportunities in the medical field often change with varying degrees of education and specialization required. This textbook allows for the integrated application of office procedures, skills, and knowledge in the classroom through the use of projects and simulations. Students learn to perform the duties of the administrative medical assistant under realistic conditions and with realistic pressures that require them to organize the work and set priorities.

This edition features two new co-authors, Nenna Bayes of Ashland Community and Technical College and Bonnie Crist of Harrison College. The changes to the book are based on their experiences in the classroom, along with extensive market feedback.

HERE'S WHAT YOU AND YOUR STUDENTS CAN EXPECT FROM THE NEW EDITION OF *MOP*:

- The table of contents has been restructured to reflect today's courses, including more integrated coverage of HIPAA, coverage of electronic health records, and a brand-new chapter (9) on preparing for employment.
- It contains a brand-new interior design, along with vibrant four-color photos.
- Each chapter has been matched up with the appropriate ABHES and CAAHEP competencies, which are listed on the chapter opener.
- The pedagogy has been updated to make the text even easier to use, including the learning outcomes. The learning outcomes are revised to reflect Bloom's Taxonomy, and the major chapter heads are structured to reflect the learning outcomes (and are numbered accordingly).
- New HIPAA tips are included, as well as Soft Skills Success discussions, which include critical-thinking questions.
    - The end-of-chapter material now includes a tabular summary, tied to the learning outcomes, new Using Terminology questions, and new multiple-choice questions. The Thinking It Through questions, which encourage critical-thinking skills, have been updated.
        - The chapter projects have been updated and aligned with the new organization of the book.
        - The updated Working Papers are both at the back of the book and available electronically at the book's Online Learning Center, www. mhhe.com/bayes7e.
            - *Medisoft*® *Advanced Version 16* is used for all Medisoft screen shots and the related student data file.

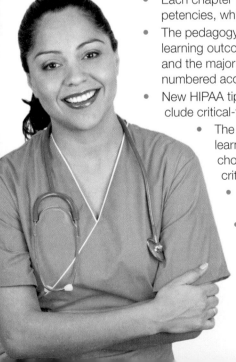

ABOUT THE COVER

Along with the many other updates in this edition of *Medical Office Procedures*, the book's cover has been redesigned to reflect what awaits today's students after they complete this course. Working in a medical office requires a balance between traditional tools and new technologies, such as EHR and other computerized systems. The cover reflects the many skills and competencies that students will learn in this course.

HERE'S HOW YOUR COLLEAGUES HAVE DESCRIBED *MOP*:

"The Bayes/Crist/Becklin text is an all-encompassing book on medical office procedures. It is complete, follows a logical order, is easy for students to understand, and has numerous activities for students to complete."
Helen W. Spain, Wake Technical Community College

"This book offers unifying themes for the students and simplifies the complexities of content in ways that enhance understanding without diluting the essential subject matter. The approach would reach most every student in our classes. Objectives are clearly stated and match the material. I find the reading and illustrations included an easy approach to complement my teaching and enhance the students' learning."
Eva Ruth Oltman, M.Ed., CPC, CMA, EMT, Jefferson Community and Technical College

"*Medical Office Procedures* is an excellent resource for any student wishing to work in a medical office. The book provides insight on the various aspects of working in a medical office, from the front office, medical assisting, chart documentation, billing and insurance, filing, transcription and medical law."
Debora A. Kaplan, MBA, Pasco-Hernando Community College

"Continuity [is a strength of the book]. The simulation pulls the whole operation of a medical office together. They [the students] are responsible for getting the entire operation correct. This is good for developing soft skills, work ethic, follow-through, etc., and also aids understanding of the entire cycle."
Pat J. Donahue, MS, Monroe Community College

"I have used *MOP* for several years and been thoroughly pleased with the textbook. Plus, the simulations are excellent—the students' knowledge, skills, and confidence grow with each simulation. When I first started teaching a medical office procedures course, I tried two other textbooks before discovering *MOP*. The first semester I used the textbook, I knew it was a perfect fit for the class. I look forward to the new and improved edition!"
Cindy Minor, Ed.M., CPS, MCAS, John A. Logan College

Medical Office Procedures
Nenna Bayes Bonnie Crist Karonne Becklin   7e

medisoft

Student Data for **medisoft** Advanced Version 16 Available Online

McGraw Hill   connect

ORGANIZATION OF *MOP*, 7E

MOP is divided into four parts:

Part	Coverage
Part 1: The Administrative Medical Assistant	Introduces the administrative medical assistant's career, defining the tasks, describing the work environments, and introducing medical ethics and medical law as they apply to the administrative medical assistant. Includes section on HIPAA as it relates to the role of the administrative medical assistant.
Part 2: Administrative Responsibilities	Introduces specific administrative responsibilities, including a chapter on managing health information with technology, and provides opportunities for practice.
Part 3: Practice Financials	Discusses procedures for preparing and organizing patients' charts and bills/insurance. Includes section on compliance and introduction to the new *ICD-10-CM* code set.
Part 4: Preparing for Employment	Prepares students for employment by covering all steps of the job-search process, from completing applications to interviews and follow-up.

NEW TO THE SEVENTH EDITION!

The following are the key changes in the seventh edition.
Each chapter has:

- CAAHEP and ABHES entry-level competencies aligned with that chapter.
- New learning outcomes written to reflect Bloom's Taxonomy.
- Updated photos.
- Updated key terms.
- Updated document samples using Word 2007.
- HIPAA Tips.
- Soft Skills Success discussions.
- Updated chapter projects.
- End-of-chapter tabular summary correlated with the learning outcomes.
- End-of-chapter matching and multiple-choice review questions.
- Updated Thinking It Through questions.
- Updated Medisoft® screenshots.

Chapter-by-Chapter

- Chapter 1: New reference to CMA (AAMA) Certification/Recertification Content Outline
- Chapter 2: Updated American Medical Association Principles of Medical Ethics; revised HIPAA material from the appendix has been inserted as Section 2.3
- Chapter 3: New Section 3.1 on the communication cycle; new Section 3.2 on nonverbal communication; material from the former Chapter 6—Written Communications—with revised sample documents using Word 2007; material from the former Chapter 4—Telephone Skills; material from the former Chapter 6—Processing Incoming Mail and Preparing Outgoing Mail; new information on best practices for safe mail handling issued by Homeland Security

- Chapter 4: New chapter title—Managing Health Information; revised material from the former Chapter 3 (removed hardware information but maintain software information); updated documentation format information to include CHEDDAR format; updated material in Section 4.4 Ownership, Quality Assurance, and Records Retention from the former 7.4; new Section 4.6, which includes screen shots on electronic health records; new Section 4.8 on technologies for material input; and moved transcription guidelines to an appendix (available at www.mhhe.com/bayes7e)
- Chapter 5: New Section 5.1 on how to manage the physical environment of the medical office; includes new Section 5.2 on different areas to manage, such as stress and time management; revised material from former Chapter 11 and new material on different management styles
- Chapter 6: Revised material (such as new coding icons) from the former Chapter 6; new Section 6.5 covering *ICD-10* with a sample crosswalk for learners
- Chapter 7: Revised material from the former Chapter 9; new knowledge application exercises within the chapter; updated CMS-1500 claim form and updated completion guidelines along with a revised project and a new project for CMS-1500 claim form completion using electronic CMS form
- Chapter 8: Revised material from the former Chapter 10; removed dated pegboard information but left rationale for balancing, and the manual balancing accounts project is now optional; new Section 8.2 on the Red Flag Requirements as they relate to the medical office; new project covering payroll
- Chapter 9: new chapter, which takes the learner through the employment process from assessing tasks and skills, locating employment opportunities, and completing an application/cover letter/résumé/interview to composing a follow-up thank-you letter—projects and Thinking It Through scenarios are included to reinforce chapter material

For a detailed transition guide between the sixth and seventh editions of *MOP,* visit www.mhhe.com/bayes7e.

TO THE INSTRUCTOR

McGraw-Hill knows how much effort it takes to prepare for a new course. Through focus groups, symposia, reviews, and conversations with instructors like you, we have gathered information about what materials you need in order to facilitate successful courses. We are committed to providing you with high-quality, accurate instructor support.

Simulations

A two-day simulation appears at the end of Chapter 4; three-day simulations appear at the ends of Chapters 7 and 8. The text provides instructions for the completion of the simulation. In each simulation, the student listens to the *Simulation Recordings* that accompany the program (available at www.mhhe.com/bayes7e). The recordings contain conversations between Linda Schwartz (the doctor's administrative medical assistant, with whom the student will identify) and Dr. Karen Larsen, various patients, and other office callers. (*Note:* The student may use the simulation recordings individually, or they may be assigned for use by the class as a whole. A complete transcript of the Simulation Recordings appears in the *Instructor's Manual* at www.mhhe.com/bayes7e.)

Student Resource Materials

In the *Working Papers* section at the back of the text, forms, medical histories, handwritten drafts, incoming correspondence, and other communications needed to complete the projects and the simulations are provided. Additional *Project Resource Materials* are provided on the student side of the Online Learning Center Web site, www.mhhe.com/bayes7e. This includes patient information forms and statements, as well as the letterhead for the physician's practice used in the projects and simulations.

medisoft

Using *Medisoft® Advanced Version 16* with *MOP*

MOP features *Medisoft® Advanced Version 16* patient accounting software with some of the projects and Simulations. McGraw-Hill has partnered with Medisoft from the very beginning, going back 15 years to when the software was DOS-based! The support you receive when you are using a McGraw-Hill text with Medisoft is second to none.

Your students will need the following:

- Minimum system requirements
  - Pentium III
  - 500 MHz (minimum) or higher processor
  - 500 MB available hard disk space
  - 512 MB RAM
  - 32-bit color display (minimum screen display of 1024 X 768)
  - Windows XP Professional SP3 or higher 32-bit
  - Windows Vista Business SP1 or higher 32-bit
  - Windows 7 Ultimate
- External storage device, such as a USB flash drive, for storing backup copies of the working database
- Medisoft Advanced Version 16 patient billing software
- Student data file, available for download from the book's Online Learning Center, www.mhhe.com/bayes7e

Instructor's Software: *Medisoft® Advanced Version 16* CD-ROM

Instructors who use McGraw-Hill Medisoft-compatible titles in their courses receive a fully working version of *Medisoft Advanced Version 16* software, which allows a school to place the live software on the laboratory or classroom machines. Only one copy is needed per campus location. Your McGraw-Hill sales representative will help you obtain Medisoft for your campus.

Medisoft-compatible titles available from McGraw-Hill

- Sanderson, *Computers in the Medical Office (CiMO),* 7e
  0073374601, 9780073374604
- Sanderson, *Case Studies for Use with Computers in the Medical Office,* 6e
  007337489X, 9780073374895
- Valerius/Bayes/Newby/Seggern, *Medical Insurance: An Integrated Claims Process Approach,* 5e
  0073374911, 9780073374918
- Valerius, *Workbook for Use with Medical Insurance: An Integrated Claims Process Approach,* 5e
  0077364333, 9780077364335
- Bayes/Crist/Becklin, *Medical Office Procedures,* 7e
  0073401986, 9780073401980

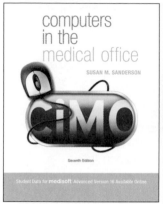 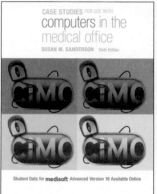 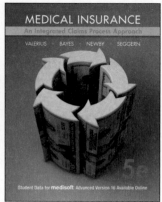

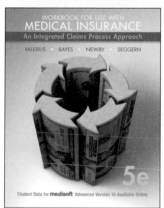 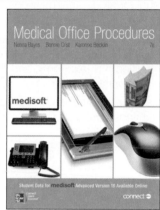

The McGraw-Hill Guide to Success for *Medisoft® Advanced Version 16*

We want your transition to *Medisoft Advanced Version 16* to be a snap! In *The McGraw-Hill Guide to Success for Medisoft Advanced Version 16,* the following topics are addressed:

- Software installation procedures for both the Instructor Version and the Student At-Home Version of Medisoft
- Student data files installation procedures
- Use of flash drives
- Backup and restore processes
- Frequently asked questions (FAQs)
- Instructor resources
- Technical support

Ask your McGraw-Hill sales representative to send you a copy, or visit www.mhhe.com/bayes7e to review the materials online.

Instructor Resources

You can rely on the following materials to help you and your students work through the exercises in the book:

- Instructor Edition of the Online Learning Center at www.mhhe.com/bayes7e. Your McGraw-Hill sales representative can provide you with access and show you how to "go green" with our online instructor support.
    - Instructor's Manual with course overview; lesson plans; sample syllabi; transition guides; answer keys for end-of-chapter questions; and correlations to competencies from several organizations, such as ABHES and CAAHEP. More details can be found in the IM and at the book's Web site, www.mhhe.com/bayes7e.
    - A PowerPoint slide presentation for each chapter, containing teaching notes correlated to Learning Outcomes. Each presentation seeks to reinforce key concepts and provide a visual for students. The slides are excellent for in-class lectures.
    - Test bank and answer key for use in classroom assessment. The comprehensive test bank includes a variety of question types, with each question linked directly to its Learning Outcome, Bloom's Taxonomy, and difficulty level. Both a Word version and a computerized version (EZ Test) of the test bank are provided.
    - Conversion Guide with a chapter-by-chapter breakdown of how the content has been revised between editions. The guide is helpful if you are currently using *MOP* and moving to the new edition, or if you are a first-time adopter.
    - Instructor Asset Map to help you find the teaching material you need with a click of the mouse. These online chapter tables are organized by Learning Outcomes, and allow you to find instructor notes, PowerPoint slides, and even test bank suggestions with ease! The Asset Map is a completely integrated tool designed to help you plan and instruct your courses efficiently and comprehensively. It labels and organizes course material for use in a multitude of learning applications.
    - *Connect Plus:* McGraw-Hill *Connect Plus* is a revolutionary online assignment and assessment solution, providing instructors and students with tools and resources to maximize their success. Through *Connect Plus*, instructors enjoy simplified course setup and assignment creation. Robust, media-rich tools and activities, all tied to the textbook Learning Outcomes, ensure you'll create classes geared toward achievement. You'll have more time with your students and spend less time agonizing over course planning.
    - McGraw-Hill LearnSmart for Medical Insurance, Billing, and Coding: LearnSmart diagnoses students' skill levels to determine what they're good at and where they need help. Then it delivers customized learning content based on their strengths and weakness. The result: Students get the help they need, right when they need it—instead of getting stuck on lessons or being continually frustrated with stalled progress.

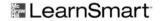

McGraw-Hill Higher Education and Blackboard have teamed up. What does this mean for you?

1. **Your life, simplified.** Now you and your students can access McGraw-Hill's *Connect Plus* and Create right from within your Blackboard course—all with one single sign-on. Say goodbye to the days of logging in to multiple applications.
2. **Deep integration of content and tools.** Not only do you get single sign-on with *Connect Plus* and Create, but you also get deep integration of McGraw-Hill content and content engines right in Blackboard. Whether you're choosing a book for your course or building *Connect Plus* assignments, all the tools you need are right where you want them—inside of Blackboard.

3. **Seamless gradebooks.** Are you tired of keeping multiple gradebooks and manually synchronizing grades into Blackboard? We thought so. When a student completes an integrated *Connect Plus* assignment, the grade for that assignment automatically (and instantly) feeds your Blackboard grade center.

4. **A solution for everyone.** Whether your institution is already using Blackboard or you just want to try Blackboard on your own, we have a solution for you. McGraw-Hill and Blackboard can now offer you easy access to industry-leading technology and content, whether your campus hosts it, or we do. Be sure to ask your local McGraw-Hill representative for details.

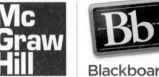

Need Help? Contact the Digital Care Support Team

Visit our Digital CARE Support Web site at www.mhhe.com/support.
Browse the FAQs (frequently asked questions) and product documentation, and/or contact a CARE support representative. The Digital CARE Support Team is available Sunday through Friday.

To the Student

You have chosen a fascinating, challenging profession. The field of healthcare is growing at a rapid pace, providing many opportunities for the trained professional. Welcome to an educational program designed to prepare you for immediate and long-range success as an administrative medical assistant. In this course, you will use *MOP* not only as a source of practical information but also as an instrument for realistic practice in applying what you have learned. Throughout the chapters, you will be asked to apply your newly acquired knowledge—not simply to tell how or why you would use the information on the job. You will then repeatedly apply the information throughout the text.

As you complete the designated projects within the text, you will accumulate many of the medical records and correspondence needed in the simulations that occur after Chapters 4, 7, and 8. You will be asked to assume the role of Linda Schwartz, an administrative medical assistant. During each simulation, you will handle various tasks assigned by the physician, the patients, and other office callers after listening carefully to recorded conversations. With some instructor guidance, you will perform your duties in an appropriate manner. You will be performing a variety of closely related administrative medical office tasks in the simulations: answering the telephone, scheduling appointments, taking messages, filing, preparing bills, and so on. You will gain proficiency in performing a wide range of administrative activities and in coping with a variety of problems and pressures in the medical office. All these activities will help you strive to organize work, set priorities, relate one task to another, and manage time. After completing these simulations, you will find that you are well prepared for the transition from classroom to office.

Starting with Part 2, you will be "working" for Dr. Karen Larsen, a family practitioner. As directed, save your work from the chapter projects. This work will form the basis for your "office files." In the simulations, you will use and add to these files. Essential patient data and forms are provided either in the Working Papers or at the book's Online Learning Center, www.mhhe.com/bayes7e. You will also need the following supplies:

- File folder labels and 31 file folders
- A ring binder or a file folder to serve as your appointment book if you are not using the Medisoft software
- An expandable portfolio to serve as your file cabinet; all your office files can be stored in this portfolio
- Paper for printing
- Computer disks to store the projects as directed
- Miscellaneous items—rubber bands, a note pad, pens, pencils, paper clips, and so on

MAKE SURE *MEDISOFT® ADVANCED VERSION 16* IS INSTALLED ON YOUR SCHOOL'S COMPUTER

Before you can complete several projects and simulations in this text, you must make sure that *Medisoft Advanced Version 16* (the actual software program) is installed on your school's computer. It is possible that *Medisoft Version 16* has already been installed on the computer you are using. If this is the case, you do not need to install it again.

How Do I Know If *Medisoft Advanced Version 16* Is Installed?

1. Click the **Start** button, select **All Programs**, and look for the Medisoft folder. If you find a Medisoft folder, click Medisoft Advanced to launch the program.
2. To determine which version of Medisoft is installed, click **Help** on the menu bar, and then click **About Medisoft**. Look in the window that appears, which lists the version number of the program.

3. If you see Version 16, skip to the section below, titled *Make Sure the Student Data File Is Loaded.*

Install *Medisoft Advanced Version 16* If Your School's Computer Does Not Have It

If you are working on a school computer, please check with your instructor on how to have the program installed. *Instructors*: If you need help, please request a copy of *The McGraw-Hill Guide to Success for Medisoft Advanced Version 16* from your sales representative. You can find more information about this guide at the book's Online Learning Center Web site at www.mhhe.com/bayes7e.

Homework Version of Medisoft

An OPTIONAL Student At-Home version of Medisoft is available for purchase. The Student At-Home CD contains a fully functional limited version of the *Medisoft Advanced Version 16* program. To purchase a copy of the Medisoft 16 Student At-Home CD, check with your instructor. Once you have purchased a copy of the CD, refer to the installation instructions for the Student At-Home version at the book's Web site: www.mhhe.com/bayes7e. On the opening screen, you will see this statement: *Students, click here for help if you need to load Medisoft or the Student Data File.*

Make Sure the Student Data File Is Loaded

The student data file contains all the patient data needed to complete the Medisoft projects and simulation tasks in this text. Before you begin the first Medisoft project, you must make sure the student data file is loaded.

Check to See If the "MOP7e" Student Data File Is Installed

1. Start Medisoft Version 16 by double-clicking on the desktop icon.
2. Look at the title bar that contains the words "Medisoft Advanced." If the "*MOP7e*" student data file has already been installed, you should see "*MOP7e*" to the right of "Medisoft Advanced." You are ready to begin the Medisoft activities.

Load the "MOP7e" Student Data File If Your Computer Does Not Have It

1. Go to the book's Web site at www.mhhe.com/bayes7e.
2. On the opening screen, you will see this statement: *Students, click here for help if you need to load Medisoft or the Student Data File.*
3. This will take you directly to the Medisoft Student Resources page in the student center with the "*MOP7e*" Student Data File.
4. Click the link labeled *MOP7e* Student Data File Instructions.pdf, and download the file. When it has finished downloading, open the file on your computer and print it.
5. Click on the link for the *MOP7e* Student Data File.zip file, and download the file to your computer desktop. This installer provides the patient database you will use to complete the Medisoft tasks in this book.
6. Follow the instructions in the *MOP7e* Student Data File Instructions.pdf document to extract the zip file and install the *MOP7e* Student Data File on the computer.

BACKING UP AND RESTORING DATA IN MEDISOFT

If you are in a school environment, it is important to make a backup copy of your work after each Medisoft session. This ensures that you can restore your work during the next session and are able to use your own data even if another student uses the computer after you or if, for any reason, the files on the school computer are changed or corrupted. For detailed instructions on how to do this, please visit Appendix A: Introduction to Medisoft at the end of this book.

NEED HELP? CONTACT THE DIGITAL CARE SUPPORT TEAM

Visit our Digital CARE Support Web site at www.mhhe.com/support. Browse the FAQs (frequently asked questions) and product documentation, and/or contact a CARE support representative. The Digital CARE Support Team is available Sunday through Friday.

Guided Tour

CHAPTER OPENER The **chapter opener** sets the stage for what will be learned in the chapter.

Learning Outcomes are written to reflect the revised version of Bloom's Taxonomy and to establish the key points the student should focus on in the chapter. In addition, major chapter heads are structured to reflect the Learning Outcomes and are numbered accordingly.

Key terms are first introduced in the chapter opener so the student can see them all in one place.

List of the relevant **ABHES and CAAHEP** competencies provide a visible correlation between chapter material and the requirements of certifications, for initial lesson planning and later skill-strengthening.

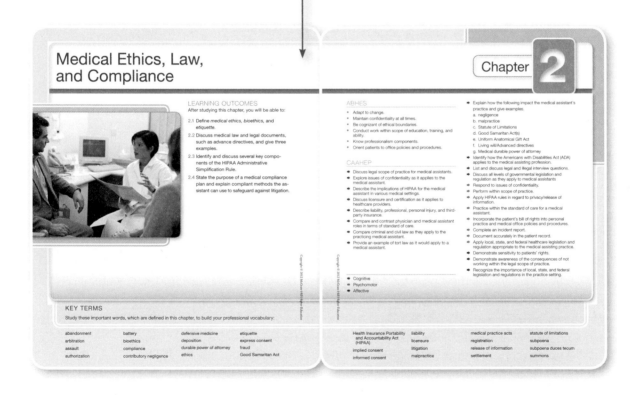

LEARNING AIDS

Key Terms

Key terms are **italicized**, so that students will become familiar with the language necessary to perform administrative tasks in the medical office. These are reinforced in the **Glossary** at the end of the book.

Tips and Guidelines

Compliance Tips and HIPAA Tips are included to highlight this important information for the students.

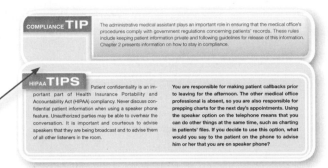

COMPLIANCE TIP The administrative medical assistant plays an important role in ensuring that the medical office's procedures comply with government regulations concerning patients' records. These rules include keeping patient information private and following guidelines for release of this information. Chapter 2 presents information on how to stay in compliance.

HIPAA TIPS Patient confidentiality is an important part of Health Insurance Portability and Accountability Act (HIPAA) compliancy. Never discuss confidential patient information when using a speaker phone feature. Unauthorized parties may be able to overhear the conversation. It is important and courteous to advise speakers that they are being broadcast and to advise them of all other listeners in the room.

You are responsible for making patient callbacks prior to leaving for the afternoon. The other medical office professional is absent, so you are also responsible for prepping charts for the next day's appointments. Using the speaker option on the telephone means that you can do other things at the same time, such as charting in patients' files. If you decide to use this option, what would you say to the patient on the phone to advise him or her that you are on speaker phone?

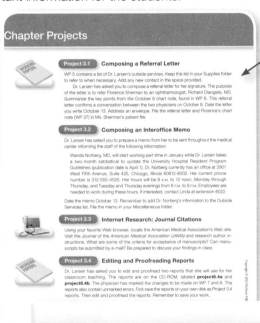

Chapter Projects

Project 3.1   Composing a Referral Letter

WP 5 contains a list of Dr. Larsen's outside services. Keep this list in your Supplies folder to refer to when necessary. Add any new contact in the space provided.

Dr. Larsen has asked you to compose a referral letter for her signature. The purpose of the letter is to refer Florence Sherman to an ophthalmologist, Richard Diangelis, MD. Summarize the key points from the October 8 chart note, found in WP 6. This referral letter confirms a conversation between the two physicians on October 8. Date the letter you write October 13. Address an envelope. File the referral letter and Florence's chart note (WP 37) in Ms. Sherman's patient file.

Project 3.2   Composing an Interoffice Memo

Dr. Larsen has asked you to prepare a memo from her to be sent throughout the medical center informing the staff of the following information:

Wanda Norberg, MD, will start working part-time in January while Dr. Larsen takes a two-month sabbatical to update the University Hospital Resident Program Guidelines (publication date is April 1). Dr. Norberg currently has an office at 2901 West Fifth Avenue, Suite 425, Chicago, Illinois 60612-9002. Her current phone number is 312-555-4525. Her hours will be 9 A.M. to 12 noon, Monday through Thursday, and Tuesday and Thursday evenings from 6 P.M. to 9 P.M. Employees are needed to work during these hours. If interested, contact Linda at extension 6022

Date the memo October 13. Remember to add Dr. Norberg's information to the Outside Services list. File the memo in your Miscellaneous folder.

Project 3.3   Internet Research: Journal Citations

Using your favorite Web browser, locate the American Medical Association's Web site. Visit the *Journal of the American Medical Association* (*JAMA*) and research author instructions. What are some of the criteria for acceptance of manuscripts? Can manuscripts be submitted by e-mail? Be prepared to discuss your findings in class.

Project 3.4   Editing and Proofreading Reports

Dr. Larsen has asked you to edit and proofread two reports that she will use for her classroom teaching. The reports are on the CD-ROM, labeled **project6.4a** and **project6.4b**. The physician has marked the changes to be made on WP 7 and 8. The reports also contain unmarked errors. First save the reports on your own disk as Project 3.4 reports. Then edit and proofread the reports. Remember to save your work.

PROJECTS AND SIMULATIONS

Projects are opportunities for your student to have hands-on practice that mirrors work in a real practice.

In-text callouts refer the student to **Projects** at the end of each chapter, providing more ways to apply the lessons learned in the chapter.

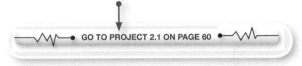

GO TO PROJECT 2.1 ON PAGE 60

Simulations appear after Chapters 4, 7, and 8 to give students hands-on experience with realistic medical office tasks.

Simulation 1

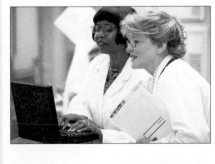

YOUR ROLE

Welcome to the practice of Dr. Karen Larsen! Today, you begin to apply the skills you have learned in this text as you assume the role of Linda Schwartz, Dr. Larsen's administrative medical assistant.

Simulation 1 is the first of three simulations in the text. These simulations provide practical experience in working in a physician's office. You will discover how various tasks relate to each other. The daily events in the office are narrated on the Simulation Recordings that accompany the text. As you listen to the recordings, you will handle various assignments as the assistant. Your simulation work will include making and canceling appointments, preparing messages, creating communications, preparing various medical forms, and following through on daily tasks.

Simulation 1

MATERIALS

You will need the following materials to complete Simulation 1. If these materials are not already in the proper folders, obtain them from the sources indicated.

Materials	Source
Appointment calendar	
Supplies folder:	
Appointment cards	WP 35
Letterhead	CD-ROM
Notepad	You provide.
Plain paper	You provide.
Patient information forms	WP 51 & 52
Records release form	WP 53
Telephone log	WP 54
Telephone message blanks	WP 9–16
To-do list	WP 55

To-Do Items

Note: If you have completed all the projects and do not have the following listed items, discuss the missing items with your instructor.

Day 1 folder:
Place patients' charts for October 14.

Day 2 folder:
Place patients' charts for October 15.

Miscellaneous folder:
Wanda Norberg, MD—message (Project 3.5) and interoffice memo (Project 3.2)

Patients' folders:

The following patients' folders (charts) should contain the chart note, patient information form, and any other items listed.

Armstrong, Monica
Baab, Thomas
Babcock, Sara—message   (Project 3.5)
Burton, Randy
Casagranda, Doris
Castro, Joseph
Dayton, Theresa
Grant, Todd
Jonathan, Charles III
Kramer, Jeffrey—message   (Project 3.5)
Matthews, Ardis
Mendez, Ana
Morton, Sarah
Murrary, Raymond
Phan, Marc
Richards, Warren
Roberts, Suzanne
Robertson, Gary
Sherman, Florence—referral letter,   (Project 3.1)
    chart note, and envelope
Sinclair, Gene
Sun, Cheng
Villano, Stephen

EVALUATION

You will be evaluated as follows:

1. Good judgment in establishing priorities—did you use good judgment? Did you accomplish the most important tasks?
2. Work of good quality—are tasks accurate and neat?
3. Quantity—did you complete a reasonable amount of work? Would a physician be satisfied with your rate of accomplishment?

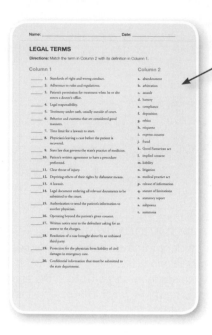

Working Papers at the end of the book provide data and forms for the students to use with the projects and simulations.

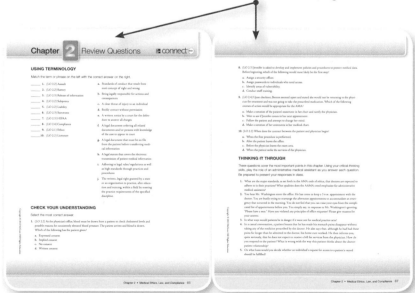

END-OF-CHAPTER RESOURCES

Chapter Summary

The **Chapter Summary** is in a tabular, step-by-step format with page references to help with review of the materials.

Soft Skills Success

The **Soft Skills Success** material discusses key soft skills for students to learn, along with critical-thinking questions to reinforce the material.

Chapter Review

The **Chapter Review** contains terminology exercises tagged by learning outcomes; multiple-choice exercises tagged by learning outcomes; and Thinking It Through exercises to test students' critical-thinking skills.

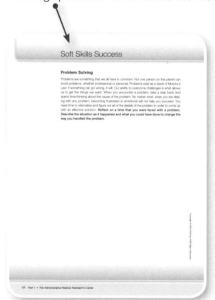

Acknowledgments

Suggestions have been received from faculty and students throughout the country. This is vital feedback that is relied upon with each edition. Each person who has offered comments and suggestions has our thanks. The efforts of many people are needed to develop and improve a product. Among these people are the reviewers and consultants who point out areas of concern, cite areas of strength, and make recommendations for change. In this regard, the following instructors provided feedback that was enormously helpful in preparing the seventh edition of *MOP.*

WORKSHOPS

In 2009 and 2010, McGraw-Hill conducted 15 allied health workshops, providing an opportunity for more than 600 faculty members to gain continuing education credits as well as to provide feedback on our products.

BOOK REVIEWS

Many instructors reviewed the sixth edition once it was published and provided valuable feedback that directly affected the development of this seventh edition. A number of people also reviewed the new seventh edition manuscript.

Judy K. Anderson
MAEd, Coastal Carolina Community College

Karen M. Arnold
UK, Newbridge College

Shasta Bennett
MSEd., Olney Central College

Cindy Jo Bersani
Morrisville State College

Tammie Bolling
Ed.D., MBA/HCM, CBCS, CMAA, CHI, Tennessee Technology Center at Jacksboro

Barbara Jane Cerna
CMA, Highline Community College

Jean M. Chenu
MS, Genesee Community College

Angela M. Chisley
AHI, RMA, College of Southern Maryland

Catherine Brooks Combs
BS, Tennessee Technology Center At Morristown

Georganne Maki Copeland
M.Ed., Centralia College

Deborah K. Cresap
MS, RMA, West Virginia Northern Community College

Linda F. Davis
MS, Copiah-Lincoln Community College

Rhonda J. Davis
CMA, RMA, GXMO, Southern State
Community College

Pat J. Donahue
MS, Monroe Community College

Lovie A. Dunn
Central Texas College

Yolande B. Gardner
CPS, CAP, Lawson State Community
College

Jacquelyn Harris
CMA (AAMA), AHI, MPCI, Bryan College

Toni R. Hartley
BS, Laurel Business Institute

Jane A. Jones
Mountain Empire Community College

Debora A. Kaplan
MBA, SPHR, HRM, Pasco-Hernando
Community College

Shanna Legleiter
MS, BS, Barton County Community
College

Brady K. LeVrier
PhD, MS, BS, Acadiana Technical
College

Constance Lieseke
CMA (AAMA), MLT, PBT (ASCP),
Olympic College

Emily Martin
MS Faulkner State Community College

Nikki May
MBA, ATC-CB, Louisiana Technical
College

Marla S. Mayer
M.Ed., BS, Orlando Tech

Amy McAnally
Central Texas College

Selinda McCumbers
Brighton College

Cindy Minor
Ed.M., CPS, MCAS, John A. Logan
College

Katrina Boyette Myricks
Holmes Community College

Eva Oltman
M.Ed., CPC, CMA, EMT, Jefferson
Community and Technical College

Barbara Parker
BS, CMA (AAMA), CCS-P, CPC,
Olympic College

Tatyana Pashnyak
COI, Bainbridge College

Jorge Perez Lopez
San Antonio College

David Allan Rice
RMA, CCPR, Milan Institute

Mary Schermer
CCA, MA, Harrison College

Helen W. Spain
MSEd, Wake Technical and
Community College

Patricia A. Stich
MSEd., Waubonsee Community
College

Deborah Sulkowski
CMA, Pittsburgh Technical Institute

Nina Thierer
CMA (AAMA), BS, Ivy Tech Community
College

Traci Thompson
MS, BS, Kilgore College-Longview

Mazie E. Will
CPS/CAP, Sul Ross State University

Jane F. Yakicic
CMA, CCS-P, Cambria-Rowe Business
College

TECHNICAL EDITING/ACCURACY PANEL

A panel of instructors completed a technical edit and review of all content in the book page proofs to verify its accuracy, along with the supplements.

Judy K. Anderson
MAEd, Coastal Carolina Community College

Tatyana Pashnyak
COI, Bainbridge College

Jacquelyn Harris
CMA (AAMA), AHI, MPCI, Bryan College

Toni R. Hartley
BS, Laurel Business Institute

Patricia A. Stich
MSEd., Waubonsee Community College

SURVEYS

Nearly 100 people participated in a survey about this course and the proposed organization for the new edition.

Gail Albert
CMA (AAMA), Berks Technical Institute

Judy K. Anderson
MAEd, Coastal Carolina Community College

Diane R. Benson
CMA (AAMA), BSHCA, MSA, CFP, ASE, NSC-SCFAT,CDE, CMRS, CPC, AHA BLS-I, FA-I, PALS, ACLS, CAAM-I, Wake Technical Community College, University of Phoenix

Cindy Bergenstock
LPN, AAS, Berks Technical Institute

Amy L. Blochowiak
MBA, ACS, AIAA, AIRC, ARA, FLHC, FLMI, HCSA, HIA, HIPAA, MHP, PCS, SILA-F, Northeast Wisconsin Technical College

Carol E. Charie
CPC, The Salter School

Jean M. Chenu
MS, Genesee Community College

Joyce Combs
CMA (AAMA), MS, Bluegrass Community and Technical College

Georganne Maki Copeland
M.Ed., Centralia College

Lovie A. Dunn
Central Texas College

Theresa Errante-Parrino
CMA (AAMA), EMT-P, BMXO, CPhT, M.Ed., Indian River State College

Tamela Freeman
BS, CMAA, CEHRS, Sierra Nevada Job Corps

H. Roger Fulk
Wright State University

Anne D. Gailey
CMA (AAMA), Ogeechee Technical College

Tammy Gant
RHIT, CPC, CMA, AHI, Surry Community College

Jen Gouge
RT, MA, Peninsula College

Claudia Guillen
RMA, LPN, Middlesex Community College

Sheila Guillot
CAP/CPS, Lamar State College-Port
Arthur

Toni R. Hartley
BS, Laurel Business Institute

Traci Hotard
RHIA, SCL Technical College

Michele L. Howard-Swan
CMA, MS, Asnuntuck Community
College

Maryann Kania
MBA, Quinsgamon Community
College

Debora A. Kaplan
MBA, SPHR, HRM, Pasco-Hernando
Community College

Barbara Marchelletta
AS, BS, CMA (AAMA), CPC (AAPC),
Beal College

Cindy Minor
Ed.M., CPS, MCAS, John A. Logan
College

Terri L. Moore
BS, Louisiana Technical College

Eva Oltman
M.Ed., CPC, CMA, EMT, Jefferson
Community and Technical College

Gail M. Ouattara
Certified Technical Instructor, Seattle
Vocational Institute

Barbara Parker
BS, CMA (AAMA), CCS-P, CPC,
Olympic College

Susan L. Russell
BS, MIT, Bluegrass Technical and
Community College

Bobbi Schommer
BSHCA, Moraine Park Technical
College

Marilyn Selliers
CPC, Lone Star College

Helen W. Spain
MSEd, Wake Technical and
Community College

Christine Sproles
BSN, MS, RN, CMT, Pensacola
Christian College

Patricia A. Stich
MSEd., Waubonsee Community
College

Tammy L. Stone
CPC, Anthem Education Group

Mary Valencia
CPC, CMC, CMOM, University of
Texas, Texas Southmost College

Wendy J. Vonhold
BA, MS, EDA, Rochester Educational
Opportunity Center

Karen Welch
AS, BS, CPS, Tennessee Technology
Center at Jackson

Linda C. Wenn
Central Community College

Jane F. Yakicic
CMA, CCS-P, Cambria-Rowe Business
College

ACKNOWLEDGMENTS FROM THE AUTHORS

To the students and instructors who use this book, your feedback and suggestions have made *MOP* a better learning tool for all.

We especially want to thank the editorial team at McGraw-Hill—Liz Haefele, Natalie Ruffatto, Raisa Kreek, and Michelle Flomenhoft—for their enthusiastic support and their willingness to go the extra mile to get this book revised. We would also like to thank freelance editors Melinda Bilecki and Nicolle Schieffer for their contributions.

The EDP staff was also outstanding; senior designer Srdj Savanovic created a terrific new design, which was implemented through the production process by Rick Hecker, lead project manager, Michael McCormick, senior buyer, Carrie Burger, photo research coordinator, and Cathy Tepper, media project manager.

This book would not be in its seventh edition were it not for the tireless efforts of Roxan Kinsey, executive marketing manager, who kept *MOP* in people's minds in the big gap between editions.

We would also like to give special thanks to Robin Bolton at Harrison College for preparing the supplements with Bonnie.

And to our families…

Nenna Bayes and Bonnie Crist

A COMMITMENT TO ACCURACY

You have a right to expect an accurate textbook, and McGraw-Hill invests considerable time and effort to make sure that we deliver one. Listed below are the many steps we take to make sure this happens.

OUR ACCURACY VERIFICATION PROCESS

First Round—Development Reviews

STEP 1: Numerous **health professions instructors** review the current edition and the draft manuscript and report on any errors that they may find. The authors make these corrections in their final manuscript.

Second Round—Page Proofs

STEP 2: Once the manuscript has been typeset, the **authors** check their manuscript against the page proofs to ensure that all illustrations, graphs, examples, and exercises have been correctly laid out on the pages, and that all codes have been updated correctly.

STEP 3: An outside panel of **peer instructors** completes a technical edit/review of all content in the page proofs to verify its accuracy. The authors add these corrections to their review of the page proofs.

STEP 4: A **proofreader** adds a triple layer of accuracy assurance in pages by looking for errors; then a confirming, corrected round of page proofs is produced.

Third Round—Confirming Page Proofs

STEP 5: The **author team** reviews the confirming round of page proofs to make certain that any previous corrections were properly made and to look for any errors they might have missed on the first round.

STEP 6: The **project manager,** who has overseen the book from the beginning, performs **another proofread** to make sure that no new errors have been introduced during the production process.

Final Round—Printer's Proofs

STEP 7: The **project manager** performs a **final proofread** of the book during the printing process, providing a final accuracy review.
In concert with the main text, all supplements undergo a proofreading and technical editing stage to ensure their accuracy.

RESULTS

What results is a textbook that is as accurate and error-free as is humanly possible. Our authors and publishing staff are confident that the many layers of quality assurance have produced books that are leaders in the industry for their integrity and correctness. *Please view the Acknowledgments section for more details on the many people involved in this process.*

1st Round:
Author's Manuscript

Multiple Rounds of Review by Health Professions Instructors

2nd Round:
Typeset Pages

Accuracy Checks by:
- Authors
- Peer Instructors
- 1st Proofreader

3rd Round:
Typeset Pages

Accuracy Checks by:
- Authors
- 2nd Proofreader

Final Round:
Printing

Accuracy Check by:
Final Proofreader

Supplements:
- Proofreading
- Accuracy Checks

PART 1

The Administrative Medical Assistant's Career

CHAPTER 1
The Administrative Medical Assistant

CHAPTER 2
Medical Ethics, Law, and Compliance

Welcome to *Medical Office Procedures*! This program has been written specifically to provide you with the skills and knowledge you will need to succeed. In Part 1, you will learn about the role of the administrative medical assistant, as well as legal and ethical aspects of the career.

CONSIDER THIS: Physicians' offices, hospitals, clinics, and other employers hire administrative medical assistants. *In what type of medical setting do you intend to pursue employment?*

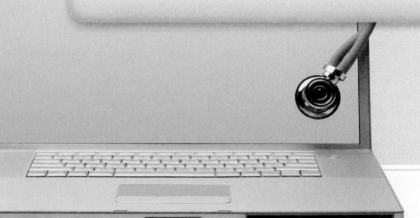

The Administrative Medical Assistant

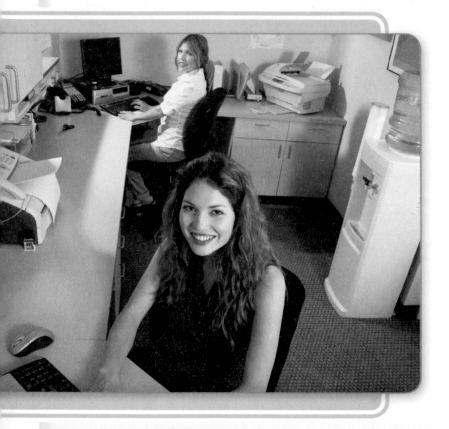

LEARNING OUTCOMES

After studying this chapter, you will be able to:

1.1 Describe the tasks and skills required of an administrative medical assistant.

1.2 List and define at least three personal attributes essential for an administrative medical assistant.

1.3 Describe the employment opportunities in various medical settings and specialties and nonmedical settings.

1.4 Identify and define at least six positive work attitudes that contribute to the work ethic and professionalism of an administrative medical assistant.

1.5 List three advantages of professional affiliation and certification.

1.6 Apply elements of good interpersonal communication to relationships with patients and others within the medical environment.

KEY TERMS

Study these important words, which are defined in this chapter, to build your professional vocabulary:

AAMA	certification	good judgment	punctuality
accuracy	confidentiality	honesty	self-motivation
administrative medical assistant (AMA)	dependability	IAAP	tact
	efficiency	initiative	team player
AHDI	empathy	maturity	thoroughness
AMT	ethnocentrism	problem-solving	work ethic
assertiveness	flexibility	professional image	

Chapter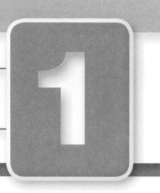

ABHES

- Adapt to change.
- Maintain confidentiality at all times.
- Project a positive attitude.
- Be cognizant of ethical boundaries.
- Express a responsible attitude.
- Conduct work within scope of education, training, and ability.
- Professionalism components.
- Orient patients to office policies and procedures.
- Adapt what is said to the recipient's level of comprehension.
- Adaptation for individualized needs.
- Instruct patient with special needs.
- Locate resources and information for patients and employers.
- Use proper telephone techniques.
- Be courteous and diplomatic.
- Serve as a liaison between the physician and others.
- Exercise efficient time management.
- Receive, organize, prioritize, and transmit information expediently.
- Show a responsible attitude.

CAAHEP

➡ Identify styles and types of verbal communication.
➡ Recognize communication barriers.
➡ Identify techniques for overcoming communication barriers.
➡ Recognize the elements of oral communication using a sender/receiver process.
➡ Identify resources and adaptations that are required based on individual needs, i.e., culture and environment, developmental life stage, language, and physical threats to communication.
➡ Recognize the role of patient advocacy in the practice of medical assisting.
➡ Discuss the role of assertiveness in effective professional communication.
➡ Identify time management principles.
➡ Use reflection, restatement, and clarification techniques to obtain patient history.
➡ Instruct patients according to their needs.
➡ Apply active listening skills.
➡ Demonstrate sensitivity appropriate to the message being delivered.

➡ Cognitive
➡ Psychomotor
➡ Affective

INTRODUCTION

As the population ages, new healthcare reforms are implemented, and newer technologies, medicine, and treatments are introduced into the healthcare industry, the opportunities for rewarding careers in medical environments increase. These changes also pose new challenges for healthcare professionals. Legal and ethical issues abound. Following procedures that comply with government regulations concerning patients' privacy is also critical.

Because of rapid changes and the increasing complexity of the industry, continuing education is necessary to succeed in performing the role of an administrative medical assistant. Equally important is exhibiting the personal attributes and work ethic that contribute to the smooth and efficient operation of the medical practice team.

Medical assistants are medical office professionals who capably perform a number of tasks in a wide variety of settings. Administrative tasks are those procedures used to keep the offices in medical practices running efficiently. Clinical tasks are those procedures the medical assistant may perform to aid the physician in the medical treatment of a patient. A committee was formed in 1996 by the American Association of Medical Assistants. The committee's goal was to revise and update standards for the accreditation of programs that taught medical assisting. Findings of the committee were published in 1997 as the "AAMA Role Delineation Study: Occupational Analysis of the Medical Assisting Profession." The Role Delineation Chart outlines the areas of competence you must master as an entry-level medical assistant. The chart was further updated in 2003 and 2009 to include additional competencies. The Medical Assistant Role Delineation Chart provides the basis for medical assisting and evaluation. All students in an accredited medical assisting program are required to master three areas of competence: clinical, administrative, and general. The AAMA Role Delineation Chart is also a good reference source that identifies the skills, duties, and procedures that medical assistants (administrative and clinical) are educated to perform. For more information on the **AAMA**, please visit http://www.aama-ntl.org.

This textbook concentrates on administrative responsibilities, which involve the personal traits and technical skills required in most medical office careers. Throughout the text, the **administrative medical assistant** is often referred to as the "assistant," or as the **AMA** rather than by the full title.

Administrative Medical Assisting Tasks

The administrative medical assistant (AMA) is a professional office worker dedicated to assisting in the care of patients. To effectively perform all the required tasks, an assistant must be proficient in a number of skills.

The following are the major categories of tasks performed by an administrative medical assistant:

- Front desk procedures
- Scheduling
- Records management
- Administrative duties
- Billing and insurance

Front Desk. The administrative medical assistant greets patients and other visitors, such as family members and pharmaceutical representatives. The assistant also verifies and updates personal data about patients, explains the fees that will be charged for services, collects payments, and guides patients through their medical office encounters.

Scheduling. The administrative medical assistant answers the telephone; schedules either by phone or in person future office appointments and out-of-office encounters, such as hospital admissions, laboratory testing, and referrals to specialists; and forwards telephone calls according to office procedures.

Records Management. The administrative medical assistant creates and maintains patient medical records (sometimes referred to as charts); stores and retrieves the records for use during encounters with physicians; and files other kinds of documents. In offices using electronic health records, the assistant begins the electronic chart by inputting patient demographic and financial information into the electronic database. As many offices begin the process of converting to electronic health records, the assistant may assume the responsibility for scanning hard copy charts into the electronic health record's database.

Administrative Duties. The administrative medical assistant opens and sorts incoming mail, composes routine correspondence, and may transcribe physicians' dictation. The assistant also maintains physicians' schedules, which involves keeping track of the time required for office encounters with patients, meetings, and conferences, as well as coordinating patients' hospital admissions and surgical procedures.

Billing and Insurance. The administrative medical assistant codes or verifies codes for diagnoses and procedures; processes and follows up on insurance claims, posts payments and prepares patients' bills; assists with banking duties; guides patients to available financial arrangements for payment; and maintains financial records.

Administrative Medical Assisting Skills

The work of an administrative medical assistant, which requires many technical and personal skills, is interesting and varied. The role of the AMA differs from that of the clinical medical assistant in that the clinical portion deals exclusively with the performance of medical tasks, such as taking blood samples and preparing a patient for a medical procedure. AMAs focus on administrative tasks ("front office skills"), such as those listed below.

Communication Skills. The assistant must understand and use correct English grammar, style, punctuation, and spelling in both writing and speaking. These skills enable the assistant to handle correspondence, medical records, and transcription and to interact well with other staff members, patients, and other medical personnel.

Electronic communications is the most common and efficient mode of communication for many messages. Even though this method of communication is fast, it requires proper grammar, punctuation, and structure. Taking the time to proofread any document prior to transmission is extremely important. Errors lead to misinformation which can lead to mistreatment.

Our nonverbal communication style is as important, sometimes more important, in the communication cycle as our verbal message. Body posture, voice tonality, and facial expressions are just a few examples of our nonverbal communications techniques. We will discussion communication skills more in depth in a future chapter.

Communicating with other medical personnel requires the knowledge, correct spelling, and proper use of medical terminology including nationally recognized medical abbreviations. Both correct pronunciation and written usage of the medical language are essential communication skills within the medical environment.

Mathematics Skills. The assistant must have good math skills to be able to maintain correct financial records, bill patients, and order and arrange payment for office supplies. Many questions asked of the medical office assistant involve a patient's financial responsibility—for example, what will be the patient's balance after insurance has paid its portion. Addition, subtraction, and percentage calculations are three math skills the assistant needs. Extracting payment information from insurance data and correctly posting to patient accounts are another area of responsibility for the AMA.

Organizational Skills. Controlling the usually hectic pace of work requires the assistant to have the skills of managing time and setting priorities. Systematic work habits, the willingness to take care of details, and the ability to handle several tasks at the same time (multitasking) are essential. Scheduling, updating and maintaining records, and keeping an orderly office require strong organizational skills. The most organized individual may still encounter many

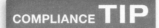
days when established priorities must be rearranged. Flexibility is another essential organizational skill needed by the medical office assistant.

Data Entry Skills. Accuracy in keying data and proficiency in proofreading are vital skills in the medical office. Patient personal and financial information is keyed into the electronic database and assimilated with the medical data to produce health claim forms and patient billings, as well as many other types of integrated reports. Errors in keyed information can have drastic effects on financial and medical information. As an example, a physician prescribes .025 mg of a medication and the information is keyed erroneously as 0.25 mg. The patient may suffer serious or fatal complications, and the practice could incur legal consequences.

AMAs must posses strong keyboarding and word processing skills, including mastery of the alpha, numeric, and symbols keys and functions, such as mail merge, in order to effectively process medical data. Producing professional letters, manuscripts, envelopes, and reports sends a nonverbal message about the professionalism of the office. Templates for chart notes and other commonly used formats save time and provide fewer opportunities for errors.

Computer and Equipment Skills. A basic understanding of a variety of technologies and the ability to use computers with mastery are essential workplace skills. Computers are used in every kind of healthcare setting for many different tasks. Computer programs handle word processing, financial spreadsheets, databases, and charts and visuals for speeches and presentations. With practice management programs, the assistant may handle billing, scheduling, account updating, records management, integrated reports (such as aging reports for patients and payors), and other tasks. Electronic scheduling is a popular feature because of its ease of searching and time-saving convenience.

Wireless technologies allow healthcare professionals who are away from their offices or hospitals to contact staff members and computers from any location. They also have constant accessibility to patient records through electronic health records programs, which are currently being defined by the federal government. Voice-recognition technology enables the physician to dictate notes using voice commands. The use of e-mail to communicate is as widespread as telephone communication, both within the medical practice and among medical practices, hospitals, and insurance companies.

To assist effectively in patient care, the medical assistant must be able to use a computer to:

- Process claims and bills and perform other routine financial tasks.
- Maintain the office schedule.
- Edit, revise, and generate documents.
- Scan and send documents to other locations.
- Communicate through e-mail within and outside the workplace.
- Research and obtain information from computer sources, such as the Internet.

Knowing how to use basic technologies, such as copiers and fax machines, has long been a requirement for every office professional. Scanners, calculators, and multiple-line telephone systems are also standard office equipment. Records must be kept on service agreements, in addition to warranties, repair records, and instructional materials for each piece of equipment. Knowing where and whom to call when equipment malfunctions is critical to the efficient flow of the office environment. Continuing to develop computer skills and learning new technological applications are crucial to the effectiveness and career advancement for administrative medical assistants.

Interpersonal Skills. Excellent interpersonal skills often come from a genuine desire to work with people. This desire and these interpersonal skills are essential for the administrative medical assistant, who is usually the patient's first contact with the medical office. That contact sets the tone for the patient's visit and influences the patient's opinion of the physician and the practice.

Many patients need someone to assist them with understanding the medical jargon sent to them from parties such as an insurance carrier. The medical office assistant serves as a liaison for the patient to help him or her translate the insurance language into everyday language and explain other medical office information.

The assistant skilled in positive communication with patients is warm, open, and friendly. Patients appreciate attention and concern—for their schedules and their comfort. Effective interpersonal skills involve looking directly at the person being spoken to, speaking slowly and clearly, listening carefully, and checking for understanding of the communicated message.

Respect for and openness to the other person are often shown by a pleasant facial expression and a genuine, natural smile. At the heart of interpersonal skills is sensitivity to the feelings and situations of other people.

1.2 ADMINISTRATIVE MEDICAL ASSISTING PERSONAL ATTRIBUTES

In addition to essential office skills, the success of the administrative medical assistant depends on a positive attitude toward work and a cheerful personality. *Personality* has been defined as the outward evidence of a person's character. Many aspects of personality are important in dealing with patients and other medical professionals.

Because patients entering a healthcare setting may be anxious, fearful, or unwell, most of them value a friendly, pleasant personality as the most important attribute of a medical assistant. The qualities discussed here are components of a pleasant personality and are useful professional and personal skills.

Genuine Liking for People

A genuine enjoyment of people and a desire to help them are keys to success in a medical assisting career. These qualities are expressed in the way you communicate with people through speech and body language.

Because patients may worry that they will be viewed only as numbers and notes on their patient charts, it is important that they feel recognized as individuals. In communicating with patients, your warmth and attentiveness help reassure patients and signal your desire to help. Looking directly at the patient and listening with attention communicate acceptance of the person. A pleasant facial expression, a natural smile, and a relaxed rather than rigid body posture are all body language signs that express openness and acceptance.

Viewing yourself and colleagues as integral medical office team members creates an atmosphere of cooperation and respect for individual differences. At times, personalities may seem to be in conflict; however, the individual who has a genuine liking of people will be able to respect differences within the team environment and accentuate the positiveness of cooperation through differences. Individuals change or lose positions more frequently due to the inability to get along with others than they do for lack of skills. Never underestimate the value of an open mind and of "playing nicely."

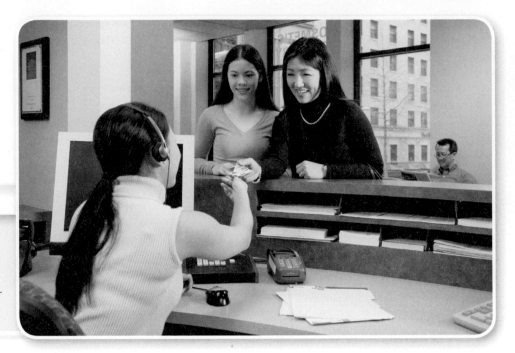

Figure 1.1

The administrative medical assistant enjoys working with people. *How do assistants show their care and concern for patients?*

Cheerfulness

The ability to be pleasant and friendly is an asset in any career. Lifting patients' spirits helps build goodwill between them and the physician. A pleasant assistant can frequently head off difficulties that occur when patients become worried, anxious, confused, or irritable.

> **EXAMPLE**
>
> It is five o'clock, normal closing time for the office. The doctor is behind schedule because of several difficult cases, and there are two patients yet to be seen in the waiting room. One of the patients approaches the assistant.
>
> **Patient:** I've been waiting a long time to see the doctor. How much longer will I have to wait?
>
> *Despite feeling tired at the end of the day and ready to go home, the assistant remains cheerful and explains the situation without frustration.*
>
> **Assistant:** Dr. Larsen has had several difficult cases today that have caused this delay. She will see you next, but it may be another 20 to 30 minutes.

In the above example, the patient may be feeling forgotten or ignored. Frequently, delays do occur. Patients should be kept apprised of delays and given the opportunity to choose to continue to wait or to reschedule their appointment.

Empathy

Many of the personal traits needed to be a successful medical assistant spring from **empathy**, a sensitivity to the feelings and situations of other people. Empathy enables you to understand how a patient feels because you can mentally put yourself in the patient's situation. Empathetic phrases such as "Insurance forms can be confusing" or "You seem confused, may I help?" may be used to show the patient you are concerned about his or her situation. Phrases that emphasize yourself or give false impressions, such as "I completely understand how you feel," should be avoided. Everyone has had some personal experience with an illness or with not feeling perfectly well. Reminding yourself of how you felt and of how you wanted to be treated in that situation will help you treat patients with kindness.

> **EXAMPLE**
>
> **Assistant:** Mr. Strauss, I realize you are not feeling well after your surgery yesterday. Would you feel more comfortable lying down while you wait?
>
> Understand that nervous patients may not be listening clearly to your instructions. Offering to repeat them and answering questions are other examples of empathy.

1.3 EMPLOYMENT OPPORTUNITIES

The U.S. Department of Labor projects this field will grow much faster than the average, ranking medical assistants among the fasting growing occupations for the 2008–2018 decade. In 2008, the Department of Labor reported 483,600 persons employed as medical assistants, with a projected 647,500 employed in 2018, a 34 percent increase. Fueling the rapid growth are advances in technologies, an aging population, and healthcare reform. Job opportunities are predicted to be excellent, especially for those with formal training, experience, and/or certification. Administrative medical assistants have opportunities to advance into management positions, such as office manager or compliance officer. There are many organizations, institutions, and companies that operate in areas within or closely related to healthcare. Workers familiar with the healthcare environment are of value and in demand.

A thorough training in technical skills, the development of good interpersonal skills, and ongoing professional development help ensure a successful career for administrative medical assistants. Because the healthcare industry is booming, a well-trained medical assistant has a wide variety of opportunities in many different settings.

Physician Practice

The most common place of employment for the administrative medical assistant is in a physician practice. The majority of physicians are associated with a group practice—in which space, staff, and physical resources, such as equipment and laboratory facilities, are shared. A group practice may consist of physicians who are all generalists or who all have the same specialty, or it may be a combination of generalists and specialists.

There are many advantages to both doctors and patients in these larger practices. Doctors may better control spiraling overhead costs of operating an office. Such practices also give new physicians the opportunity to join an established practice and to acquire new patients to add to their clientele. Because of the large volume of patients, the administrative medical assistant may specialize in a task area, such as patient scheduling, or may perform a variety of duties.

Some administrative medical assistants work in a small office where one or two physicians practice. The assistant acts as the doctor's right hand, taking care of all administrative tasks. Working in a small office gives the assistant a great deal of responsibility, variety in the tasks to be done, and an opportunity to develop close ties with patients and the physician.

There are job opportunities for assistants in a wide range of practices. Many such medical specialties are listed and defined in Figure 1.2. In addition to these specialties, the American Medical Association (AMA) lists 170 others. Many of the specialties on this expanded list are surgical practices related to the specialties shown in Figure 1.2. However, there are also specialties that deal with new areas, such as undersea and aerospace medicine. Other specialties reflect the increased use of new technologies to treat illness. Interventional radiology is an example of such a specialty; it uses tools guided by radiologic imaging to perform procedures that are less invasive than those required with surgery.

Figure 1.2 Examples of Medical Specialties and Subspecialties

Addiction Medicine: An addiction medicine specialist is a physician who diagnoses and treats the complications of substance abuse addiction, including the physical and psychological complications.

Allergy: An allergist diagnoses and treats adverse reactions to foods, drugs, and other substances.

Anesthesiology: An anesthesiologist maintains pain relief and stable body functions of patients during surgical procedures.

Bariatric: A bariatric physician specializes in the causes, treatment, and prevention of obesity.

Chiropractic: This discipline studies the disease process as a result of deviations/changes to the normal workings of the nervous system. Common treatment options include body manipulation and other forms of therapy.

Dentistry: A dentist is concerned with the care and treatment of teeth and gums, especially prevention, diagnosis, and treatment of deformities, diseases, and traumatic injuries.

Subspecialties include the following:

An **endodontist** specializes in root canal work.

A **forensic** dentist applies dental facts to legal issues.

An **oral surgeon** specializes in jaw surgery and extractions.

An **orthodontist** straightens teeth.

A **pedodontist** provides dental care for children.

A **periodontist** specializes in gum disease.

A **prosthodontist** specializes in dentures and artificial teeth.

Dermatology: A dermatologist diagnoses and treats diseases of the skin and related tissues.

Emergency Medicine: An emergency room physician provides immediate treatment of accidents and illnesses.

Family Practice: A family practice physician provides total healthcare for the family.

Geriatrics: This field of medicine diagnoses and treats conditions and diseases that are specific to the older population.

Hospice: This field of medicine renders interdisciplinary care to individuals with life-threatening conditions. Physical (pain management), psychological, and spiritual services are given to the patient and the family. The primary focus of hospice care is quality of life.

Gynecology: A gynecologist is concerned with the diseases of the female genital tract, as well as female endocrinology and reproductive physiology.

Internal Medicine: An internist diagnoses a wide range of nonsurgical illnesses. Subspecialties include the following:

Cardiovascular Medicine: A cardiologist diagnoses and treats diseases of the heart, blood vessels, and lungs.

Endocrinology: An endocrinologist diagnoses and treats endocrine gland diseases.

Gastroenterology: A gastroenterologist diagnoses and treats diseases of the digestive tract and related organs.

Gerontology: A gerontologist treats the process and problems of aging.

Hematology: A hematologist diagnoses and treats diseases of the blood.

Immunology: An immunologist diagnoses and treats symptoms of immunity, induced sensitivity, and allergies.

Infectious Disease: A specialist in infectious disease diagnoses and treats all types of infectious diseases.

Nephrology: A nephrologist diagnoses and treats disorders of the kidneys and related functions.

Oncology: An oncologist diagnoses and treats cancer.

Pulmonary Disease: A pulmonologist diagnoses and treats lung disorders.

Rheumatology: A rheumatologist is concerned with the study, diagnosis, and treatment of rheumatic conditions.

Neurology: A neurologist diagnoses and treats disorders of the nervous system.

Obstetrics: An obstetrician provides care during pregnancy and childbirth.

Occupational Medicine: A specialist in occupational medicine works with companies to prevent and manage occupational and environmental injury, illness, and disability and to promote health and productivity of workers and their families and communities.

Ophthalmology: An ophthalmologist cares for the eyes and vision.

Osteopathology: This field of medicine specializes in the diagnosis and treatment of the neuromusculoskeletal system.

Orthopedics: An orthopedic surgeon or orthopedist provides treatment of the musculoskeletal system.

Otorhinolaryngology: A physician in otorhinolaryngology specializes in the diagnosis and treatment of illnesses of the ears, nose, and throat (ENT).

Pathology: A pathologist investigates the causes of disease using laboratory techniques.

Pediatrics: A pediatrician specializes in the comprehensive treatment of children.

Physical Medicine/Rehabilitation: A physiatrist evaluates and treats all types of disease through physical means, such as heat.

Plastic Surgery: A plastic surgeon repairs and reconstructs body structures through surgical means.

Psychiatry: A psychiatrist diagnoses and treats mental, emotional, and behavioral disorders.

Radiology and Nuclear Medicine: A radiologist uses radioactive materials to diagnose and treat disease.

Thoracic Surgery: A thoracic surgeon uses surgery to diagnose or treat diseases of the chest.

Urology: A urologist diagnoses and treats diseases of the urinary tract.

Clinics

The administrative medical assistant may be employed by a clinic. A clinic may specialize in the diagnosis and treatment of a specific disorder—back pain, headache, mental health, or wound treatment, for example—and is considered an outpatient setting. Many clinics have a number of specialties within one building. The specialties may be related, so that the patient moves from department to department for extensive examination and specialty consultations.

Hospitals and Medical Centers

Hospitals and the large physical complexes that make up medical centers employ many administrative support personnel, particularly those skilled in specific medical office management tasks. Assistants may work in the admissions department in several areas of a hospital or medical center—the main admitting office, where patients are received for a stay in the hospital; admissions to the emergency room; or admissions for patients in same-day surgery clinics. Departments such as patient education, insurance, billing, social services, and medical records also need skilled and knowledgeable assistants. Career opportunities for assistants in these facilities will continue to grow along with the technological advances in diagnosis and treatment and the size of the aging population.

Care Facilities

There are many facilities specializing in the short-term care of patients recovering after hospital stays. There are also patients who enter rehabilitation centers to improve the functioning of their back, arms, legs, hips, or hands. Other facilities provide long-term care for patients with chronic mental or physical illnesses. All of these facilities rely on skilled personnel who understand patients and their care.

Insurance Companies

The healthcare industry is subject to great pressure because of high health costs and the reality that people are living longer and often require greater care as they age. Insurance companies and government health insurance programs must ensure that claims from healthcare providers are "clean claims"—in other words, the claim forms are correct and complete. They employ administrative medical assistants who are skilled in handling medical documents and understand medical procedures. Assistants may work for the following:

- Large insurance companies specializing in healthcare, such as Blue Cross Blue Shield and CIGNA
- Government-sponsored programs, such as Medicare, Medicaid, and Tricare
- Other insurers, some of which are sponsored by clubs, unions, and employee associations
- Managed care organizations

All areas of employment have complex needs and require the handling of tasks such as completing and checking reports received from doctors, coding diagnoses and procedures, adjusting claims, sending payments of claims, and renewing contracts.

1.4 WORK ETHIC AND PROFESSIONALISM

Positive personality traits are developed into habits and skills that help the administrative medical assistant deal effectively with tasks and people. These habits and skills, which form a **work ethic**, greatly enhance employees' value in any medical work setting.

Work Ethic

Employers responding to research surveys about employees rank certain habits and skills the highest. These habits and skills make the employee valuable to the practice. They are also often predictors of success in a medical office setting.

For centuries, work ethics, the outward display of an employee's values and standards, has been one of the foundation stones of business. Businesses have either been successful or failed as a direct result of employees' work ethics. We will discuss several areas in which employees outwardly display work ethic.

Accuracy. Because even a minor error may have major consequences for a patient's health, physicians rank **accuracy** as the most important employee trait. Although physicians may give exact instructions, they may not oversee tasks to completion. The physician counts on the assistant to perform tasks with complete correctness, including constant attention to detail.

Thoroughness. The careful and complete attention to detail required for accuracy is known as **thoroughness**. The thorough assistant produces work that is neat, accurate, and complete. This trait involves

- Listening attentively.
- Taking ample notes.
- Paying attention to details, such as who, what, when, why, where, and how.
- Verifying information.
- Following through on details without having to be reminded.

The physician and other team members should be able to depend on the assistant to accomplish any task in a complete, accurate, and timely manner.

Dependability. The administrative medical assistant who finishes work on schedule, does required tasks without complaint (even when they are unpleasant), and always communicates willingness to help is said to be a dependable employee. **Dependability** is closely related to accuracy and thoroughness. The dependable assistant

- Asks questions and repeats instructions to avoid mistakes.
- Asks for assistance with unfamiliar tasks.
- Enters all data, such as insurance claim information and lab values, carefully.
- Takes clear and complete messages.

Others can depend on the assistant to accomplish tasks effectively and as efficiently as possible. When an emergency situation occurs and the AMA must miss work, contact the designated staff member, such as the office manager, immediately so tasks and responsibilities can be completed on time.

HIPAA TIPS

Patient confidentiality is an important part of Health Insurance Portability and Accountability Act (HIPAA) compliancy. Never discuss confidential patient information when using a speaker phone feature. Unauthorized parties may be able to overhear the conversation. It is important and courteous to advise speakers that they are being broadcast and to advise them of all other listeners in the room. If there is a possibility of being overheard by patients or visitors, the speaker phone should not be used. The voice should be kept sufficiently low even when not using a speaker phone.

You are responsible for making patient callbacks prior to leaving for the afternoon. The other medical office professional is absent, so you are also responsible for prepping charts for the next day's appointments. Using the speaker option on the telephone means that you can do other things at the same time, such as charting in patients' files. If you decide to use this option, what would you say to the patient on the phone to advise him or her that you are on speaker phone?

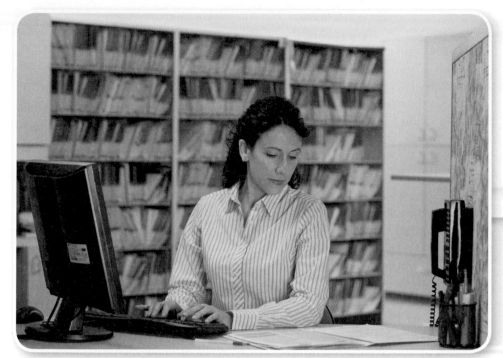

Figure 1.3

The administrative medical assistant shown here is completing an insurance claim form. *How can assistants ensure accuracy in their work?*

Efficiency. Effective individuals accomplish tasks, but efficiency has higher value in the work environment than effectiveness alone. Using time and other resources to avoid waste and unnecessary effort when completing tasks is the defining mark of **efficiency**. An example of an efficient administrative medical assistant is one who plans the day's work in advance, makes a schedule for completion, and assembles the materials and resources necessary to complete the tasks. Efficiency also includes the organizational ability to divide large, complex tasks into smaller, more manageable components. Rearranging resources to complete tasks efficiently may require change. Flexibility is a key component when working within a medical office environment.

Flexibility. The ability to adapt, to change gears quickly, and to respond to changing situations, interruptions, and delays is **flexibility**. The flexible assistant is able to respond calmly to last-minute assignments to meet deadlines under pressure, and to handle several tasks at once. The ability to grasp new situations and new concepts quickly is an important aspect of flexibility. Being able to implement new ideas and good suggestions with self-confidence is a mark of flexibility.

The medical office is a changing environment. The introduction of computer technology and implementation of the Health Insurance Portability and Accountability Act (HIPAA) require extreme flexibility by all medical office team members. Government-mandated implementation of electronic health records and a new coding system (ICD-10) are quickly approaching as the next new horizon of change. Flexibility and good judgment will be key contributors to a smooth transition.

Good Judgment. The quality of **good judgment** involves the ability to use knowledge, experience, and logic to assess all the aspects of a situation in order to reach a sound decision. Frequently, good judgment is expressed by the administrative medical assistant who knows when to make a statement and when to withhold one. For example, choosing the right time and right words when making a suggestion to an employer or to other staff members shows good judgment. It may also be good judgment to decide that the suggestion should not be made because, based on your objective and honest evaluation of past experience, the suggestion will not be accepted.

Honesty. Telling the truth is **honesty**. It is expressed in words and actions. It is the quality that enables the physician to trust the administrative medical assistant at all times. The trustworthy assistant understands the serious nature of the physician's work and the confidential nature of the patient's dealings with the physician. The assistant can be trusted not to reveal any of a patient's data, any conversations, or any details, which must always remain confidential. Honesty is central to the integrity that allows the assistant to effectively represent the profession. Finally, the honest assistant demonstrates initiative by quickly reporting mistakes without attempting to cover them up or blame others.

Initiative. To take action independently is to show **initiative**. The administrative medical assistant works with certain routine administrative activities every day. Dealing with these often requires the assistant to take action without receiving specific instructions from the physician. The assistant's ability to move work forward and to resolve issues by using initiative is a valuable skill in a busy office.

Initiative also involves making unsolicited offers of help that mark a valued employee, one who goes beyond the job's regular responsibilities. For example, offering to stay late to help the physician or coworkers finish extra work is always appreciated. To give patients additional help, you may offer to call for a taxi after an appointment, obtain a wheelchair when needed, write out instructions, or send a reminder card before the next appointment. Medical office assistants who demonstrate initiative also have critical-thinking skills and problem-solving abilities.

Problem-Solving Ability. **Problem-solving** involves logically planning the steps needed to accomplish a job. Asking for advice when appropriate and acting wisely also demonstrate the ability to solve problems effectively. The administrative medical assistant who is adept at solving problems also has a basic understanding of the goals and requirements of the work environment. Critical-thinking skills and problem-solving skills work together to establish steps and reach solutions. Just as problem-solving involves logically planning steps, the assistant who uses critical-thinking skills looks at all possible resources to build the steps. Critical thinkers use past experiences and present resources and knowledge to form future solutions. In other words, they think "in and outside their box." Brainstorming, listing all possible ideas, with others allows the assistant to gather information that otherwise may not have been considered. Being able to produce solutions in a timely manner should be one of the goals of a problem-solving team.

Punctuality. Being on time—**punctuality**—is important for the administrative medical assistant because of the physician's schedule and the need to complete routine duties before patients arrive. A medical office is often open for the staff a half hour before patient appointments. This is not a time for employees to use in getting from home to work. It is a time for planning the day's work, organizing tasks, and greeting patients who arrive before the start of business hours. It is common for an answering service to continue answering calls during this time to allow the assistant and other team members time to prepare. Given enough time, the self-motivated employee may prepare the next day's tasks prior to leaving at the end of the work shift.

Self-Motivation. The quality of **self-motivation** is expressed by a willingness to learn new duties or procedures without a requirement to do so. The administrative medical assistant who helps with work that needs to be done and learns new aspects of job responsibilities is self-motivated. Alertness is an aspect of self-motivation. This alertness enables the assistant to see and undertake jobs that need to be done and to anticipate the patient's and the physician's needs. A mix of self-motivation and tact should be used when seeking areas to assist fellow team members.

Tact. The ability to speak and act considerately, especially in difficult situations, is known as **tact**. Working with people in ways that show you are sensitive to their possible reactions helps you achieve the purpose at hand smoothly and without giving offense. Tactful manners and speech create goodwill with patients and other members of the medical office team.

Being a Member of the Team. Those who have the positive attitude of a **team player** are generous with their time, helping other staff members when necessary. A good team player observes stated office policies and quickly learns the unwritten rules of office life, such as

- When it is acceptable to sit at another employee's desk
- Whether it is acceptable to eat or drink at your desk
- How to time a break and determine how long it should be
- When and in what manner it is acceptable to converse with coworkers

Being a good team player also involves the simple courtesies: avoiding personal activities, phone calls, and text messaging; knocking before entering an office, even if the door is open; being careful about sharing details of your personal life in ordinary polite conversation; and avoiding the use of profanity and coarse language. Team players, moreover, are always careful to observe confidentiality by not discussing patients or commenting in any way about them or any other staff members.

Working outside the traditional office environment, such as processing medical insurance claims from home, still requires the staff member to work as part of and consider the needs of the medical office team. Missing a deadline or keeping materials longer than anticipated can cause a ripple effect. Aggressive behavior within a team promotes ill feelings and a lack of cooperation; however, professionally assertive behavior among those working together as a team can promote positive attitudes toward daily responsibilities and a willingness to cooperate to accomplish goals.

Assertiveness. **Assertiveness** is the ability to step forward to make a point in a confident, positive manner. In some ways, assertiveness is the result of having acquired many of the habits, attitudes, and skills discussed here. Administrative medical assistants who are accurate, dependable, and honest, who understand and perform tasks with intelligence and good judgment, are confident employees. They are able to step forward and contribute to a more efficient, more cordial work environment. Assertiveness is always a positive force. It is unlike aggressiveness, which is a hostile and overbearing attitude. Assertiveness assumes that the assistant not only is competent but also has established cordial and cooperative working relationships.

Professional Image

Few professions are as much respected as the medical profession. It has an image of health, cleanliness, and wholesomeness. If you choose to work in a healthcare setting, your appearance and bearing must reflect this image. Patients expect your positive personality and pleasing manner to be reflected in your appearance through healthful habits, good grooming, and appropriate dress.

Being in style, as advertisements and magazines define style, is not the same thing as projecting a **professional image**. Style is about reflecting a personal vision of who you are in the way you act, dress, and groom, such as hairstyle and nail care. In the workplace, however, you reflect not your own personal vision but the employer's preferences about how the practice should be seen by patients and the community.

Physical Attributes. Good health is the result of maintaining good posture, eating a properly balanced diet, getting sufficient rest, and exercising regularly. These good health

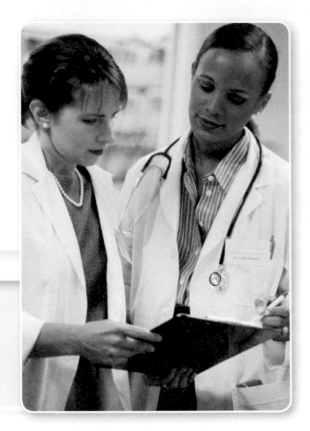

Figure 1.4

The administrative medical assistant projects a professional image.
What habits, grooming, and dress styles show professionalism?

habits show in the energy of your body when you move, walk, or communicate; in the healthful glow of your skin; in the alertness and clarity of your eyes; and even in the shine of your hair and the health of your nails.

Habits that promote good health are essential to maintaining a professional image. These good health habits are complemented by good grooming habits. Although cleanliness is the basis of good grooming, grooming means more than cleanliness. A daily bath or shower, the use of deodorant, regular dental care along with daily dental brushing and flossing, and a neat overall appearance are all elements of good grooming. Also included in good grooming habits are the following:

- Nails should be manicured, so that the hands look cared for. Employees should avoid bright or unusual nail polish colors and stenciled nails. Nails should not be so long that they pose a threat to others or interfere with working at the keyboard. Office policy on artificial nails should be followed.
- Hair requires frequent shampooing and should be arranged in a conservative style that will not require a great deal of attention during working hours.
- The patient and assistant should be able to look at each other eye to eye; therefore, hair should not cover the eyes or interfere with sight.
- Male employees should shave daily or have neatly trimmed facial hair.
- Perfumes or colognes should be avoided in the office. Staff members and patients may be irritated by fragrances, especially those with a floral base. Lotions should also be unscented.
- Makeup should be used moderately and should complement the assistant's skin type and color.
- Clothes must always be freshly laundered and pressed. If you are required to wear a white uniform, it must be kept *snow* white and should never be worn over dark underclothes. If street clothes are worn in the office, they should be simple and should fit well. Tight or revealing clothes are not appropriate.
- Shoes should be comfortable and in good repair.

- Jewelry and hair ornaments are not good accompaniments to uniforms. Jewelry that is worn with street clothes in the office should be small and unobtrusive. Large bangles and bracelets with dangling parts are often noisy and get in the way of work.
- Most professional work environments have a stated policy concerning the amount and type of jewelry that may be worn—for example, one ring per hand (engagement ring/wedding band is considered one). Piercings and tatoos are common in today's society and office policy will state what may be worn and/or shown. Common policies state that no more than two earrings per ear are permitted and that no other piercings may have jewelry, such as tongue, nose, eyebrow, or lip. Tatoos should be covered.

Maturity. Many administrative and personal skills contribute to the achievement of **maturity**. And maturity *is* an achievement. It takes great determination to acquire and practice the attitudes, habits, and skills that contribute to maturity.

Emotional and psychological maturity is not dependent on age. It is made up of many aspects of personality and of many skills. The mature person is able to work with supervisors and under pressure, even in unpleasant or frustrating conditions. The mature person sees a job through and gives more than is asked. Maturity enables a person to gather and use information to make good decisions. Maturity is reflected by independence of judgment as well as by ambition and determination. As maturity becomes evident in the administrative medical assistant, it inspires the confidence of managers, patients, and coworkers.

1.5 PROFESSIONAL GROWTH AND CERTIFICATION

When an employee stops being willing to learn, he or she stops growing professionally and becomes less valuable to their employers and other colleagues. Learning and growing in the field allow the administrative medical assistant to become more successful and to enjoy an enviable professional status. Once assistants have completed specific requirements, they are eligible to join several national associations. By passing examinations, medical assistants may become certified. **Certification** is the indication given by certain associations that a person has met high standards and has achieved competency in the knowledge and tasks required. Through continuing education, seminars, conferences, and meetings with other professionals in the field, these organizations provide opportunities to grow as office professionals and to advance in a chosen career.

AAMA. The American Association of Medical Assistants (**AAMA**) is a major nationwide organization. The AAMA recommends to the Commission on Accreditation for Allied Health Education Programs (CAAHEP) those formal education programs that have met AAMA curriculum standards. Further, the AAMA sponsors the national certification examination for medical assistants in three areas: general, administrative, and clinical. As stated earlier in the chapter, specifics within each of the three areas are outlined at the AAMA Web site (http://www.aama-ntl.org). Those who pass the examination are certified and receive the designation of Certified Medical Assistant (CMA).

The AAMA requires CMAs to be recertified every five years. This practice ensures that medical assistants keep up with developments in the field. There are hundreds of continuing education courses sponsored by the AAMA to help assistants keep current and become recertified.

Although medical assistants need not be certified to be employed as assistants, certification improves the chances of career advancement and provides motivation for continued professional growth.

AMT. The American Medical Technologists (**AMT**) is another nationwide organization offering certification for medical assistants. Successful completion of this examination earns the credential of Registered Medical Assistant (RMA). A certification exam to become a Certified Medical Administrative Specialist (CMAS) is also offered through AMT.

AHDI. The Association for Healthcare Documentation Integrity (**AHDI**), formerly known as the American Association of Medical Transcription (AAMT), is a nationwide organization that promotes professional standards and growth for those who have a special interest in transcription and wish to be certified. AHDI offers the Certified Medical Transcriptionist (CMT) certification exam. It is recommended that individuals wishing to take this exam have at least two years of transcription experience in acute care transcribing. Also offered by the AHDI is the Registered Medical Transcriptionist (RMT) exam. Individuals with less than two years of transcription experience (such as a recent graduate) may sit for this exam. Part One consists of multiple-choice questions from six content areas: medical terminology, English language and usage, anatomy and physiology, disease process, healthcare records, and professional development. Part Two is a medical transcription work simulation.

Even with the use of voice-recognition technology, medical transcriptionists will continue to be in demand. The technology cannot yet handle all the nuances of English. The transcriptionist's skill in English usage, grammar, and style ensures the competent editing and correction of materials. Taking advantage of certification and opportunities for continued study in this field, as in medical assisting, helps in career advancement.

IAAP. The International Association of Administrative Professionals (**IAAP**), previously known as Professional Secretaries International (PSI), is a worldwide nonprofit organization working with career-minded administrative professionals to promote excellence through education, community building, and leadership development. Core values of IAAP include integrity, respect, adaptability, communication, and commitment. This organization sponsors two comprehensive examinations—the Certified Professional Secretary (CPS) and the Certified Administrative Professional (CAP). Individuals successfully completing the CPS demonstrate competence in office technology, office systems and administration, and management. Those passing the CAP demonstrate competence in the three areas of the CPS exam plus one additional area, advanced organizational management. The organization, which maintains chapters all over the country, makes professional contacts easy. The IAAP provides study materials and information about available review courses.

There are companies that offer salary incentives to those who become certified secretaries. In this area, as in all other areas of most professions, certification improves the chances for advancement.

AAPC and AHIMA. The American Academy of Professional Coders (AAPC) and the American Health Information Management Association offer certification in areas related to coding health information management. AAPC offers the credentials of Certified Professional Coder (CPC), Certified Professional Coder-Outpatient Hospital (CPC-H), Certified Professional Coder-Payer (CPC-P), and Certified Interventional Radiology Cardiovascular Coder (CIRCC). Credential exams are also available in many speciality areas, such as dermatology.

AHIMA offers three certifying exams in coding—CCA (Certified Coding Association), CCS (Certified Coding Specialist), and CCS-P (Certified Coding Specialist-Physician Based). Four exams are offered to allow individuals to demonstrate their competency in areas dealing with health information and the medical records. RHIT (Registered Health Information Technician) and RHIA (Registered Health Information Administrator) both deal exclusively with the the quality of medical records. Knowledge of medical, administrative, ethical, and legal requirements as they pertain to medical record information is required. Applicants will also be asked to demonstrate their competence in computer information systems.

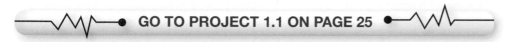 **GO TO PROJECT 1.1 ON PAGE 25**

1.6 INTERPERSONAL RELATIONSHIPS

The administrative medical assistant is usually the first person the patient comes into contact with when making an appointment or going to the doctor's office. The way in which the assistant receives and welcomes the patient, whether by phone or physically in the office, establishes the tone of the visit, the professionalism of the office, and the patient's feelings about the doctor and the treatment.

The responsibility to make patients feel that they are important and that enough time is available to them for treatment is of major concern for the medical assistant. Although the office may be busy, and both the doctor and the patients may want to speak to the assistant at the same time, the assistant must remain calm, reassuring, and pleasant to everyone.

Taking Care of Patients

Greeting a patient by name, if possible, contributes to making that patient feel important. If you are away from the desk when a patient arrives, acknowledge the patient with a smile and a greeting as soon as you return.

Every person is to be shown the same degree of respect and concern without regard to race, age, gender, or socioeconomic situation. Every doctor's office accepts patients who receive care for a nominal fee or even completely free. The physician's aim in all cases is the same: to make the person well in the shortest possible time. The assistant's aim in all cases is to treat all patients with the same amount of sympathy, concern, and attention.

Familiarity

A physician may choose to establish a less formal tone in the office in order to make patients feel more comfortable. Even when this is the case, the office is still a professional setting. Certain ways of expressing familiarity, either with the physician or with the patients, are not appropriate.

The doctor should always be referred to and spoken to by title and last name: "Dr. Larsen will see you now." This courtesy is observed even if the physician and administrative medical assistant are relatives or have a personal relationship. Conversation in front of patients should never indicate anything other than a professional relationship.

Patients may have preferences about the way they are addressed. It shows respect to address the patient by the appropriate title and last name: "Mr. /Mrs. /Ms. /Miss /Reverend /Lopez." If a patient wishes to be addressed in some other way, such as by a first name or nickname, that patient will invite you to do so. The assistant should make a notation of the preference for future use. Names that are difficult for the assistant should have the pronunciation noted. It is acceptable to call children by their given name.

> **EXAMPLE**
>
> **Assistant:** Mrs. Haynes, Dr. Larsen is ready to see you now.
>
> **Patient:** Thank you, Linda, but please call me Margaret. I'm not used to being called Mrs. Haynes.

Social Relationships

In many offices, the policy discourages, or may even forbid, a social relationship between a patient and a staff member. Such a policy reflects the physician's belief that these relationships are not consistent with a professional atmosphere and may interfere with the proper medical management of the patient's case. Under no circumstances should you make a social engagement with a patient without first checking office policy and discussing the situation with your employer.

Conversation with Patients

If the administrative medical assistant has to spend considerable time with a patient, the patient is the one who decides whether or not to start a conversation. If the patient wishes to talk, the patient should also choose the subject. The assistant should listen and respond courteously. General subjects, such as the weather, sports, hobbies, or local events, may be ideal topics. Try to avoid controversial subjects, such as politics or religion. Keeping the conversation to general topics should also ensure that you are never in a situation where you argue with a patient or try to persuade a patient that a certain view is correct.

Because the patient identifies the administrative medical assistant with the doctor, the patient also believes that the assistant carries the doctor's authority. For this reason, the assistant should never offer a patient medical advice or comment on the patient's treatment. Very few patients have a substantial knowledge of medicine, anatomy, or physiology. They may easily misunderstand a remark made by the assistant, especially if the remark contains a technical term. If the patient seeks advice or asks a question related to treatment, the medical assistant should respond tactfully: "That is a question the doctor should answer for you. Be sure to ask about that during your examination."

Difficult Patients. The best test of interpersonal skills may be the successful handling of difficult, unreasonable, or unpleasant patients. The patient's self-control may be undermined by the pain and worry that accompany the illness. Dealing with short-tempered or irritable patients requires the medical assistant to show patience, understanding, and restraint. Calmly repeating instructions to an uncooperative patient may be difficult, but it may prevent having to ask a patient to redo a procedure or task or having to repeat the instructions later.

EXAMPLE

Assistant: Mr. Rosen, here are the instructions for the x-ray you are going to have on Monday. Let me go over them with you again to make sure you understand them and to see whether you have any questions. If you think of any questions at a later time, you may call me. I have written my name and telephone number here and will be happy to help answer your questions.

A patient who has had to wait a long time to see the doctor may become restless or impatient. In such instances, the medical assistant should make some gesture of attention. Introduce a general topic of conversation or reassure the patient that you are aware of the lateness of the schedule and thank the person for understanding.

There are times when patients become angry. A mistake in an insurance payment, a long wait to see the doctor, or even the patient's physical pain or discomfort may trigger an outburst of bad temper. The medical assistant must remain calm and courteous. A gentle tone and soothing voice sometimes help calm a patient. Separate facts from feelings and never argue. Politely offer to help correct a situation in any way you can. The offer by itself may help eliminate the patient's anger.

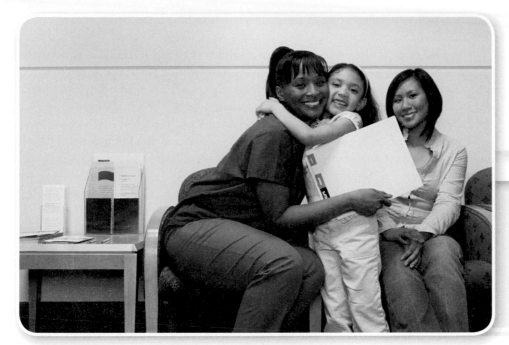

Figure 1.5

The administrative medical assistant ensures that patients leave the office with a feeling of goodwill. *What actions and attitudes cause patients to feel positive about their office visits?*

Every patient should leave the doctor's office with a feeling of goodwill. Frequently, the medical assistant will have an opportunity to talk to the patient as the patient prepares to leave the office. Calling the patient by name, if possible, and extending a pleasant good-bye will have beneficial results. A patient who leaves the office on a positive note may tell others about a good experience with the staff.

Terminally Ill Patients. If a patient whom you know to be terminally ill engages you in conversation, be sensitive to the situation by avoiding certain questions that you might ordinarily ask, such as "How are you?" Try to keep the conversation short and general. Terminally ill patients usually are willing and eager to discuss topics such as children and/or grandchildren, spouses/partners, or other individuals of whom they are proud. Many patients have hobbies, such as gardening or music, about which they are excited to share. Select topics that are short-term in nature instead of long-term topics, such as plans for the next New Year's celebration. The bottom line is to be empathetic to the patient's condition and emotional state.

Confidentiality

Maintaining the **confidentiality**, or privacy, of patients' medical information is a legal requirement. A doctor who gives information about a patient without a patient's permission, except to another doctor, can be prosecuted under the law, and the doctor's license may be revoked. Similar legal requirements and penalties apply to employees in the doctor's office.

Patient Sign-in Log. Documentation of a patient's visit, in his or her own handwriting, is provided when the patient signs in on the log. The patient's privacy is to be protected at all times, which includes the check-in and waiting area.

Traditionally, a patient arrives at the office and signs his or her name and other pertinent information, such as arrival time, appointment time, and doctor to be seen, on a check-in or visitor's log. Leaving this information available to be viewed by others is a violation of HIPAA. Many offices still use this format; however, as soon as the patient arrives, the name is marked through with a broad, dark marker. The problem with this method is that the written documentation of the patient's visit in his or her own handwriting has been eliminated.

Currently, one of the preferred sign-in methods is a label method. Patients arrive and place their name on a label on the sign-in log. Information about the arrival time and appointment time, as well as other generic information, are checked off by the patient. The label containing the patient's name is then removed by the administrative medical assistant and placed into the patient's chart as evidence of the patient's arrival.

Assigning numbers to patients on their arrival is another method of protecting patient confidentiality. Their number, instead of their name, is used when addressing them in the waiting area.

Sometimes patients will verbally check in on their arrival. The assistant will make a notation of their arrival on a preprinted daily schedule.

Medical Histories. Medical histories of patients contain a great deal of confidential information, not only about the patients but also about their families and perhaps other contacts, such as friends. Employees may not disclose any information about a patient's illness, personal history, or matters relating to family or others.

Confidentiality about medical records is also to be observed in any conversations the medical assistant has with the patient. It is not the medical assistant's place to share with the patient the doctor's diagnosis or prognosis. The doctor is the sole judge of what information is to be given to, or withheld from, the patient. The assistant must refuse to discuss the patient's case and should refer the patient to the doctor for information.

Many people other than the patients themselves may ask the medical assistant for information about a patient's case. There are some patients who are curious about other patients whom they may know or may have seen in the doctor's office during their own visits. There are some curious patients who may try to obtain personal information about the doctor, staff, or other patients. Friends or relatives of a patient may inquire about the doctor's opinion, the method of treatment, or the duration of the illness. A courteous but firm refusal, such as "I'm sorry, but that information is confidential," should prevent further attempts to get information.

Record Security. The medical assistant must be aware of the location of the front desk and of various work areas in relation to public spaces, such as the lobby or waiting room. Location is important in safeguarding the confidentiality of records because they may be read if left where other patients, staff members, or visitors can see them. Because patient records, schedules, and billing information are now often computerized, the locations of computer screens at the front desk and in work areas are also important. Sensitive information should not remain on the screen when you need to be away from the desk. Screen savers should be used when away from the computer area, and access to computer data should be password protected. Screens should not be able to be viewed by patients, either on their arrival or their departure. Monitor protectors that allow data to be viewed only from the front may also prevent accidental disclosure of medical information.

Hardcopy medical charts are often placed outside the exam room for the physician to review prior to entering the room. As other patients pass this area, they can see the name on the chart. This is illegal disclosure of protected medical information and a violation of HIPAA. A very simple solution is to turn the chart around, so that the name and any other medical information are not exposed.

In areas close to the waiting room or lobby, caution should also be exercised in conversations, whether over the phone or face to face. Conversations between a patient and the assistant or among employees may easily be overheard. Unless sound-proof glass is being used, simply sliding the glass window closed does not prevent information from being heard.

In general, nothing that happens in the office should be repeated at home or to friends. A patient can sometimes be identified by the circumstances of the case or by some other detail, even when the patient's name is not mentioned.

There is wisdom in the adage "What you see here, what you hear here, must remain here when you leave."

Cultural Diversity

People's beliefs, value systems, and language, as well as their understanding of the world, grow out of the culture into which they were born and in which they were raised. It is important to understand that, just as the elements of your culture are formative for you, so the cultures of others are formative for them. Although each culture is different, no one culture is superior in any way to any other culture. However, it is important to understand that people in cultures different from yours may express themselves and present themselves in a different way from what your own culture has taught you to expect. **Ethnocentrism** is the tendency to believe that one's own race or ethnic group is the most important and that some or all aspects of its culture are superior to those of other groups. This, in and of itself, can be a barrier within the office team environment and in interactions with patients. Be respectful of people of all cultures and backgrounds. This does not mean that you accept the beliefs and customs of the culture as your own, but that you are considerate of each individual's right to express individualism within cultural practices, such as dress. Never assign patients to stereotypes that are racial, ethnic, or religious.

Language Barriers. Although most aspects of other cultures do not present barriers, a great cultural barrier may occur when the patient and staff do not speak the same language. The ideal solution is to be able to speak to a family friend or relative who accompanies the patient and can act as an interpreter. If this is not possible, you may want to have several foreign language phrase books on hand in the office. Sometimes, using drawings and hand signs will help. When communicating through language barriers, maintaining the privacy and confidentiality of patients' medical health information is essential. Diversification of patient populations is increasingly common. Office personnel should examine their patients' primary communication languages and determine if there is a need for an interpreters within the medical team. A team member with English as a second language could prove to be a valuable asset, not only to the administrative team but also to the clinical team members. Not having appropriate cultural resources to meet the needs of the day's patients can create a disruption in the schedule, just as not having the appropriate medical instruments can stop the day's schedule. Following are guidelines for communicating with patients who do not speak English:

- Speak slowly and clearly.
- Do not raise your voice above an ordinary conversational tone. Speaking louder does not improve understanding.
- Use simple words, not technical terms.
- Be brief.
- Have key phrases, such as "your next appointment is" or "thank you," translated into languages used by patients within the practice. Staff members should practice the phrases and be ready to use them when needed.

Another form of language barrier may occur in the office when the assistant must communicate with patients who are deaf. Following are tips for communicating successfully with deaf patients.

- Determine the patient's preferred form of communication: signing, writing, or speech/lip reading. Make note in the patient's chart, and be prepared when the patient arrives.
- Head nodding by the patient does not necessarily means understanding. The patient may be relying on another individual to explain the details.

- Larger, quicker, more forceful motions by the deaf individual may be an expression of heightened emotions.
- Body language, especially facial expressions, of the administrative assistant are keenly observed by the patient.
- Key phrases, such as "good morning" or "your copayment today is," should be learned and practiced by the staff member.

When the communication mode is lip reading,

- Make sure you have the patient's complete attention prior to beginning the communication process. A simple statement such as "Are you ready to begin?" will ensure that both parties are ready to communicate.
- Maintain direct face-to-face contact with the patient at all times during the communication process.
- Clear your mouth and mouth area of all items that may be intrusive to communication, such as gum or candy.
- Provide adequate lighting in the area and ensure that no shadows will interfere with lip reading. This should be checked with another office member prior to communication with the patient.

If the patient's mode of communication is writing, provide writing tools, such as a white board and marker or pen and paper. Many patients, both deaf and hearing, communicate faster with electronic devices. A small computer may be used to communicate between the administrative assistant and the patient. Whether the preferred mode of communication is signing, writing, or speech/lip reading, the privacy and confidentiality of the patient's medical information must be protected.

Nonpatients

All visitors to the doctor's office should be treated courteously. Often, a patient's friend or relative may accompany the patient.

Visitors on business, such as pharmaceutical company sales representatives, call on the office frequently. The doctor may not wish to take time away from the patient schedule and may ask the administrative medical assistant to get information on the product, obtain samples, and keep the business cards on file. Some offices schedule a specific time each week and/or month for pharmaceutical representatives. This gives the representative an opportunity to present materials to the physician and allows the physician to devote time exclusively to the representative.

> **EXAMPLE**
>
> **Sales representative:** I'm here to see Dr. Larsen about a new antibiotic from my company.
>
> **Assistant:** Dr. Larsen has scheduled the first Monday of each month from noon to 2 P.M. as the time she will see sales representatives. Shall I enter your name on the calendar for next month?

There may be other visitors who take up the doctor's time unnecessarily, and most doctors appreciate an assistant who screens them and tells them that the doctor is not interested.

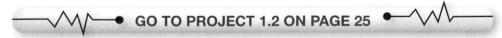
GO TO PROJECT 1.2 ON PAGE 25

Project 1.1 **Internet Research: Professional Organizations**

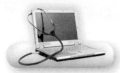

Using the Internet, research the Web sites of the AAMA, AMT, AHDI, and IAAP. Write down the student membership requirements of each and the advantages of belonging to each.

Project 1.2 **Work Ethic and Interpersonal Relationships**

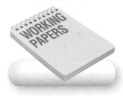

On WP 1 in the back section of this text-workbook, match each of the terms in Column 2 with its definition in Column 1.

Chapter Summary

1.1 Describe the tasks and skills required of an administrative medical assistant.
Pages 4–7
	• The administrative medical office assistant has task responsibilities in the following areas:
	  — Front office procedures
	  — Scheduling
	  — Records management
	  — Administrative duties
	  — Billing and insurance
	• These tasks require skills in the following areas:
	  — Communication
	  — Mathematics
	  — Organization
	  — Computers
	  — Interpersonal relationships

1.2 List and define at least three personal attributes essential for an administrative medical assistant.
Pages 7–9
	• Personal attributes needed for the successful administrative medical assistant are equally as important as required tasks and skills. Among the personal attributes needed are
	  — Genuine liking for people: enjoying people and having a desire to help them.
	  — Cheerfulness: the ability to be pleasant and friendly.
	  — Empathy: sensitivity to the feelings and situations of other people.

1.3 Describe the employment opportunities in various medical settings and specialties and nonmedical settings. Pages 9–11	• Employment opportunities for administrative medical assistants are increasing in physician practices (single and multi-physician practices), clinics, hospitals and medical centers, care facilities, and insurance companies. Other opportunities are increasing in the field of education and accounting firms.

1.4 Identify and define positive work attitudes that contribute to the work ethic and professionalism of an administrative medical assistant.
Pages 11–17
	• Habits and skills that make up the work ethic of an administrative medical assistant include
	  — Accuracy: the ability to be correct, clear, and thorough.
	  — Thoroughness: the ability to apply careful and complete attention to detail.
	  — Dependability: the ability to be relied upon to fulfill instructions and to complete tasks on time.

— Efficiency: the ability to use time and other resources in such a way as to avoid wasted efforts.
— Flexibility: the ability to respond quickly to changed situations, last-minute assignments, and delays; the willingness to accept and implement new ideas.
— Good judgment: the ability to use knowledge, experience, and logic to assess all the aspects of a situation in order to reach a sound decision.
— Honesty: the ability to always tell the truth and to quickly assume responsibility for mistakes.
— Initiative: the ability to take action independently.
— Problem-solving: the ability to use logic to plan needed steps to accomplish a goal.
— Punctuality: the ability to be on time.
— Self-motivation: the ability to express a willingness to learn new duties and/or procedures without a requirement to do so.
— Tact: the ability to speak and act considerately, especially in difficult situations.
— Team membership: the ability to work positively with others, to be generous with his or her time, to assist others, to be courteous, and to observe rules of confidentiality.
— Assertiveness: the ability to step forward to make a point in a confident, positive manner.
— The professional image of the administrative medical assistant is that of a friendly, capable professional who inspires confidence. From the assistant's manner, speech, posture, and appearance, patients and others have the impression of someone who is mature and dedicated to competent service.

1.5 List three advantages of professional affiliation and certification.
Pages 17–19
	• Certification
	  — Often favorably influences an employer's opinion.
	  — Contributes to career advancement.
	  — Fosters professional growth by the need to be recertified, continuing education programs, seminars, webinars, conferences, and the opportunity to network with others in the same profession.

1.6 Apply elements of good interpersonal communications to relationships with patients and others in the medical environment. Pages 19–24	• Administrative medical assistants should treat patients, physicians, colleagues, and others with courtesy, always maintaining a calm, pleasant, reassuring manner. • They should refrain from revealing confidential information and they have a professional relationship with the physician(s), colleagues, patients, and visitors in the office. • Medical team members need to create an atmosphere of interest in others by using positive nonverbal communications—body language, facial expressions, eye contact, etc.

Self-Awareness

Do you ever find time to think about who you are, your strengths and weaknesses, or your personality? What about your habits and values? Many people are not inclined to spend much time on self-reflection; consequently, many of us have a pretty low level of self-awareness. This is unfortunate because self-awareness can improve, and it can help us identify opportunities for professional development and personal growth. **Describe your level of self-awareness. What do you think needs to be changed in your life to improve your self-awareness?**

Self-Confidence

Self-confidence is extremely important in almost every aspect of our lives. People who lack self-confidence can find it difficult to become successful. Self-confident people have qualities that everyone admires, and they inspire confidence in others. Gaining the confidence of others is one way in which a self-confident person finds success. The good news is that self-confidence can be learned and built on. **How can you work to build up your level of self-confidence? Why is self-confidence so important to success?**

Multicultural Sensitivity

Learning about others; laughing with them about some of the things they were taught as kids; celebrating similarities while accepting differences—when we have lots of resources, people seem more generous and accepting. Race and ethnicity are difficult subjects to discuss, but culture can be joked about, discussed, and embraced. **How can you promote multicultural sensitivity?**

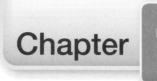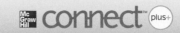
USING TERMINOLOGY

Match the term or phrase on the left with the correct answer on the right.

_____ 1. (LO 1.2) Empathy

_____ 2. (LO 1.6) Ethnocentrism

_____ 3. (LO 1.4) Thoroughness

_____ 4. (LO 1.5) AHDI

_____ 5. (LO 1.5) Certification

_____ 6. (LO 1.4) Accuracy

_____ 7. (LO 1.4) Problem-solving

_____ 8. (LO 1.4) Initiative

_____ 9. (LO 1.4) Dependability

_____10. (LO 1.4) Tact

a. Completing tasks with correctness and attention to detail

b. A trait that results in complete, neat, and correct tasks

c. Sensitivity to other people's feelings and situations

d. A trait characterized by working independently and offering to help others

e. Recognition given by associations that an individual has met high standards and has demonstrated competency in given knowledge and tasks

f. Provides certification opportunities for medical transcriptionists

g. Believing that one's own race, ethic group, and/or culture is superior to all other groups

h. The ability to speak and act considerately in various situations

i. Logically and systematically planning steps to accomplish a task

j. Finishing tasks on schedule, without complaining, and offering to assist others

CHECK YOUR UNDERSTANDING

Select the most correct answer.

1. (LO 1.6) Nenna worked as an administrative medical assistant but was dismissed from her AMA position after numerous patients complained about how they were greeted. Nenna claims she always used an appropriate verbal greeting with each patient. Which of the following may have contributed to the miscommunication between Nenna and the patients?

   a. Lack of professional certification
   b. Not enough reading material in the waiting area
   c. Nonverbal facial expressions and tone of voice
   d. An unclean uniform

2. (LO 1.4) During his first six months at a local medical clinic, Aaron completed and submitted insurance claims to various carriers. He used a software program to check and process his claims prior to submitting them for payment. This demonstrated that he accurately completed claims using very few resources. Which of the following was he demonstrating?

   a. Tact
   b. Ethnocentrism
   c. Assertiveness
   d. Efficiency

3. (LO 1.5) While searching online for a medical coding position, Maria noticed that several opportunities required CCS-P, CPC, or other current coding credentials. Which of the following key words or phrases could she use to search for their meaning on the Internet?

   a. Certification
   b. Interpersonal relationship skills
   c. Computer skills
   d. Records management skills

4. (LO 1.3) Addison would like to work in a medical-related administrative field but is not interested in a medical office setting. Which of the following may offer the best choice of a career for Addison?

   a. Food management
   b. Education
   c. Home health sales
   d. Both b and c are correct.

5. (LO 1.1) During her interview, Ashley stated she has worked within the physical medical office setting and from the home setting using electronic health records and insurance claim processing programs. Her records show she received high evaluations and was frequently given more administrative authority. She had demonstrated competence in

   a. Communication skills within the team environment.
   b. Organizational skills.
   c. Computer skills.
   d. All of the above are correct.

6. (LO 1.2) After he finishes his shift at the Flatwoods Medical Clinic for Burned Children, Andrew volunteers his time with the local equestrian program for physically challenged children. Which of the following personal attributes is Andrew demonstrating most clearly?

   a. Dependability
   b. True and genuine liking of other individuals
   c. Resourcefulness
   d. Cheerfulness

7. (LO 1.4) An AMA should always be aware of the impression and professional image given by his or her actions and presentation because

   a. The physician and practice are represented through the AMA.
   b. It is part of the job description.
   c. It may lead to an increase in salary or wages.
   d. None of the above are correct.

THINKING IT THROUGH

These questions cover the most important points in this chapter. Using your critical-thinking skills, play the role of an administrative medical assistant as you answer each question. Be prepared to present your responses in class.

1. What qualities and skills are needed by the assistant who is responsible for the front desk? Why are these critical skills?

2. How can imagining yourself in someone else's situation help you develop empathy for patients?

3. Do you think that assistants working in various medical settings have the same type of assignments? Might some employers assign assistants a single task or related tasks, such as processing insurance claims, while in other settings the assistant is likely to perform a variety of tasks?

4. Why is it important to be a team player in the office?

5. What qualities project a professional image in an administrative medical assistant?

6. An assistant is asked by another employee why the assistant decided to meet the requirements to become certified. What might the assistant answer?

7. How should an assistant communicate with non-English-speaking patients and with patients who are visually and/or hearing impaired?

Medical Ethics, Law, and Compliance

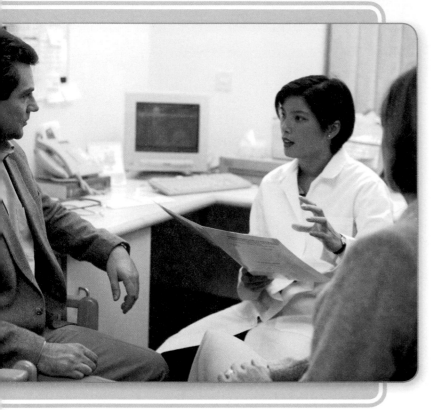

LEARNING OUTCOMES
After studying this chapter, you will be able to:

2.1 Define *medical ethics, bioethics,* and *etiquette.*

2.2 Discuss medical law and legal documents, such as advance directives, and give three examples.

2.3 Identify and discuss several key components of the HIPAA Administrative Simplification Rule.

2.4 State the purpose of a medical compliance plan and explain compliant methods the assistant can use to safeguard against litigation.

KEY TERMS
Study these important words, which are defined in this chapter, to build your professional vocabulary:

abandonment	battery	defensive medicine	etiquette
arbitration	bioethics	deposition	express consent
assault	compliance	durable power of attorney	fraud
authorization	contributory negligence	ethics	Good Samaritan Act

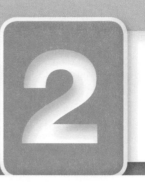

Chapter 2

ABHES

- Adapt to change.
- Maintain confidentiality at all times.
- Be cognizant of ethical boundaries.
- Conduct work within scope of education, training, and ability.
- Know professionalism components.
- Orient patients to office policies and procedures.

CAAHEP

- Discuss legal scope of practice for medical assistants.
- Explore issues of confidentiality as it applies to the medical assistant.
- Describe the implications of HIPAA for the medical assistant in various medical settings.
- Discuss licensure and certification as it applies to healthcare providers.
- Describe liability, professional, personal injury, and third-party insurance.
- Compare and contrast physician and medical assistant roles in terms of standard of care.
- Compare criminal and civil law as they apply to the practicing medical assistant.
- Provide an example of tort law as it would apply to a medical assistant.

- Explain how the following impact the medical assistant's practice and give examples.
  - a. negligence
  - b. malpractice
  - c. Statute of Limitations
  - d. Good Samaritan Act(s)
  - e. Uniform Anatomical Gift Act
  - f. Living will/Advanced directives
  - g. Medical durable power of attorney
- Identify how the Americans with Disabilities Act (ADA) applies to the medical assisting profession.
- List and discuss legal and illegal interview questions.
- Discuss all levels of governmental legislation and regulation as they apply to medical assistants
- Respond to issues of confidentiality.
- Perform within scope of practice.
- Apply HIPAA rules in regard to privacy/release of information.
- Practice within the standard of care for a medical assistant.
- Incorporate the patient's bill of rights into personal practice and medical office policies and procedures.
- Complete an incident report.
- Document accurately in the patient record.
- Apply local, state, and federal healthcare legislation and regulation appropriate to the medical assisting practice.
- Demonstrate sensitivity to patients' rights.
- Demonstrate awareness of the consequences of not working within the legal scope of practice.
- Recognize the importance of local, state, and federal legislation and regulations in the practice setting.

- Cognitive
- Psychomotor
- Affective

Health Insurance Portability and Accountability Act (HIPAA)	liability	medical practice acts	statute of limitations
	licensure	registration	subpoena
implied consent	litigation	release of information	subpoena duces tecum
informed consent	malpractice	settlement	summons

INTRODUCTION

Daily news headlines reflect legal and ethical questions: Should life support be ended for a patient when there are no signs of brain function? May a patient sue the physician for an unsuccessful treatment? When may a healthcare provider refuse to treat a patient? All consumers of healthcare services are interested in these legal and healthcare issues. As healthcare professionals, administrative medical assistants have an even greater interest in such issues. Understanding the legal and ethical aspects of healthcare helps them act according to the highest professional standards. Such knowledge also helps assistants resolve issues of confidentiality and patients' rights.

2.1 MEDICAL ETHICS

All professions, as well as people's lives, are governed by standards of conduct. The standards of conduct that grow out of one's understanding of right and wrong are known as **ethics**. The medical ethics that govern the healthcare professions are usually found in written policies or codes for each profession. These standards are not laws. A person acting within the law may nevertheless do something that is not ethical. A person may also do something right, or ethical, while breaking the law. Ethics are statements of right and wrong behaviors that hold members of the profession to a high degree of behavior.

Principles of Medical Ethics

Hippocrates, a Greek physician who lived during the fourth and fifth centuries B.C.E., is called "the father of medicine." He made the first statement of principles governing the conduct of physicians. This statement, known as the Hippocratic oath, is the foundation of modern medical ethics. In part, the oath requires the physician to pledge the following:

> I will follow that method of treatment which, according to my ability and judgment, I consider for the benefit of my patients, and abstain from whatever is deleterious [harmful] and mischievous. . . . Whatever, in connection with my professional practice or not in connection with it, I may see or hear in the lives of men which ought not to be spoken abroad, I will not divulge, as reckoning that all such should be kept secret.

Today, physicians follow the principles of medical ethics developed by the American Medical Association (AMA). It is easy to see from reading the code, shown in Figure 2.1, that these principles can be traced back to the Hippocratic oath. The code requires physicians, among other rules, to practice high standards of patient care, to respect patients' rights, to treat patients with compassion, and to safeguard patient confidences.

The Medical Assistant's Ethical Responsibility

Most other associations that regulate healthcare professions also have codes of ethics to set levels of competence and patient care. The American Association of Medical Assistants (AAMA) has developed the Code of Ethics and Creed, which outlines moral and ethical behaviors for the medical assistant in relation to the medical professional and specifically to the career field of medical assisting. Because the administrative medical assistant is considered an agent of the physician while performing tasks related to employment, the AAMA code is based on AMA standards.

Medical assistants, in their role and within the boundaries of their job responsibilities, are also required to treat all patients with respect, to maintain confidentiality, to improve their knowledge and skills, and to contribute to the community. As an example, many medical offices organize teams to walk or run in community charity events to raise money for medical research. Attending continuing education workshops, seminars, and conferences that update skills and knowledge within the AMA field is another way to uphold the AMA code of ethics. In addition, assistants should endeavor to merit the respect of the

> **Figure 2.1 AMA Principles of Medical Ethics (2001)**
>
> *Preamble*: The medical profession has long subscribed to a body of ethical statements developed primarily for the benefit of the patient. As a member of this profession, a physician must recognize responsibility to patients first and foremost, as well as to society, to other health professionals, and to self. The following Principles adopted by the American Medical Association are not laws, but standards of conduct which define the essentials of honorable behavior for the physician.
>
> I. A physician shall be dedicated to providing competent medical care, with compassion and respect for human dignity and rights.
>
> II. A physician shall uphold the standards of professionalism, be honest in all professional interactions, and strive to report physicians deficient in character or competence, or engaging in fraud or deception, to appropriate entities.
>
> III. A physician shall respect the law and also recognize a responsibility to seek changes in those requirements which are contrary to the best interests of the patient.
>
> IV. A physician shall respect the rights of patients, colleagues, and other health professionals, and shall safeguard patient confidences and privacy within the constraints of the law.
>
> V. A physician shall continue to study, apply, and advance scientific knowledge, maintain a commitment to medical education, make relevant information available to patients, colleagues, and the public, obtain consultation, and use the talents of other health professionals when indicated.
>
> VI. A physician shall, in the provision of appropriate patient care, except in emergencies, be free to choose whom to serve, with whom to associate, and the environment in which to provide medical care.
>
> VII. A physician shall recognize a responsibility to participate in activities contributing to the improvement of the community and the betterment of public health.
>
> VIII. A physician shall, while caring for a patient, regard responsibility to the patient as paramount.
>
> IX. A physician shall support access to medical care for all people.
>
> The Principles of Medical Ethics constitute the Preamble to the much longer *Code of Medical Ethics*. The Code of Medical Ethics and opinions of the Council on Ethical and Judicial Affairs (CEJA) may be found on the *Code of Medical Ethics and CEJA Reports* page.

public and of the medical profession. The creed emphasizes the qualities of effectiveness, loyalty, compassion, courage, and faith.

Medical coders can find their respective code of ethics at either the Web site for the American Academy of Professional Coders (aapc.com) or the Web site for the American Health Information and Management Association (ahima.org).

Bioethics

The area of **bioethics** deals with the ethics of medical treatment, technology, and procedure. Advances in the sciences, rapid developments in technology, and new kinds of treatment have dramatically increased the number of bioethical issues and questions. Professional guidelines in these areas may still need to be established. These issues are associated with abortion, the definition of *death*, patients' rights, and types of medical care. The response to bioethical issues may require a restatement or a new application of existing ethical guidelines.

Issues. Because physicians have always faced life-and-death situations, they have also faced difficult decisions. Today, their ethical responses have been made even more difficult by the increased power of technology and scientific knowledge. Consider the ethical aspects of these questions:

- What rights are involved with using a human fetus?
- Should genetic engineering—the altering of cells to produce physical traits or to eliminate disease—be encouraged? Suppose one of the outcomes is the cloning of a human being?

- How should scarce usable body organs be fairly allocated throughout the United States?
- When is it acceptable to remove a patient from life support? Who makes that decision?
- Should the physician be criminally responsible for assisting a terminally ill patient in his or her own suicide?

The ability to create, sustain, or end life is a major concern for individuals and society. Many people who fear that their lives may be sustained without their consent have made living wills. In a living will, a person states clearly the intent to refuse certain life-sustaining measures and specifies the length and methods of these measures. Should that person become unable to make that decision, another person may be appointed to carry out the requirements of the will. The person's wishes may also be stated with regard to organ donation. The living will, which is valid in most states, is one response to a bioethical issue.

Moral Values. The link between moral values, or concepts of what is good, and professional behavior is shown in ethics by the use of words such as *compassion, honesty, honorable,* and *responsibility*. The primary ethical obligation of the physician is to put the benefit of the patient first. Moral values may dictate that physicians take certain actions and refrain from others. For example, considering the patient's well-being, the physician may agree to perform an abortion. However, every physician also has the right, based on his or her moral views, to refuse to perform abortions. Physicians also make moral choices about treatment based on how the treatment will benefit the patient. Some patients may request a particular treatment for their illness. A physician may ethically refuse to use the requested treatment if it does not meet the recognized standard of acceptable care.

Many times, physicians find moral values contained within the laws of the state where they practice; these laws must be obeyed. For example, violence to children must be reported in many states. However, even if the law does not require this notification, the physician must respond ethically to report such cases. The physician's own belief system, good judgment, and decision-making skill all contribute to the ethical practice of the profession.

Etiquette

Etiquette is defined as those behaviors and customs that are standards for what is considered good manners. While codes of ethics specify standards for capable patient care, *etiquette* is a broad term for behaviors that mark courteous treatment of others.

Proper office etiquette should be used by the AMA at all times—including when upholding the respective code of ethics. Consider the following scenario and the application of etiquette.

SCENARIO

Patient A comes into the office and presents medical coverage through a state assistance program. Patient B checks in and presents a Blue Cross Blue Shield card for medical coverage. The AMA addresses the BCBS patient with a friendly, warm tone and a smile. Patient A is not acknowledged with a verbal greeting and the AMA uses hand sanitizer while looking at Patient A.

The AMA exhibited poor etiquette by treating Patient A as a lesser patient by a refusal to offer a warm, friendly greeting and by the implied behavior that Patient A is unclean. The AMA code of ethics says patients will be treated with human dignity. The AMA did not uphold the code of ethics.

Frequently, an employer's rules of etiquette are found in the policy and procedures manual of the medical practice. Examples of good manners in the office include

- Dressing appropriately to show respect for others and for the profession.
- Using proper forms of address for both the physician and patients.
- Cheerfully greeting all who visit the office.
- Using good telephone techniques.
- Observing the use of polite everyday phrases: "Please," "Thank you," "Excuse me."

Etiquette forms the basis of effective communication and fosters satisfying interactions in all cultures and settings. Using good manners and following those aspects of etiquette that may be unique to the workplace help create a pleasant environment in an efficient office.

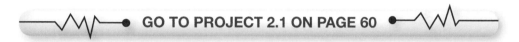

GO TO PROJECT 2.1 ON PAGE 60

2.2 MEDICAL LAW

Law is a set of rules made and enforced by a recognized authority. For example, federal, state, and city laws require some actions and forbid others. Law protects citizens and helps society work smoothly. Physicians and other healthcare professionals may be affected by the law—both criminal and civil statutes. The law, then, as it applies to standards of acceptable care, is known as *medical jurisprudence*, or *medical law*.

Law and the Right to Practice

Medical law regulates the right to practice and the granting of various licenses and certifications. Each state governs the practice of medicine within its borders through laws known as **medical practice acts.** These acts

- Define *medical practice.*
- Explain who must be licensed to give healthcare.
- Set rules for obtaining a license.
- State the duties imposed by the license.
- Cover the grounds on which the license may be revoked.
- List the statutory reports that must be sent to the government.

Medical practice acts also protect users of healthcare services. To do this, the acts set forth the penalties for practicing medicine without a valid license. The acts also define *misconduct*, including conviction of a felony, such as insurance fraud; unprofessional conduct, such as sexual behavior with a patient; and personal or professional incapacity, such as mental illness; inappropriate use, or overprescribing, of drugs. The penalty for such acts may be the suspension or revoking of a license.

Licensing. The license to practice medicine, called **licensure**, is granted by a board established in each state. Licenses are issued to applicants once they have completed the educational requirements and have successfully passed an examination. Licenses may also be issued as a result of reciprocity, the recognition by one state of another state's requirements for licensure. Those who have passed the examination given by the National Board of Medical Examiners receive licenses from the state through what is called *endorsement.*

Relicensure is required either annually or every other year. Those who hold licenses may be relicensed by paying a fee and providing proof, such as certificates of course completion, that they have met continuing education requirements. As an example, for a medical coder holding the CPC credential through AAPC to renew certification, membership must be maintained and at least 36 approved continuing education units (CEUs) must be completed every two years. To renew the CMT credential through AHDI, at least 30 approved CEUs must be completed every three years.

Certified Specialization. The American Board of Specialties determines the competency of, and then certifies, those doctors who intend to practice a medical specialty. The board requires additional academic in-hospital training in which the medical student, known as a *resident*, concentrates on a specialty and takes a comprehensive examination. Fulfilling the requirements, the candidate becomes *board-certified*. This certification is an essential minimum standard of competence in a particular medical specialty.

Narcotics Registration. A physician in clinical practice who will have occasion to prescribe or dispense drugs must register for a permit. This **registration** (permit) issued by the registration branch of the Drug Enforcement Administration (DEA) grants these permits, which must be renewed annually.

The Physician's Practice

In today's complex healthcare environment, the physician's practice has many elements of both a health service and a business, such as providing good patient care, scheduling, performing billing and insurance procedures, hiring and training staff, and maintaining the physical resources of the office, such as equipment and the office premises. Every part of the practice is affected by legal and ethical considerations.

Because the physician's primary responsibility is to practice an acceptable standard of patient care, the laws, responsibilities, and ethical considerations that surround the physician-patient relationship are of great importance.

Contracts. The relationship between the physician and the patient starts when the patient goes to the physician for care. The contract is implied; it is not expressed in either words or writing. The physician does not say, "I am here to offer you care." The patient does not say, "I am requesting care." The patient usually has a complaint, and the physician treats it. The physician's behavior, in having a practice open to patients, and the patient's behavior, in going to the physician's office, together establish an implied contract. At times a written, or express, contract is provided, and both physician and patient sign a document. The physician may provide a standard written contract to allow a patient to pay for services over an extended period of time, for example.

Once the physician-patient relationship is established, the physician is legally required to

- Possess the ordinary skill and learning commonly held by a reputable physician in a similar locality. The patient has the right to believe that the physician is so qualified. Accordingly, the physician's license should be displayed in the office.
- Use his or her learning, skill, and best judgment for the benefit of the patient.
- Preserve confidentiality.
- Act in good faith.
- Perform to the best of his or her ability.
- Advise against needless or unwise treatment.
- Inform and advise the patient when the physician knows a condition is beyond his or her scope of competency.

The physician is not legally required to

- Accept as patients all those who seek his or her services.
- Restore a patient to the same condition that existed before illness occurred.

- Obtain recovery for every patient.
- Guarantee successful results from an operation or a treatment.
- Be familiar with all possible reactions of patients to various medicines.
- Be free from errors in complex cases.
- Possess the maximum amount of education possible.
- Continue care after a patient discharges himself or herself from a hospital, even if harm could come to the patient.

In the physician-patient relationship, the patient also has certain responsibilities. The patient must give the information necessary for the physician to make a correct diagnosis; follow the physician's instructions and any orders for treatment, provided that these are within the bounds of similar standards of care for physicians who practice in that area of medicine; be, in general, cooperative; and pay for all services rendered.

Consent. When a patient goes to a physician's office for treatment, that patient's consent to treatment, like the contract itself, is not stated outright. This **implied consent** applies to routine treatment only. For more complicated procedures, especially surgery, diagnostic tests, and x-ray treatments, it is important to have **express consent.** The patient may express consent either in writing or orally. It is standard practice for the patient to give written consent by signing a special consent form before any special procedure is performed. An exception to this practice is the patient who is incapable of giving consent when an emergency requires immediate action. Express consent is important to avoid later lawsuits or, even more seriously, criminal accusations.

When oral consent is acceptable, it may be given in a phone conversation, provided that the call is a three-way conversation involving the patient and two office personnel. Both office employees then must sign as witnesses to the conversation in which the patient expressed consent.

There is another aspect of patient consent, whether implied or express. The patient must give **informed consent**, meaning that the patient has had the illness or problem explained by the physician in simple, understandable language. The patient has also been given options for treatment and for the refusal of treatment, with the individual benefits and risks of each, along with the physician's prognosis. Also, the medical team personnel must give the patient an opportunity to ask questions and provide time, if needed, for the patient to discuss the plan with his or her family or advisors. Patients also have the right during informed consent to have their questions answered to their satisfaction—not necessarily to their liking, but to their satisfaction. Also, a check on the patient's comprehension should be conducted. The physician will know what he or she intended the patient to understand, but the physician must check to be sure the patient actually received and processed the information as intended. Also addressed during informed consent are the likelihood of success, treatment alternatives, and the potential outcome without treatment. In other words, the patient has been given enough information to make a knowledgeable decision. A sample consent form is shown in Figure 2.2.

Adults who are *legally competent* are able to give informed consent. The law requires that, in order to be competent, a person must have attained legal *majority* (adult age as defined by law) and must be of sound mind. When a patient is not able to give consent, that consent must be given by the next of kin, the legal guardian, or a court-appointed guardian, such as a court-appointed surrogate or proxy. A **durable power of attorney** may have been executed by the patient. A durable power of attorney (DPA) gives someone else, of the patient's choosing, the right to make decisions for the patient. Specifically, a medical DPA gives another individual the legal right to make decisions relating to a patient's medical issues such as long-term care. Copies of all legal documents must be on file in the patient's record prior to granting permission for another to given informed medical consent.

Figure 2.2

Informed Consent Form

CONSENT FOR INFLUENZA (FLU) VACCINE
Office of Karen Larsen, MD

Purpose of the Influenza Vaccine

Influenza is a highly contagious respiratory tract infection. Symptoms may include chills, fever, headache, cough, sore throat, and muscle aches. Generally, the illness lasts several days to a week or more. The flu may be severe or even life-threatening for some people.

Each year the influenza vaccine is updated because viruses that cause the flu often change.

Influenza Vaccine

The flu vaccine contains inactive (dead) influenza viruses selected by the U.S. Food and Drug Administration. Because it is an inactive virus vaccine, the vaccine will not give you the flu.

Protection from the flu vaccine develops within 2 weeks after receiving the vaccine and may last up to a year.

Risks and Side Effects

The risk of the flu vaccine causing serious problems is very small. Mild side effects may include soreness, redness, and swelling of the injection site; fever; and muscle aches. If any side effects occur, they may begin upon receiving the vaccine injection and last 1 to 2 days.

NOTE: People who have an allergy to eggs, chicken, or chicken feathers should not receive the influenza vaccine. Also people who currently have an active infection should not receive the vaccine.

If you have any questions or concerns, please check with your physician before receiving the flu vaccine.

Freedom of Consent

The influenza vaccine is a voluntary injection. You are free to deny this consent.

Patient's Consent

I have read this form. I understand the purpose of the influenza vaccine and the risks and benefits of the vaccine. I have expressed any questions or concerns about the flu vaccine to my physician.

_____   _____
Patient receiving the vaccine (Please print)   Date of birth

_____   _____
Signature of patient or guardian   Date

Those who have not reached the adult age required by law, and are therefore minors, may give legal consent in certain cases:

- A minor who is in the military service
- A minor who is living away from his or her parents and is managing his or her own financial affairs
- A college student who is living away from home
- A minor who is married or divorced

The following are the kinds of care that minors may usually consent to:

- Pregnancy tests
- Prenatal care
- The diagnosis and treatment of a sexually transmitted disease
- The diagnosis and treatment of alcohol or drug abuse

Figure 2.3

Consent for Videotaping
Form

CONSENT FOR VIDEOTAPING

I, _____*Anita Melendez*_____ , give my consent for the videotaping of my appointment with Karen Larsen, MD, including medical history and examination on this date.

I understand that I have a right to private, confidential medical consultation and treatment, and I voluntarily waive that right so that the videotape may be used for teaching purposes at the University Medical School.

I am in agreement that my medical history, which is related to the taped examination, may be disclosed during the described use of the videotape for _____*teaching purposes*_____.

I further understand that at any future time I may request in writing that certain parts or the entire recording may be deleted and not used.

Signature _____*Anita Melendez*_____   Date _____*7/10/20—*_____
Witness _____*Joanne Diaz*_____   Date _____*7/10/20—*_____

Although there is no one consent form required by law, the informed consent that the patient signs should usually contain the following:

- The name of the patient and the date
- The name of the procedure to be performed
- The name of the physician performing the procedure
- An explanation of the procedure
- A statement of risks and benefits
- A statement that the patient signs to signify understanding of the procedure and the information given in the form
- The patient's signature
- The signature of a witness (optional) testifying to the patient's signature

In addition to written, informed consent for procedures, there are other reasons for obtaining patient consent. For example, if a physician wishes to videotape a patient visit or procedure for training purposes, the physician must obtain the patient's written consent. An example of this type of consent form is shown in Figure 2.3.

In addition to consent forms, the medical chart for a patient should contain all legal documents that may be used for the care of the patient. Advanced directives are legal documents stating the patient's wishes for medical care, should he or she not be able to make these decisions. A living will states whether the patient wants medical personnel to administer or sustain life by artificial means, such as life support measures. When a patient

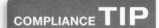

does not want to be resuscitated, a DNR (Do Not Resuscitate) should be executed and on file with the medical office. Copies of a durable power of attorney should also be filed in the patient's record. When a patient is admitted to the hospital, each of these documents should also be forwarded to the hospital.

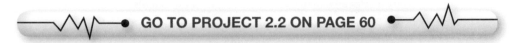
GO TO PROJECT 2.2 ON PAGE 60

Medical Liability and Communications

Liability means legal responsibility. In many areas of life, people are liable, or legally responsible, for actions (or nonactions) and their consequences. The owner of a home may be liable for an injury caused to a guest in the home.

Physicians have liability in their roles as providers of healthcare and as owners of a practice. Vicariously, physicians are also responsible for the actions of their staff. If the medical coder releases information on a healthcare claim that is not directly related to the services rendered on the claim, the physician is ultimately responsible for the breach of confidentiality. In general, physicians are responsible not only for the quality of the care they give to patients but also for

- *The safety of employees.* An office policy and procedures manual will often contain regulations that relate to observing state laws for safety, including the handling of discarded waste and hazardous materials.
- *The safety of the premises.* Rules that help ensure protection from injury, theft, and fire need to be specified. This is important not only for patients and employees but also for the safety of records.

Physicians, wishing to protect themselves from lawsuits brought by patients, sometimes practice **defensive medicine**. This means that physicians order additional tests and follow-up visits to confirm a diagnosis or treatment result. The physician's liability as it relates to patient care is discussed below.

Malpractice. **Malpractice** is the improper care or treatment of a patient by a physician, hospital, or other provider of healthcare as a result of carelessness, neglect, lack of professional skill, or disregard for the established rules or procedures. In spite of vigilance on the part of the physician and the office staff, accidents may occur during treatment. Some patients may be dissatisfied with the care they have received. In cases such as these, a patient may file a malpractice suit against the physician. A patient who files a suit is required to prove that there is an injury, as the law defines *injury*, and that the physician's inadequate care was the direct cause of the injury.

Termination. As discussed earlier, the contractual agreement between the patient and the physician calls for the physician to furnish care to the patient for a particular illness as long as care is required. At times, a physician may choose to terminate, or end, the physician-patient relationship because a patient does not follow treatment instructions or because the patient has stated (either orally or in writing) an intent to seek care from another physician. The physician may also terminate the relationship if the patient fails to pay for services.

The physician is required to notify the patient of the decision to terminate and to allow the patient a reasonable amount of time to obtain another physician. The notification should be in the form of a letter, sent to the patient, that states the reason the physician is ending the relationship, the date of the termination, and the physician's willingness to continue treatment temporarily if the patient needs further care.

After a withdrawal letter has been sent, the physician should provide the patient's name to the administrative medical assistant who schedules appointments. If the patient calls and requests an appointment, the call should be transferred to the physician, who will explain to the patient what needs to be done to reestablish care.

Abandonment. Unless the patient is discharged in an appropriate way, either because the treatment was completed or because the physician followed the procedure for termination, the patient may sue the physician for **abandonment.** Good documentation is essential to proving that the physician did not abandon the patient.

EXAMPLE

Notations in patient medical record:
4/6/—   Patient cancelled appointment. Rescheduled for 4/13/—.
4/13/—   Patient did not show up for follow-up appointment.

As a precaution, patients should be notified of any absences of the physician from the office—for vacation, conferences, or emergencies. The name and telephone number of the substituting physician should be made available to patients. The assistant may post a notice of the physician's absence or mail a notice to patients. The notice or letter should be kept on file. As electronic health records are implemented in the medical field, notices of absence and coverage during the absence should also be posted at the Web site for the physician.

The following example could constitute medical abandonment.

EXAMPLE

Patient A had a surgical procedure scheduled with Dr. Smith on Tuesday. The patient arrived at the hospital and registered. After several hours, the surgical unit phoned the physician's office and received a recorded message that Dr. Smith was out of town and would not return for three weeks. Information for coverage was not given. No patients were notified of his absence. Dr. Smith has also missed scheduled patient appointments in the past.

Assault and Battery. The clear threat of injury to another is called **assault.** Any bodily contact without permission is called **battery**. In medical law, *battery* is interpreted to include surgical and medical procedures performed without the patient's consent or procedures that go beyond the degree of consent that was given.

A badly damaged uterus is removed during exploratory surgery, even though the patient had not signed a consent for the removal.

In this example, even though the procedure may have been in the best interest of the patient, the physician may be sued for battery. Unless a physician acts in a grave emergency, he or she may well lose a suit in court as a result of not having proper patient consent.

Fraud. An intentionally dishonest practice that deprives others of their rights is called **fraud**. Depending on the laws of the state where the physician practices, the penalty may range from reprimand to the revoking of a license.

A wide range of activities is included under the definition of fraud:

- Making false statements to a patient about the benefits of a particular drug or treatment.
- Falsifying diplomas or licenses
- Submitting false or duplicate claims for payment to the federal government or an insurance company.

All members of the medical office team should be cautious about making fraudulent claims (verbal or written) or claims that may be interpreted as fraudulent. Changing the date a service was rendered for purposes of gaining an insurance payment is considered fraud and should not be done!

Litigation. The bringing of lawsuits, or **litigation**, against the physician is not uncommon. Many lawsuits arise out of civil law. Civil law deals with crimes against persons committed by other persons or institutions, such as the government or a business. While criminal law handles the actual commission of a crime, civil law gives a person the right to sue. For example, a physician may be convicted of battery in a criminal court and then may be sued by the patient in civil court for injuries resulting from the battery. The civil court may decide to award the patient a certain amount of money for the injuries.

One common type of civil suit that patients may bring is for malpractice. However, the law also covers many other aspects of the physician's practice, such as the hiring process, drug testing of employees, equal opportunity, sexual harassment, fair labor laws, and workers' compensation.

If called to court, follow the directions and advice of the practice's attorney. It is not advisable to go to court without legal representation. If the practice does not have an attorney on retainer, contact other practices that do and retain his or her services. Additionally, medical office personnel may purchase liability insurance.

Steps in Litigation

Once a lawsuit is begun, there are several steps involved in resolving it:

- *Summons.* A written notice—the **summons**—is sent to the person being sued (the *defendant*), ordering the defendant to answer the charges made. The summons is sent by the court along with a copy of the complaint filed by the other party (the *plaintiff*).
- *Subpoena.* A **subpoena** is a legal document in which the court orders that all documents relevant to the case be delivered to the court. A subpoena may also require any person who has information related to the case to appear in court.
- *Deposition.* A sworn statement to the court before any trial begins, and usually made outside of court, is called a **deposition**.

The Physician's Response to Litigation

Complete, accurate documentation is critical in physician-patient disputes. The documentation may provide the physician with evidence of **contributory negligence**. A patient's refusal to have tests, x-rays, or vaccinations or a patient's failure to follow the physician's instructions may be considered contributory negligence. The physician's notations in the patient record, made at the time of the patient's actions, would protect the physician against a later claim that reasonable precautions had not been taken. Any contact by telephone or letter regarding laboratory or x-ray reports should also be indicated.

> **EXAMPLE**
>
> Notation in patient's medical record:
>
> 3/12/—   Patient refused to have chest x-ray. Patient did accept medication.

Alternatives to Trial

The complaint may be heard in court at a trial. However, the case may also be resolved through settlement or arbitration. In a **settlement**, the plaintiff and the physician's insurance company reach an agreement and the case does not go to court. In **arbitration**, through a process fair to both sides, an *arbitrator* (an unbiased third party) is chosen. This person, rather than a judge, hears evidence and helps both sides resolve the dispute or makes a decision if the two sides cannot agree. Because the defendant and the plaintiff agree beforehand to abide by the arbitrator's decision, the arbitration also ends the case before it reaches court.

Statute of Limitations

A law that sets a time limit for initiating litigation is called a **statute of limitations**. This time limit varies from state to state. The time span during which a lawsuit for malpractice may be brought may begin when the claimed negligence first occurred, when the claimed negligence was first discovered, or when the physician-patient relationship ended. In pediatric cases, the time span may begin after the patient reaches majority. When children are treated, physicians should retain records long enough to cover this span of time. Information about particular state laws is available from state offices and their Web sites.

Good Samaritan Act

The purpose of a **Good Samaritan Act** is to protect the physician from liability for civil damages that may arise as a result of providing emergency care. Because there are minor variations from state to state, the medical assistant's role in emergency situations is defined by the state in which the assistant is employed.

Medical Communications—Access to Information. All information a patient gives a physician is confidential. Administrative medical assistants who process physicians' correspondence and work with patients' records are authorized to read this information. However, no patient information may be conveyed to anyone outside of the practice without permission from the patient. Under the federal law known as the *final privacy rule*, patients must provide a general consent to the sharing of information for the purposes of carrying out treatment or submitting insurance claims. They must also provide written **authorization** for specific items that are not covered by the general consent.

Patients have the right to see their medical records. Preferably, this is to be done with the physician's participation, so that the information can be interpreted for the patient in a meaningful way. The physician must always be notified when patients request to review their records.

Release of Information

It is often necessary to release information from patients' medical records to insurance companies, other medical facilities, or other physicians. These releases are connected to patient care, proper treatment, and accurate billing. The strictest confidentiality must be maintained while providing requested data. The medical office follows a procedure to make sure that the party asking for the data has the right to receive it, and that proper authorization to release the information has been granted, and that appropriate methods and security precautions are used to transmit the data.

Figure 2.4

AUTHORIZATION TO RELEASE MEDICAL INFORMATION

Original Authorization MUST be attached to the patient's permanent medical record. A copy of this Authorization should be attached to the forwarded medical record.

DATE: _____

TO: Karen Larsen, MD
2235 South Ridgeway Avenue
Chicago, IL 60623-2240
312-555-6022, 312-555-0025 fax

RE: Patient name _____
Patient street address _____
Patient city, state, ZIP _____
Patient telephone _____
Patient date of birth _____

The undersigned hereby requests and authorizes Karen Larsen, MD, to release to (INSERT NAME OF RECIPIENT OF PATIENT RECORDS) or any of his/her/their assigned representatives, copies of any and all records and documents regarding the undersigned's past and current medical treatment, medical condition(s) and medical expenses. The information to be released includes any and all medical and hospital records currently within your possession, including, but not limited to, any and all x-ray films, pathology slides, laboratory reports, medical histories, consultation reports, prescriptions, medical correspondence, consent forms, employment information, and billing information.

In addition to authorizing the release of the above stated medical records and documents, the undersigned expressly authorizes Karen Larsen, MD, to release the following information to the designated individual or entity: (Please initial the items below for release, if appropriate)

____ Psychiatric information ____ Drug/Alcohol information ____ HIV-related information

The physician is instructed to comply with this request by providing copies of my records only, with the understanding that my original medical record will be maintained within the possession of Karen Larsen, MD.

A copy of this authorization **shall not** be used in lieu of an originally signed authorization.

This authorization may be revoked by the undersigned at any time by a written notice to the physician except to the extent that action has already been taken.

This authorization will expire sixty (60) days from the date of this request OR _____ (specify other date) and will be null and void thereafter.

_____   _____
Signature of patient   Date

Patient is a minor, or patient is legally unable to sign because _____

_____   _____
Signature of authorized person   Date

_____   _____
Print name of authorized person   Relationship to patient

Disclosure statement: This information is being disclosed to you from records whose confidentiality is protected by federal and state law. Federal and state law prohibit you from making any further disclosure of this information without the specific written authorization of the person to whom it pertains, or as otherwise permitted by law.

The administrative medical assistant can ensure the proper transfer of information by following the office's procedure carefully, double-checking the source and validity of the request, and verifying that the patient has given permission in writing to release the information. This written permission is in the form of an authorization for **release of information**, sometimes simply called a *release*. The authorization for release of information must meet several legal requirements in order to be valid. A sample authorization form is shown in Figure 2.4. The release must contain:

- The name of the facility releasing the information.
- The name of the individual or facility requesting and receiving the information.
- The patient's full name, address, and date of birth.
- The specific dates of treatment.
- A description of the information to be released.
- The signature of the patient.
- The date the form was signed.

Helping Ensure Confidentiality

The assistant can help protect confidentiality by

- Avoiding any conversation, either in person or on the telephone, with a patient or others, about any aspect of treatment, patient records, or financial arrangements. When speaking on the phone, also avoid using the caller's name or the name of any patient.
- Being careful when calling patients about test results—never leaving a message on the answering machine or with any other person except to request a return call from the patient.
- Always keeping documents shielded from view in areas where fax machines, copy machines, and printers are located.
- Always removing documents from these areas and shredding them, rather than putting materials in the trash.
- Protecting computerized records and other information. Do not leave information showing on any unattended screen. Be careful of access to the network if the computer shares programs and data files.

Exceptions to Confidentiality. Under some circumstances, the physician is required to file reports containing confidential information to state departments of health or social services. These are called *statutory reports*. The government needs this information to protect the health of the whole community. Each state has its own requirements for statutory reports. Each state is responsible for making and enforcing the laws related to the reports it needs. The following are examples of circumstances requiring statutory reports:

- Births
- Deaths
- Abuse of a child, a vulnerable or elderly adult, or a battered person; state law requires teachers, physicians, and other licensed healthcare workers to report cases of suspected abuse, and any private citizen may, at any time, file a complaint with a protective agency
- Injuries resulting from violence, such as gunshot or stab wounds, or any other evidence of criminal violence
- Occupational illnesses, such as chemical poisoning
- Communicable diseases, including acquired immune deficiency syndrome (AIDS), hepatitis, neonatal herpes, Lyme disease, rabies, and sexually transmitted diseases
- Cases of food poisoning

Transmission of Information Electronically. In today's medical practice, it is very common to transmit information electronically. To ensure that health information is protected from misuse, a federal law, the **Health Insurance Portability and Accountability Act**, or **HIPAA** (pronounced hip-uh), regulates how electronic patient information is stored and shared. HIPAA will be covered in more detail later in the text. The administrative assistant must be conscientious about the following:

- If information is faxed, the assistant should carefully check the fax number and then call to confirm receipt.
- The assistant should use a cover page for the fax, requesting the return of the information if it has reached the wrong person.

COMPLIANCE TIP

The physician's office may only forward information about a patient that is part of the patient's care in that office. Information about patients that comes from hospital or clinic records cannot be forwarded by the physician's office. Such information must be requested from the source that generated it.

COMPLIANCE TIP

To comply with the HIPAA Privacy Rule, medical offices must give each patient a copy of their Notice of Privacy Practices at the patient's first encounter. The written notice explains how patients' information may be used or disclosed and describes their privacy rights. Patients must then sign an acknowledgment showing that they have read and understand the document.

- The assistant should not send confidential information by e-mail. Most e-mail networks are not secure.

The following section (2.3) discusses HIPAA in detail.

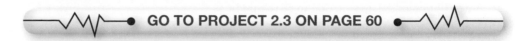

GO TO PROJECT 2.3 ON PAGE 60

2.3 HIPAA

HIPAA (the Health Insurance Portability and Accountability Act of 1996) became Public Law 104-191 in 1996. A major provision of HIPAA, known as Administrative Simplification, affects medical practices as well as hospitals, health plans, and healthcare clearinghouses. Its rules have gradually been passed and then implemented in the healthcare industry.

Implementing HIPAA has changed administrative, financial, and case management policies and procedures. There are now strict requirements for the uniform transfer of electronic healthcare data, such as for billing and payment; new patient rights regarding personal health information, including the right to access this information and to limit its disclosure; and broad new security rules that healthcare organizations must put in place to safeguard the confidentiality of patients' medical information.

There are three parts to HIPAA's Administrative Simplification provisions:

1. **HIPAA Electronic Transaction and Code Set Standards Requirements**
   National standards for electronic formats and data content are the foundation of this requirement. HIPAA requires every provider who does business electronically to use the same healthcare transactions, code sets, and identifiers.
2. **HIPAA Privacy Requirements**
   The privacy requirements limit the release of patient protected health information without the patient's knowledge and consent beyond that required for patient care.
3. **HIPAA Security Requirements**
   The security regulations outline the maximum administrative, technical, and physical safeguards required to prevent unauthorized access to protected healthcare information. The security standards help safeguard confidential health information during the electronic interchange of healthcare transactions.

Who Must Comply?

Covered Entities. There are three categories of what are termed "covered entities"—health providers, health plans, and healthcare clearinghouses—that must comply with HIPAA.

- *Healthcare providers.* "Healthcare provider" includes any person or organization that furnishes, bills, or is paid for healthcare in the normal course of business. Providers include, among many others, physicians, hospitals, pharmacies, nursing homes, durable medical equipment suppliers, dentists, optometrists, and chiropractors. A healthcare provider is a covered entity under the HIPAA Privacy Rule only if it conducts any HIPAA standard transactions electronically or if another person or entity conducts the HIPAA standard transactions electronically on its behalf (such as a billing service company and a hospital billing department).
- *Health plans.* A health plan is an individual or a group plan that provides or pays for the cost of medical care. Health plans include employee welfare benefit plans as defined under the Employee Retirement Income Security Act of 1974 (ERISA), including insured and self-insured plans, except plans with fewer than 50 participants that are self-administered by the employer.

- *Healthcare clearinghouses.* Healthcare clearinghouses are companies that "translate" or "facilitate" translation of electronic transactions between the providers of healthcare and the healthcare plans. In other words, they are a "go between," electronically formatting the provider's claim and billing information in the HIPAA-approved electronic standards needed by the healthcare plan and transmitting the information to the healthcare plan.

Almost all physician practices are included under the HIPAA standards. A practice is *not* a covered entity only if it does not send any claims (or any other HIPAA transaction) electronically *and* does not employ someone else, such as a billing agency or clearinghouse, to send electronic claims or other electronic transactions to payers or health plans on its behalf. Since the Centers for Medicare and Medicaid Services (CMS) refuse to pay any Medicare claims that are not filed electronically from all but the smallest groups, those that have fewer than 10 full-time employees, noncompliance is not practical for physician practices.

Business Associates. HIPAA also indirectly affects many others in the healthcare field. For instance, software billing vendors and third-party billing services that are not clearinghouses are not required to comply with the law; however, they may need to make changes in order to be able to continue to do business with someone who is a covered entity. Through business associate agreements, healthcare providers are responsible for making sure that the software they use, or the third-party biller or clearinghouse they use to help process claims, is able to produce HIPAA-compliant transactions. Business associates must also provide the covered entity satisfactory assurances that it will appropriately guard information as required by HIPAA. Examples of business associates include software vendors, lawyers, transcriptionist services, and accounting firms.

HIPAA Transaction and Code Set Standards

The HIPAA Transaction and Code Set Standards require standardization in healthcare e-commerce. These standards enable any provider to fill out a claim for a patient—regardless of the payer—and submit that claim electronically in the same format. Every payer must accept the standard format and standard codes and send electronic messages back to the provider, also in standard formats, advising the provider of claim status, remittance, and other key information necessary for payment to proceed.

Standard Transactions. The HIPAA transactions standards apply to exchanges for the most common provider-to-health plan messages between providers and payers, greatly expanding the amount of health information that is exchanged electronically as well as the types of patient information involved in electronic communications.

Technically described as X12, standards for eight electronic transactions have been adopted:

- Claims or encounters X12 837P for physicians and X12 847I for hospitals (equivalent to the paper CMS-1500, UB-92, and ADA Dental Claim forms)
- Claim status inquiry and response X12 276/X12 277, respectively
- Eligibility inquiry and response X12 270/X12 271, respectively
- Enrollment and disenrollment in a health plan X12 834
- Referral authorization inquiry and response X12 278
- Payment and remittance advice X12 835
- Health plan premium payments X12 820
- Coordination of Benefits (COB) X12 837; uses the same number as the healthcare claim because it sends a claim to both the primary and the secondary healthcare plans

In the future, standards for First Report of Injury and claim attachments must be adopted, also due to HIPAA mandate.

Standard Code Sets. Under HIPAA, a code set is any group of codes used for encoding data elements, such as tables of terms, medical concepts, medical diagnosis codes, or medical procedure codes. Medical data code sets used in the healthcare industry include coding systems for diseases, impairments, other health-related problems, and their manifestations; actions taken to diagnose, treat, or manage diseases, injuries, and impairments; and any substances, equipment, supplies, or other items used to perform these actions.

Code sets for medical data are required for data elements in the administrative and financial healthcare transaction standards adopted under HIPAA for diagnoses, procedures, and drugs. The following are the HIPAA standard code sets:

- *For diseases, injuries, impairments, and other health-related problems:* International Classification of Diseases, 9th edition, Clinical Modification (ICD-9-CM), Volumes 1 and 2.
- On January 19, 2009, HHS adopted its two final rules. One of the two rules modifies the code set for medical coding of diagnoses. This modification adopts ICD-10-CM (International Classification of Diseases, 10th revision, Clinical Modification) for diagnostic coding for physician coding. The new set will replace ICD-9-CM, Volumes 1 and 2. Implementation date, as of the date of this publication, is October 1, 2013.
- *For procedures or other actions taken to prevent, diagnose, treat, or manage diseases, injuries, and impairments:*
  - *Inpatient hospital services:* International Classification of Diseases, 9th edition, Clinical Modification, Volume 3: Procedures. On January 16, 2009, HHS adopted a revision of the code data sets. ICD-10-PSC (International Classification of Diseases, 10th Revision) will be the standard transaction code set for inpatient procedural coding. This will replace ICD-9-CM, Volume 3. Implementation date, as of the date of this publication, is October 1, 2013.
  - *Dental services,* Code on Dental Procedures and Nomenclature (CDT-4)
  - *Physicians' services:* Current Procedural Terminology, 4th edition (CPT)
- *Other hospital-related services:* Healthcare Common Procedures Coding System (HCPCS)

HIPAA Privacy Rule

The HIPAA Privacy Rule provides the first comprehensive federal protection for the privacy of health information. It is designed to provide strong privacy protections that do not interfere with patient access to, or the quality of, healthcare delivery. It creates for the first time national standards to protect individuals' medical records and other personal health information. The privacy rule is intended to

- Give patients more control over their health information.
- Set boundaries on the use and release of health records.
- Establish appropriate safeguards that healthcare providers and others must achieve to protect the privacy of health information.
- Hold violators accountable, with civil and criminal penalties that can be imposed if they violate patients' privacy rights.
- Strike a balance when public responsibility supports disclosure of some forms of data—for example, to protect public health.

Before the HIPAA Privacy Rule, the personal information that moves across hospitals, doctors' offices, insurers or third-party payers, and state lines fell under a patchwork of federal and state laws. This information could be distributed—without either notice or authorization—for reasons that had nothing to do with a patient's medical treatment or healthcare reimbursement. For example, unless otherwise forbidden by state or local law, without the privacy rule patient information held by a health plan could, without the patient's permission, be passed on to a lender, who could then deny the patient's application for a home mortgage or a credit card, or to an employer, who could use it in personnel decisions. The privacy rule establishes a federal floor of safeguards to protect the confidentiality of medical information. State laws that provide stronger privacy protections will continue to apply over and above the federal privacy standards.

Protected Health Information (PHI). The core of the HIPAA Privacy Rule is the protection, use, and disclosure of protected health information (PHI). Health information (HI) means any information, whether oral or recorded in any form or medium, that is created or received by a healthcare provider, a health plan, a public health authority, an employer, a life insurer, a school or university, or a healthcare clearinghouse and that relates to the past, present, or future physical or mental health or condition of an individual; the provision of healthcare to an individual; or the past, present, or future payment for the provision of healthcare to an individual.

Protected health information (PHI) means individually identifiable health information that is transmitted or maintained by electronic (or other) media. The privacy rule protects all PHI held or transmitted by a covered entity, in any form or media, whether electronic, paper, or oral, including verbal communications among staff members, patients, and/or other providers. Under this definition, a report of the number of people treated by a physician who have diabetes is not PHI, but the names of the patients are protected. PHI includes many facts about people, such as names, addresses, birth dates, employers, telephone numbers, Social Security numbers, bioidentifiers (such as a fingerprint or voiceprint), and health plan beneficiary numbers, any of which could be used to identify them.

Provider Responsibilities. The HIPAA Privacy Rule recognizes that medical offices and payers must be able to exchange PHI in the normal course of business. The rule says that there are three everyday situations in which PHI can be released *without* the patient's permission: treatment, payment, and operations (TPO).

- *Treatment* means providing and coordinating the patient's medical care. Physicians and other medical staff members can discuss patients' cases in the office and with other physicians. Laboratory or x-ray technicians may call to clarify requests they cannot read because of the physician's handwriting. This information can be provided by the physician or another medical staff member.
- *Payment* refers to the exchange of information with health plans. Medical office staff members can take the required information from patients' records and prepare healthcare claims that are transmitted to health plans.
- *Operations* are the general business management functions needed to run the office.

  For the average healthcare provider or health plan, the privacy rule requires activities such as

1. Notifying parents about their privacy rights and how their information can be used.
2. Adopting and implementing privacy procedures for its practice, hospital, or plan.
3. Training employees, so that they understand the privacy procedures.
4. Designating an individual to be responsible for seeing that the privacy procedures are adopted and followed.
5. Securing patient records containing individually identifiable health information, so that they are not readily available to those who do not need them.

Medical office staff should be careful not to discuss patients' cases with anyone outside the office, including family and friends. Avoid talking about cases, too, in the practice's reception areas, where other patients might overhear comments. Close charts on desks when they are not being worked on. When leaving a chart outside the examination room for the physician to review, place the patient's chart so that the name or number it not visible to other patients who are passing by that room. Simply stated, place the chart backwards. A computer screen displaying a patient's records should be positioned so that only the person working with the file can view it. Using a filter over the monitor will provide more protection from unauthorized disclosure of information. Files should be closed when the computer is not in use.

A covered entity must disclose protected health information in only two situations: (1) to individuals (or their personal representatives) specifically when they request access to, or an accounting of disclosures of, their protected health information and (2) to HHS when it is undertaking a compliance investigation or review or enforcement action.

The privacy rule must be followed by all covered entities—health plans, healthcare clearinghouses, and healthcare providers—even if they contract with others to perform some of their essential functions. These outside contractors are called business associates, defined as a person or an organization that performs certain functions or activities for a covered entity that involve the use or disclosure of individually identifiable health information. When a covered entity uses a contractor or other non-workforce member to perform *business associate* services or activities, the rule requires that the covered entity include certain protections for the information in a business associate agreement. In the business associate contract, a covered entity must impose specified written safeguards on the individually identifiable health information used or disclosed by its business associates.

Acknowledgment of Receipt of Notice of Privacy Practices.

To comply with the HIPAA Privacy Rule, medical offices, as well as other providers and health plans, must give each patient an explanation of privacy practices at the patient's first contact or encounter. To satisfy this requirement, medical offices give patients a copy of their Notice of Privacy Practices and/or display a copy of the Privacy Practices in the waiting area. It must be visible for patients to view. The notice explains how patients' PHI may be used and describes their rights. The office must also ask patients to review this notice and sign an Acknowledgment of Receipt of Notice of Privacy Practices, showing that they have read and understand the document.

Minimum Necessary.

When using or disclosing protected health information, a provider must make reasonable efforts to limit the use or disclosure to the minimum amount of PHI necessary to accomplish the intended purpose. Minimum necessary means taking reasonable safeguards to protect a person's health information from incidental disclosure. State laws may impose more stringent requirements regarding the protection of patient information.

These minimum necessary policies and procedures also reasonably must limit who within the entity has access to protected health information, and under what conditions, based on job responsibilities and the nature of the business. The minimum necessary standard does not apply to disclosures, including oral disclosures, among healthcare providers for treatment purposes. For example, a physician is not required to apply the minimum necessary standard when discussing a patient's medical chart information with a specialist at another hospital.

Treatment, Payment, and Healthcare Operations.

Patients' medical care information can be shared (used and disclosed) by providers, without a written release of information from the patient for treatment of the patient, to obtain payment for services and to conduct the healthcare operation of the medical provider, such as transmitting daily information to the entity's certified public accountant (CPA). *Use* of information refers to the entity's internal sharing of medical data, such as the medical coder asking a question of the physician in regard to a patient's diagnosis. *Disclosure* of information refers to the entity's external sharing of medical data, such as sending medical treatment and diagnostic information on a claim form to a healthcare plan.

Patient Rights. Under HIPAA, patients have an increased awareness of their health information privacy rights, including the following:

- The right to access, copy, and inspect their health information
- The right to request an amendment to their healthcare information
- The right to obtain an accounting of certain disclosures of their health information
- The right to alternative means of receiving communications from providers
- The right to complain about alleged violations of the regulations and the provider's own information policies

For the healthcare provider, these rights apply to the patient's designated record set, which includes medical and billing records maintained for the patient. However, mental health information, psychotherapy notes, and genetics information are not included in the designated record set. For the healthcare plan, the designated record set includes items such as enrollment, claim decisions (such as denials and payments), and the medical management system of the healthcare plan.

For use or disclosure of PHI other than for treatment, payment, or operations (TPO), the patient must sign an authorization to release the information. For example, information about alcohol and drug abuse may not be released without a specific authorization from the patient. The authorization document must be in plain language and include the following:

- A description of the information to be used or disclosed
- The name or other specific identification of the person(s) authorized to use or disclose the information
- The name of the person(s) or group of people to whom the covered entity may make the disclosure
- A description of the purpose of each requested use or disclosure
- An expiration date
- The signature of the individual (or authorized representative) and date

Patients who observe privacy problems in their providers' offices can complain either to the medical office or to the Department of Health and Human Services (HHS). Complaints must be put in writing, on paper or electronically, and sent to the Office of Civil Rights (OCR), which is part of HHS, usually within 180 days. The office must cooperate with an HHS investigation and give HHS access to its facilities, books, records, and systems, including relevant protected health information.

Exceptions to the Privacy Rule. There are a number of exceptions to the privacy rule. All these types of disclosures must also be logged, and the release information must be available to the patient who requests it.

- *Release under court order.* If the patient's PHI is required as evidence by a court of law, the provider may release it without the patient's approval upon judicial order. In the case of a lawsuit, a court sometimes decides that a physician or medical practice staff member must provide testimony. The court issues a subpoena, an order of the court directing a party to appear and testify. If the court requires the witness to bring certain evidence, such as a patient's medical record, it issues a **subpoena** *duces tecum*, which directs the party to appear, to testify, and to bring specified documents or items.
- *Workers' Compensation cases.* State laws may provide for release of records to employers in workers' compensation cases. The law may also authorize release to the state workers' compensation administration board and to the insurance company that handles these claims for the state.
- *Statutory reports.* Some specific types of information are required by state law to be released to state health or social services departments. For example, physicians must make such statutory reports for patients' births and deaths and for cases of abuse.

Because of the danger of harm to patients or others, communicable diseases (such as tuberculosis, hepatitis, and rabies) must usually be reported.

- *HIV and AIDS.* A special category of communicable disease control is applied to patients with diagnoses of human immunodeficiency virus (HIV) infection and acquired immunedeficiency syndrome (AIDS). Every state requires AIDS cases to be reported. Most states also require reporting of the HIV infection that causes the syndrome. However, state law varies concerning whether only the fact of a case is to be reported, or if the patient's name must also be reported. The medical office's guidelines will reflect the state laws and must be strictly observed, as all these regulations should be, to protect patients' privacy and to comply with the regulations.

- *Research data.* PHI may be made available to researchers approved by the practice. For example, if a physician is conducting clinical research on a type of diabetes, the practice may share information from appropriate records for analysis. When the researcher issues reports or studies based on the information, specific patients' names should not be identified.

- *De-identified health information.* There are no restrictions on the use or disclosure of "de-identified" health information that does not identify an individual.

HIPAA Security Rule

The regulations of the security rule work in concert with the final privacy standards and require that covered entities establish administrative, physical, and technical safeguards to protect the confidentiality, integrity, and availability of health information covered by HIPAA. The security rule specifies how they must secure such protected health information (PHI) on computer networks, the Internet, disks and magnetic tape, and extranets.

The security rule also mandates that

- A security official must be assigned the responsibility for the entity's security.
- All staff, including management, must receive security awareness training.
- Organizations must implement audit controls that record and examine workers who have logged into information systems that contain PHI.
- Organizations must limit physical access to facilities that contain electronic PHI.
- Organizations must conduct risk analyses to determine information security risks and vulnerabilities.
- Organizations must establish policies and procedures that allow access to electronic PHI on a need-to-know basis.

HIPAA National Identifiers

The HIPAA law requires identifiers for the following:

- Providers
- Employers
- Health plans
- Patients

CMS has issued rules only for two: the Employer and National Provider Identifiers.

Employer Identifier. The HIPAA Employer Identifier standard was needed because employers are frequently sponsors of health insurance for their employees. The identifier is used to identify the patient's employer on claims to the plan. In addition, employers must identify themselves in transactions when they enroll or disenroll employees in a health plan or make premium payments to plans on behalf of their employees. The final regulation establishes the Employer Identification Number (EIN) issued by the Internal Revenue Service as the HIPAA standard.

Healthcare Provider Identifier. The National Provider Identifier (NPI) rule provides a unique provider identifier for each provider. It is a 10-position numeric identifier with a check digit in the last position to help detect keying errors. In May 2008, the NPI officially replaced all other identifying numbers for providers, such as the previously used UPIN numbers from providers. Claim forms have been modified to accommodate the NPI numbers.

Patient and Health Plan Identifiers Not Issued. Due to the public concern over privacy, a patient identifier standard has not yet been adopted. Because of the central importance of health plans in the provision and administration of healthcare services, HIPAA requires the development of a Health Plan Identifier. CMS has not proposed such an identifier, and it is not certain when one will be issued.

2.4 MEDICAL COMPLIANCE PLANS AND SAFEGUARDS AGAINST LITIGATION

Medical practices must take steps to reduce the risk of accusations of fraud and abuse when submitting claims to insurance companies and federal agencies, such as Medicare. The processes involved in coding and billing are complicated, and there is much room for error. Although many errors are not intentional, medical practices are required to show their resolve to behave with **compliance**, or adherence to rules and regulations.

To assist in this process of ensuring that procedures are in compliance, the Office of the Inspector General (OIG), an agency of the U.S. Department of Health and Human Services (HHS), has issued *Compliance Program Guidance for Individual and Small Group Physician Practices*. This voluntary plan is a positive step toward helping physicians protect themselves and their practices from violations related to claims and reimbursements. Using the guidance provided by the OIG, physicians can develop an effective compliance plan for their practices.

There are specific risk areas in practices that a medical compliance plan addresses:

- *Coding and billing.* The risks include billing for services not rendered, submitting claims for equipment or medical supplies that are not reasonable, and double billing, which results in duplicate payment.
- *Reasonable and necessary services.* The practice must offer the patient only necessary procedures and treatments that meet Medicare's definitions and may not offer more complex and more expensive methods when simpler, less expensive alternatives exist.
- *Documentation.* Great care is to be taken in entering data and maintaining and retaining all information related to treatment, claims, and reimbursements.
- *Improper inducements, kickbacks, and self-referrals.* Neither the physician nor anyone on staff may accept payment for awarding contracts or for purchasing anything (*inducements*). Neither may anyone knowingly offer, pay, solicit, or receive bribes to influence getting business that is reimbursable by federal government programs (*kickbacks*). The physician may not refer a patient to any health service with which the physician or any member of the physician's immediate family has a financial relationship (*self-referral*).

The Medical Compliance Plan

The major purpose for creating and implementing a compliance plan within the practice is to prevent the submission of erroneous claims or unlawful conduct involving the federal healthcare programs.

The OIG *Program Guidance* suggests seven basic elements for any compliance plan set up within the practice:

- *Written policies and procedures.* There should be written policies and procedures for patient care, billing and coding, documentation, and payer relationships.
- *Designation of a chief compliance officer.* The officer may be an office manager or a biller. The officer's duties include monitoring the plan, conducting audits periodically, and investigating reports or allegations of fraud.
- *Training and education programs.* Education is an essential component because the physician relies on staff members to follow procedures that reduce the practice's vulnerability to fraud. Topics such as fraud, waste, and abuse should be covered on a continuing basis. Documentation of all training (i.e., topics, participants, dates, length of training) should be placed in the Compliance Manual. All employees should receive training on how to perform their jobs according to the standards and regulations of the practice. Employees should also understand through their training programs that compliance is a condition of their continued employment.
- *Effective line of communication.* The practice should create an environment where there is an open-door policy and employees feel encouraged to report mistakes promptly and to report any potential problems without fear of retribution.
- *Auditing and monitoring.* An audit should be conducted at least once a year by a designated staff member or an outside consultant. The audit includes checking for data entry errors and confirmation that all orders are written and signed by a physician.
- *Well-publicized disciplinary directives.* Every staff member should understand the penalties for noncompliance. Disciplinary guidelines should include the circumstances under which someone would receive any one of a range of penalties, from a verbal warning to dismissal to referral for criminal prosecution.
- *Prompt corrective action for detected offenses.* Corrective action should be taken within 60 days from the date on which the problem is identified. Problems must be investigated at once; a policy on overpayments must be clear and enforced.

The Administrative Medical Assistant's Role in Compliance

The potential for accusations of fraud is always present in the complex areas of patient care, billing and coding, and documentation. If fraud is detected and not reported or corrected, the reputation and legal standing of the practice are put at grave risk. The assistant has job responsibilities related to all of these areas and plays a central role in helping to ensure that the practice is in compliance.

The assistant who is working efficiently and effectively is key to the success of a compliance plan. In the following areas of responsibility, the assistant helps the practice stay in compliance:

- *Accurate data entry.* Accurate work speeds the correct payment of claims and lessens the chances of federal audit.
- *Accurate documentation.* Good documentation reduces the chances for mistakes and provides an excellent trail if proof of corrective action is required. In addition to protecting the practice, accurate documentation contributes to improved patient care.
- *Timely filing and storing of records.* Keeping records in good order and for an appropriate length of time can show the physician's good faith efforts to apply the principles of compliance.
- *Prompt reporting of errors or instances of fraudulent conduct.* The assistant has the ethical and professional responsibility to help the physician correct mistakes and investigate instances of unlawful behavior.

Safeguards Against Litigation

The assistant needs to be aware that liability for negligence is recognized by law to include not only the physician's actions but also the actions of the physician's employees. An assistant who is performing tasks within the job description and as a proper assignment is considered to be the agent of the physician. It is the physician's responsibility to define the assistant's job properly, to state and regulate office policies, to assist in teaching the policies, and to see that policies and procedures are implemented. It is the assistant's responsibility to understand thoroughly his or her job description and the office policies. The assistant, then, must act responsibly within the scope of his or her job and according to office policies.

It is easier to prevent a malpractice claim than to defend one. Assistants who maintain good interpersonal relationships with patients and other staff members help reduce the likelihood of litigation. In particular, the following guidelines are useful:

- Keep everything that you hear, see, and read about patients completely confidential.
- Never criticize a physician to a patient.
- Do not discuss a patient's condition, diagnosis, or treatment with the patient, with other patients, or with staff members. What the physician tells the assistant about a patient is to be kept confidential, even from the patient.
- Do not diagnose or prescribe, even though you feel sure you know what the physician would prescribe. There are often circumstances of which you are unaware. Prescribing constitutes the practice of medicine and is unlawful unless you are licensed.
- Notify the physician if you learn that a patient is under treatment by another physician for the same condition.
- Inform the physician of all information given by the patient, such as when the patient has questions, appears confused, or seems not to understand directions or instructions given.
- Also inform the physician about any unpleasant incident that may have occurred between the patient and any staff member. In this case, the assistant writes a notation to the physician, which does not become part of the patient's record.
- Notify the physician if the patient mentions that he or she has no intention of returning to the office or complying with the treatment plan.
- Be available to assist the patient and the physician.
- Obtain proper authorizations for release of information and consents. File these with the patient's records.
- Keep complete and accurate records, including notations about a patient's failure to keep an appointment, cancellation of an appointment, or failure to follow treatment instructions.
- Be selective in giving information over the telephone. Many practices accept requests for information only when they are written.
- Observe the confidentiality of computerized records by shielding computer screens from the view of patients or other staff members, protecting passwords, and following practice security guidelines when using e-mail transmitting information.
- Keep prescription pads and medications in a secure place.
- Be safety conscious. See that all equipment is in safe working condition, and be alert to potential safety hazards.

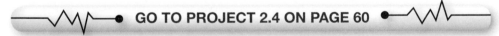

GO TO PROJECT 2.4 ON PAGE 60

Chapter Projects

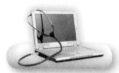

Project 2.1 **Internet Research: Bioethical Topics**

Using the Internet, research articles on two different bioethical issues of interest to you. Read both articles on each issue. Upon completion of your research, submit a written document regarding what you have learned. Also be prepared to contribute the results of your reading in class.

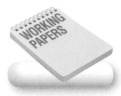

Project 2.2 **Physician's Obligations and Medical Law**

WP 2 contains statements that refer to the obligations of the physician and/or medical law. Mark each statement with either "T" for *true* or "F" for *false*. For each *false* answer, please document on a separate sheet of paper what makes the statement *false*. Also, be prepared to share your answers in class.

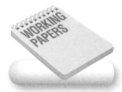

Project 2.3 **Medical Liability and Communications**

WP 3 contains statements that refer to the obligations of the physician and/or medical law. Mark each statement with either "T" for *true* or "F" for *false*. For each *false* answer, please document on a separate sheet of paper what makes the statement *false*. Also, be prepared to share your answers in class.

Project 2.4 **Legal Terms**

In WP 4, match each legal term in Column 2 with the correct definition in Column 1. Be prepared to give your answers in class.

2.1 Define *medical ethics*, *bioethics*, and *etiquette*. Pages 36–39	• Ethics are the standards of conduct that grow out of one's understanding of right and wrong. Medical ethics require physicians to practice high standards of patient care; respect patients' rights; treat patients with compassion; and safeguard the privacy of patients' communications. • Bioethics deals with the ethical issues involved with medical treatments, procedures, and technology. • Etiquette involves following medical manners and customs, such as using proper form of address for the physician, greeting cheerfully all visitors to the office, and using good telephone techniques.
2.2 Discuss medical law and legal documents, such as advance directives, and give three examples. Pages 39–50	• Advance directives are legal documents prepared in advance by the patient, stating the patient's wishes for receiving or not receiving certain medical care, should the patient be unable to make decisions at that time. Advance directives give the medical team specific directions as to the type of care to render. • Advance directives include DNRs (Do Not Resuscitate), living wills, and medical durable power of attorney.
2.3 Identify and discuss several key components of the HIPAA Administrative Rule. Pages 50–57	• HIPAA defines three categories of covered entities: — Healthcare providers: individuals or entities that render services — Healthcare plans: entities that provide payment for healthcare services — Clearinghouses: entities that electronically process health claim information from providers and transmit data to plans • Both health information and protected health information contain health information and health payment information about a patient's past, present, and possible future. Both can be used by covered entities and business associates to conduct business. • Health information is any information used by a covered entity, but protected health information could be the same information, only it would contain information that would allow the individual to whom the health information refers to be identified.

	- The purpose of an Acknowledgment of Receipt of Notice of Privacy Practices is to
	  — Inform the patient of how his or her protected health information may be used and/or disclosed by the covered entity.
	  — Describe the patient's rights concerning his or her protected health information.
	- There are exceptions to the privacy rule as it relates to the patient's protected health information
	  — Court-ordered release of information
	  — Workers' Compensation cases
	  — Statutory reports
	  — HIV and AIDS reports
	  — Research data submission
	  — De-identified health information
	- Another provision of the Administrative Simplification Act under HIPAA describes how protected health information is to be protected through security guidelines. Administrative, physical, and technical policies and procedures are implemented to protect the confidentiality, integrity, and availability of protected health information. Six of the safeguards the covered entities are to implement are
	  — Assigning an officer to oversee the security measures
	  — Training all personnel on the policies and procedures for PHI security
	  — Auditing controls to document who has accessed PHI
	  — Limiting physical access to facilities containing PHI
	  — Conducting risk analyses to identify areas of risk and vulnerability
	  — Establishing written policies and implementing procedures that limit access to and protect PHI

2.4 State the purpose of a medical compliance plan and explain compliant methods the assistant can use to safeguard against litigation. Pages 57–59	- The purpose of the implementation of policies and procedures stated in a compliance plan is to prevent the submission of erroneous claims or unlawful conduct involving federal programs. - The administrative medical assistant can contribute to compliance in several ways: — Entering data accurately, and documenting thoroughly

- — Maintaining the flow of records, especially if the provider is using hardcopy patient records
- — Reporting errors or the instances of fraudulent/abusive situations promptly
- It is easier to prevent a malpractice suit and litigation than to defend one. Some of the ways all members of the medical team can help prevent litigation are
  - — Keep all patient PHI confidential and all information to yourself.
  - — Refer all medical questions to the clinical personnel.
  - — Keep any critical thoughts of others, including the physician, away from patients.
  - — Notify the physician if you learn of a patient who is seeking treatment for the same condition from another source.
  - — Forward information to the physician when a patient seems confused or has not understood the physician's instructions.
  - — Inform the physician of any unpleasant situations between the patient and a medical team member.
  - — Notify the physician if the patient states he or she has no intention of returning or of following the treatment plan. This should be documented in the patient's record.
  - — Be available to patients and to others in the medical team.
  - — Obtain and document all needed forms and authorizations, such as release of information and advance directives.
  - — Keep thorough and updated documentation in all patient records. Remember, if it is not documented, it wasn't done.
  - — Attempt to get all requests for PHI in writing and keep a list of all disclosures of PHI.
  - — Implement security safeguards to protect confidentiality.
  - — Keep prescription pads and medications secured.
  - — Maintain a safe work/patient environment.

Soft Skills Success

Problem Solving

Problems are something that we all have in common. Not one person on this planet can avoid problems, whether professional or personal. Problems exist as a result of Murphy's Law: if something can go wrong, it will. Our ability to overcome challenges is what allows us to get the things we want. When you encounter a problem, take a step back and spend time thinking about the cause of the problem. No matter what, when you are dealing with any problem, becoming frustrated or emotional will not help you succeed. You need time to rationalize and figure out all of the details of the problem in order to come up with an effective solution. **Reflect on a time that you were faced with a problem. Describe the situation as it happened and what you could have done to change the way you handled the problem.**

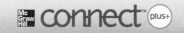
USING TERMINOLOGY

Match the term or phrase on the left with the correct answer on the right.

_____ **1.** (LO 2.2) Assault

_____ **2.** (LO 2.2) Battery

_____ **3.** (LO 2.3) Release of information

_____ **4.** (LO 2.2) Subpoena

_____ **5.** (LO 2.2) Liability

_____ **6.** (LO 2.3) Summons

_____ **7.** (LO 2.3) HIPAA

_____ **8.** (LO 2.4) Compliance

_____ **9.** (LO 2.1) Ethics

_____ **10.** (LO 2.2) Licensure

a. Standards of conduct that result from one's concept of right and wrong

b. Being legally responsible for actions and consequences

c. A clear threat of injury to an individual

d. Bodily contact without permission

e. A written notice by a court for the defendant to answer all charges

f. A legal document ordering all related documents and/or persons with knowledge of the case to appear in court

g. A legal document that must be on file from the patient before transferring medical information

h. A legal statute that covers the electronic transmission of patient medical information

i. Adhering to legal rules/regulations as well as high standards through practices and procedures

j. The written, legal right granted by a state or an organization to practice, after education and training, within a field by meeting the practice requirements of the specified discipline.

CHECK YOUR UNDERSTANDING

Select the most correct answer.

1. (LO 2.2) At the physician's office, blood must be drawn from a patient to check cholesterol levels and possible reasons for consistently elevated blood pressure. The patient arrives and blood is drawn. Which of the following has the patient given?

   a. Expressed consent

   b. Implied consent

   c. No consent

   d. Written consent

2. (LO 2.2) When the results of the blood work in Question 1 were returned, the physician decided to schedule the patient for a heart catherization. Other courses of treatment had been tried, unsuccessfully, to lower the blood pressure and cholesterol levels. Which of the following must the patient give prior to the procedure?

   a. Expressed consent
   b. Implied consent
   c. Informed consent
   d. Both a and c are correct.

3. (LO 2.1) During a recent political campaign, the candidates stated varying positions on stem cell research. Under which category does this topic fall?

   a. Ethics
   b. Etiquette
   c. Compliance
   d. Bioethics

4. (LO 2.2) When Bruce was diagnosed with Alzheimer's disease, he decided he might need another individual to make informed medical decisions, should he not be able to make them for himself. Which document would he need to complete?

   a. Medical durable power of attorney
   b. Expressed consent form
   c. Certificate of deposit
   d. Deposition

5. (LO 2.3) Of the following, which is NOT a covered entity?

   a. Clearinghouse
   b. Healthcare providers
   c. Office supply delivery service
   d. Healthcare plans

6. (LO 2.3) The following information was displayed on the computer screen containing electronic health information data: Sandy Smith, Social Security number 555-55-5555, DOB 07-07-1959. Upon checkout, Sandy's neighbor saw the data on the screen and later called Sandy to ask why she was seeing an OB/GYN. This is a breech of confidentiality because

   a. Protected health information was disclosed without permission.
   b. Health information was disclosed.
   c. The phone number was incorrect.
   d. The blood type was not listed.

7. (LO 2.3) How an office will contact a patient to remind him or her of an appointment should be stated within the

   a. Informed consent
   b. Disclosure log
   c. Release of information
   d. Acknowledgment of Receipt of Notice of Privacy Practices

8. (LO 2.4) Jennifer is asked to develop and implement policies and procedures to protect medical data. Before beginning, which of the following would most likely be the first step?

   a. Assign a security officer.
   b. Assign passwords to individuals who need access.
   c. Identify areas of vulnerability.
   d. Conduct staff training.

9. (LO 2.4) Upon checkout, Benton seemed upset and stated she would not be returning to the physician for treatment and was not going to take the prescribed medication. Which of the following courses of action would be appropriate for the AMA?

   a. Make a notation of the patient's statement in her chart and notify the physician.
   b. Wait to see if Jennifer comes to her next appointment.
   c. Follow the patient and attempt to change her mind.
   d. Make a notation of her comments in her medical chart.

10. (LO 2.2) When does the contract between the patient and physician begin?

   a. When the first procedure is performed.
   b. After the patient leaves the office.
   c. Before the physician leaves the exam area.
   d. When the patient seeks the services of the physician.

THINKING IT THROUGH

These questions cover the most important points in this chapter. Using your critical-thinking skills, play the role of an administrative medical assistant as you answer each question. Be prepared to present your responses in class.

1. What are the major standards, as set forth in the AMA code of ethics, that doctors are expected to adhere to in their practices? What qualities does the AAMA creed emphasize for administrative medical assistants?

2. You hear Mr. Washington enter the office. He has come to keep a 3 P.M. appointment with the doctor. You are busily trying to rearrange the afternoon appointments to accommodate an emergency that occurred in the morning. You do not feel that you can raise your eyes from the complicated list of appointments before you. You simply say, in response to Mr. Washington's greeting, "Please have a seat." Have you violated any principles of office etiquette? Please give reasons for your answer.

3. In what ways would patients be in danger if it were not for medical practice acts?

4. In a casual conversation, a patient boasts that he has made his stomach pains disappear without taking any of the medicine prescribed by the doctor. He also says that, although he had had these pains far longer than he admitted to the doctor, his home cure worked. He then informs you, quite seriously, that he does not expect to receive a bill for services from the physician. How do you respond to the patient? What is wrong with the way this patient thinks about the doctor-patient relationship?

5. On what basis would you decide whether an individual's request for access to a patient's record should be fulfilled?

6. A request for a patient's medical record is sent by fax to the office. The fax cover sheet contains the letterhead of a nearby medical facility. You do not recognize the name of the physician, fax number, or telephone number stated for the physician's office. How do you respond to the request?

7. Payment from an insurance company has just arrived at the office. In processing the paperwork, you notice that an error has been made in coding the procedure. The error has resulted in an overpayment to the practice. The error is only the latest mistake in a growing number of errors, all made by the same staff member. What are your responsibilities in this situation?

8. In a dispute between a patient and the doctor, both parties have agreed to an alternative to trial. What happens in an arbitration? What advantages may arbitration have over a court trial?

9. What are the aspects of an administrative medical assistant's behavior and attention to procedure that help the practice avoid litigation?

PART 2

Administrative Responsibilities

CHAPTER 3
Office Communications

CHAPTER 4
Managing Health Information

CHAPTER 5
Office Management

Part 2 discusses the important duties of the administrative medical assistant concerning oral and written communications. It also presents the tasks involved with scheduling the physician's appointments and handling mail. Aspects of office management include how to manage the physical environment and one's personal stress.

CONSIDER THIS: Communication skills are at the heart of successful relations with the medical staff, patients, and others in the physician's practice. *What steps can you take to improve your effectiveness in speaking and writing?*

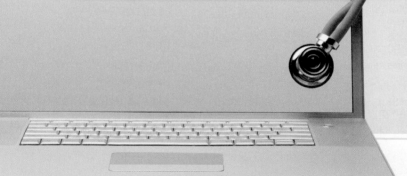

Office Communications

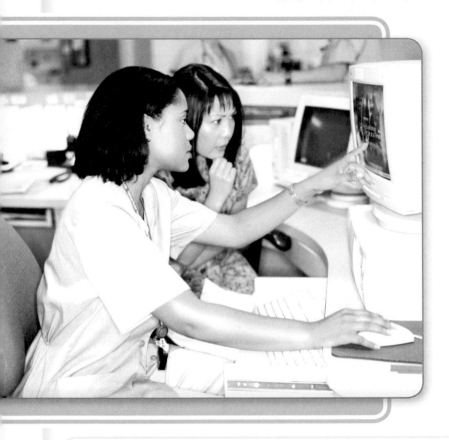

LEARNING OUTCOMES

After studying this chapter, you will be able to:

3.1 List the steps of the communication cycle and give an example of a barrier to each step.

3.2 Explain how the verbal message is affected by nonverbal communication.

3.3 Apply effective written communication techniques to compose written medical office correspondence.

3.4 Explain how proper triage of patients during a phone conversation can assist the office environment.

3.5 Recall and explain two different types of scheduling options and provide examples of practices that would be most suited to each of the schedules.

3.6 Recall the steps in processing incoming mail and discuss related safety recommendations.

KEY TERMS

Study these important words, which are defined in this chapter, to build your professional vocabulary:

annotate
bibliography
block-style letter
Bound Printed Matter
Certificate of Mailing
Certified Mail
channel
chief complaint (CC)
cluster scheduling
Collect on Delivery
decoding

Delivery Confirmation
double-booking appointments
editing
encoding
endnotes
emergency
established patient (EP)
Express Mail
feedback
first-class mail

first draft
footnote
insured mail
Media Mail
message
modified-block-style letter
new patient (NP)
noise
no shows
optical character reader (OCR)

open/fixed office hours
open punctuation
Parcel Post
POSTNET
Priority Mail
proofreading
registered mail
Restricted Delivery
return receipt
screening calls

Signature Confirmation of Delivery
Special Handling
standard punctuation
telephone etiquette
title page
triage
urgent
wave scheduling
ZIP
ZIP+4

Chapter 3

ABHES

- Adapt to change.
- Maintain confidentiality at all times.
- Project a positive attitude.
- Be cognizant of ethical boundaries.
- Evidence a responsible attitude.
- Conduct work within scope of education, training, and ability.
- Application of electronic technology.
- Apply computer concepts for office procedures.
- Be courteous and diplomatic.
- Serve as a liaison between the physicians and others.
- Receive, organize, prioritize, and transmit information expediently.
- Fundamental writing skills.
- Use appropriate guidelines when releasing records or information.
- Professional components.
- Monitor legislation related to current healthcare issues and practices.
- Orient patients to office policies and procedures.
- Adapt what is said to the recipient's level of comprehension.
- Adapt information for individualized needs.
- Instruct patients with special needs.
- Locate information and resources for patients and employers.
- Use proper telephone techniques.
- Be courteous and diplomatic.
- Exercise efficient time management.

- ➡ Cognitive
- ➡ Psychomotor
- ➡ Affective

CAAHEP

- ➡ Recognize elements of fundamental writing skills.
- ➡ Discuss applications of electronic technology in effective communication.
- ➡ Organize technical information and summaries.
- ➡ Identify styles and types of verbal communication.
- ➡ Recognize communication barriers.
- ➡ Identify techniques for overcoming communication barriers.
- ➡ Recognize the elements of oral communication using the sender-receiver process.
- ➡ Identify resources and adaptations that are required based on individual needs, i.e., cultural and environmental, developmental life stage, language, and physical threats to communication.
- ➡ Recognize the role of patient advocacy in the practice of medical assisting.
- ➡ Discuss the role of assertiveness in effective professional communication.
- ➡ Identify time management principles.
- ➡ Report relevant information to others succinctly and accurately.
- ➡ Explain general office policies.
- ➡ Instruct patients according to their needs to promote health maintenance and disease prevention.
- ➡ Compose professional/business letters.
- ➡ Use office hardware and software to maintain office systems.
- ➡ Use reflection, restatement, and clarification techniques to obtain patient history.
- ➡ Demonstrate telephone techniques.
- ➡ Analyze communications in providing appropriate responses/feedback.
- ➡ Demonstrate empathy in communicating with patients, family, and staff.
- ➡ Apply active listening skills.
- ➡ Demonstrate sensitivity appropriate to the message being delivered.
- ➡ Demonstrate recognition of the patient's level of understanding in communication.

INTRODUCTION

In the healthcare profession, an important part of the administrative medical assistant's job is interacting with patients, building relationships with coworkers, and representing the physician and the quality of the practice.

These are all good reasons to develop outstanding communication skills. It is not only in interpersonal relationships but also in letters, memos, reports, and e-mail that the assistant represents the practice. Success as an assistant is due as much to written and oral communication skills as to technical skills.

3.1 THE COMMUNICATION CYCLE

Have you ever played the game of telling one person something and the message is passed on to others until finally the last person says what he or she heard and it is nothing like the original message? Communication between individuals or groups is what creates the web of our lives. Everything we do is interactive, even if we are interactive with only ourselves, and our communications have a ripple effect on others, which alters the context in which we live. Understanding this interactivity is crucial to healthy communication. How efficiently we use the communication cycle and how well we identify barriers to effective communication will contribute to the effectiveness of our communications.

The Circular Communication Cycle

In order for communications to be sent, received, and understood as intended, each step of the communication cycle must be completed. If not, misunderstanding and conflict can create a nonproductive atmosphere in the work environment and in our personal lives. Time will be lost and productivity will decrease when the cycle breaks down. Each step is interconnected with the other steps.

Origination of Message by the Sender. At the beginning of the communication cycle, the sender must organize the message. The communicator should ask questions such as

- What and why do I want to communicate? The sender will formulate ideas he or she wants to communicate. These ideas, known as the **message**, can be influenced by the sender's background, physical well-being, and beliefs, as well as the context in which the message is formulated.
- Who is my receiver, or audience? The audience may be one or a group of individuals. When preparing the message, the sender must consider the background of those who will be receiving the message. The educational level, professional field, and cultural background of the receiver are just a few of the items to consider when composing a message.
- What is the best method to communicate the message? Some messages are best delivered verbally; some can be effectively communicated through written methods. The chosen method for transmitting the message is called the **channel**.
- When should I communicate the message? The timing of the delivery is critical to the effectiveness of the communication. The receiver's perception of the message can be greatly influenced, positively or negatively, by the time at which the message is delivered and received. One example is giving a patient pre-surgery instructions when the patient is giving you the medical chart and charge sheet from the visit. The patient is not ready to receive the information.

Encoding of the Message by the Sender. Expressing ideas through words and gestures is known as **encoding**. Words and gestures have different meanings to individuals in different cultures. Concrete words should be used in place of relative terms. A patient may need to arrive 30 minutes prior to the scheduled procedure time. If the assistant tells the patient to arrive early for the procedure, the patient's perception of early may be only 5 minutes.

Other items to consider when encoding a message are the receiver's background knowledge of the message, physiological considerations (such as hearing loss), and language barriers.

Transmitting the Message Through a Channel. It is vital to transmit clearly what you want to say and, as mentioned earlier, to properly time your message. Consider the following before transmitting a message:

- Are there any barriers that will disrupt the communication process? Anything that can break down the communication transmission process is known as **noise**. Noise can come from external sources, such as cell phone static, others talking, equipment running, or even typographical errors in a message. Internal noise, such as other thoughts or illness, can disrupt the cycle as well.
- Is the receiver ready to accept the message? As discussed previously, timing of the message can help or hinder the receiver's interpretation of the message.
- Does the nature of the message lend itself to a particular channel of communication? Messages that are general in nature, such as providing an appointment, are effectively transmitted through verbal or written channels. Messages of a more sensitive nature should be evaluated for the most effective channel. Disciplinary actions or warnings should be delivered using a face-to-face channel, not by phone or e-mail. Current channels of communication include written (such as reports and letters), visual (photos), electronic (including e-mail and fax), and telephone.

Receiving and Decoding the Message by the Receiver. Perception is a person's reality, and the way a message is received and perceived is the meaning of the message for the receiver. Factors such as different backgrounds, noise, and knowledge base often make successful communication difficult. **Decoding** is the receiver's application of meaning to the transmitted message. A patient may be greeted with "Good Morning" but the voice tone is angry and short. The words transmitted are verbally correct but the accompanying nonverbal cues may cause the patient to decode the message as "Good morning, but leave me alone."

Checking for Understanding Through Feedback. **Feedback**, the receiver's responses, helps the sender determine if successful communication has occurred. Responses include both verbal and nonverbal reactions. A slightly tilted head or a perplexed look may indicate the receiver is confused. A receiver should ask questions for clarification. As the sender, ask the patient to repeat information. You may also restate information or question the patient to check for understanding.

Barriers to the Communication Cycle

Many factors can create a barrier within and to the communication cycle. The best-planned message may not be received properly if barriers have not been considered. Each message sent and received must pass through a cultural, personal, and ethical bias base. This filtering process can hinder the intended message from being received.

Physical barriers can make it difficult to send and/or receive an intended message. Noisy surroundings, poor acoustics, and dim lighting can negatively affect the message. Hearing loss, fatigue, and illness also make it difficult to send and/or receive messages.

Selecting the proper wording can enhance the meaning and interpretation of the message. Using words that are unfamiliar to the receiver, such as medical insurance jargon, can destroy the message. Use words that create a receptive environment for the message. It is important to remember that most individuals think much faster than they speak, up to three times faster. As you verbally send a message, concentrate on the current message and words and refrain from thinking ahead. This can cause receivers to become bored with the message and their minds to wander.

Another barrier to effective communication is inactive listening. As a sender and receiver, we become involved in the cycle. The fast pace of society has conditioned many individuals to fake attention to messages and simply wait for the sender to stop talking, so that they can begin talking! This can cause miscommunication and failure to hear all the facts. When someone else is speaking (sending a message), we need to stop talking and begin listening, even if we don't agree with the message. This is the first step to becoming an active listener. Try to listen objectively and patiently before responding. Judging a message based on the sender's appearance is another contributor to inactive listening. If you must judge, judge the message, not the sender's appearance.

3.2 NONVERBAL COMMUNICATION

We have all heard the old saying "Actions speak louder than words," and it is no more true in any area than communication. Since communication is interactive and contributes largely to the web of life in which we live, we must be very aware of not only our verbal messages but also the nonverbal communication we send with it. Our verbal message may have all the right elements, which we discussed earlier in this chapter, but our nonverbal message may say something different.

Facial expression, tone of voice, eye contact, body movement and posture, our use of space, and appearance all contribute to our unspoken message. When our verbal message says one thing but our body language communicates another, we confuse our audience and lose credibility. When a listener must choose between the spoken message and the nonverbal one, the nonverbal message wins!

Facial Expression

The face is one of the most visible and expressive parts of the body. It is capable of many expressions, which reflect our thoughts and emotions. Few people have a true "poker face," which doesn't display their emotions. Most individuals have a wide variety of facial expressions, which they use many times during a conversation. A smile, a frown, pressed lips, and a wrinkled brow are just a few of the ways people can express emotions. It is common for a medical office to employ individuals with varying cultural backgrounds. Gestures may have different meanings to individuals, even within a small grouping. In American culture, a smile is considered a gesture of approval, satisfaction, or happiness. However, other cultures perceive a smile as an expression of nervousness or embarrassment.

Tone of Voice

This may, on the surface, seem to be a verbal communication barrier. However, when the words of a message give one meaning but the sender's tone of voice gives another, the tone of voice becomes a nonverbal communication cue. Feelings can be hurt by the tone of voice used by another. For example, you discover an error in a patient's account and realize it was your error. Right away, you go to the office manager and inform him of the error and your intent to correct it. He says, "That's fine," but his tone of voice is very sharp and loud. Do you believe it is fine and he is not upset? The tone in his voice says he is and that is the conveyed message.

Eye Contact

Confidence and interest are expressed nonverbally by making and keeping eye contact with an audience. Whether the audience is an individual or a group, maintaining eye contact allows the sender and receiver to be attentive and show respect for the other. When direct eye contact is maintained, a level of trust may be established. For most individuals, it is difficult to look someone directly in the eyes and lie. These characteristics are true of the American culture. However, in other cultures, direct eye contact can be offensive and make the communicators uncomfortable.

Body Movement and Posture

Gestures, or movements we make with our body, attach meaning to a message. The ways in which we sit, talk, and stand tell their own tale. Leaning toward a person conveys interest in the message, while stepping away conveys a perception of distrust or offense. Leaning back in a chair can convey the message of being relaxed, while tapping a finger or pencil signifies that the conversation should end. Standing tall and straight is associated with high position, but slumping of the shoulders and lowering of the head make us appear shy or lacking in self-confidence. Our posture should support our verbal message and can be a powerful nonverbal cue.

Each culture has its own values associated with body movement. As a medical assistant, you should know the different cultures represented among your patients and colleagues and use body movement and posture accordingly.

Space

Just how close should you stand to another person while communicating? Have you ever invaded someone's space? The spaces, or zones, around us have meaning and serve as social areas for interaction with others. The public zone (12 feet or more from your audience) is used for most public speaking events. A social zone is used for communications within 4 to 12 feet of our audience. Many individuals begin to feel uncomfortable when others enter their personal zone, which is 1.5 to 4 feet away, and become extremely uncomfortable with people in their intimate zone (1 to 1.5 feet). Too close, and our message will take second place to the discomfort the listener is feeling from our invasion of their zone. Too far away, and we send the message of being aloof and cold. In some cultures, however, it is considered rude not to stand extremely close (within the American intimate zone) when talking with an individual.

Try this role-playing exercise. Ask a fellow student if he or she can tell you what the last assignment was for class. Listen intently and then pretend you did not hear. Move into the student's personal zone and ask the question again. Notice any changes in the other individual, such as moving away from you or changing his or her tone of voice.

Appearance

Clothing and grooming send their own message about the communicator. Professional clothing in the medical office environment helps create a positive atmosphere for patients and colleagues. Scrubs should be clean and wrinkle free. Underlying clothing should not be visible through the scrubs. If scrubs are not worn, casual office or professional office clothing should be worn. No holes or tears should be visible in clothing. Even on "dress-down or casual days," clothing should be professionally presentable.

Hygiene and grooming also convey a nonverbal message. Nails should be kept to a minimal length and clean; hair should be washed and neat; and most individuals need to shower every day. Cleanliness, or lack thereof, affects our ability to be taken seriously. It is true that, "we never get a second chance to make a first impression."

3.3 WRITTEN COMMUNICATION

Writing and speaking effectively have these points in common:
- The communication has an appropriate tone—a way of phrasing ideas, announcements, directions, and requests that is pleasant, positive, and reassuring.
- The communication has a clear purpose, aim, or goal.

- The message is directed to a person, or "listener," who is to receive it.
- Correct English is used—including acceptable grammar, spelling, and punctuation.
- Complete information is given in a direct, concise, and courteous way.

This section focuses on preparing written communications and the office procedures that deal with receiving and sending correspondence. However, the qualities of positive tone, clear purpose, a sense of the intended audience, good use of the English language, and a direct and courteous delivery of complete information are necessary whether you are speaking or writing.

Reasons for Written Rather Than Oral Communication

Because there are so many issues of law, ethics, and confidentiality in medical offices, written communication may often be preferable to a conversation or phone call. Written communication may be required for many reasons, including the following:

- *Giving complex directions or instructions.* Patients who are anxious or distracted may need to read information at a time when they are calm. Repeating the physician's instructions or other information in writing may be more effective than oral communication.
- *Being efficient.* Writing a brief message may not require the time and effort of a phone call or face-to-face conversation.
- *Documenting an event or a fact.* The written documentation of aspects of patient care and practice management helps protect the practice from legal problems.
- *Providing for confidentiality.* It may be difficult or improper to use the telephone for certain communications with a patient.

Formatting

Before dealing with the content of correspondence, it is necessary to consider the appearance of the letter on the page. When a letter from your office is received, it should be pleasing to the eye and invite the reader's attention.

The arrangement, or format, of the letter on the page may be one that your employer has selected and is shown in the office procedures manual. For example, the preferred office style for a letter may be to place the subject line above the greeting, rather than below the greeting, or a double space may be used between the reference initials, enclosure notation, and copy notation. If this is not the case, you will need to choose one of the accepted formats for correspondence. There are two frequently used letter formats that give the letter a well-balanced and attractive appearance—block and modified-block style. The actual formatting features of the letter depend on the word processor being used. In addition to the two letter styles, two formatting styles are now being used—those prepared in a contemporary style using a word processing software such Word 2007 or a similar word processor, and those prepared in a traditional format. Documents prepared in the newer formatting style are the preferred layout, and examples in this chapter have been prepared using this format.

Block Style. The major rules for a **block-style letter** prepared in the new format, shown in Figure 3.1(*a*), are

- Place the dateline at 2" (enter/tap three times) or place the dateline at least 0.5" below the letterhead. If preferred, center a one-page letter vertically, from top to bottom, on the page.
- Enter (tap) twice (taps) beneath the date and key in the letter address. Single space the letter address by removing the 1.5 spacing from the address.
- Enter (tap) twice and key in the salutation and enter (tap) twice after the salutation to being the body of the letter.
- Use normal spacing (1.5) for the body of the letter. Tap once between paragraphs.

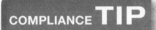

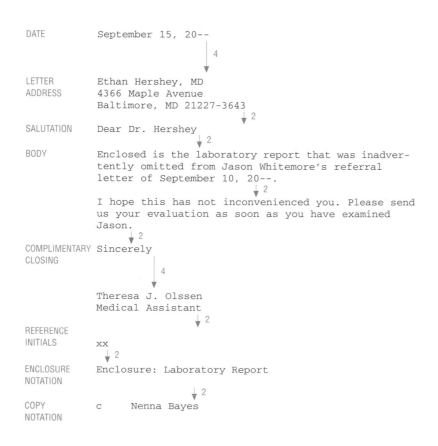

Figure 3.1(a)

Block-Style Letter with Open Punctuation

- Place the complimentary closing one tap/enter below the body of the letter and capitalize only the first word of the closing (e.g., Very truly yours).
- Enter twice and key in the writer's name and title.
- Key reference initials, lowercase, one tap/enter below the writer's name if you are not the author of the document.
- Tap/enter once to key in Enclosure or Enclosures. To list and align enclosures, tab to 1.0".
- Place a copy notation (c) one tap/enter below enclosures. If multiple names are listed, align the names using the Tab key.

Modified-Block Style. The major rules for a **modified-block-style letter**, shown in Figure 3.1(b), are similar to those for a block letter, but with these two exceptions:

- Position the date line, complimentary closing, and signature line at a Tab stop placed at 3.25".
- Begin all other lines at the left margin or, if you wish, indent new paragraphs 0.5".

Copyright © 2012 McGraw-Hill Higher Education

Chapter 3 • Office Communications **77**

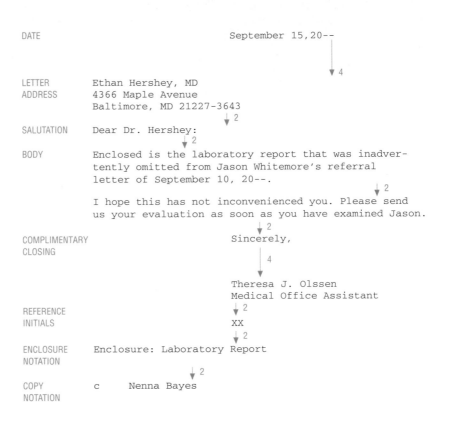

Punctuation

There are two styles of punctuation used in business letters:

- **Mixed/Standard punctuation.** Place a colon after the salutation and a comma after the complimentary closing. This is also referred to as closed punctuation.
- **Open punctuation.** Do not use *any* punctuation after the salutation or complimentary closing. This is the currently preferred style of punctuation for business letters.

Continuation Pages

When a letter has more than one page, always use blank stationery of the same quality as that of the first page. Do not use stationery with a letterhead, even when the first page has a letterhead. Use a top margin of 1" on pages after the first page, and add an appropriate heading, which includes the name of the recipient, page number, and date.

Valuable resources are a good dictionary and a copy of a comprehensive reference manual, such as *The Gregg Reference Manual*, tribute edition, by William A. Sabin (Glencoe/McGraw-Hill, Columbus, Ohio, 2011).

Types of Correspondence

The assistant is responsible for composing letters about many different office matters. The kinds of correspondence frequently initiated by the assistant, or written at the request of the physician, include the following:

- Letters of acknowledgment
- Letters of information
- Referral and consultation letters
- Follow-up letters
- Interoffice memorandums
- E-mail

Letters of Acknowledgment. The receipt of certain letters, materials, gifts, or requests for information requires a letter of acknowledgment. Such a letter may be written and signed by the assistant or written by the assistant for the physician to sign. The letter of acknowledgment should include the date on which the item or request was received and a description of what was received. If the letter is a request for a response or decision, the assistant should acknowledge the inquiry but make no promises in the name of the physician about the exact date or nature of the response unless information was obtained from the physician.

The main purpose of a letter of acknowledgment is to let the sender know as soon as possible that a request is being handled. In the case of a gift, the letter states that the gift has been received and is appreciated. Because writing letters of acknowledgment is a frequent task, a form letter may be used. Such form letters are easy to create with the templates found in word processing programs.

Letters of Information. Letters of information must have clear and complete information. Concise statement of the information is also appreciated by the recipient. If the information contains instructions related to treatment, the letter usually has the physician's signature, although the physician may ask the assistant to compose the letter.

Referral and Consultation Letters. Referral letters are used when a physician transfers part or all of a patient's care to another physician. For example, a general practitioner may refer a patient with a heart condition to a cardiologist for an extended period of treatment. Requests for a consultation happen when the physician asks another physician to examine a patient and report back findings on a specific question. For example, a general practitioner may ask a gastroenterologist to perform a colonoscopy and report the results of that examination as part of a patient's comprehensive physical examination.

Some practices send a brief letter thanking the physician who sent the patient when a patient is referred. The note is usually sent once the patient has been seen, so that a brief medical report can be included. Figure 3.2 is an example of this type of letter and may be used as a guide in drafting a referral letter. If a referred patient does not make or keep an appointment, a letter should be sent to the referring physician, explaining that the patient did not appear, after a reasonable period of time has passed.

Many medical insurance plans require patients to see a general practitioner before they can see a specialist. In these plans, the patient receives a referral letter or form from the general practitioner and takes it to the specialist's office. The referral contains an authorization number, which the assistant records as part of the patient's information. This type of referral may be handled differently by the medical office and generally does

Figure 3.2

Letter Thanking a
Physician for the Referral
of a Patient

KAREN LARSEN, MD
2235 South Ridgeway Avenue   312-555-6022
Chicago, IL 60623-2240   Fax: 312-555-0025

August 14, 20--

Hugh Arnold, MD
Suite 440
2785 South Ridgeway Avenue
Chicago, IL 60647-2700

Dear Dr. Arnold:

RE: FRANZ GUEHN   DOB: 08/05/----

Thank you for referring Franz Guehn to me. I have
just completed his examination. Mr. Geuhn was first
examined by me on June 4. His diagnosis at that
time was otitis externa, bilaterally; defective
hearing, mixed type, bilaterally. The results of
the audiogram are enclosed.

In July, Mr. Guehn had another audiogram (results
are also enclosed). At that time, a considerable
loss of high tones indicated a beginning degeneration of the auditory nerve, associated with
severe tinnitus.

Thank you for referring this patient to me.

Sincerely,

Karen Larsen, MD

nb

Enclosures: June Audiogram
               July Audiogram

COMPLIANCE TIP

Remember that, if medical
records are attached to
correspondence, the
patient must sign a re-
lease form.

not require a thank-you note. The administrative medical assistant must learn the policies of the office for these situations.

To make a referral or ask for a consultation, the physician who is sending the patient usually writes or phones the other physician, giving the reason for the request and a summary of the results of the pertinent tests or treatments the patient has had. If the referral is discussed on the phone, a letter confirming the conversation is sent. The other physician then knows that a patient is expected and has a brief history of the patient's problem. The referring office may also schedule an appointment for the patient with the other physician. Figure 3.3 is an example of this type of letter and may be used as a guide in drafting a referral letter.

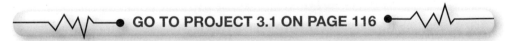

GO TO PROJECT 3.1 ON PAGE 116

Follow-Up Letters. Sometimes it is necessary to follow up on a request or a letter that has not received a response. In writing such a letter, be courteous, give the recipient the details of the original request and include a duplicate of the original request, and be clear about what action you wish the recipient to take.

Figure 3.3

Letter Informing a
Physician of the Referral
of a Patient

KAREN LARSEN, MD
2235 South Ridgeway Avenue   312-555-6022
Chicago, IL 60623-2240   Fax: 312-555-0025

August 16, 20--

Lynn Corbett, MD
Professional Building, Suite 300
8672 South Ridgeway Avenue
Chicago, IL 60623-2240

Dear Dr. Corbett

RE: JANET SCHMIDT   DOB: 09/30/----

Janet Schmidt, a four-year-old female, has had a
heart murmur since birth and recently has had
extreme pressure on her chest. I am referring Janet
to you for examination.

Enclosed is Janet's complete medical history, along
with the results of her latest tests, including all
lab work.

Janet's mother is to call you for an appointment
within the next two weeks. She has been given a
preauthorization number from her insurance carrier.

I would appreciate receiving your evaluation.

Sincerely

Karen Larsen, MD

nb

Enclosures: Medical History
                     Test Results

Interoffice Memorandums.

Informal messages exchanged within an organization may be written as interoffice memorandums, usually referred to as "memos." Memos are written on stationery that may have a preprinted heading, such as *Interoffice Memorandum* or the name and logo of the practice.

There may be preprinted guide words near the top of the page, such as *TO:*, *FROM:*, *DATE:*, and *SUBJECT:*. If you require more guide words, such as *DEPARTMENT:* or *EXTENSION:*, you may use two columns, so that the memo heading does not take too much space.

If the memo is being sent to a number of people, after the guide word *TO:*, you may wish to key the words *See Distribution*. On the second line below the writer's initials at the end of the memo, key the word *Distribution* followed by a colon. Leave one line blank, and then type the names of those to whom the memo is to be sent, arranging the names either by rank or alphabetical order.

Memos do not usually contain an inside address or complimentary closing, as a letter does. When memos are announcements to a number of people, there is no salutation. However, if the memo concerns only one individual, a salutation followed by a colon may be used, such as *Dear Tom:* or the name *Tom:* alone.

Figure 3.4

Interoffice Memorandum

```
                        INTEROFFICE MEMORANDUM


        TO:         Department Managers

        FROM:       Karen Larsen, MD

        DATE:       September 15, 20--

        SUBJECT:    Outside Laboratory Usage


        After careful study, I have decided that Penway
        Laboratory will be our outside resource labora-
        tory for the next three months. They have
        contracted to provide us with fast, reliable
        service. They are certified by Medicare to
        provide all necessary lab test results.

        Our contact person at Penway will be Gina
        McPherson. She will bill us directly for any
        outside services we use with Penway. Also, she
        will send us monthly reports on our usage of
        their facility. Gary, I want you to keep an
        accurate report of turnaround results and other
        possible problems encountered with the lab
        tests we send to Penway.

        During the week of December 20, we will have a
        meeting to discuss our usage of Penway. You and
        Gina will meet with me to discuss the continued
        usage of Penway Laboratory.

        nb

        Distribution:

                    Gary Libinski
                    Susan Solosky
                    Nancy Westing
```

A signature may or may not appear above the name of the sender, depending on the procedures followed in your office. The keyboarder's initials should appear two lines below the writer's name or initials or two lines below the body of the message. An example of an interoffice memo is shown in Figure 3.4.

E-mail. Recently, the most exciting form of communication has been e-mail. Preparing an e-mail is similar to preparing an interoffice memorandum. An e-mail address is keyed into the *TO:* field. Since a *FROM:* field is not included in the heading, many professionals include their name after the body of the message or compose a closing to be attached to each outgoing e-mail. Dates and time are automatically included with the e-mail.

A *SUBJECT:* line should be included. Mixed case may be used (capitalize the first letter of all words except prepositions and conjunctions), or the line may be keyed in all caps. Whichever format is used, the *SUBJECT:* line should be concise.

> **EXAMPLES**
>
> Outside Laboratory
> Outside Laboratory Usage

The second example gives more detail of the message. If a subject line is not used, the recipient may perceive the e-mail as unimportant, and not open it.

When composing the body of an e-mail, the standard protocol is to address only one topic and keep the e-mail to one page. Many writers include the recipient's name as a salutation or use the name in the first line of the body. If you use a salutation, such as Dear Nancy:, also include the writer's name in the closing.

Even though e-mail communication may be considered less formal than letters, it is still important to present a professional written image. Correct grammar, punctuation, and structure should be used. Always proofread an e-mail prior to hitting SEND. It is a good practice not to send anything through e-mail you do not want made public. Imagine your message being posted on the front page of your local paper or read on the evening news. Because of their ease, e-mails are often composed when the writer is angry or frustrated. If this is the case, go ahead and compose the e-mail but minimize it and allow yourself a cool-down period before hitting SEND. After you have allowed yourself this cool-down period, you may want to delete the e-mail or revise it before sending it to the recipient.

Always ask permission from the sender prior to forwarding an e-mail. Messages received may be intended only for the recipient. The sender may want to send a second e-mail with alternate wording, send an e-mail directly, or simply make a phone call.

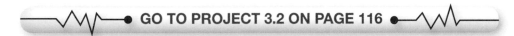

GO TO PROJECT 3.2 ON PAGE 116

Preparing Professional Reports

Many physicians are involved in writing articles, books, or reports on the results of research. They may also need to prepare speeches or presentations. Helping prepare reports is often a duty of the administrative medical assistant.

Preparing Draft Manuscript. The manuscript that will eventually be submitted to a publisher starts out as a draft. Some writers begin with an outline, jotting down headings and subheadings. The rough draft may then be filled in with notes added to the outline. Other writers make many notes, ask the assistant to key the notes, and write from these.

The **first draft** is the first complete keying of the manuscript. All text should be spaced to allow ample room for corrections and additions. The manuscript may go through many drafts before it is final. Each draft should be identified by number—*Draft 1, Draft 2*, and so on. Before saving a draft to the computer file, be sure that you have labeled it with its correct draft number or used the word processor's automatic draft-numbering feature.

After each round of corrections, additions, and deletions, the physician will ask you to key the changes and to proofread and edit the draft. Suggestions for proofreading and editing are given later in this chapter.

Preparing Final Manuscript. The purpose of the writing determines the final format selected. The purpose of some reports is to share information; these reports may be meant for distribution only within the organization. Such reports may have an informal format and may even be prepared as a letter or memo. There are several templates for formats provided in word processing applications. If the procedures manual in your office does not dictate a format, you may want to choose one of these templates.

Formal reports, usually more complex and longer than informal reports, are often written for readers outside the organization. Documents meant as professional reports or manuscripts for publication often have special features, such as a table of contents, list of illustrations, summary, and list of sources consulted by the writer. The publisher of a journal article can give rules for format and style to help the assistant prepare the manuscript. A manuscript may be rejected by the publisher if the appropriate format such as MLA (Modern Language Association) or *AMA (American Medical Association) Manual of Style* is not used. For other kinds of formal reports, the specifications for both a traditionally prepared report and a report prepared with Word 2007 are given here.

- *Title page*

    Traditional: On the first manuscript page, called the **title page**, key the title of the report in all-capital letters. Key the subtitle, if there is one, in capital and small letters, double-spaced below the title. Boldface should be used for the title and subtitle. Key *Prepared by* 12 lines below the subtitle. Then double-space to key the writer's name and credentials; writer's title, if appropriate; and writer's affiliation on separate lines. Key the date of the report 12 lines below the affiliation. Center all the text horizontally and vertically on the page.

    Current format: Within the word processing software, select to insert a cover page and select the desired cover page style. Key in the requested information in the provided fields, such as "Key in the document title." Figure 3.5 *(a)* shows the title page of a formal report prepared with Word 2007.

- *Text*

    Traditional: The text of the report should be double-spaced, with the first line of each paragraph indented 0.5 inch. There should be 1-inch margins on all sides.

    Current format: Accept the preset default selection, usually 1.5, for spacing and the default font.

- *Numbering*

    Traditional and current format: The title page should not be numbered; all other pages should be numbered in the upper right-hand corner. Pages are numbered consecutively, starting with the number 1, from the beginning to the end of the manuscript.

Figure 3.5(a)

Title Page of a Formal Report

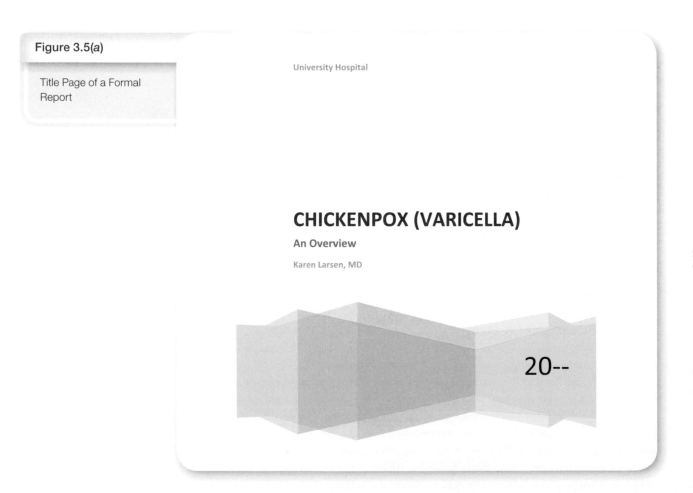

University Hospital

CHICKENPOX (VARICELLA)

An Overview

Karen Larsen, MD

20--

- *Headings*

    Traditional format: Section headings, such as *SUMMARY, INTRODUCTION,* and *CHAPTER 1,* should be keyed in all-capital letters in boldface type. Each section should start on a new page, with a 2-inch top margin, and there should be two blank lines below the section heading. Main text headings, which alert readers to new subjects within a section, should be keyed in all-capital letters and placed flush with the left margin on a separate line. Text subheadings should be keyed in capital and small letters, indented 0.5 inch, and followed by a period; text should follow right after the subheading on the same line. Boldface should be used for text headings, and there should be one blank line above headings.

    Current format: Side heading should be keyed at the left margin with the first letter of all main words capitalized. Select a heading style, such as Heading 1, and key in the heading. After the heading, enter/tap one time.

- *Italics and underscoring:* Words within the text that are to be emphasized may be underscored or italicized. Although foreign words should also be italicized or underscored, medical terms that are foreign words but are in common use should not be either italicized or underscored.

- *Quotations:* If quotations are brief, they may be set in quotation marks and appear as part of the text. Longer quotations (four or more lines) should be single-spaced for traditional format or default normal spacing for current format and indented 0.5 inch from the left and right margins.

- *Notes:* Writers use notes in a report to (1) add parenthetical comments or (2) provide the sources for information or quotations. A raised number appears in the text at the point of reference for the note; the note itself is also numbered. Notes that are positioned at the bottom of the page on which the reference appears are called **footnotes**. Notes that are grouped together at the end of the report are called **endnotes**. Most word processing programs have a notes feature that enables the keyboarder to create footnotes and endnotes.

- *Illustrations:* If a manuscript that is to be sent to a publisher or printer contains photographs, tables, charts, or graphs, these illustrations may be submitted as digital computer files or as reproduction copy. If digital files are needed, a scanner can be used to create a computer file of the illustration. The file name should describe the illustration. If reproduction copy is to be submitted, each illustration should be mounted on a separate sheet of blank, letter-size paper and identified by a title, caption, or brief description written on the sheet of paper. The manuscript page number containing the reference to the illustration should also be noted on the paper. Every photograph submitted should be a glossy print. Care should be taken not to write on either the front or the back of the photograph.

- *Bibliography:* All the works consulted by the writer, including items given in notes, are listed, alphabetically by author, in a **bibliography** at the end of the report. The publisher or an appropriate reference manual should be consulted for the format and style required. The University of Chicago's *Chicago Manual of Style*, the *Publication Manual of the American Psychological Association*, the American Medical Association's *Manual of Style*, and *Scientific Style and Format: The CBE Manual for Authors, Editors, and Publishers*, published by the Council of Biology Editors, are manuals that the writer may wish to consult for detailed descriptions of how to style and format notes and bibliographies.

    An example of the first page of an informal report prepared with Word 2007 is shown in Figure 3.5(b).

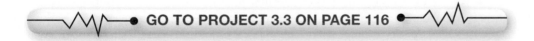

GO TO PROJECT 3.3 ON PAGE 116

Figure 3.5(b)

```
                    CHICKENPOX (VARICELLA)

                      By Karen Larsen, MD,
                      University Hospital,

                       January 25, 20——

DEFINITION

    Chickenpox is a highly contagious, acute infection causing pruritic
rash, slight fever, malaise, and anorexia.

ETIOLOGY

    Herpes virus varicella-zoster causes chickenpox. It is transmitted by
direct contact (respiratory secretions more prominently than skin lesions)
and by indirect contact (air waves). The highest communicable period is
the early stages of skin lesion eruption. Incubation period ranges from 13
to 17 days.

CLINICAL SYMPTOMS

    The prodrome of chickenpox generally begins with slight fever, malaise,
and anorexia. The pruritic rash begins within 24 hours as erythematous
macules, then progresses to papules, and then to clear vesicles. The vesi-
cles turn cloudy and break. Scabs then form. The rash begins on the trunk
and scalp. After the vesicles become cloudy and break, the rash spreads
to the face but rarely spreads to the extremities.

TREATMENT

    The patient should remain in isolation for at least one week after the
onset of the rash. Local or systemic antipruritics, calamine lotion, cool
soda baths, and antihistamines should be used for relief of symptoms. If
a bacterial infection develops, an antibiotic should be prescribed.
Varicella-zoster immune globulin (passive immunity) can be given to sus-
ceptible patients within 72 hours of exposure to varicella.
```

Proofreading and Editing

High quality in written communications is necessary because both internal and external correspondence represent your employer and the practice. The professional image of the practice depends in part on the impressions others form through the correspondence they receive. Incorrect, careless, or unclear communications may be damaging.

Two processes used to ensure accuracy and clarity are proofreading and editing. **Proofreading** is the careful reading and examination of a document for the sole purpose of finding and correcting errors. **Editing** is the assessment of a document to determine its clarity, consistency, and overall effectiveness. The good proofreader asks, Is this document entirely correct? The good editor asks, Does this document say exactly what the writer intended in the best way possible?

Proofreading Methods. Frequently, only one person reads a document for accuracy, comparing it to the original document. A single proofreader is all that is required for most routine correspondence and reports. For complex documents or highly technical materials, two proofreaders may work as partners. One person reads the original document aloud, including all punctuation and significant style and format elements; the other person examines the new copy carefully and makes the required corrections.

If you are the writer of the original document, proofreading is more difficult because there is no document against which to check for accuracy. For this task, an excellent working knowledge of English grammar, word usage, punctuation rules, and spelling is required. In cases where someone else has written the document, both the proofreader and the author should proofread the document.

Proofreading on the Computer Screen

Proofreading documents on the computer screen is an essential skill. You may want to use a piece of paper held against the screen to show only one line, so that you concentrate line by line on the text. Once you have examined the document line by line for errors and have corrected these, proofread your corrections carefully. Now you are ready to print and send a correct document.

Using Spell and Grammar Checkers

It is all too easy when you are proofreading on the screen to believe that the spell-check and grammar features in the word processing program have found all the errors for you. However helpful these features are, they simply cannot find many types of errors.

Spell checkers have a dictionary of a certain number of words. Specialized words that are used frequently can be added to the spell checker's dictionary. The software will always highlight or underscore a word it does not recognize. You will then need to decide whether the word is correct. Specialized dictionaries, such as an electronic medical dictionary, are frequently installed to help minimize the number of errors recognized by the word processor. For example, without the installation of a medical dictionary, the word *hyperglycemia* would be noted as a misspelled word in most spell checkers. When words are manually added to a spell checker, proofread the word to be sure it is spelled correctly. If words are added to the electronic dictionary and they are misspelled, the spell checker will not catch the misspelling.

The spell checker does not usually alert you to a word that is spelled correctly but may be misused. In some word processing programs, ordinary mistakes of this kind are underscored by the grammar checker. For example, using *their* where *there* should be used will be underscored by the software. However, certain other words that are frequently misused are not underscored. In the following examples, the mistakes may not be underscored by the software: "There are *too* of them (using *too* instead of *two*)"; "He did not *except* the gift (using *except* instead of *accept*)." The spell-check and grammar features are not adequate substitutes for a knowledgeable, alert reader.

Proofreading Symbols. Proofreaders and editors use standard symbols to indicate specific corrections to documents. If the document is to be published, the symbols will guide those who print the document. When corrections are made on the computer, these symbols on the paper copy guide the person keying the corrections. These proofreaders' marks, shown in Figure 3.6, should always be used when making corrections. Some physicians, however, may choose to use correction marks and symbols on hardcopy documents (e.g., transcribed reports) they have composed themselves.

Proofreading Techniques. It is always necessary to read every document several times. There are many elements in any written document and therefore many opportunities for error. Each time you read a document, you are concentrating on a different element:

1. Read for content. Does the document agree *exactly* with the original? Have any words been omitted? Have any words been repeated, especially at the ends of lines?
2. Read for correct grammar, spelling, usage (both words and numbers), and keyboarding errors. In addition to reading, use the spelling and grammar checkers but do not totally rely on them.
3. Check the format. Has everything been keyed with correct spacing, margins, headings, centering, and page numbers? Is the format consistent throughout the document?
4. When you are reading for consistency, check that the writer always uses the same style for phone numbers and dates—for example, either *(212) 555-7952* or *212-555-7952*, and either *10/19/2003* or *10-19-2003*
5. When proofreading for clarity, be sure that the most appropriate and concise words are used to communicate the idea. For example, do not use *demonstrate* for *show* or *utilize* for *use.*
6. In a separate step, proofread all numbers once again. Be sure that the number of digits in items such as addresses and ZIP codes is correct. Be sure there are no transposed numbers.

Figure 3.6

Proofreaders' Marks

∧	Insert word or letter.......	add it	∧#	Insert a space...............	addso it
✎	Omit word.....................	and so it	⟨	Insert a space...............	andso it
····	No, don't omit..............	and so it	⊂	Omit the space.............	10 a. m.
╲	Omit stroke..................	and sood it	─Ⓤ⒮	Underscore this...........	It may be
╱	Make letter lowercase...	And so it	◌	Move as shown..............	it is not
≡	Make a capital..............	if he is	‿	Join to word.................	the port
≡	Make all capitals	I hope so	word	Change word................	and if he
⌐┘	Move as indicated........	and so ┘	∘	Make into period...........	to him
=	Line up horizontally	TO: John	◯	Don't abbreviate	Dr. Judd
‖	Line up vertically	‖ If he is	◯	Spell it out.....................	1 or 2 if
ss⌐	Use single spacing........	and so it	⁋	New paragraph.............	If he is
∪	Transpose.....................	nad it so	⌄	Raise above line............	Hale1 says
ds⌐	Use double spacing......	and so it	+#↑	More space here..........	It may be
=⁄	Insert a hyphen.............	white hot	_#↑	Less space here	If she is
s┘	Indent — spaces...........	s┘ If he is	2#	2 line spaces here.........	It may be
∿	Bold.............................	He is not	─	Italicize........................	It may be

7. Carefully check and confirm important data, such as the correct spelling of names, addresses, all numbers, and the use of titles, such as *Dr.* or *Rev.*

8. Read the document again after you have made all the corrections. Be sure that, in making required corrections, you have not introduced any new errors.

9. Use the spell-check and grammar features available in word processing, but keep a good dictionary, medical dictionary, and English reference manual close at hand.

Common Errors. The following is a list of common errors you may find when you proofread documents:

- Keyboarding mistakes, such as the omission or repetition of words and other typographical errors; misstrokes of keys—for example, keying *slepp* instead of *sleep*
- Errors of transposition in both letters and numbers—for example, keying *flies* instead of *files* or *appointment on October 13* instead of *appointment on October 31*
- Spacing errors, including not spacing correctly between words, such as keying *patientdoes* instead of *patient does*; incorrect spacing within a word, such as keying *the re* instead of *there*; too much spacing between lines

Editing Techniques. If you are the person who originates the document, you may find it difficult to assess your own work. However, you do have a thorough understanding of your purpose. When you are editing a document created by someone else, you need to be careful that you understand the writer and the situation well enough that you do not make inappropriate changes.

When you edit a document, you are judging clarity, organization, and consistency of format and style. In editing, you also use your proofreading skills. You have the overall objective of making the document as effective as possible. To assess the document,

1. Read the whole document first to get a sense of its organization and purpose.

2. Look at sentence structure to determine that it is correct. Look at sentences to be sure that they are not awkwardly constructed.

3. Assess the correctness of spelling, grammar, punctuation, and English usage.
4. Look for problems in the tone of the letter. Is the tone appropriate for the intent of the letter?
5. Determine that the content is complete and clear. If you have any questions, be sure to get clarification from the writer.

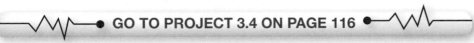

GO TO PROJECT 3.4 ON PAGE 116

3.4 TELEPHONE SKILLS

The main channel of communication between the patient and physician is the telephone. Almost all patients make their first contact with the physician by phone. Urgent and emergency cases are also reported by phone. The assistant must learn to recognize the situation in each type of call and handle it correctly. Often, the physician is engaged with another patient's care, and the assistant must be able to reassure the caller without interrupting the physician.

Attitudes are contagious. Patients judge the care they receive by the attitude of office personnel (reflected by the speaker's tone of voice and choice of words in telephone situations) as well as by the actual medical service provided by the physician. The caller should be paid the same attention given a person in a face-to-face conversation.

Telephone calls may be incoming, outgoing, or interoffice. Since administrative medical assistants typically handle all incoming calls to medical offices, they should use each call as an opportunity to present a positive image for the physician and the practice. An assistant must

- Follow proper **telephone etiquette** (conduct).
- Screen calls according to the office's policy.
- Take complete and accurate messages.

Telephone Etiquette

When answering the telephone, try to visualize the person with whom you are talking. Think about who the caller is, what the caller is asking, how the caller feels, and whether he or she is a patient. If you do this, your voice will sound alert, interested, and concerned during the conversation.

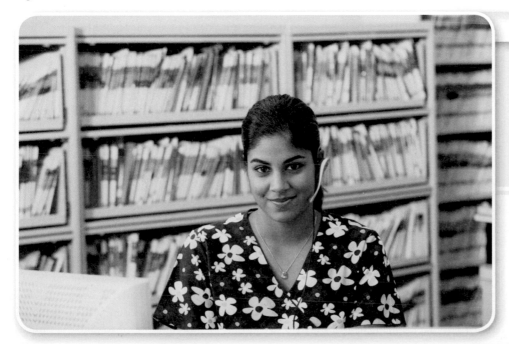

Figure 3.7

When answering the phone, the administrative medical assistant presents an image of the physician and the office. *How can the assistant present a positive image to callers?*

Use a pleasant tone that conveys self-assurance, along with a genuine desire to be understanding and helpful. This is what is meant by the phrase *using a "voice with a smile."*

Use variations in pitch and phrasing to avoid sounding monotonous, and never indicate impatience or annoyance through the sound of your voice. Hold the mouthpiece of the phone about an inch from your mouth to avoid distortion or faintness of voice. Speak clearly and distinctly; do not run words together or mumble. Even if you answer the phone with the same greeting many times a day, say the words slowly enough for the caller to understand. Always speak at a moderate pace throughout the conversation, giving the caller time to think about and understand what you have said.

When concluding a conversation, say, "Good-bye," and use the caller's name. Refrain from using the phrase "bye-bye," which does not demonstrate professionalism. Thank the caller for calling. Remember, the caller had a choice of whom to call! This will leave the caller with a pleasant impression. Allow the caller to hang up first. Finally, replace the receiver gently when you hang up.

Promptness.   Courtesy begins with promptness in answering the call. The ideal time to answer a call is on the second ring. This allows the caller a moment of preparation time to begin the conversation (the caller will expect to hear at least one ring before there is an answer). If you must place the caller on hold, always ask permission and briefly say why you must place him or her on hold.

> EXAMPLE
>
> **Dr. Larsen's office.** I have another incoming call. May I place you on hold?
>
> *or*
>
> **Dr. Larsen's office.** I am on another call. May I place you on hold?

Again, always ask permission prior to placing a caller on hold and thank the person for holding when you return. If you must keep the individual on hold for more than 30 seconds, go back on the line and ask if the caller wants to continue holding or if you may take the caller's number and promptly return the call.

If the call is long-distance, attempt to have another office team member respond to the call. If this is not possible, explain to the caller your need to complete another call and ask the person if he or she wishes to continue holding or to call back. However, if you have phone service that includes a large number or unlimited long-distance calling, offer to return the phone call yourself.

Greeting and Identifying.   There are many ways to answer the phone, but the preferred method is to answer with the name of the physician or clinic followed by the assistant's name. Using "Hello" as a greeting in an office environment is considered too casual and nonprofessional. Answering with "Good morning" or "Good afternoon" adds a personal touch but may be inefficient in a busy office. It may be more important to take the time to say the name of the office slowly and distinctly. If the physician has a common surname, the physician's full name may be used to avoid confusion.

> **EXAMPLE**
>
> **Assistant:** Dr. Karen Larsen's office, Linda speaking.

In large clinics, the person who is operating a switchboard may answer the call by identifying the name of the clinic and asking how the call should be directed. After a call has been transferred, employees in individual departments will then identify themselves.

> **EXAMPLE**
>
> **Assistant:** Northeast Clinic. How may I direct your call?
>
> **Patient:** I'd like to make an appointment with Dr. Nasser.
>
> **Assistant:** I will transfer you to Sharon at the appointment desk.
>
> **Second assistant:** Appointment desk. This is Sharon. How may I help you?

Following are some other tips to remember as part of proper telephone etiquette:
- Identify the nature of the call, so that it can be properly handled. For example, calls may be categorized as routine versus emergency.
- Use courteous phrases, such as "please," "thank you," and "you are welcome."
- Actively listen to the caller. Engage yourself in the communication process by totally concentrating on the call and asking questions and/or repeating information back to the caller. Set your own thoughts aside while in the conversation. Listen objectively without judging the caller. By nature, when we hear something to which we object, we tend to miss information. Active listening is not a natural tendency—it needs to be practiced.
- Use words appropriate to the situation, but avoid using technical words.
- Offer assistance as necessary but, as an assistant, do not offer medical advice.
- Avoid unnecessarily long conversations.
- Avoid using colloquial or slang expressions, such as *you know*, *ain't*, and *uh-huh*. Dialects are different and the "rule of thumb" is to respect local dialect but speak proper English.
- If necessary, repeat information at the close of the call.
- Avoid overly personal conversations, even if initiated by the patient.

Screening Calls

Most incoming calls concern matters that can be handled by an administrative medical assistant guided by the preferences of the physician. Some physicians prefer to speak to patients no matter what the circumstances. However, this routine is likely to be inefficient because it can cause interruptions to the patients who are being seen at the time by the physician. Also, medical records are probably not available for the physician's reference at the time of the call. In some offices, a nurse is available to answer patients' questions. Other offices have a policy that nonemergency calls are returned by the physician or nursing staff during preset hours, such as after 4 P.M.

Screening calls, or evaluating calls to decide on the appropriate action, is often a difficult problem for the beginner, who may be afraid to assume the responsibility of making decisions. It is important to discuss this aspect of the job with the physician at the very beginning and to ascertain to what extent the administrative medical assistant will handle calls alone, what information should be given out, when messages should be taken, and when the patient should be told that the physician or nurse will return the call. A call screening sheet, such as the one shown in Figure 3.8 can help you screen and transfer calls.

Figure 3.8

Call Screening Sheet

CALL SCREENING SHEET

Purpose of Incoming Call	Doctor	Nurse	Message	Other
MEDICAL				
Emergency: Dr. in				Come in. In case of life-threatening emergency, call 911 and send medical emergency personnel to the caller's location.
Emergency: Dr. out of office				Send to ER
Seriously ill		✓		
Test results from lab			✓	
Information; advice; test results			✓	
Rx renewal			✓	
Doctor	✓			
Hospital: ER, ICU	✓			
Other				
NONMEDICAL				
Appointment				Appt. desk
Medical records				Arlene
Insurance				Tina
Billing/charges				Tina
Personnel				Gary

The administrative medical assistant must be guided by the physician in deciding whether to handle a call or to transfer it to the physician. The first priority is to determine the name of the caller and nature of the call. You will then have a good idea of how to handle it.

Sometimes it may be hard to find out who is calling or what the call concerns. Phrases such as "May I please tell Dr. Larsen who is calling?" and "May I tell the nurse what you are calling about, please?" help you ascertain the information you need to complete or transfer the call.

Message-Taking Situations. Many calls can be handled by taking a message. The following are some examples:

- An ill new patient wants to talk with the physician about treatment.
- A patient already under treatment wants to talk with the physician.
- A patient's relative requests information about the patient.
- A personal friend or relative of the physician calls for the physician.
- Attorneys, financial planners, hospital personnel, and so on call about business.
- A patient calls with a satisfactory or unsatisfactory progress report (for example, a patient was told at the time of an appointment to call back with how a medication or treatment is working).
- Lab or x-ray results are called in.
- Prescription refills are requested.

The following calls are usually put through to the physician:

- Calls from other physicians
- Emergency calls—for example, calls from the intensive care unit or the emergency room of the hospital.
- Calls from patients the physician has already identified (for example, out-of-town patients, the family of a seriously ill patient calling to check on the patient's condition, or a patient in labor).
- Calls from a patient with an acute illness, such as a severe reaction to a medication.

If there is a nurse in the office, many of these calls can be routed to the nurse, who will then decide whether to interrupt the physician in an examination room.

Some examples of various screening situations follow.

EXAMPLE: CALL TO SCHEDULE AN APPOINTMENT

Assistant: Dr. Karen Larsen's office, Linda speaking.

Caller: I would like to speak to Dr. Larsen.

Assistant: Dr. Larsen is with a patient. May I help you?

Caller: Well, I need to make an appointment for next week.

Assistant: Mary, at the appointment desk, will be able to help you. Would you like me to transfer your call to her?

or

I can schedule an appointment for you. Are you a patient of Dr. Larsen's?

The assistant can then proceed to schedule an appointment for the patient.

EXAMPLE: CALL TO DISCUSS A MEDICAL QUESTION

Assistant: Dr. Larsen's office, Linda speaking.

Caller: I need to talk to Dr. Larsen.

Assistant: Dr. Larsen is with a patient. May I help you?

Caller: I'm a patient of Dr. Larsen's, and I have some questions about my medications.

Assistant: May I ask who is calling?

Caller: This is Wendy Chen.

Assistant: I will transfer you to the nurse, Ms. Chen. She should be able to help you.

or

The nurse should be able to help you with those questions, but she will need to pull your medical records. Let me take a message and ask her to return your call.

Transferring Calls. Telephone systems are provided with buttons for transferring a call to another line within the office. When calls are transferred, the system automatically puts the outside caller on hold. This means that the two people within the office can speak privately if necessary before one of them returns to the outside caller. For example, the administrative medical assistant can ask a question and relay the answer to the caller without having the physician or nurse speak to the patient, or the assistant can ask the physician or nurse to pick up the call and speak with the caller directly.

If a call must be transferred to another individual or department, be considerate of the caller. Explain that the call can best be handled by someone else, give the caller the name and extension (if available) of the party to which the call will be transferred, and offer to transfer the call.

Emergency Calls. An emergency call may come at any time. The caller will probably be upset, and people who are excited often forget to give the most important information. It is imperative that the assistant remain calm and handle the call efficiently, reassuring the caller that help will come as quickly as possible. The importance of obtaining the name, address, and phone number of the patient cannot be emphasized too strongly. The more information you can obtain, the better.

A physician who is in the office when an emergency call comes through will speak with the patient. However, the person answering the phone should screen the call to determine if it is urgent. Great tact and excellent judgment are needed to do this. These qualities are developed through training by the physician or office manager in what is a real emergency as the practice defines it and how to handle the calls.

Telephone calls from emergency departments are normally routed straight to the physician. In most offices, it is professional protocol also to directly route other physicians' calls straight to the physician.

Nonmedical Screening Situations. One of the most difficult situations to handle over the telephone is the person who refuses to state the purpose of the call, saying that it is a "personal call" or a "personal matter." A personal friend does not hesitate to state that fact. Similarly, a legitimate caller will give a name and state the reason for the call. The administrative medical assistant may explain that the physician will not return the call unless the nature of the call is known, if the physician has given such instructions. If the caller absolutely refuses to give information, it is permissible to suggest that a letter be written and marked "Personal," so that the physician can become acquainted with the matter and give a response. A confident, pleasant voice will help you make the physician's position clear while avoiding needless disputes. When such situations occur, always keep the physician informed of the call and the attempted resolution.

Taking Messages

Because most calls cannot be taken immediately by a medical staff member, the assistant must take clear messages, so that the calls can be returned later.

Remember the following procedures for taking efficient, informative telephone messages:

- Always have pen and message pad on hand or have the electronic message center on the computer screen.
- Make notes as information is being given.
- Ask politely to have important information repeated.
- Verify information such as names, spellings, numbers, and dates for accuracy. You might ask, "Would you spell that prescription's name, please?" or "Let me repeat that to be sure I have noted it correctly."
- Make inquiries tactfully. A tactful question might be "Will Gary know what this is about?" or "Could I tell Sue what this is about?" or "Is this a medical matter? If so, the physician will need your medical record."

The more information you include in the message, the better. Be brief yet thorough.

When taking a phone message, do not say, "I will have the physician call you." This makes a commitment on behalf of the physician. It is better to say, "I will give the message to the physician," or "I will ask the physician to call you."

After taking a message regarding a patient's care, the assistant should obtain the patient's chart. The phone message should be attached to the chart with a paper clip and placed in the message center for the nurse or the physician. The message slip, or a transcription of it, as

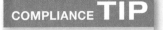

Correctly maintaining patients' medical records requires all communications from patients, including phone calls, to be properly documented. Correct documentation is legible, signed, and dated.

Copyright © 2012 McGraw-Hill Higher Education

Figure 3.9

MESSAGE

TO _Dr. Larsen_ **DATE** _7/23_ **TIME** _4 p.m._

FROM _Clara Wicks_

PHONE _555-3455_

☑ **PLEASE CALL** ☐ **RETURNED YOUR CALL** ☐ **WILL CALL AGAIN**

REGARDING _pt Dan Hanley. Chief complaint: difficulty hearing._

Ears checked by nurse? wax.

TAKEN BY _tjo_

well as the physician's or nurse's actions, will be permanently documented in the patient's medical record.

Message Slips. Printed phone message slips are available from stationers for writing down messages efficiently and fully. See Figure 3.9 for an example of such a slip. Telephone message slips have blanks for noting basic information about the phone call, such as the date, time, to and from information, and subject of the call. In some offices, the computer system is used to enter and send messages to the physician.

Some physicians design their own telephone message slips and have them printed. A message slip customized for a physician's office will list the standard symptoms related to a given physician's specialty or field of practice. When a patient calls, the administrative medical assistant can take a message by checking off the symptoms that pertain to the patient. Figure 3.10 shows an example of a telephone message slip customized for a physician's office.

Verifying Information. When you are taking messages, it is a good idea to repeat important details, such as the date and time of an appointment or a telephone number. Verifying information reassures both parties of the call. If you are not sure of the correct spelling of a name, say, "I'm sorry. Will you spell your name again, please?" or "I want to get your name correctly. Will you please repeat that?" Sometimes questions about a message need to be asked or information needs to be clarified. Each message, whether electronic or handwritten, should include the initials or name of the individual taking the message. Taking ownership of the message demonstrates professionalism and confidence in your abilities.

Using Speakerphones. In a busy office, speakerphones give the assistant a method of hands-free communication with the caller. When taking messages electronically, either a headset or speakerphone is necessary. While the speakerphone has many advantages, it does have limitations.

In an office with a noisy environment, speakerphones are not the best choice for receiving and placing calls. Also, in a medical office, protected health information (as discussed in

Figure 3.10

Customized Telephone Message Slip

TELEPHONE MESSAGE

DATE	TIME	PHYSICIAN
10/8/--	1:30	Larsen

PATIENT	AGE	PHONE
Patricia Strand	18 months	555-7643

Mother—Betty

__ Abdominal pain	__ Earache	__ Sore throat
__ Cough	__ Headache	__ Swollen glands
__ Cramps	__ Nasal congestion	✔ Temperature _100 R_
✔ Diarrhea	__ Rash	__ Urinary
__ Dizziness	__ Runny nose	✔ Vomiting

REGARDING: Patricia sick x 24 hours. Keeps some clear liquids down. Just finished 10 days of Septra DS.

tjo

Chapter 2) is discussed during phone conversations. Using a speakerphone can allow a breach of confidentiality and the unintentional disclosure of PHI.

When using a speakerphone, there are a few things to remember:

- Always ask the caller's permission prior to conversing over a speakerphone or let the person know he or she is on a speakerphone.
- Ask the caller if the conversation reception is clear.
- Refrain from creating noise, such as moving papers or rolling chairs.
- Inform the caller if someone else is in the area and can hear the conversation.

Answering Services. Many physicians' offices use commercial answering services or answering machines for phone coverage when the office is closed. Commercial answering services can answer the office's calls from a remote location. All unanswered calls are forwarded to an operator during nonoffice hours. This operator takes messages for routine calls or contacts the physician or appointed nurse if the call is an emergency. The physician or administrative medical assistant checks in with the answering service for any messages after returning to the office. An answering machine connected to the office telephone line plays a prerecorded message to the caller. It tells the caller what to do when the call is urgent or routine. The message can be changed according to the circumstance. Remember that the answering machine needs to be turned off when the staff are in the office. When recording the message, speak at a reasonable speed in a pleasant, variable tone. Listeners should have time to record the information, such as a contact phone number or instructions. Repeating the contact information will give the caller extra time to record it and will provide an accuracy check.

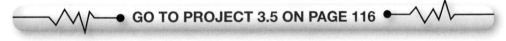

GO TO PROJECT 3.5 ON PAGE 116

Outgoing Calls

In addition to answering calls, administrative medical assistants place calls for the medical practice to patients, hospitals, clinics, and laboratories, as well as to insurance companies, suppliers, banks, and other businesses.

Planning the Call. Plan the conversation before making a call by gathering important papers (such as the patient's medical record), obtaining necessary information, and outlining questions to ask. Know the specifics of the call before you dial. Ask yourself who, what, where, when, and why, and make appropriate notations. Be aware of the following:

- Whom to call and ask for once the phone is answered
- What information to give or obtain
- Questions to ask
- When to call
- Possible situations that might arise during the call (what-if situations)

> **EXAMPLE**
>
> **Dr. Larsen:** Linda, please call Dr. Martin and ask him to see Lucy Barlow.

To complete the call requested in the preceding example, Linda will need to ask Dr. Larsen the following:

- What is Lucy's diagnosis (if applicable)?
- When should Lucy be seen by Dr. Martin?
- What are the contingency plans (what-ifs)? For example, what is the alternative if Lucy must be seen today but Dr. Martin is not in the office today?

Always obtain the necessary information and have it on hand before scheduling services (such as referrals, laboratory and x-ray procedures, surgery, and hospital admissions). Insurance information should also be given to the provider. Under HIPAA's TPO provision, release of information from the patient is not needed when scheduling an appointment for continuity of the patient's care.

Using Resources. Numerous resources are available to help the assistant place calls and manage the flow of calls in a medical office.

Telephone Directories

An alphabetic directory, or white pages, lists telephone customers by name in alphabetic order. The white pages usually contain other information as well, such as directory-assistance numbers, billing information, long-distance calling procedures, and area code maps. In large cities, information concerning government agencies, including phone numbers, is often listed in the blue pages section of the alphabetic directory.

A classified directory, or yellow pages, lists telephone subscribers under headings for types of businesses, such as "Office Supplies or Laboratories—Medical." Classified directories also contain advertising for subscribing businesses and sometimes contain local street maps and ZIP code listings.

There are also many directory services available on the Internet—for example, AOL NetFind, Switchboard.com, YellowPages.com, B2B (Business to Business) Yellow Pages, 555-1212, and many more. These directories use search engines to locate phone numbers, addresses, and e-mail addresses locally, in the United States, and in some foreign countries.

A personal directory is used for phone numbers that are frequently called by the office staff. The personal directory should be kept near the phone for easy access and would probably include a list of the following phone numbers:

- Hospitals
- Insurance companies
- Laboratories
- Medical supply companies
- Pharmacies
- Hospital emergency room
- Specialists for referrals made to patients

Figure 3.11

Telephone systems use computer technology to improve office efficiency. *What telephone system features are helpful in a medical office?*

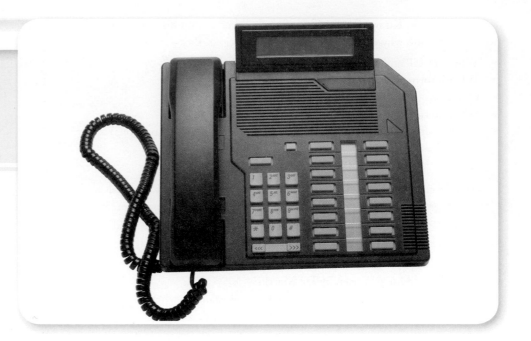

Most phone systems are equipped with an automatic speed-dial feature that allows the user to store 20 or 30 numbers electronically. A frequently dialed number can be stored under one or two digits to save time in dialing. If speed-dial numbers are used, they can be listed in a separate column or table in the personal directory.

Other Automated Features

Desk phone systems today, such as the one shown in Figure 3.11, are designed to provide automated features such as call pickup, call forwarding, call transfer, automatic hold recall, and automatic call distribution. They can also be programmed to place a call at a set time or to notify the user when a previously dialed busy line is open. One day, automated phone systems may be used to carry out routine functions in a medical office, such as turning on the lights or the heating system at a preprogrammed time or locking the door when the office is closed.

Placing the Call. When you have the proper information and are prepared to place a call, use the following procedures:

- Identify yourself and the physician's office. If you are calling for the physician, identify the physician.
- State the reason for the call.
- Provide the necessary information.
- Ask tactfully for information.
- Listen carefully and make notes as needed.
- Verify information.
- If the person you are trying to reach is unavailable, leave a message for that person to call you back. Remember to follow the confidentiality guidelines of the office.

Using the Fax Machine. A facsimile (fax) machine may be used to send or receive information about patients immediately. The physician must develop and follow guidelines for faxing information about patients. A patient's confidentiality must be protected—the fax machine should be located where only authorized personnel have access to it. Federal and state laws must be followed for maintaining medical records. Generally, follow these guidelines:

- Contact the receiver before transmitting the information.
- Send a release of information with a facsimile cover letter (see the example in Figure 3.12).

Figure 3.12

Facsimile Cover Letter
with Return Receipt

KAREN LARSEN, MD

2235 South Ridgeway Avenue
Chicago, IL 60623-2240

312-555-6022
Fax: 312-555-0025

FACSIMILE COVER LETTER

DATE: _____ TIME: _____ a.m./p.m.

TO: _____
(name)

_____
(facility)

_____
(address)

FAX NUMBER: _____

RE: _____

FROM: _____
(name/department)

   KAREN LARSEN, MD

Number of pages including cover letter: _____

NOTICE OF CONFIDENTIALITY: The faxed document or documents contain confidential information. The information is only for use by the above-named receiver. Use of the information in any form is strictly prohibited if you are not the intended receiver. Please notify our office immediately if you received this fax in error. Contact our office by telephone to arrange for the return of the original fax document.

_____

RETURN RECEIPT: Please complete the following statement and return it to the above-stated fax number.

I, _____, verify that I have received _____ pages
   Authorized Receiver

from _____.
   Sending Facility

- File the original cover letter in the chart.
- Request a signed return receipt of the faxed information.
- Photocopy documents received on thermal fax paper before placing them in a patient's chart because thermal fax paper deteriorates over time.

Even with faxing safeguards in place, the advances in software capabilities create challenges when verifying the authenticity of a faxed request. Consider the following:

Your male patient is in the process of a divorce. Because of the past relationship, both parties know a substantial amount of personal information and history about the other, such as medical and financial issues. The wife phones the office, posing as her husband's attorney, and requests that his medical records be faxed to "her" office. She is advised that a faxed release of information from the husband is needed before the data may be released. The wife creates a fake letterhead using an online template, and she forges her husband's signature. After reviewing the faxed request, the office manager gives the approval for the records to be faxed to the "attorney" using the fax number on the release. Through this illegal disclosure of information, the wife learns that the husband had contracted a sexually transmitted disease and had disclosed the name of a partner from whom he may have received the disease. It was not his wife.

Double-checking with the patient prior to faxing the information and checking the authenticity of the law firm may have prevented the disclosure. Also, using a predetermined password for releasing information may deter illegal requests. For example, when completing registration paperwork, include a field called "Release of Information Password." All requests for disclosure of PHI must contain this password. Additionally, the implementation of electronic health records will help eliminate the need to fax sensitive medical information. Electronic health records will be discussed in more detail in a later chapter.

Faxing may be done using stand-alone equipment—not connected to any other machine—or through fax software on a computer. Some printers function both as printers and stand-alone fax machines. Whatever type of fax machine is used, a telephone line must be available. Most medical practices have dedicated fax lines, which means that the fax machine is connected to a separate phone line reserved only for sending and receiving faxes. With a dedicated fax line, the fax machine is available 24 hours a day to receive or send faxes.

Following Through on Calls. Proper handling of telephone calls does not end after the phone is hung up. The administrative medical assistant must follow through on all requests made and instructions provided in the conversation. See Figures 3.13 through 3.15 for examples of follow-through methods.

Figure 3.13

Follow-Through Notation Made Directly on a Telephone Message Slip

MESSAGE

TO ___Nurse_____ DATE ___10/6___ TIME ___10:20___

FROM ___Laura Paulson_____ 11:00 Told to come for cultures for all family members.

PHONE ___555-7261_____ Sue, R.N.

☑ **PLEASE CALL** ☐ **RETURNED YOUR CALL** ☐ **WILL CALL AGAIN**

REGARDING ___Jason has strep. Andy + Eric now have sore throats. Should family___
___come in for cultures?_____

_____

_____

TAKEN BY ___tjo_____

Figure 3.14

Follow-Through Memo Summarizing a Telephone Call

```
MEMO TO:  Karen Larsen, MD
FROM:     University Hospital
DATE:     September 25
SUBJECT:  Dr. Dean Ashcroft's seminars

The University Hospital telephoned at 4 p.m. today about a series
of four seminars titled "Educating Caregivers."
    1. Early Care: Prenatal
    2. Prevention of Accidents Involving Household Poisons
    3. Early Abusive Behaviors
    4. Addicted Caregivers
Dr. Ashcroft is the sponsor of the series. Please let me know if
you would like to register for any of these seminars.

TJO
```

All telephone messages (and other messages) from or concerning a patient should be entered into the patient's medical record. In such cases, the message slip can be taped or filed inside the chart after it has been acted on. Another option is to make a chart notation of the telephone call information or the physician may make a chart entry. All entries must be signed and dated. If using electronic medical records, the message should be transferred or recorded into the patient's electronic record. Some offices have a page in the patient's record specifically for messages (see Figure 3.16 for an example).

TO-DO LIST

Date _____7/23_____

RUSH	ITEMS TO DO	DONE
	~~Send records to Dr. Peters re: Jill Sommers.~~	7/26
	~~Reserve conference room 7/31 at 8 a.m.~~	7/26
	Remind Dr. Larsen to get slides for 7/31.	
*	Call Brent Ashwood 7/23 re: disability form at 555-7287.	

Figure 3.15

Follow-Through Notation on a To-Do List

CHART NOTE

Hanley, Dan   312-555-3455
DOB: 07/27/19--   Age: 59

July 23, 20--, 8:30 a.m.
TELEPHONE CALL

From Clara Wicks, RN, at Wilcox Nursing Home. Patient complained of difficulty hearing. Nurse Wicks checked his ears and found them to be plugged with wax. Called for directions. I told the nurse to irrigate the patient's ears. If the patient is not better in a day, an appointment should be made.

Karen Larsen

K. Larsen, MD/tjo

Figure 3.16

Telephone Message Notation Made on a Patient's Chart

Using Electronic Mail (E-mail). Messages and files can be transmitted in digital form from computer to computer through an electronic mail system, commonly known as e-mail. E-mail saves time, conveys messages rapidly, and promotes flexibility. Users may access the system outside the office to send or receive messages and files from home or other locations. Electronic voice mail operates in the same manner, storing voice messages. It is critical to note that e-mail must be subject to the same strict privacy rules as other forms of communication. The medical office adopts guidelines to protect the confidentiality of patients' electronically transmitted medical data. Currently, e-mail is not the preferred method of communicating medical information. The potential for unintentional disclosure of PHI is high. Current government initiatives are supporting the implementation of electronic health records, which will be discussed in a later chapter, and the transmission of electronic medical data. A much higher level of electronic security will need to be developed before e-mailing of medical information is considered secure.

3.5 SCHEDULING

Scheduling appointments is one of the principal duties of the administrative medical assistant. To be able to do so efficiently and intelligently is an important skill. Appointments must be entered into an appointment book or computer scheduling software. The assistant is responsible for collecting the necessary data for an appointment, such as the patient's name, phone number, and reason for making the appointment.

To help in juggling patients' appointment preferences with the policies of the physician and the availability of office personnel and equipment, a number of scheduling methods are used. Changes in scheduled appointments, such as cancellations, must be indicated and the time slot used for another patient whenever possible. The physician's outside appointments should be listed and, if necessary, the physician reminded of them in advance. Clear and accurate communication between the administrative medical assistant and the physician yields beneficial results for both the practice and the patients.

Following the Physician's Policy

The physician's policy for seeing and treating patients is the initial guideline in scheduling. Policy may be affected by the physician's office hours, the physician's specialty, how quickly the physician works, the treatment or procedure to be performed, the available office personnel and equipment, and the type of facility.

Office Hours. Before appointments can be made, the administrative medical assistant must know the basic schedule of the physician's office. The physician probably will have to make rounds of patients at one or more hospitals on certain days and at certain hours. Office hours, therefore, may vary on different days. Some physicians have office hours in the evenings and on weekends. If there are several physicians in the practice, the hours of each physician may be different. The administrative medical assistant should be aware of each physician's hours as well as how and where each physician can be reached at other times. While office hours may differ depending on the requirements of the practice, a thorough understanding of specific policies within a practice contributes to greater efficiency.

Length of Time Required for Appointments. The length of time required for different types of appointments is based on the procedure, the equipment used, and the amount of time usually spent with a patient. The assistant must be aware of the range of possibilities. A complete physical examination takes longer than a routine blood pressure checkup, for example. The physician may also specify to the assistant when certain types of procedures are best scheduled. For example, the physician may ask the assistant to schedule lengthy appointments, such as complete physicals, as the first appointment

COMPLIANCE TIP

In most practices, changes that patients make to scheduled appointments, such as cancellations, are documented in the patient's medical record.

available in the morning or afternoon, or not to schedule them on certain days or at certain times of the day.

Other Policies, Preferences, and Obligations of the Physician. Most physicians treat patients only in their immediate field of practice. The assistant must be familiar with the types of patients the physician sees. For example, the physician might not see patients under age 16. Other preferences the physician has that affect the daily schedule may include a preferred lunch time, as well as times for meetings or appointments attended on a regular basis. A primary consideration in scheduling is allotting time for the physician's hospital rounds. Hospital visits at set hours should be noted.

Once the basic schedule of the office is set, specific guidelines are used to schedule appointments for patients.

Types of Scheduling

An efficient scheduling system reduces the waiting period for patients, makes the best use of the physician's time, and takes advantage of available personnel and facilities. Many providers have added evenings and weekend appointment times to their schedules in order to accommodate the changing work needs of their patient population. Scheduling methods must also provide flexibility during high-patient season, such as seasonal allergy periods and the beginning of school. A number of scheduling systems are commonly used.

Scheduled Appointments. Many physicians' offices and clinics use a scheduling system in which each patient is given a set appointment time—that is, an approximate time the patient will be seen by the physician. This system decreases the waiting time for the patient and gives the office staff more control over the flow of patients in the office. Also, because the reason for each patient's visit is known in advance, the staff can make the best use of office facilities, equipment, and medical staff time. Abbreviations for the **chief complaint (CC)**, the reason for the visit, are used when making appointments. Equipment, time, and other resources necessary to provide medical care can be prepared when the CC is known prior to the patient's arrival.

Open/Fixed Office Hours. Many clinics have **open/fixed office hours** during which the physician is in the office and available to see patients—from 10 A.M. to noon, for example. Patients sign in with the receptionist and are seen in the order in which they arrive. Other patients are scheduled at specific/fixed appointment times. This system allows patients the freedom to come to the clinic when they wish, but it also has several drawbacks:

- The reason for the patient's visit is not known until the patient arrives at the office.
- It is difficult to control the flow of patients. Thus, many patients may arrive at the same time, causing crowding and long waits. Patients who arrived at the same time and have a longer waiting period may become irritated. At other times, there may be no patients, causing the physician's and staff's time to be used inefficiently.
- Equipment and office facilities may be used inefficiently.

Wave Scheduling. One way to avoid these problems is to combine open/fixed office hours with scheduled appointments. This system is called **wave scheduling** (also known as **cluster scheduling**). In an office using wave scheduling, the administrative medical assistant arranges for a certain number of patients (such as six) to come between 9 A.M. and 10 A.M., then arranges for the next six patients who call to arrive between 10 A.M. and 11 A.M., and so on throughout the day. Wave scheduling gives patients the flexibility of open office hours while allowing the assistant more control over the flow of patients. This method works well in practices such as dermatology and endocrinology, in which the physician often does not need laboratory and x-ray results in order to diagnose and treat the patient.

Another version of wave scheduling is to schedule a patient with a complex problem on the hour (for example, 10:00 A.M.) and to schedule short routine exams for the remainder of the hour.

Double-Booking. When the schedule is full and there are more patients who need to be seen, some offices use the method of **double-booking appointments**. The extra appointments are entered in a second column beside the regularly scheduled appointments. In some cases, triple columns are used for triple-booking of appointments. Double-booking can be done efficiently; however, most double-bookings occur simply because too many patients were scheduled in a given time frame, which is the result of an inefficient scheduling method. Knowing the chief complaint of the patient and the resources, including room, equipment, and personnel to provide for the encounter, will help the assistant know when and how many patients to schedule in a given time. Following is an example of efficient double-booking. An allergist sees both new and established patients in his practice. Eight rooms and two nurses are available. Each new patient takes approximately 2 hours to assess, and a follow-up visit takes 15 minutes. New patients are scheduled as the first appointment and every half hour beginning at 9 A.M. Follow-up visits are also scheduled during the same time frame. After the 9 A.M. new patient is taken to the exam room and accessed, the first follow-up appointment arrives at the scheduled 9:15 A.M. appointment. By this time, the nurse has finished taking the new patient's history and is now available to prepare the follow-up patient. Only four new patients are scheduled in the morning and four in the afternoon. Follow-up patients are scheduled each 15 minutes during the same time frame.

See Figure 3.17 for examples of appointment books using these various scheduling methods.

Computer Scheduling. A variety of computer scheduling software programs are used in medical offices. Most scheduling software allows the user to search for the next available slot for the amount of time needed and other resources such as a specific room and/or equipment, desired location (such as an outreach clinic), or requested physician. For example, if the assistant must schedule a complete physical, the computer searches for the next available one-hour appointment. After this slot has been located, the assistant can confirm that the date and time are acceptable to the patient and then enter the appropriate information to fill the slot.

In addition to a printout of the daily schedule, most scheduling software can generate reports of cancellations and no shows. A **no show** is a patient who, without notifying the physician's office, fails to show up for an appointment. Figure 3.18 shows a screen from the scheduling program Office Hours from NDCmedisoft™ (the patient billing program used as an example in this text). Most scheduling programs can also be used to generate patient registration information, as well as chart labels for patients' records.

Screening Patients' Illnesses

When scheduling an appointment, the administrative medical assistant must use good judgment to determine how soon a patient needs to be seen. This process is called screening, or **triage** (tree-áhj). Some patients must come to the office *stat* (the term used in healthcare to mean "immediately"), some may be scheduled for later the same day or the following day, and others may be scheduled at a later time that is convenient for both the physician and the patient.

Figure 3.19 lists the appointment scheduling guidelines that are to be used throughout this text. Many offices have their own protocol for scheduling; thus, an administrative medical assistant on the job must adapt to that office's scheduling guidelines.

The difference between stat and today appointments depends on the severity of the condition, which is determined by questions and the answers received when triaging the caller.

Monday, September 29

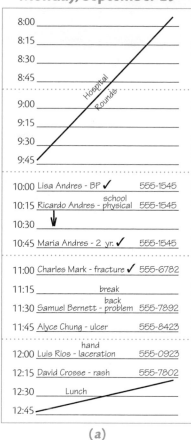

Time		
8:00		
8:15		
8:30		
8:45		
9:00	*Hospital Rounds*	
9:15		
9:30		
9:45		
10:00	Lisa Andres - BP ✓	555-1545
10:15	Ricardo Andres - physical (school)	555-1545
10:30	↓	
10:45	Maria Andres - 2 yr. ✓	555-1545
11:00	Charles Mark - fracture ✓	555-6782
11:15	break	
11:30	Samuel Bernett - problem (back)	555-7892
11:45	Alyce Chung - ulcer	555-8423
12:00	Luis Rios - laceration (hand)	555-0923
12:15	David Crosse - rash	555-7802
12:30	Lunch	
12:45		

(a)

Monday, September 29

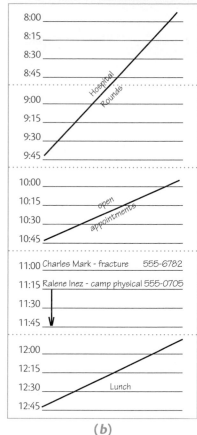

Time		
8:00		
8:15		
8:30		
8:45		
9:00	*Hospital Rounds*	
9:15		
9:30		
9:45		
10:00		
10:15	*open appointments*	
10:30		
10:45		
11:00	Charles Mark - fracture	555-6782
11:15	Ralene Inez - camp physical	555-0705
11:30	↓	
11:45		
12:00		
12:15		
12:30	Lunch	
12:45		

(b)

Monday, September 29

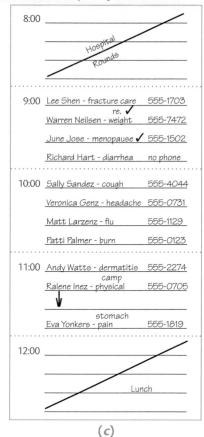

Time		
8:00		
8:15	*Hospital Rounds*	
8:30		
8:45		
9:00	Lee Shen - fracture care	555-1703
	Warren Neilsen - weight re. ✓	555-7472
	June Jose - menopause ✓	555-1502
	Richard Hart - diarrhea	no phone
10:00	Sally Sandez - cough	555-4044
	Veronica Genz - headache	555-0731
	Matt Larzenz - flu	555-1129
	Patti Palmer - burn	555-0123
11:00	Andy Watts - dermatitis	555-2274
	Ralene Inez - physical (camp)	555-0705
	↓	
	Eva Yonkers - stomach pain	555-1819
12:00		
	Lunch	

(c)

Monday, September 29

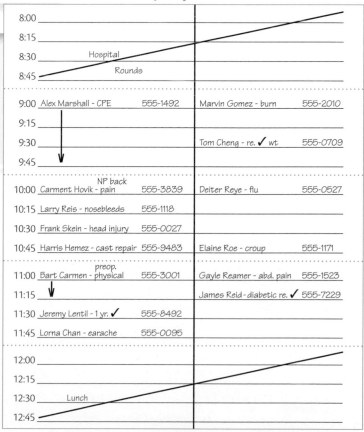

Figure 3.17

Appointment Books Showing *(a)* Scheduled Appointments, *(b)* Open/Fixed Appointment Hours, *(c)* Wave Schedule, and *(d)* Double-Column Schedule

8:00				
8:15				
8:30	Hospital			
8:45	Rounds			
9:00	Alex Marshall - CPE	555-1492	Marvin Gomez - burn	555-2010
9:15	↓			
9:30			Tom Cheng - re. ✓ wt	555-0709
9:45				
10:00	Carment Hovik - pain (NP back)	555-3839	Deiter Reye - flu	555-0527
10:15	Larry Reis - nosebleeds	555-1118		
10:30	Frank Skein - head injury	555-0027		
10:45	Harris Hemez - cast repair	555-9483	Elaine Roe - croup	555-1171
11:00	Bart Carmen - physical (preop.)	555-3001	Gayle Reamer - abd. pain	555-1523
11:15	↓		James Reid - diabetic re. ✓	555-7229
11:30	Jeremy Lentil - 1 yr. ✓	555-8492		
11:45	Lorna Chan - earache	555-0095		
12:00				
12:15				
12:30	Lunch			
12:45				

(d)

Figure 3.18

medisoft® Office Hours
Appointment Scheduler

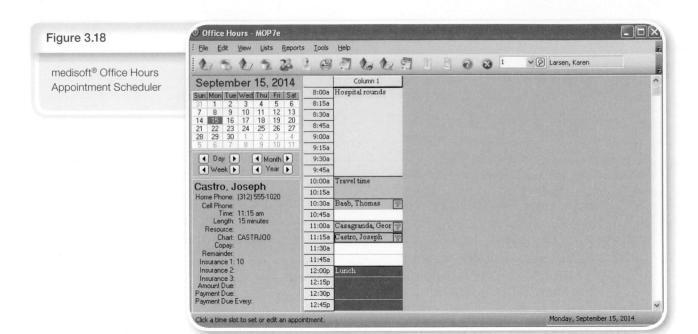

Figure 3.18

medisoft® Office Hours
Appointment Scheduler

Figure 3.19

Guidelines for Scheduling

The following guidelines for scheduling appointments are to be used throughout this text. Note that, to offer more convenient appointments to patients, many facilities have adopted same-day appointments (SDA); therefore, the following breakdown is just a general guideline.

The difference between stat and today appointments is the severity of the condition, which is known from the questions and answers received when talking with the caller. For example, a nosebleed that is bleeding profusely would be seen sooner than an occasional nosebleed. It is also always better to make an appointment sooner than to leave a critical condition until later.

STAT and/or TODAY	TOMORROW	LATER
abdominal pain	blood in stools	elective procedures
blurry vision	cast repair	follow-ups
breathing difficulty	dermatitis symptoms	physicals
burn	flu, unless severe or in	rechecks
chest pain	a child	well checks
croup	hemorrhoids	
foreign bodies	hernia	
head injury	rash unless other symptoms	
laceration	vaginal discharge	
migraine/severe headache	vague complaints	
nausea and vomiting		
nosebleed		
pain when urinating		
possible fractures		
pregnancy with		
cramps/bleeding		

It is imperative to understand that a tomorrow appointment can change to an emergency situation with the addition of another symptom; for example, cast repair would become a today appointment if the patient stated that there was swelling around the cast, change in the color of skin, and/or moisture drainage.

Many offices use a flowchart method of triage, similar to the method used by 911 dispatchers. When a patient calls the office, the assistant will begin with a low-complexity medical question, such as "How high is your fever?" or "Are you having difficulty breathing?" Based on the patient's answer to each question, the assistant will progress to the next question or appropriate response. At all times, the assistant must remember that he or she is administrative, not clinical, personnel and cannot practice medicine by giving medical instructions. If, after triage, the situation is considered an emergency, the patient should be immediately brought to the office, instructed to call 911, or sent directly to the emergency department.

Considering Patients' Preferences

The trend is to offer more convenient appointments to patients. As a result, many facilities have adopted same-day appointments (SDA). Figure 3.19 provides a general guideline. Be aware that an appointment for tomorrow can change into an emergency situation with the addition of another symptom. For example, skin rash would become a today appointment if the patient stated that there was a sudden temperature spike and onset of vomiting.

Some patients prefer to be seen at a certain time or on a certain day of the week. Work schedules vary from the traditional "9 to 5" schedule. Physicians must consider the demographics of their patients and service area. In a community with a high factory-employee population, the practice may offer more evening hours. In a "college town," Saturday and Sunday hours may be more popular than morning hours. Try to schedule appointments according to patients' preferences if the schedule allows, taking into consideration the urgency of the appointment situation. Some physicians have office hours on certain evenings, such as every other Thursday evening, to better accommodate their patients' work schedules.

Necessary Data

When patients' appointments are scheduled, all necessary data should be collected and recorded. In general, this includes some or all of the following information:

- Patient's first and last names
- Telephone number
- Address
- Date of birth (DOB)
- Reason for the appointment
- Patient status: **new patient**, or **NP** (a patient who has not seen the physician or a physician of the same specialty in the same practice in the last three years), **established patient**, or **EP** (a patient who has seen the physician or a physician of the same specialty in the same practice in the last three years), or referred by another physician
- Referring physician
- Insurance provider
- Notations regarding any laboratory tests or x-rays required before the examination

Always verify the patient's name and its spelling and repeat telephone numbers. A practice may have patients with duplicate names. Careful attention must be used to be sure the correct patient is scheduled. In cases such as twins, the patient should be asked for an individually identifiable piece of information, such as the last four digits of a Social Security number. Confirm the appointment time by repeating it to the patient—for example, "Sara, your appointment with Dr. Larsen is for Wednesday, July 16, at 2:15." When the patient arrives in the office, the information taken when the appointment was scheduled should be verified. New patients are asked to arrive at least 15 to 30 minutes early to complete the registration process. To save time, the forms may be mailed or e-mailed to the patient prior to the appointment. The patient should bring the completed form(s) with him or her. Established patients are asked at least once a year whether any information previously given

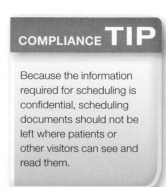

COMPLIANCE TIP

Because the information required for scheduling is confidential, scheduling documents should not be left where patients or other visitors can see and read them.

has changed. If the information has changed, the patient should be asked to fill out updated registration forms. If the information is the same, the patient should be asked to sign and date a verification, stating that the information has not changed.

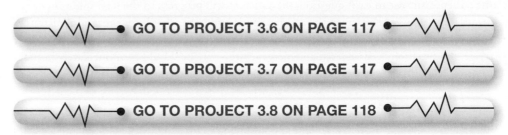

GO TO PROJECT 3.6 ON PAGE 117

GO TO PROJECT 3.7 ON PAGE 117

GO TO PROJECT 3.8 ON PAGE 118

Keeping to the Schedule

Any number of situations arise in the course of a day that require the administrative medical assistant to cancel and reschedule appointments or to work an appointment into the existing schedule. In addition, the assistant must adjust the schedule for any emergencies that arise, as well as set up next appointments for patients currently in the office who need a follow-up encounter with the physician.

Irregular Appointments. Occasionally, a patient walks in without an appointment. If the physician is busy and it is judged that the walk-in patient should be seen at that time, you may explain that the physician will see the patient for a few minutes when the patient can be worked into the schedule.

A patient with a true **emergency** (if medical care is delayed for a serious injury or illness, the patient's life or body part may be threatened) should be seen on arrival. The administrative medical assistant should notify the nurse or physician of the emergency and escort the patient to an available examination room. The assistant must tactfully explain the presence of walk-in and emergency patients to other waiting patients who have made appointments that will now be delayed. If a physician outside the office calls to request that a patient be seen that day by one of the physicians in your office, that patient must also be worked into the day's schedule.

On days when the schedule is full, and after the assistant has completed triage, the office nurse may help determine whether a patient is truly an emergency case and will ask the physician for further instructions or whether the case is **urgent** (a nonlife-threatening medical injury or illness, needing prompt medical attention with 24 hours to prevent serious decline of the patient's condition) and the patient may wait to see the physician. In some cases, the physician may request that emergency patients who telephone be referred to the emergency room. Do not refer the patient to another physician or clinic unless you are directed to do so by your physician or employer.

In addition to appointments for patients, physicians have hospital commitments, seminars, lectures, meetings, and personal appointments that may change at the last minute. All these changes must be logged into the appointment calendar to avoid schedule conflicts later on.

Late Patients

The entire schedule may be thrown out of balance because a patient is late. Patients who are late for appointments may have to be asked to wait until the physician has seen the next patient or until a treatment room is available. It is not the administrative medical assistant's place to criticize a patient for tardiness, but most physicians wish to be notified of a patient who is habitually late because it is an inconvenience to other patients. Sometimes the patient who is late must be asked to reschedule.

For patients who are habitually late, a notation should be entered in the patient's record. Such patients should be scheduled either in the last appointment slot for the morning or during the last appointment slot of the day. It is also a good practice to give habitually late patients an appointment time 15 to 20 minutes prior to their scheduled appointment.

Extended Appointments

Schedules also fall behind when either the physician or the patient loses track of the time during an examination, causing the appointment to go past the allotted period. The physician may have to be reminded if the visit runs over the scheduled time. The administrative medical assistant can use the intercom or knock on the examination room door and hand the physician a written reminder when the physician comes to the door. For physicians who use electronic methods for recording patient data, an electronic message may be sent, reminding the physician that the next patient is ready. The physician can then decide whether or not to conclude the visit with the patient.

Out-of-Office Emergencies

The schedule may also be disrupted when the physician is called out of the office for an emergency. Certain specialties, such as an OB/GYN, tend to have more out-of-office situations than other specialties. The administrative medical assistant should explain the situation to waiting patients and ask patients whether they wish to wait for the physician or reschedule their appointments.

> **EXAMPLE**
>
> **Assistant:** Dr. Larsen has been called out on an emergency. She is not likely to be back for at least an hour. Would you like to wait for her to return, or shall I reschedule your appointment?

As a courtesy, patients should also be informed if the physician is running late as a result of unforeseen interruptions. The administrative medical assistant might explain as follows: "Dr. Larsen is running behind schedule by about 30 minutes. Would you like to wait, or shall I reschedule your appointment?" Do not offer to reschedule if the schedule is behind by only a few minutes.

Registering Arrivals. Registering new patients (asking them to sign in) on arrival at a physician's office or clinic is the duty of the administrative medical assistant. The assistant should then verify the patient's name, address, and other information with the patient's record. If a computerized scheduling program is being used, it is all the more important to verify the spelling of each patient's name, since an exact spelling will help locate the patient's appointment time and information quickly.

When an appointment is made for a new patient, many offices ask the patient to arrive a few minutes early to complete information forms. At this time, the practice's payment policy is explained to the patient. Preparing new patient packets with information about the practice, insurance coverage accepted, payment policy, privacy practices, and similar items will save time in the schedule.

Patients' identities, which are part of their PHI, must be protected. This includes the sign-in methods used for registering patients' arrivals. A simple way to protect PHI is by using a dark, broad-tipped marker to strike out the patients' names. Another method is to use peel-off labels. The goal is to protect the name (PHI) of the patients.

When the patient has signed in, the administrative medical assistant leaves the medical file for the nurse or physician's assistant, indicating that the patient is ready to be seen. If an appointment book is used, a check mark is entered to show that the patient has arrived. It is the assistant's responsibility to see that the patient's chart is in order and that all forms are completed before the physician sees the patient.

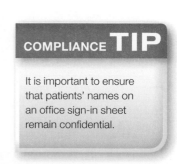

COMPLIANCE TIP

It is important to ensure that patients' names on an office sign-in sheet remain confidential.

The registration record can be checked periodically against the appointment schedule to make sure that a patient who has arrived has not forgotten to sign in. Many offices post a sign, asking that patients notify the front desk if they are still waiting 20 minutes past their appointment.

Canceling and Rescheduling Appointments. Almost every patient will cancel an appointment at one time or another; some patients make a habit of doing so. When a patient calls to cancel an appointment, a new appointment time should be suggested. A notation regarding the cancellation is also entered into the patient's medical record (especially if the cancellation is made on the same day as, or the day before, the scheduled appointment).

If a manual schedule is kept, cancellations are noted by drawing a line through the appointment and entering a new one. In computer scheduling systems, the medical assistant must perform a number of steps to locate the appointment and reschedule it. The appropriate cancellation code should be used to show the reason for the cancellation and whether it was rescheduled. As changes in the appointment book are made throughout the day, the assistant must remember also to make the changes on the workstation schedule used by the physician and nurse.

The office policy for cancellations and rescheduled appointments should be posted in areas accessible to patients, such as the waiting area or examination room. Registration packets for new patients should also contain the written policy. If a patient habitually cancels appointments (e.g., three sequential appointments), the physician may dismiss the patient from his or her care. A certified letter should be sent, informing the patient of the dismissal.

No Shows. The administrative medical assistant should also make a notation in a patient's medical record if the patient fails to keep an appointment and does not call to cancel. Since medical records are legal documents, all notations of no-show appointments should be entered into the record, signed, and dated. Figure 3.20 shows an example of a chart note recording a no-show appointment.

The physician will decide what action to take if a patient repeatedly makes appointments but does not keep them. Specialty practices sometimes charge patients for no-show appointments or canceled appointments when notification is not made 24 hours in advance. Collection of no-show charges is difficult and typically causes bad public relations. However, it is the physician's decision to pursue the collection of no-show fees.

Next Appointment. Before a patient leaves the examination room, the physician will tell the patient when to return. When the patient stops at the checkout area, the administrative medical assistant should inquire whether another appointment is needed. In many offices, the need for another appointment—often referred to as a "recall"—is noted on the encounter form or in the patient's medical record, which the patient gives the assistant after the appointment.

In most cases, the physician will give the patient instructions such as "Return in 10 days" or "Return in 3 weeks." The assistant should schedule the patient's next appointment for a convenient time as close as possible to the suggested return date.

Figure 3.20

Chart Notation for a No-Show Appointment

```
August 14, 20——
Patient failed to show for appointment. Called the nurs-
ing home and left a message for the head nurse to call
our office.
```

Figure 3.21

_____ Bill Fleming _____

YOUR APPOINTMENT IS:

_July 1_____ AT _10:30_____

SPECIAL INSTRUCTIONS:

_____

_____

KAREN LARSEN, MD
2235 South Ridgeway Avenue
Chicago, IL 60623-2240
312-555-6022

PLEASE CALL IF YOU CANNOT KEEP THIS APPOINTMENT.

Never trust an appointment time to memory with the intention of entering it later, no matter how hectic the office is. Make it a habit to enter the information into the appointment book or computer immediately, and then write an appointment card, which will serve as a reminder for the patient. See Figure 3.21 for an example of an appointment card.

Many offices use a system of follow-up telephone calls to remind a patient of an appointment for the next day. If the follow-up appointment is several months in the future, the patient may be asked to complete a postcard with the patient's address before leaving the office, so that the card can be sent as a reminder to the patient. If the office uses a computerized scheduling system, the computer can print reminders to be sent to patients scheduled for follow-up visits.

As electronic medical records begin to increase in use, the ability to contact patients electronically will become the norm. Currently, variations of the electronic format for patient communications are being used. Web-based, automated, practice-initiated message delivery systems, such as MedFusion, are being used to notify patients of appointments. Other forms of secure messages include health maintenance information, lab results, and financial information, such as past due notices. Nonsecure information, such as flu shot notices, may also be accessed by the patient.

Open Slots for Catching Up. No matter how carefully appointments are scheduled, crowding is sometimes unavoidable and appointments fall behind schedule. Leaving a 15- or 20-minute interval free in the late morning and again at the end of each day will help you straighten out a delayed schedule. If no delays occur, these open slots can be used to catch up with other work. Open slots also allow time for emergency patients and unscheduled patients.

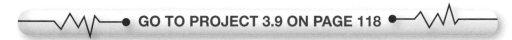

GO TO PROJECT 3.9 ON PAGE 118

Out-of-Office Appointments

Appointments that may be scheduled outside the office include hospital admissions, surgery, and diagnostic or other special procedures. Follow basic scheduling procedures for such appointments, obtaining the necessary patient data required for each type of appointment.

Hospital Admissions. The following information is needed for hospital admissions:

- Complete name of patient
- Patient's information: age, DOB, address, and telephone number
- Diagnosis or problem
- Preferred date of admission

- Preferred accommodations
- Previous admissions
- Insurance coverage information

Surgical and Diagnostic Procedures. The following information is needed for surgery or for diagnostic or other procedures:

- Surgery or other procedure to be performed
- Length of time needed for surgery (if known)
- Approximate date and time desired
- Specific surgical assistants required
- Type of anesthesia to be used and person administering it
- Special requirements, such as diagnostic testing required before the patient undergoes the procedure

Other considerations for scheduling are:

- Scheduling the appropriate time required by the physician in each situation.
- Giving patients clear and simple instructions for hospital admission.
- Scheduling fasting tests in the morning so the patient does not need to go without eating longer than necessary. Inform patients about any preparations that are required before undergoing a surgical or diagnostic procedure (for example, informing them that they are to have nothing to eat or drink after midnight of the night prior to the procedure and/or how and when to complete pre-testing, such as x-rays).
- Confirming that any requested assistants and/or anesthesiologists are available.

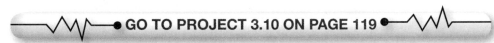

GO TO PROJECT 3.10 ON PAGE 119

 ## PROCESSING INCOMING MAIL AND PREPARING OUTGOING MAIL

Every physician receives an enormous amount of mail every day, so the efficient handling of correspondence is vital. As an assistant, you must learn to distinguish quickly between the types of mail most often received. You must use sound judgment to sort mail according to its importance. The mail generally falls into these categories:

- Important items, such as those sent by Express or Priority Mail, or mail that is registered or certified (or sent via overnight services, such as Federal Express)
- Regular first-class mail
- The physician's personal mail
- Periodicals and newspapers
- Advertising materials
- Samples

Processing Guidelines for Incoming Mail

Use the following guidelines to process incoming mail. Sort the items by category, depending on their importance.

1. Open all letters except those marked "Personal" or "Confidential," unless you are authorized to open all mail. If a mailing marked "Personal" or "Confidential" is opened accidentally, the assistant should reseal the correspondence with clear tape, note "Opened by Mistake" on the envelope, and place his or her initials by the notation.
2. Check the contents of each envelope carefully.

3. Stamp the date on each item to show when it was received.
4. Attach enclosures to each item.
5. Carefully put aside checks from patients to be recorded and deposited later.
6. Check to be sure the envelope is empty and is not needed before discarding it. If evidence of a postmark is needed, retain the envelope.
7. Write a reminder on the calendar or in the follow-up (tickler) file about material that is being sent separately.
8. Attach the patient's chart to correspondence regarding the patient. Place such correspondence in a high-priority area on the physician's desk.
9. If a business letter responds to a request, pull the relevant file and attach the letter to it.
10. Set aside correspondence that can be answered without the physician's seeing it, such as payments needing receipts, insurance forms or questions, bills, and other routine business matters.

In some offices, the assistant is required to **annotate** communications. That is, the assistant skims an item and writes necessary or helpful notes in the margin or on an attached self-stick note.

It may save time if the items that require the physician's attention are placed on the desk in the order of importance. Medical journals are placed on the physician's desk with other mail. Medical samples should be unpacked and placed in the physician's supply cabinet if they can be used. If they cannot be used, follow the office policy, which may include saving them for a charity. Samples should not be thrown in the trash.

Best Practices for Safe Mail Handling

Since the anthrax mailings in 2001 and subsequent suspicious mailings since then, businesses have realized they may be at risk for mail threats and have implemented steps to protect the mail handlers and the business. The U.S. Department of Homeland Security has issued *Best Practices for Safe Mail Handling*, which sets in place best practice procedures for federal agencies. The following are some of the standards issued by Homeland Security. The complete document can be found at *www.oca.gsa.gov*.

- *Centralize mail handling.* Centralizing mail handling and processing operations contains the risk to the business or provider.
- *Wear personal protective equipment.* Gloves should be worn when sorting mail. Surgical gloves are readily available in the provider's office and should be used. Other protective equipment includes masks, protective/safety glasses, and smocks. It is during the initial contact with incoming mail that suspicious items can be identified.
- *Maintain a list of suspicious indicators for handlers.* Establish and use a listing of suspicious package indicators, such as a "grainy" feel to the contents of the envelope. Personnel should receive initial and ongoing training to help them identify suspicious mailings.
- *Develop isolation/emergency procedures.* Policies and procedures regarding the steps to isolate a suspicious mailing should be posted in the centralized incoming mail area, so that they can be read easily and quickly. Emergency procedures should also be posted. Included in the emergency procedures should be emergency phone numbers, including the phone number and/or contact number for the local hazardous materials (HAZMAT) team.

As with most situations, it is better to be prepared and proactive than to be unprepared and reactive.

Preparation of Outgoing Mail

Outgoing mail consists of professional, business, and personal correspondence. Professional correspondence concerns patients, clinical matters, and research. Business correspondence relates to the management of the office and may concern insurance companies, lawyers, supply houses, and bills to patients. Personal correspondence pertains to the physician's personal rather than professional life, such as notes to friends or letters about the physician's personal business interests.

Mail Classifications. For mail to be handled in the most efficient and cost-effective way, the assistant must know the various classifications of mail and services offered. The United States Postal Service (USPS) provides excellent information in easy-to-use formats.

The USPS Web site (www.usps.com) has a complete listing and description of services and rates. The site is an easy reference for ZIP codes and correct state abbreviations, as well as for all domestic rates and fees; it has postal rate calculators and information on new rates and mailing rules. The local post office can also supply leaflets describing USPS services. The assistant must always be aware of current postal rates, requirements, and services.

The following are mail classifications specified by the USPS:

- *First-class Mail*: **First-class mail** includes all correspondence, whether handwritten or typewritten; all bills and statements of accounts; and all materials sealed against postal inspection and weighing 13 ounces or less.
- *Priority Mail*: **Priority Mail** offers two- to three-day service to most domestic destinations. Items must weigh less than 70 pounds. This is the fastest way to send heavier items. Rates depend on the weight when the charge is calculated by postal zone. Another option is to use the one low charge to send any item or items that fit into the priority shipping container and pay one low fee.
- *Express Mail*. The fastest service, **Express Mail**, offers overnight delivery to most destinations. Express Mail deliveries are made 365 days a year, including Saturdays, Sundays, and holidays. All items must weigh less than 70 pounds and be less than 108 inches in combined length and girth. Up to $100 in insurance is included with Express Mail. If a signature verifying receipt is needed, a return receipt service can be added. The charge depends on weight. There is pickup service. For all materials that can be sent in a flat-rate envelope (provided by the USPS), there is one low charge.
- *Parcel Post*: **Parcel Post** is used for mailing certain items—books, catalogs, other printed matter, or merchandise—not weighing more than 70 pounds and no more than 130 inches in length and girth. The charge depends on weight, distance, and shape of the container. Many extra services, such as a **Certificate of Mailing** and a **Signature Confirmation of Delivery**, can be added to Parcel Post.
- *Media Mail*: **Media Mail** is used for mailing items such as books, catalogs, sound recordings, video recordings (e.g., a video tape), and media that can be read by a computer, including DVDs. This classification may not be used for advertising. Items must be 70 pounds or less and the cost is based on weight and size.
- *Bound Printed Matter*: **Bound Printed Matter** classification of mail is used for any material permanently bound by materials such as glue, staples, or spiral binding. At least 90 percent of the mailed materials must be imprinted materials generated by a means other than handwriting or typewriting. Items may weigh up to 15 pounds and the cost is determined by weight, distance, and shape.

Mail Services. The following services are available through the USPS:

- *Certified mail*: **Certified Mail** provides the sender with a mailing receipt. The USPS keeps a record of delivery. This service is available with First-class or Priority Mail. The USPS issues unique article numbers, which allow senders to track online the delivery status of the mailing. The recipient's signature is required upon delivery and is maintained by the USPS. When it is important to verify the mailing of materials, such as a patient termination letter, Certified Mail may be used to maintain evidence that the correspondence was mailed.

- **Insured Mail** is used to cover mailings for loss or damages. Coverage is available for up to $5,000. First-class mail, Parcel Post, and Media Mail may all be insured for rates determined by the amount of coverage desired.
- **Registered Mail** provides the greatest security for valuables. The sender gets a receipt at the time of mailing, and a delivery record is kept by the USPS. The mailing post office also maintains a record of mailing. Only first-class and Priority Mail may be registered. Postal insurance is provided for articles with a declared value of $25,000. The charge is determined according to the declared value of the item(s).
- **Collect on Delivery** allows the sender to have the USPC collect the recipient's payments and, if necessary, postage. Currently, the USPC will accept payment either by personal check or cash. Items are insured up to $1000. COD may be used on domestic deliveries; however, it may not be used on mailings sent to military post office addresses (APO/FPO).
- **Delivery Confirmation** provides proof by the date, ZIP code, and time of delivery. If the delivery was not successful, the date and time of the attempt are recorded. This service can be purchased both in the traditional, hardcopy detail format or through the electronic tracking system.
- **Special Handling** should be used when mailing are unusual or requires extra care such as live poultry. Items which are breakable normally do not require special handling. Adequate packing should be used and "FRAGILE" should be marked on the package. There are special services that may also be of use.
- **Return Receipt** provides the sender with evidence of delivery. It is available for most kinds of mail classifications when mail is insured for $50 or more.
- **Certificate of Mailing** is a certificate which provides only proof of an item's having been mailed. It does not provide proof of delivery. It must be purchased at the time of mailing and is kept by the sender.
- **Signature of Confirmation** is used to provide proof (confirmation) of the date and time of delivery or attempted delivery. This service may be purchased only at the time of mailing.
- **Restricted Delivery** permits a sender to authorize delivery only to the addressee or the addressee's authorized agent. The addressee must be specified in the address by name.

ZIP Codes. Before sending any outgoing mail, the ZIP Code or the ZIP+4 should be placed as the last item in the mailing address. **ZIP** (Zone Improvement Plan) is a standardized, numerical code which is assigned by the USPS and designates a special delivery area. In 1983, the USPS expanded the ZIP system to include a four-digit extension to the original ZIP code. This system is known as **ZIP+4**. The four-digit extension provides very specific details for delivery, such as a building number, floor number, office number, or other identifying unit which could be used to pinpoint more precisely the delivery destination.

Though the use of ZIP+4 is not mandatory, it provides more efficient delivery of mail by reducing the number of handlings. Fewer handlings by humans and/or machines reduce the number of inaccurate deliveries and, consequently, reduce cost. Though mail can be processed by humans, cards and other first-class mail are primarily processed by an **optical character reader (OCR)** which reads the address. **POSTNET** (a bar code consisting of a series of long and short vertical lines) is placed on the lower portion of the mailing. POSTNET is an interpretation of the ZIP code or the ZIP+4. Most word processing software packages have the ability to print the POSTNET onto the envelope.

If you do not know the ZIP or ZIP+4, visit the ZIP Locator at HYPERLINK "http://www.usps.gov"www.usps.gov.

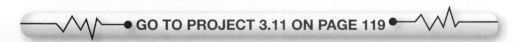
GO TO PROJECT 3.11 ON PAGE 119

Chapter Projects

Project 3.1 **Composing a Referral Letter**

WP 5 contains a list of Dr. Larsen's outside services. Keep this list in your Supplies folder to refer to when necessary. Add any new contact in the space provided.

Dr. Larsen has asked you to compose a referral letter for her signature. The purpose of the letter is to refer Florence Sherman to an ophthalmologist, Richard Diangelis, MD. Summarize the key points from the October 8 chart note, found in WP 6. This referral letter confirms a conversation between the two physicians on October 8. Date the letter you write October 13. Address an envelope. File the referral letter and Florence's chart note (WP 37) in Ms. Sherman's patient file.

Project 3.2 **Composing an Interoffice Memo**

Dr. Larsen has asked you to prepare a memo from her to be sent throughout the medical center informing the staff of the following information:

> Wanda Norberg, MD, will start working part-time in January while Dr. Larsen takes a two-month sabbatical to update the University Hospital Resident Program Guidelines (publication date is April 1). Dr. Norberg currently has an office at 2901 West Fifth Avenue, Suite 425, Chicago, Illinois 60612-9002. Her current phone number is 312-555-4525. Her hours will be 9 A.M. to 12 noon, Monday through Thursday, and Tuesday and Thursday evenings from 6 P.M. to 9 P.M. Employees are needed to work during these hours. If interested, contact Linda at extension 6022.

Date the memo October 13. Remember to add Dr. Norberg's information to the Outside Services list. File the memo in your Miscellaneous folder.

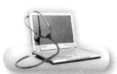

Project 3.3 **Internet Research: Journal Citations**

Using your favorite Web browser, locate the American Medical Association's Web site. Visit the *Journal of the American Medical Association (JAMA)* and research author instructions. What are some of the criteria for acceptance of manuscripts? Can manuscripts be submitted by e-mail? Be prepared to discuss your findings in class.

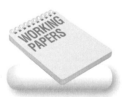

Project 3.4 **Editing and Proofreading Reports**

Dr. Larsen has asked you to edit and proofread two reports that she will use for her classroom teaching. The reports are on the CD-ROM, labeled **project6.4a** and **project6.4b**. The physician has marked the changes to be made on WP 7 and 8. The reports also contain unmarked errors. First save the reports on your own disk as Project 3.4 reports. Then edit and proofread the reports. Remember to save your work.

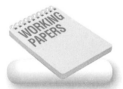

Project 3.5 **Taking Messages**

Today's date is October 13, and Dr. Larsen is not available for telephone calls. Using WP 9–16, take complete messages for the following situations:

- Andrew Kramer at 312-555-1913 calls at 9:30 A.M., stating that his eight-year-old son, Jeffrey, a patient of Dr. Larsen's, has been complaining about a sore throat and an earache for two days. They are unable to come to the office for an appointment today. Jeffrey has no fever, is on no medications, and has no allergies. Is there any over-the-counter medication they can use until they can make an appointment?

- Sara Babcock, an established patient, calls at 9:45 A.M. Her telephone number is 312-555-5441. She would like to have her Ortho Tri-cyclen® birth control medication refilled at Consumer Pharmacy (312-555-1252). It was last filled one year ago.
- At 9:50 A.M., Wanda Norberg, MD, calls to set up an appointment with Dr. Larsen. Dr. Larsen has hired Dr. Norberg to work part-time, starting in January. She can be reached after 5:30 P.M. at 312-555-1322.

Put the remaining message slips in your supplies folder.

Project 3.6   Scheduling Decision Making

Using WP 17, choose the appropriate answer for each situation. Be prepared to discuss your answers in class.

Project 3.7   Setting Up Dr. Larsen's Practice

The icon to the right precedes certain projects and simulations throughout this textbook. The icon indicates that all or part of a task can be done in Medisoft® using the Student Data File that accompanies this text and which is available at the text's Online Learning Center (OLC). Make sure to read Appendix A before you begin using Medisoft®. (Remember, not every part of every project can be done in Medisoft®. Follow the instructions below.)

Dr. Larsen's practice is already set up and stored in the Student Data File at the OLC. Appendix A provides instructions on downloading and installing the Student Data File on your computer. After the file is installed, click the Appointment Book option on the Activities menu to open Office Hours, and enter October 13, 2014, as the date. Then go to the following dates on the calendar and enter the following appointments using the Break Entry shortcut button:

- October 16, 2014, from 5 to 6 P.M., University Meeting
- October 23, 2014, from 5 to 6 P.M., Dinner Meeting
- October 28, 2014, from 7 to 8 P.M., Lecture

Enter the appropriate information in the Name and Length boxes, and click the Save button. Print Dr. Larsen's schedule for all three days (October 16, 23, and 28).

The icon to the right accompanies instructions for completing the project *without the use of Medisoft®*.

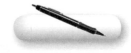

Information about Dr. Larsen's appointment schedule is found on WP 18. WPs 19–34 are Dr. Larsen's appointment calendar pages.

You will use WPs 18–34 throughout most of the course, entering, canceling, and rescheduling patients' appointments, as well as Dr. Larsen's other appointments. Remove these pages, and secure them in your appointment calendar. Place WP 18 as the first page of the binder or folder you will use for your appointment calendar.

Today's date is October 10. Check the calendar for the week of October 13, noting that Dr. Larsen is attending an all-day seminar at the university on October 13. Some appointments have been preset on your calendar.

Enter Dr. Larsen's following commitments on the appropriate pages:

- October 16, University Hospital Accreditation Meeting from 4 to 6 P.M., Whitman Hall, Rosewood Room
- October 23, 5 P.M., University Hospital Dining Room, dinner meeting with Wanda Norberg, MD
- October 28, 7 P.M., lecture on resident requirements, Dr. Margo Matthews at University Hospital, Whitman Hall, Room 203

Project 3.8 Scheduling Appointments

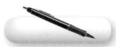

Today's date is October 10, 2014. Using Office Hours, enter the following appointments on Dr. Larsen's schedule and then print out the schedule for each day (October 14–15 and 20–22). Appointments are 15 minutes long unless otherwise noted. Complete the Chart and Length fields only. (Note: For new patients, leave the Chart field blank and fill in the Name and Phone fields. The Name field is the unlabeled field to the right of the Chart box.)

Today's date is October 10. On your appointment calendar, enter the following appointments. Dr. Larsen's policy is to enter the first and last names of the patient, the reason for the visit, and the patient's telephone number. The amount of time needed for the appointment (15 minutes, unless otherwise noted) is blocked out with arrows.

Appointments

- October 14, 10:30 A.M., David Kramer, new patient, kindergarten physical, 312-555-8153, mother Erin Mitchell
- October 14, 10:45 A.M., Erin Mitchell, new patient, backache, 312-555-8153
- October 14, 11:00 A.M., Gary Robertson, established patient, urinary problems, 312-555-9565
- October 14, 11:15 A.M., Laura Lund, established patient, cramps, 312-555-4106
- October 14, 11:45 A.M., Charles Jonathan III, established patient, knee pain, 312-555-3097
- October 15, 10:30 A.M., Ardis Matthews, established patient, nausea, 312-555-3178
- October 20, 10:30 A.M., Thomas Baab, established patient, CPE (1 hour), 312-555-3478
- October 20, 11:45 A.M., Doris Casagranda, established patient, rash, 312-555-1200
- October 21, 11:00 A.M., Sara Babcock, established patient, CPE (1 hour), 312-555-5441
- October 22, 11:15 A.M., Ana Mendez, established patient, neck pain, 312-555-3606

Project 3.9 Rescheduling Appointments

Today's date is October 13. Reschedule each of the following patients according to the instructions given below.

Using Office Hours, cancel and reschedule the following appointments. Then print out the new schedules.

Dr. Larsen's policy is to draw a single line through canceled appointments. Reschedule the following appointments:

Appointments

- Thomas Baab calls to ask if he can cancel his appointment on October 20 at 10:30 A.M. and reschedule it for this week, same time, Wednesday. You inform him that 11:00 A.M. on Wednesday, the 15th, is available. He agrees to that time. Make the appropriate changes.
- Charles Jonathan III stops in to change his October 14 appointment. You reschedule him for October 21 at 10:45 A.M. Complete an appointment card using the form on WP 35. Make the appropriate changes. Place the unused appointment cards in your Supplies folder.

Project 3.10   Out-of-Office Scheduling

Using WP 36, choose the appropriate answer for each situation. Be prepared to discuss your answers in class.

Project 3.11   Communications Terms

On WP 37, match the communications term in Column 2 with its definition in Column 1.

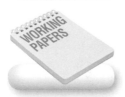

Chapter 3 Summary

3.1 List the steps of the communication cycle and give an example of a barrier to each step. Pages 72–74	• The communication cycle has five steps: — Origination of the message by the sender. In this step, the sender analyzes the receiver and formulates the message. Barriers to consider are the knowledge base of the receiver and the physical environment. — Encoding of the message by the sender. In this step, the sender attaches words and gestures to the message. A barrier to consider would be a language barrier. — Transmission of the message. The sender determines the best channel for the message and sends the message to the receiver. A barrier to consider would be noise that disrupts the channel and the message. — Receiving and decoding of the message by the receiver. In this step, the receiver interprets the message. A barrier to consider is the inactive listening by the receiver. — Checking for understanding through feedback. In the last step, the sender verifies the receiver has interpreted the message as intended using techniques such as questioning and asking the receiver to paraphrase. A barrier to this step would be a judgmental assumption by the sender.
3.2 Explain how the verbal message is affected by nonverbal communication. Pages 74–75	• Nonverbal communication has a greater impact on the receiver of a message than the verbal message. Most of our communication is through nonverbal channels. When the verbal message sends a communication but the nonverbal message, such as facial expression or body language, says something different, the nonverbal message is the one received.
3.3 Compose an effective and efficient written business communication. Pages 75–89	• Written correspondences are a reflection of the medical practice and its employees. Documents should be prepared with proper grammar and word usage, sentence structure, and format. Prior to sending out any document, it should be carefully proofread and edited using personal knowledge and electronic methods, such as spell and grammar checkers.

3.4 Explain how proper triage of patients during a phone conversation can assist the office environment. Pages 89–102	• When patients call the medical office, they must be properly assessed in order to meet their needs. By asking a predetermined sequence of questions (triage), the assistant can determine if the situation is an emergency. • By having the information available, the patient can be given proper instruction, such as "Go directly to the emergency department" or "Make an appointment in the near future." • Assessing/triaging better uses office resources by determining the time, equipment, and personnel needed to assist and properly direct the patient.
3.5 Recall and explain two types of scheduling options and provide examples of practices that would be most suited to each of the schedules. Pages 102–112	• Two methods of scheduling appointments are open/fixed and wave hours. — Open/fixed scheduling: the physician is in during fixed hours, such as noon to 2 P.M. to see patients. Patients are seen in the order they arrive. During the remaining hours, the physician sees patients by appointment. Outreach clinics are well suited for open/fixed hour scheduling. — Wave scheduling: groups of patients are asked to arrive usually on the hour. For example, 10 patients are asked to arrive at 9 A.M., and another group of 10 are asked to arrive at 11 A.M. Larger clinics with multiple physicians may use this method of scheduling.
3.6 Recall the steps for processing incoming mail and discuss related safety recommendations. Pages 112–115	• When processing incoming mail, the assistant should follow the practice's policies and procedures for handling incoming mail. Examples of the procedures are — Opening all incoming mail, except those marked "Personal" or "Confidential," and carefully removing all contents. — Date stamping each item and attaching any enclosures to the items. — Double-checking the envelope for any missed content. — Setting aside checks to be processed in a central, secure location. — Attaching the patient's chart or other office record to correspondence.

- Many best practice procedures for handling incoming mail have been implemented by Homeland Security.
  - Protective equipment, such as gloves and masks, should be worn by individuals processing incoming mail to provide for personal protection.
  - Centralizing receipt and processing of incoming mail will reduce the threat risk to the practice by localizing the possible effect.
  - Providing a list of suspicious indicators to mail handlers can reduce the possibility of a threat being carried out. This increased awareness will help them identify possible threats in the initial processing stage. As soon as a threat is suspected or confirmed, the local authorities should be notified.
  - Providing a listing of all emergency contact information and procedures will reduce the employee's response time.

Soft Skills Success

Ability to Speak

A person is only as effective as his or her communication skills. Learning how to speak effectively will increase your confidence, make you more comfortable with other people, and fine-tune your communication skills, both verbal and written. The ability to speak well often starts with a good vocabulary. Without good speaking skills, you may find yourself talking but saying virtually nothing. Speaking skills, in short, give you the ability to communicate effectively, with little or no chance for misunderstanding. This is especially important in healthcare. **Explain why the ability to speak well is so important.**

Communication

The act of communicating involves verbal, nonverbal, and paraverbal components. The verbal component refers to the content of our message, the choice and arrangement of our words. The nonverbal component refers to the message we send through body language. The paraverbal component refers to how we say what we say: the tone, pacing, and volume of our voice. Communication is one of the most important of the soft skills, and its significance is growing due to the advancement of technology. **How can nonverbal communication interfere with the patient–healthcare provider interaction?**

USING TERMINOLOGY

Match the term or phrase on the left with the correct answer on the right.

_____ 1. (LO 3.6) Certified mail

_____ 2. (LO 3.3) Block-style letter

_____ 3. (LO 3.1) Channel

_____ 4. (LO 3.1) Decoding

_____ 5. (LO 3.2) Noise

_____ 6. (LO 3.1) Encoding

_____ 7. (LO 3.4) Triage

_____ 8. (LO 3.5) Wave scheduling

_____ 9. (LO 3.5) Open/fixed hours
scheduling

_____ 10. (LO 3.1) Feedback

a. Systemically assessing a patient to determine when the patient can be scheduled

b. A method of scheduling combining scheduling appointments and fixed office hours

c. Internal and external interferences with the communication cycle

d. Chosen method of transmitting a message

e. Applying meaning to a received message

f. A method of seeing patients during a specified time without a scheduled appointment

g. Letter style in which all text is left aligned

h. Applying gestures and words to a message or an idea

i. How a recipient responds to a message

j. Provides sender with documentation of mailing materials

CHECK YOUR UNDERSTANDING

Select the most correct answer.

1. (LO 3.1) When Dr. Cary's AMA stepped toward a patient to explain the hospital preadmission procedure, the patient abruptly took a step backwards. Which of the following is the most likely reason for the patient's movement during the communication process?

   a. The AMA had bad breath.
   b. The patient's cell phone was ringing.
   c. The patient needed to sit down.
   d. The AMA had intruded into the patient's personal space.

2. (LO 3.2) Kelsey felt she was being treated rudely by the medical office receptionist. When Kelsey arrived for her appointment, the receptionist greeted Kelsey, quickly shut the glass window, and began pointing her finger toward Kelsey. The receptionist was discussing a newly discovered crack in the wall with the office manager. Kelsey felt unwelcomed because

   a. The receptionist's verbal message did not match her nonverbal message.
   b. The receptionist's verbal and nonverbal message were the same.
   c. The crack on the wall was offensive to Kelsey.
   d. The receptionist did not offer Kelsey coffee or water.

3. (LO 3.3) A copy notation in a letter is placed

   a. Immediately after the date.
   b. One enter stroke below the complimentary closing.
   c. Below the reference initials and any enclosure notation.
   d. One enter stroke below the inside address.

4. (LO 3.4) While triaging a patient over the phone, the AMA learned the patient had "a really deep cut on the inside of the upper thigh and there was blood everywhere." The patient stated he was not able to stop the bleeding. The patient should be advised to

   a. Come to the office, since the wound may become infected.
   b. Go immediately to the emergency department because he may have cut into an artery.
   c. Elevate the leg above his heart and see if the bleeding decreases.
   d. Schedule an appointment for the following morning.

5. (LO 3.5) During the monthly office meeting, the method of scheduling appointments was discussed. The patients frequently had wait times in excess of two hours and were very upset by the time the physician saw them. The practice is a large community clinic that uses wave scheduling. Which of the following scheduling methods may be a better alternative for the clinic?

   a. Scheduled appointments in the morning for call-in patients and open hours in the afternoon.
   b. Wave scheduling with double- and triple-booking of patients at the top of each hour.
   c. There is no better scheduling method.
   d. See fewer patients.

6. (LO 3.6) When processing incoming mail, the assistant should do all of the following except

   a. Date stamp the correspondence.
   b. Attach needed patient data to correspondence.
   c. Refrain from opening the physician's mail marked "Confidential."
   d. Place received checks in different locations.

7. (LO 3.6) Kendra works in an abortion clinic and has been asked to develop a proactive plan for safe mail handling. Her recommendations include receiving all mail in one location, developing a list of risk identifiers, and establishing protocol for suspicious mail. Based on *Best Practices for Safe Mail Handling*, which of the following should be added to Kendra's plan?

   a. Remove all coffee cups from the mail-receiving area.
   b. Establish a uniform time for processing mail.
   c. Open all mail, regardless of whether or not it is marked "Personal" or "Confidential."
   d. Require all mail handlers to wear protective gear, such as surgical gloves, goggles, and masks.

THINKING IT THROUGH

These questions cover the most important points in this chapter. Using your critical-thinking skills, play the role of an administrative medical assistant as you answer each question. Be prepared to present your responses in class.

1. Mrs. Jenage was seen by the physician and needs to be admitted to the hospital. She is legally deaf but does read lips. How will you communicate hospital admission instructions to Mrs. Jenage and check to be sure the instructions were received correctly?

2. In a job interview, you are asked to describe the quality of your written communication skills and state why these skills are important. How do you respond?

3. Mrs. Court, who has a history of missed appointments, has just missed her latest one. The doctor asks that you contact her about the missed appointment, to mention politely that this has happened before, and to ask her to reschedule as soon as possible. Why would you choose to write a letter rather than call the patient?

4. Prepare a draft of the body of the letter to Mrs. Court. Keep in mind the doctor's directions about the content and tone.

5. A colleague sends you this e-mail: "Please help! I need to prepare final manuscript for an article Dr. Trelando is submitting." You decide to e-mail the directions for preparing the title page and text pages for final manuscript. What does your e-mail say?

6. State four important procedures in opening and sorting the mail.

7. What steps would you take to investigate the lowest-cost shipping method for a small package that must be delivered overnight?

8. You receive a call from an assistant at Dr. Janis's office about a referral from your office. The referral is scheduled for today, but Dr. Janis cannot locate the referral letter sent by your office. How can e-mail help in this situation?

9. A patient calls at 11:15 A.M. on a Tuesday morning to say that she has slipped on the ice while going out to get her mail and may have fractured her wrist. There is a good deal of pain and swelling. Her son is available to drive her to the office. You check today's schedule and find that it is full. What is the best way to respond to the patient?

Managing Health Information

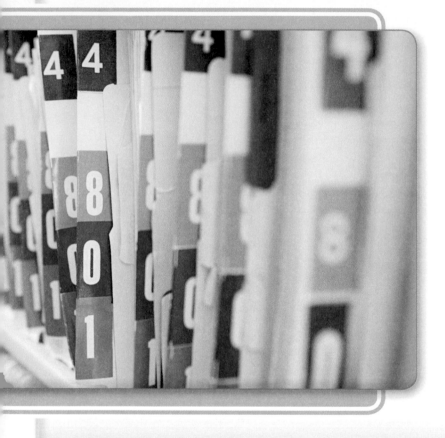

LEARNING OUTCOMES

After studying this chapter, you will be able to:

4.1 Classify various uses of computer technology.

4.2 Recall reasons for maintaining a medical chart and documents that compile the medical chart.

4.3 Identify components of a paper-based medical record and explain how the same components will be compiled in an electronic health record format.

4.4 Distinguish among active, inactive, and closed files.

4.5 Differentiate among records management systems that may be used in a medical office.

4.6 Discuss the advantages and challenges of electronic health records implementation.

4.7 List three medical abbreviations not to be used that have been targeted by JACHO.

4.8 Discuss various input technologies used to create medical documentation.

KEY TERMS

Study these important words, which are defined in this chapter, to build your professional vocabulary:

accession book

active files

AHIMA

alphabetic filing

application software

ARMA

assessment

CHEDDAR

closed files

coding

color-coding

cross-reference sheet

database

dead storage

diagnosis (Dx)

electronic health records (EHRs)

e-mail

family history (FH)

file server

folders

graphics application

guide

history of present illness (HPI)

impression

inactive files

indexing

inspecting documents

Internet

label

laptop

lateral files

mainframe

medicolegal

micrographics

minicomputer

mobile-aisle files

networking

Chapter 4

ABHES

- Adapt to change.
- Maintain confidentiality at all times.
- Project a positive attitude.
- Be cognizant of ethical boundaries.
- Evidence a responsible attitude.
- Conduct work within scope of education, training, and ability.
- Application of electronic technology.
- Apply computer concepts for office procedures.
- Be courteous and diplomatic.
- Serve as a liaison between the physicians and others.
- Receive, organize, prioritize, and transmit information expediently.
- Fundamental writing skills.
- Prepare and maintain medical records.
- File medical records.
- Use appropriate guidelines when releasing records or information.
- Monitor legislation related to current healthcare issues and practices.
- Perform medical transcription.
- Exercise efficient time management.

➡ Cognitive
➡ Psychomotor
➡ Affective

CAAHEP

➡ Recognize elements of fundamental writing skills.
➡ Discuss applications of electronic technology in effective communication.
➡ Organize technical information and summaries.
➡ Identify systems for organizing medical records.
➡ Describe various types of content maintained in a patient's medical record.
➡ Discuss pros and cons of various filing methods.
➡ Discuss the importance of routine maintenance of office equipment.
➡ Describe indexing rules.
➡ Discuss filing procedures.
➡ Identify types of records common to the healthcare setting.
➡ Report relevant information to others succinctly and accurately.
➡ Organize a patient's medical record.
➡ File medical records.
➡ Maintain organization by filing.
➡ Document accurately in the patient record.
➡ Perform routine maintenance of office equipment with documentation.
➡ Apply HIPAA rules in regard to privacy/release of information.
➡ Consider staff needs and limitations in establishment of a filing system.

numeric filing

objective

online

open-shelf files

operating system

out guide

output device

password

past medical history (PMH)

personal computer

physical exam (PE)

plan

problem-oriented medical record (POMR)

records management

releasing

retention

review of systems (ROS)

rule out (R/0)

SOAP

social history (SH)

sorting

spreadsheet programs

storing

subject filing

subjective

supercomputer

tab cuts

tabs

template

transcription

vertical files

virus

voice-recognition technology

wireless communication

word processing program

INTRODUCTION

There are three main categories of records found in medical facilities: (1) medical records of the patient's state of health, (2) correspondence pertaining to the field of healthcare, and (3) documents related to the business and financial management of the practice. Management of these records is the topic of this chapter.

4.1 COMPUTER USAGE

Today's medical environment requires a medical assistant to possess skill and knowledge of computer functions and related programs. Following are five areas where computers are commonly used in the medical office:

- Scheduling
- Creation and maintenance of patients' medical records
- Communications
- Billing, collections, claims, and financial reporting
- Clinical work

Scheduling

Many medical offices use electronic scheduling systems to set up and maintain appointments. These systems have many features that are not available with paper logbooks. For example, with an electronic scheduling system, an administrative medical assistant can print a daily list of appointments for the physician. Having such schedules available in a quick and easy-to-read format is helpful for everyone in the medical office.

Another advantage is efficient rescheduling of appointments. With a paper logbook, first the assistant locates the appointment that needs to be changed. Once the appointment is found, it has to be crossed through and a new entry made. With electronic scheduling, the assistant enters the patient's name in a search box, and the computer locates the appointment in seconds. Old appointments can be deleted with a single keystroke, and new ones keyed in within seconds. It is also easy to move an appointment to a different time, day, or month.

Another advantage of electronic scheduling is electronic searching for available time slots in a provider's schedule. For example, suppose a patient needs to schedule three 15-minute appointments during the next three weeks but is available only on Tuesday and Thursday afternoons. The assistant enters a set of criteria in the scheduler, and the computer locates the first available slots that match the criteria. This saves the assistant the trouble of leafing through several weeks of appointments in a paper log.

Electronic scheduling can also be used to keep track of providers' time away from the office, such as for medical conferences, surgical procedures performed in the hospital, and days off. Figure 4.1 shows the physician's hospital rounds and travel time noted in the electronic scheduler for Medisoft®. Reminder notices and telephone calls that need to be made to patients before appointments can also be automatically generated.

HIPAA TIPS

HIPAA regulations require medical offices to prevent unauthorized users from accessing office computers. Virus detection and elimination software, firewall technology, and intrusion detection tools will all assist in serving this purpose by keeping unauthorized users from violating HIPAA.

Why is it important to never share your password with other employees?

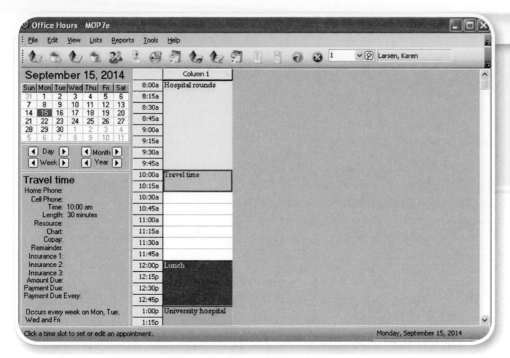

Figure 4.1

Electronic schedulers like Medisoft® Office Hours are used in many medical offices. *In what ways do such programs make the administrative medical assistant more efficient?*

Creation and Maintenance of Patients' Medical Records

A medical record contains all the office's information about a patient, such as medical history, physician notes, medical reports, x-rays, charts, and correspondence. Most medical practices use computers to handle some part of patients' medical records. In some offices, the records are completely electronic. With electronic health records, there are no actual paper records. All data about a patient, including x-ray images, lab test results, medical history, and so on, are created and stored on a computer. Electronic health records will be discussed later in this chapter.

The advantage of using electronic medical records is clear. For example, increasingly, clinical information is obtained electronically. Information such as the results of MRIs, x-rays, and blood tests can be transmitted in seconds to an electronic medical record. The time that would otherwise be required to output the results of tests, mail or fax them, and file them in a paper file is eliminated.

Perhaps one of the greatest advantages in using electronic medical records is that the data can be accessed instantly from any location. If a patient enters a hospital during an emergency, with the patient's permission, a physician can access the patient's medical record from the hospital in a matter of seconds to receive information on medical history, prior tests and lab work, medications prescribed, progress notes, and so on.

Electronic medical records also provide new opportunities for medical research. With access to large collections of patient information over a long period of time, medical researchers can look for patterns in similar cases, compare the results of treatments, and determine the best course of action.

Communications

Computers are used in the medical office to handle many communications tasks. An assistant needs to be familiar with the use of the following:

- Word processing
- E-mail
- Computer networks
- The Internet
- Wireless communication

Word Processing. A **word processing program** is used to enter, edit, format, and print documents. A word processor can handle all the written correspondence an assistant usually creates: referral letters, consultation reports, routine letters about appointments or test reports, interoffice memorandums, and standard forms and reports. In addition, the assistant may use a word processor in conjunction with a dictation machine to transcribe medical records, letters, reports, and articles.

A development in computer application programs that directly affects word processing and medical dictation is the improvement of voice-recognition software, which is discussed later in this chapter.

E-mail. A second communications tool widely used in the medical office is electronic mail, or **e-mail**, a telecommunications system for exchanging written messages through a computer network. Both the sender and receiver must have e-mail addresses. E-mail messages can be sent to someone in the same office or as far away as another country. In either case, the process is the same.

Computer Networks. A third type of communications tool used in a medical office is a computer network. A network links computers together, so that software, hardware, and data files can be shared. **Networking** provides a means of communicating, exchanging information, and pooling resources among a group of computers. A user who goes **online** is connecting to a computer network. Networks provide

- Simultaneous access to programs and files.
- A simple backup process.
- Sharing of computer devices.

Figure 4.2

This assistant is working with patients' medical records. *How can the assistant protect the confidentiality of data on a computer screen?*

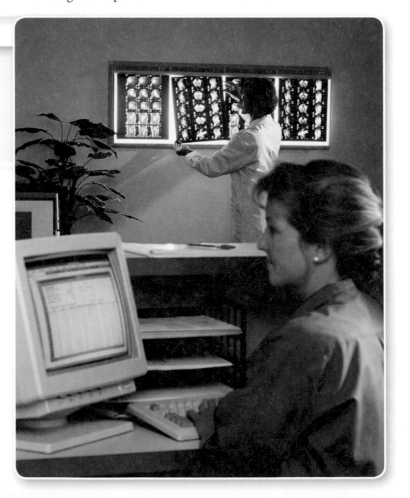

In a network, a central computer, called a **file server** (or simply a "server"), stores the computer programs and data to be shared by all the computers in the network. Network versions of software programs provide users simultaneous access to programs and data. Thus, only one version of a program and its associated data are needed for everyone on the network. This arrangement saves storage space on computers and makes it much easier to keep track of information, since all information is stored in one place. In addition, computer data, such as patient billing information, can be used by more than one person at a time. If the computers are not linked together in a network, only one person can access a file at a time. In a large office that manages a high volume of data, this would be highly inefficient. Similarly, at the end of the day, an extra copy of all data for safekeeping (a backup copy) can be obtained by creating a duplicate of the data on the file server, rather than on many separate machines. This procedure saves time and introduces fewer errors, since one person, usually the file server manager, is in charge of all backups.

Computers in a network are also able to share external devices, such as printers. Normally, every computer that does not operate within a network has its own external devices. If the computers are connected through a network, several computers can share the same equipment. This arrangement is less expensive for the office.

The Internet. An administrative medical assistant should also be familiar with the use of the Internet as a communications tool. The **Internet** is an enormous computer network that links computers and smaller computer networks worldwide. The Internet connects millions of computers around the world, making it possible to exchange information in seconds. The information that is shared can be text, graphics, sound, video, and even whole computer programs.

Uses of the Internet in the medical office continue to expand. Transmitting health claim information, researching medical data, obtaining travel fares, and ordering medical supplies are just a few of the unlimited uses of the Internet. Assistants use Internet search engines, such as Google, Bing, and Yahoo!, to locate information they need. Key words and phrases are used to retrieve data from various Internet sources. Online medical databases are used to educate physicians concerning conditions and treatment regiments. Patients are also able to research medical topics and educate themselves as consumers of healthcare.

Wireless Communication. All networks require some type of material to send data from one computer to another. In network communications, these materials are referred to as "media." Types of media currently in use include twisted-pair wire, which is made of copper, and fiber-optic cable, made of a thin strand of glass that transmits pulsating beams of light. A newer form of communications system, referred to as **wireless communication**, or wireless connectivity, uses radio waves, rather than wires or cables, as the medium for transmitting data. Cell phones and wireless Internet connections, known as WIFI, are examples of wireless communication. Wireless communication networks should be password-protected to prohibit unauthorized users from accessing the wireless network. Wireless communication will be discussed in more detail later in this chapter.

Billing, Collections, Claims, and Financial Reporting

Computers are used in medical offices to manage financial records. Computers were originally invented as tools for working with numbers. This makes them well suited for managing financial accounts. Computers are often used in the medical office for

- Billing and collections.
- Electronic transmission of insurance claims.
- Financial records relating to the operation of the office, such as employee records, payroll, accounts payable, and legal financial data.

Billing and Collections. Most medical offices use a medical billing program, such as Medisoft®, the program that is used with this text, to keep track of patients' accounts. It is important for any business to keep track of its funds. Accurate financial records are required for tax reporting and are critical for the practice's success. Without them, the business's owners do not know whether they will meet their financial obligations each month and whether the business is working at a profit or loss.

It is the assistant's job to see that every patient is billed appropriately and that insurance claims are submitted for patients who have health insurance. It is also the responsibility of the assistant to see that payments received from patients and insurance carriers are properly recorded. A medical billing program is designed to keep track of the constant flow of bills and payments between patients, the medical practice, and insurance companies. Figure 4.3 shows a Patient Ledger report generated through Medisoft®.

Although different medical offices use various types of software to keep track of patient accounts, all medical accounting systems require certain types of information. They are designed to use **databases**, which are collections of related data, such as the following:

- *Patient data.* The program's patient database contains information about each patient.
- *Transaction data.* The program's transaction database contains information about each patient's visits.

Electronic Transmission of Insurance Claims. One of the most important tasks of an administrative medical assistant is the creation of health insurance claims. When a patient with health insurance visits the office, a health insurance claim must be submitted to the patient's insurance company, describing the date of the visit, the diagnosis, the procedures performed, the cost of each procedure, payments made by the patient, and so on. On the basis of this information, the insurance company determines how much, if anything, the insurer owes the practice and/or the patient. A medical billing program, such as Medisoft®, helps the assistant generate health insurance claims and can be used to send the claims to insurance companies electronically. Filing claims electronically costs less than mailing printed forms, allows almost

Figure 4.3

Payment information from a patient's ledger is displayed by the Medisoft® program. *What kinds of numerical errors might using a computer program help eliminate?*

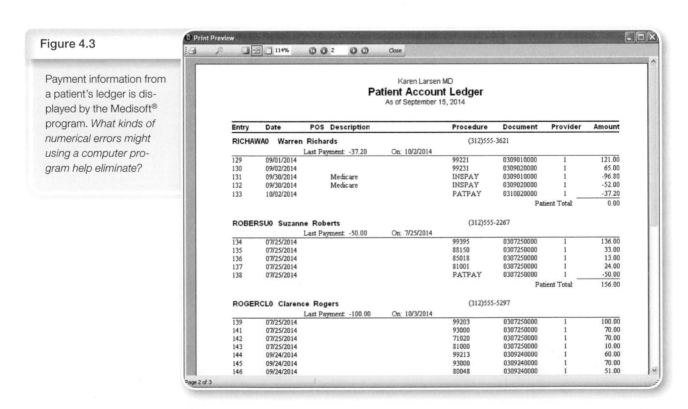

instantaneous submission, and creates an audit trail of submitted claims from the provider. The receiver (insurance payer) transmits a report of received claims back to the provider. Missing electronic claims can then be retransmitted to the insurance payer. Faster payments from insurance payers are received through electronic fund transfers (EFT) into the provider's account.

Financial Records Relating to the Operation of the Office. In addition to keeping track of patients' accounts, computer programs can be used to keep track of office operations. Like any business, a medical office must keep employee records, pay its employees (payroll) and suppliers, and maintain financial legal files. Computer programs are available to help in the creation and management of such records.

Clinical Work

Clinical usage of computers in the medical office is changing rapidly. Even simple procedures, such as recording a patient's pulse, blood pressure, or weight or conducting a simple auditory test, that used to be performed by a doctor using simple handheld instruments are now carried out with the help of computerized equipment. The variety of computers used in the field of radiology alone is staggering, from simple x-ray machines to specialized equipment designed to improve mammography (x-rays of the breast).

Medical labs, such as pathology labs and blood labs, also rely heavily on computers. Computers are required for administering tests, extracting results, and outputting test data. Indeed, the use of electronic medical records has been a natural outgrowth of the widespread clinical use of computers in the health industry.

Physician research today also takes advantage of computers. Physicians conduct research to help with patient care, to prepare papers for lectures, and to write articles for journals. In the past, physicians conducting research turned to medical textbooks, journals, case studies, and other materials found in a medical library. Today, much of the same material can be accessed with the help of a computer.

Each office should have an acceptable use policy (AUP) for equipment, time, and other resources, including the computer. Acceptable use policies should be written and included in the office's policy and procedure manual. However, the policy may be unstated. It is best practice to recognize that all hardware, software, and connectivity belong to the practice. Personal use of company-owned resources should be avoided.

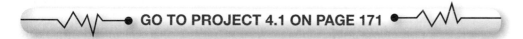

GO TO PROJECT 4.1 ON PAGE 171

Computer Categories

Many of the specifications that have usually separated one type of computer from another are becoming harder to define. The smallest computers used today have processing powers that rival the processing powers of the largest computers made less than a decade ago. The terms used to describe the major categories of computers—*supercomputer, mainframe, minicomputer,* and *personal computer*—have remained the same, but the capabilities of each group continue to change dramatically.

Supercomputers. **Supercomputers** are the most powerful computers available. Used by scientists, they are designed to process huge amounts of data. Supercomputers are extremely expensive, costing many millions of dollars.

Mainframe Computers. **Mainframes** are used in large businesses, hospitals, large clinics, and government organizations. They store massive databases, which many users can access at the same time. Mainframes are most often used in conjunction with computer terminals.

Figure 4.4

Portable electronic devices are used by many professionals in the healthcare field. *What are the advantages of using these devices?*

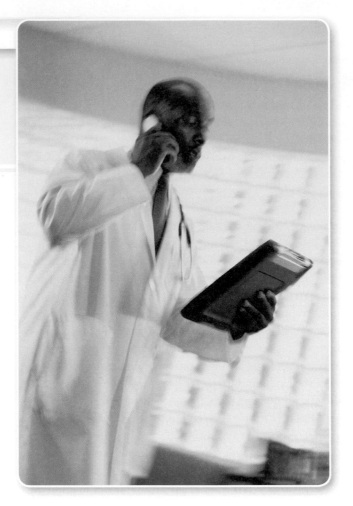

A computer terminal is a workstation that consists of a keyboard and screen. A computer terminal does not have its own processing unit or storage, since it uses the processing unit and storage of the mainframe to which it is connected, which may be feet or miles away.

Minicomputers. **Minicomputers** have less power than mainframes. Some minicomputers are designed for single users, but many operate with tens or even hundreds of terminals. In size and shape, minicomputers resemble a large file cabinet. They are popular in all kinds of businesses because they have many of the features of a mainframe but are not as big or nearly as expensive.

Personal Computers. Most computer users are more familiar with the personal computer than with any other type. **Personal computers**—PCs, or, less commonly, microcomputers—come in many sizes and shapes. Those that are designed to sit on a desk are desktop computers. To save space on the desktop, some models, called "tower models," are designed so that the system unit stands vertically on the floor. Portable models that are designed to fit into a briefcase or pocket are notebook computers, personal digital assistants, tablet PCs, or **laptops.** These mobile devices have the popular feature of being able to run on plug-in current or batteries. Figure 4.4 illustrates a physician using a portable device.

Ergonomics

Ergonomics is the science of designing the work environment to meet the needs of the human body. Ergonomics theories are finding practical application in computerized offices because of the number of injuries associated with working long hours on computers. The

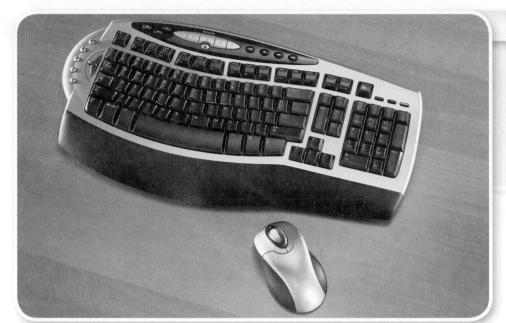

Figure 4.5

An ergonomic keyboard is designed to be more comfortable for the user. *Why is it important for the administrative medical assistant to pay attention to ergonomics when working?*

physical ailments that can result from long hours at a computer are known as cumulative trauma disorders or repetitive stress injuries.

Two hardware components—the keyboard and the monitor—are especially problematic. Figure 4.5 shows an ergonomic keyboard. A person who spends long periods at a computer performing repetitive movements should take frequent breaks. It is also a good idea to stretch the wrists and upper body at given intervals to avoid such problems as carpal tunnel syndrome and frozen shoulders. Following are a number of ergonomic tips to help computer users avoid the stress and strain that often result from working on a computer:

- Position the monitor at or below eye level, between 2 and 2.5 feet away, to avoid unnecessary neck strain and eyestrain.
- Use a copyholder to hold up any papers you need to refer to, and place it at eye level, a comfortable distance from your eyes (about 1.5 feet away), to avoid neck strain and eyestrain. Do not place papers flat on the desk, which forces you to keep your neck bent for long periods of time.
- Lower the height of the keyboard, if necessary, so that your hands are at the same level as your wrists. Your arms should be relaxed and forearms parallel to the floor. This is the best way to avoid injuring your wrists. Figure 4.6 is an example of proper keyboarding ergonomics.
- Hand and wrist supports are highly recommended to prevent the fatigue and stress to the hands and wrists that result from repetitive motions at the keyboard or with a mouse.
- Adjust the height and tilt of the chair, so that both feet are flat on the floor and your back is properly supported. Arm rests are recommended for office chairs.
- Focus your eyes on distant objects at regular intervals to avoid the eyestrain and headaches associated with focusing on a computer monitor for long periods.

Computer Software

Computer hardware, no matter how powerful, is useless without software, the instructions that tell the hardware what to do. Since there are many things a computer can do, there are thousands of types of software. Before the software performs any specialized function, however, such as word processing or mapmaking, the computer's **operating system** gets the computer running and keeps it working. **Application software,** which includes word

Figure 4.6

Maintaining the correct position for keyboarding reduces strain. *How can incorrect keyboarding techniques affect a computer user?*

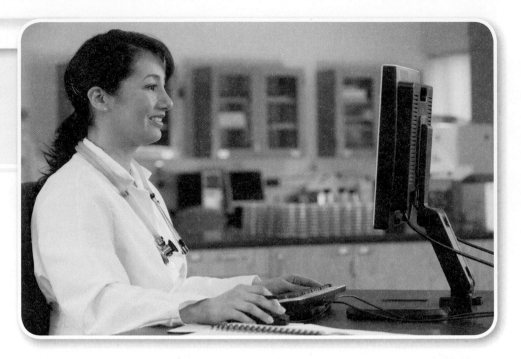

processing, graphics, spreadsheet, and database management software, applies the computer's capabilities to specific applications.

Operating System. The operating system tells the computer how to use its own components. When the computer is first turned on, the operating system runs various self-tests to check what devices are attached to the computer and whether the computer memory is functioning properly. Next, the operating system is loaded into the memory to control the basic functions of the computer, telling the computer how to interact with the user and the various input and **output devices**. The operating system continues to run in the background until the computer is turned off. The administrative medical assistant who uses computers regularly should know what operating system the computer uses, in case technical help is required. It is also important for the assistant to keep up to date with new versions of the operating system and learn how to take advantage of them.

Word Processing Programs. Most computer users are familiar with word processing programs. Microsoft Word and WordPerfect are two of the most popular examples. In addition to allowing the user to enter, edit, and format text quickly and easily, a word processor can be used to create templates. A **template** is a standard version of a document that is used over and over. It is altered slightly for each new document and saves the assistant the time required to key and format each document anew. Word processors also have features for checking spelling and grammar. Spell checkers are used to verify the spelling of words in a document before proofreading. The assistant can add words, such as uncommon medical terms for a given specialty that come up often in a physician's dictation, to a customized dictionary in the computer. The spell checker will include these words each time it checks a document for spelling errors.

Graphics Applications. A **graphics application** allows the user to manipulate images. Some graphics programs, called paint or draw programs, allow the user to create illustrations from scratch electronically. Others are designed to mix and match already created images, text, video, sound, and animation.

Another type of graphics application, which is more likely to be used in a medical office, is presentation software. PowerPoint is an example of a presentation software. It can be used to create professional-looking visual aids for presentation to an audience. These aids include photographic transparencies; paper printouts, such as cover sheets, colored graphs, and charts; and computer slide shows.

Spreadsheet Programs. **Spreadsheet programs**, such as Excel and Lotus 1-2-3, are designed to imitate paper bookkeeping ledgers. An electronic spreadsheet is a grid made up of rows and columns. Each box on the grid is a cell, and each cell has an address. For example, the address for the cell at the intersection of Column D and Row 3 is D3. By keying a combination of text labels, numerical data, and mathematical formulas into the cells, the user controls which calculations are to be carried out where in the spreadsheet. The result is that any number of calculations can be carried out at great speed. Anyone in charge of creating and maintaining a budget will find a spreadsheet program indispensable.

In a medical office, spreadsheets can be used for any activity involving numbers—for example, to keep track of supplies or to prepare budgets. Personnel departments often use spreadsheets to track wages and salaries paid to employees.

Database Management Software. Database management software helps the user enter data into a database and then sort the data into useful subsets of information. A number of database management programs are popular for personal computers, such as Access, dBase, Paradox, and R:BASE. Organizations that handle specialized data require custom-made database management programs to meet their needs. Medisoft®, the medical billing software used with this text, is an example of customized database management software. It is designed to meet the unique accounting needs of a medical practice. These include scheduling appointments, recording patient information, recording diagnoses and procedures, billing patients and filing insurance claims, and reviewing and recording payments. Medisoft® helps users accomplish all these tasks.

The four categories of application software discussed—word processing, graphics, spreadsheets, and database management—are perhaps the most widely used of all computer applications. Each type of software may be purchased separately, or an integrated software package—also called an "office suite"—may be bought. An integrated package combines several application programs.

Other categories of software generally include desktop publishing software, entertainment and education software, utilities software, and communications software. Utilities software helps with the upkeep and maintenance of the computer. Communications software is used to set up a network, for example, or connects a modem to an Internet service provider, such as America Online.

Computer Security and Patient Confidentiality

Although everyone working in a medical office must maintain the strict confidentiality of patients' medical records, proper treatment and billing often require information from these records to be released to insurance companies, other medical facilities, or other physicians. Because much of the information used in healthcare is stored and accessed using computers, special care must be taken to preserve the confidentiality of computerized patient information. Following are some steps a medical office can take to safeguard computerized information.

Screen Savers. Assistants and other office workers should not leave their desks and allow a computer screen showing information about a patient to remain visible. If a worker must be away from the desk for short periods of time regularly, a screen saver can be used to protect data from being seen by others. Screen savers are programs that display moving images on the screen if no input is received for several minutes. As soon as input resumes, the moving images disappear.

Inspection of Audit Trails. Another security measure that is used with computerized patient data is the periodic inspection of a data entry log. The inspection is usually done by the chief compliance officer or the practice manager. Whenever new information is entered or existing data in a database are changed, the computer records the time and date of the entry as well as the name of the computer operator. This computer record creates an audit trail that can be used to trace unauthorized actions to the responsible person.

Passwords for Limited Access. The use of electronic health records raises questions about who should have access to such files and how the information in them can be safeguarded, so that it does not end up where it does not belong. Often, the information in an electronic health record is highly confidential, since it contains all the details of a case, including a patient's medical history, the patient's ledger, and insurance information.

One security measure for safeguarding computerized information is the use of passwords. **Passwords** are assigned to limit the number of individuals who have access to particular computer files and to help users create a computerized audit trail.

Standard Release-of-Information Forms. Electronic health records must be kept as confidential as any other type of medical record. Therefore, a signed and dated release-of-information form must be on file before an electronic record can be transmitted. As with paper-based records, the release of information should be limited to the purpose mentioned in the request, so that only the portion of the medical records specifically requested is transmitted. Similarly, any conditions about when the permission expires, such as "permission expires in 60 days," must be carefully met.

Safeguards for Electronic Claims Transmission. Online systems should use some form of encryption to safeguard data that are being transmitted electronically. Encryption is a method of turning data into unintelligible gibberish during transmission.

Electronic signature systems should also be used to maintain the security of transmitted data in a medical practice. Electronic signature systems, which are regulated by state authorities, are used with electronic health records and electronic prescriptions, as well as for electronic claims transmission. Similar to a password system, an electronic signature system identifies the sender and the recipient of the data being sent. It locks the document, so that it can be opened only by the intended recipient, who has the unlocking key.

One way of protecting data transmitted over the Internet is to use a firewall. A firewall is a software program developed specifically to prevent outside parties from gaining access to particular areas of an organization's computer files. Another means of protecting files is the use of some combination of passwords, encryption, and electronic signatures.

Full Disclosure Policy. It is a good practice for the medical office to display a written policy on who has access to patients' medical records, as well as what that level of access is. Informing patients of such a policy protects the medical practice from potential lawsuits.

Backing Up Data. There are many unpredictable ways computer files can be lost or destroyed. A hard disk failure, power surge, or destructive computer virus can wipe out weeks of work. Every computer system should have a regular procedure for backing up data to safeguard against lost or corrupted files. On a network, the person in charge of managing the file server takes charge of backing up files. On stand-alone (independently operated) computers, each user is responsible. On a personal computer, for instance, a full backup copy of all files should be made no less than once or twice a month. Partial backups of files that have been worked on in the course of a day should be made at the end of every day. Although backing up files this often may seem extreme, it is important to consider the potential loss.

Virus Checkers. A computer **virus** is a program written with the intent of damaging another user's data, software, or computer. Generally, the virus is buried in a legitimate program or hidden on a disk. By running the program or using the disk, the user unknowingly activates the virus. Viruses can be programmed to do many things, such as destroy data or erase an entire hard disk. One way of contracting viruses is by downloading unknown programs or files on the Internet. Trojans, viruses hidden inside a seemingly safe file (like the mythical Trojan Horse), are activated when the "safe" file is used. A worm virus will "eat" its way through a computer program or system. Trojans and worm viruses are examples Malware (malicious software).

A virus checker is a utilities program that periodically searches a computer system for viruses. Antivirus software is designed to root out a virus before it does damage. Antivirus programs check every file on a storage drive and can be set up to check periodically or continuously. If they find infected files or suspicious programs, they attempt to remove them. Because so many viruses are sent through the Internet as e-mail or attached files, it is best to set up the virus checker to receive updated virus-detection information from the manufacturer's Internet site at least once per week. The virus checker automatically downloads information on new viruses that have been identified and runs the check to detect their presence on the computer system.

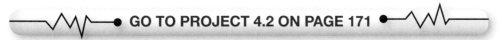

GO TO PROJECT 4.2 ON PAGE 171

4.2 THE MEDICAL RECORD

The patient medical record, also referred to as the patient's "chart" or "file," is the source of information about all aspects of a patient's healthcare. Accurate, up-to-date medical records are vital to a medical practice. Current records are necessary for enabling a continuum of care for patients, for financial and legal success, and for research purposes. It is not surprising, therefore, that one of the most important skills an administrative medical assistant can demonstrate is the ability to maintain accurate, complete medical records. In working with medical records, the assistant should be familiar with

- Medical records as legal documents.
- The types of reports and information typically found in a medical record.
- The importance of well-maintained medical records for the practice.
- The method for making corrections to a medical record.

Medical Records as Legal Documents

A patient's medical record constitutes the legal record of the medical practice. On occasion, patients' records may have to be produced in court, either to uphold the rights of the physician if the physician is involved in litigation or to substantiate a patient's claim if the physician is called as a witness. In malpractice cases, the content and quality of a medical record can be pivotal, leaving a greater impression on a jury, it is said, than even the physician's credentials, personality, or reputation. For this reason, medical files are often referred to as **medicolegal** documents, providing documentation of medical care, and they are admissible in a court of law. If the data in a medical record are incomplete, illegible, or poorly maintained, a plaintiff's attorney may be able to make even the best patient care appear negligent. Therefore, it is important for the administrative medical assistant to help the physician maintain medical records as carefully as possible. The assistant should bear in mind that any record could become a vehicle for defending a clinical course of action down the road.

What Is in a Medical Record?

A patient's medical record holds all the data about that patient. Medical records generally include the following items.

- *Chart notes:* A chronological record of ongoing patient care and progress, chart notes are entries made by the physician, the nurse, or another healthcare professional

Figure 4.7

Chart Note Regarding a
Phone Call from a Patient

CHART NOTE

```
Jackson, Alma                                    312-555-1102
DOB: 09/06/19--                                  Age: 47


8/3/20--
I received a telephone call from the patient today concerning not
knowing her lab results from last week. I checked her medical
record and noted that the lab tests were sent to an outside lab.
I explained that to the patient and told her that Dr. Larsen would
contact her with the results as soon as possible.


Karen Latter

Karen Latter, RN
```

regarding pertinent points of a given visit or communication with the patient. The chart notes for a new patient may be extensive, often containing the details of a comprehensive medical history and physical. Thereafter, chart notes may simply describe changes in the patient's condition or treatment plan. Figure 4.7 is an example of a simple chart note, entered by a registered nurse, regarding a phone call from a patient.

- *History and physical (H&P):* *History* refers to the patient's complete medical history (usually obtained by the nurse, assistant, or physician during an interview with the patient on his or her first visit); *physical* refers to the objective evaluation of relevant body areas or systems based on the patient's medical history.
- *Referral and consultation letters:* Copies of letters sent to or received from other physicians, referring the patient for specific examinations, tests, and so on, are part of the medical record.
- *Medical reports:* Lab reports, x-ray reports, and reports from procedures such as electrocardiograms are kept in the medical record. The type and number of medical reports in the file depend on the patient's condition and the specialty of the attending physician. After the physician has reviewed the medical report, he or she must sign and date it to document the physician's review of the data.
- *Correspondence:* Copies of all correspondence with the patient, including letters, faxes, and notes of telephone conversations and e-mail messages, are part of the medical record.
- *Clinical forms:* Forms such as immunization records and pediatric growth and development records are included.
- *Medication list:* A list of all medications prescribed, including dosage and dispensing instructions, as well as a list of the patient's known allergies to medications are in the medical record.

In addition to medical data, the patient's record contains administrative information, such as the patient's personal data (including insurance and billing records), as well as data on the release of information and the assignment of benefits—including insurance and billing records—and the release of information and assignment of benefits.

Reasons for Maintaining Medical Records

Medical records provide the practice with complete information regarding the patient. Thus, they are used in the following ways:

- As the main source of information for coordinating and carrying out patient care among all providers involved with the patient

- As evidence of the course of an illness and a record of the treatment being used, thereby providing a record of medical necessity
- As a record of the quality of care provided to patients
- As a tool for ensuring communication and continuity of care from one medical facility to another
- As the legal record for the practice
- As the main record to ensure appropriate reimbursement
- As a source of data for research purposes—for example, as background material for preparing a lecture, an article, or a book

Because the medical record is the basis for so many activities in a practice, every effort should be made to maintain it well. The following procedures should be used. Each time the patient is seen by a provider—such as for a blood pressure check or a return visit for a medication, whether in the office or at another location—an entry must be made in the patient's medical record. Entries must be keyed or handwritten in ink. As the sample chart note in Figure 4.7 illustrates, every entry should contain (1) patient identifying information—name, date of birth, and, if office policy states, age; (2) the date of the patient's visit or communication; and (3) the signature and title of the responsible provider or other healthcare professional. If an entry is transcribed, it is signed with the name of the dictator, followed by the initials of the transcriptionist. Two or three lines of space should be left on the record for the dictator's handwritten signature. A signature log should be maintained with the policy manual and updated as employees either leave or join the practice. Offices using electronic medical record entry methods should affix an electronic signature to all chart entries. Electronic signatures should contain the date and the timestamp of when the electronic signature was affixed to the record or document. Phrasing such as "Electronically signed by" or "Reviewed and verified by" usually accompany the electronic signature.

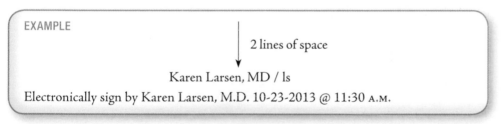

EXAMPLE

2 lines of space

Karen Larsen, MD / ls

Electronically sign by Karen Larsen, M.D. 10-23-2013 @ 11:30 A.M.

Entries should be made in a compact way, without leaving large gaps between notes. This eliminates the possibility of someone's tampering with the record later and ensures that the entries will be sequential. It is also important to make entries in a medical record promptly. Frequent delays in making entries will reflect poorly on the provider. Finally, the items should be placed within each section in a consistent chronological order, either ascending or descending.

Making Corrections

Because medical records are legal documents, it is not permissible to correct them with an eraser or correction fluid or to scribble out entries. Such methods could present the appearance of fraud. If you make an error while recording an entry or discover an error in a medical record, use the following method to correct it:

- Use the strike-through feature in the word processing program or draw a single line through the incorrect statements in the medical record (making sure the inaccurate material is still legible).
- Enter the word *error* next to the deleted statement.

COMPLIANCE TIP

Remember that no part of a record should be altered, removed, deleted, or destroyed. Only proper correction procedures may be used. Great care must be taken when entering data to ensure that they are inserted in the correct chart. If an error or a discrepancy is discovered in a medical record at a much later date, the physician may dictate an addendum to the record to correct the discrepancy. Remember, any alteration of a medical record may constitute the appearance of fraud, and proper correction procedures should always be followed.

- Write your initials and the date next to the correction.
- Enter the correct information above or below the inserted line in the medical record.

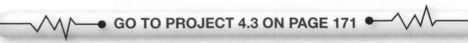

GO TO PROJECT 4.3 ON PAGE 171

4.3 DOCUMENTATION FORMATS

The **SOAP** method is the most common system for outlining and structuring chart notes for a medical record. It facilitates the creation of uniform and complete notes in a simple format that is easy to read. The acronym *SOAP* stands for the following headings that are used to structure the chart notes: *SUBJECTIVE, OBJECTIVE, ASSESSMENT,* and *PLAN*. Each of these headings contains a specific type of information, as follows. Problem-oriented medical records (POMR) is another common documentation format. **CHEDDAR** format also breaks down the components of a patient encounter into seven detail-oriented sections: chief complaint, history, exam, details of problem, drugs/dosages, assessment, and return information.

The SOAP Method

Subjective Findings. **Subjective** findings are the patient's description of the problem or complaint, including symptoms troubling the patient, when the symptoms began, external or associated factors, remedies tried, and past medical treatment. The subjective information in a SOAP record may include any or all of the subheadings that follow.

- **Chief complaint (CC):** The reason for the visit, or why the patient is seeking the physician's advice.

S O A P
Subjective Findings

Figure 4.8

During a new patient's first visit, the physician usually takes note of the patient's complete medical history. *Why is it important for patients' medical histories to be placed in their charts promptly?*

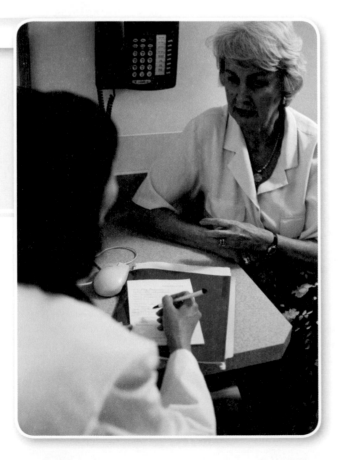

- **History of present illness (HPI):** Information about the symptoms troubling the patient—location, quality, severity, timing, duration, context, modifying factors, and any associated signs and/or symptoms. The patient should be asked questions such as when the symptoms began, what affects them (things that make the symptoms better or worse), what may have caused the symptoms, any remedies the patient has tried, and any medical treatment already given.
- **Past medical history (PMH):** A listing of any illnesses the patient has had in the past along with the treatments administered or operations performed. This history also includes a description of any accidents, injuries, congenital problems, or allergies to medicines or other substances.
- **Family history (FH):** Facts about the health of the patient's parents, siblings, and other blood relatives that might be significant to the patient's condition. For example, family history is especially important in treating hereditary diseases.
- **Social history (SH):** The patient's social history and marital history, especially if they are pertinent to the patient's treatment. Information regarding the patient's eating, drinking, or smoking habits, the patient's occupation, the patient's sexual activity, and the patient's interests may also be included in this section.
- **Review of systems (ROS):** The physician's review of each body system with the patient (for example, the respiratory system and the genitourinary system). The physician asks specific questions about the functioning of each system and reviews information in the patient's record.

In some chart notes, the three subheadings *PMH*, *FH*, and *SH* (for *past medical history, family history*, and *social history*) may be combined into one subheading, *PFSH*.

Objective Findings. The **objective** findings in a SOAP record are the physician's examination of the patient. Results of the examination may be dictated under the heading **physical exam (PE)**. The exam may be a complete physical examination, in which the findings for each of the major areas of the body are included, or it may cover only the pertinent body systems for that visit. The following subheadings cover body systems that may be included in a physical exam:

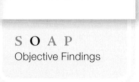

SOAP
Objective Findings

VITAL SIGNS (VS): The patient's temperature, pulse, and respirations (TPR); blood pressure (BP); and height and weight are included in this category. This heading may also be labeled CONSTITUTIONALS.

GENERAL: A general description of the patient might be, for example, "This is a well-developed, well-nourished, 27-year-old Caucasian female."

HEENT: This abbreviation stands for *head, eyes, ears, nose*, and *throat*.

NECK

HEART

CHEST

LUNGS

ABDOMEN

PELVIC

RECTAL

EXTREMITIES

NEUROLOGICAL

The results of lab tests, x-rays, and other diagnostic procedures are also part of the objective findings. These results may be included in the corresponding body system review, or they may be listed as separate entries or under a separate heading, such as *LAB*, usually after the list of body systems.

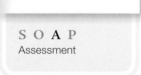

SOAP
Assessment

Assessment. The **assessment** in a SOAP record is the physician's interpretation of the subjective and objective findings. The term *assessment* is used interchangeably with the terms

Figure 4.9

Findings from the physician's examination must be recorded accurately in the patient's chart. *How can the administrative medical assistant ensure that the transcription is accurate?*

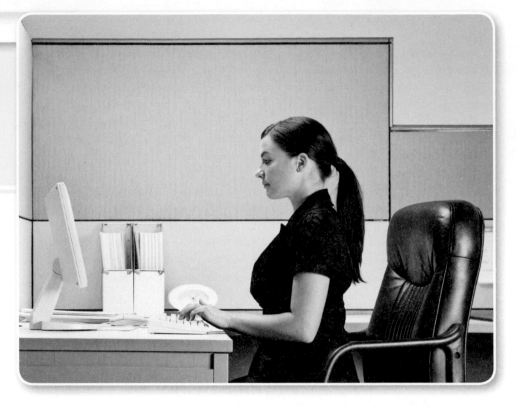

diagnosis (Dx) and **impression** and gives a name to the condition from which the patient is suffering. Sometimes the assessment is tentative, pending further developments. Occasionally, the physician uses the phrase **rule out (R/O)** before a diagnosis, meaning that the diagnosis, while possible, is not likely and that further tests will be performed for confirmation.

Plan. The **plan**, or treatment, section lists the following information regarding the physician's treatment of the illness:

S O A P
Plan

- Prescribed medications and their exact dosages
- Instructions given to the patient
- Recommendations for hospitalization or surgery
- Any tests that need to be performed

Figures 4.10 and 4.11 (on page 146) contain examples of chart notes that incorporate the SOAP format. In Figure 4.10, although not all the SOAP headings are spelled out, the entries clearly follow the SOAP format. The subjective findings begin with *CC* (chief complaint) and continue to *PHYSICAL EXAM*, which contains the objective findings. The assessment and plan follow with their own headings.

In Figure 4.11, the SOAP format is more apparent, with the addition of a *LAB* heading after the objective findings. Notice that the level of detail contained in the entries in Figure 4.10 is much greater than that in Figure 4.11. This is because the patient described in Figure 4.10 is a new patient, and therefore a complete history and physical have been performed. The patient described in Figure 4.11 is a returning patient who is visiting for help with a specific illness.

As can be seen from an examination of Figures 4.10 and 4.11, the SOAP format can accommodate many variations. The value in using the SOAP outline, or a variation of it, is that, by following the simple formula of the acronym, the person writing or dictating the note is more likely to cover all the important issues. In addition, the logic of the format lends itself well to displaying the provider's thought processes in deciding on a course of treatment.

Copyright © 2012 McGraw-Hill Higher Education

HISTORY AND PHYSICAL REPORT

Paulson, Laura
DOB: 03/01/19--   Age: 44

3/6/20--
CC: Annual female exam for this 44-year-old black patient.

PMH: Tonsillectomy at age 3; wisdom teeth pulled at age 29.

ALLERGIES: SULFA.

CURRENT MEDICATIONS: None.

FH: Father died at age 70 of multiple problems, including carcinoma of larynx,
stroke, and pneumonia. Mother, age 66, is in good health. No siblings.

SH: Laura completed high school, plus one to two years of college. Patient works
at a dry cleaner, pressing machine and front desk. Does not smoke or use alcohol.
She was never on birth control pills or any other major medication.

MARITAL HISTORY: Husband, age 46, is in good health. They have been married 24 years
and have three children in good health.

ROS:
SKIN: Negative.
HEENT: Patient wears glasses with last eye exam 3 months ago. She has occasional
sinusitis.
CHEST: No chest pain or palpitation.
RESPIRATORY: Negative.
ABDOMEN: Negative.
PELVIC: LMP 3 weeks ago. Gravida 3, para 3. Patient uses OTC birth control products.
MUSCULOSKELETAL: Occasional stiffness of elbow.
NEUROLOGICAL: Negative.

PHYSICAL EXAM:
GENERAL: Alert black female in no acute distress. BP, 116/82. Pulse, 86.
Respirations, 24. Height, 64 inches; weight, 128 pounds.
HEENT: Normocephalic. Ears, TMs normal. Eyes, PERLA; EOMs, intact. Nose, patent.
Throat, within normal limits.
NECK: Supple. Thyroid, not enlarged. Carotids, equal without bruits.
BREASTS: Fine lumps bilaterally; nothing suspicious.
HEART: Regular sinus rhythm without murmurs.
LUNGS: Clear to A&P.
ABDOMEN: Soft; without masses, tenderness, or scars.
PELVIC: Cervix, clean. Uterus, anteverted and smooth. Adnexa and vagina, WNL.
Rectovaginal confirms.
EXTREMITIES: Within normal limits with fine varicosities bilaterally.
NEUROLOGICAL: Cranial nerves II-XII, intact.

ASSESSMENT: Generally healthy female.

PLAN: 1. Schedule mammogram.
         2. Routine screen labs.
         3. UA.
         4. Hemoccults x 3.

Karen Larsen

Karen Larsen, MD/ls

Figure 4.10

Chart Note Showing a Physician's Report on a History and Physical Exam

Having such a record improves communication for all those involved in the care of the patient. It also minimizes the provider's exposure to legal risk.

The CHEDDAR Method

Another format used for medical documentation is called **CHEDDAR**. This method of entry uses the same information as the SOAP method and places it under seven headings:

C (chief complaint)

H (history of the present illness)

E (examination)

D (details of problems and complaints)

D (drugs and dosage—past and current medications)

A (assessment)

R (return visit or referral to a specialist)

Figure 4.11

Chart Note in the SOAP
Format

CHART NOTE

Benson, Harriett
DOB: 07/29/19--   Age: 23

March 6, 20--
SUBJECTIVE: Patient presents with mild urinary urgency and frequency.
Patient has also had frequent lower abdominal pain, but no abnormal
vaginal symptoms.

OBJECTIVE: Temperature, 98.6°. Pulse, 76 and regular. Respirations,
20. Abdominal exam reveals mild suprapubic tenderness; otherwise,
exam is unremarkable.

LAB: Urinalysis is negative; urine culture is pending.

ASSESSMENT: Suspect urethritis.

PLAN: Patient placed on 7-day course of ciprofloxacin 500 mg b.i.d.
She was reminded to drink at least 8 glasses of water daily. RTC if
not improving.

Karen Larsen

Karen Larsen, MD/ls

The following is an example of a chart note using the CHEDDAR documentation format:

CHART NOTE

Rodriguez, Erin
DOB: 07/31/20--   Age: 9

07/07/20--
CC : Patient's mother stated daughter has developed a red, itchy skin rash
on her right arm.

H: Patient began complaining of an "itchy" arm after returning from a
school outing two days prior in a park with poison oak. The patient fell
into the poison oak when attempting to retrieve a ball. Soon after the
itching began, the patient developed a red, pinpoint rash on the arm.
Mother stated she used OTC ointments on the rash with no relief.

E: General: Patient is a WD, WN nine-year-old female with no history of
rashes. BP 110/75; WT 82 lbs., Pulse 80
Skin: Smooth, red rash on the right inner and outer forearm. No discharge
noted.
HEENT: Normocephalic. Ears, TMs normal. Eyes, PERLA. Nose, Patent. No
deviation noted. Throat, within normal limits.

D: Patient has dark red, nonpustule rash on right inner and outer forearm.
Rash appears irritated.

D: Mother gave patient OTC Benadryl four hours prior to being examined.
Patient is currently on no other medication.

A: Dermatitis due to contact with poison oak.

R: Patient is to continue to use OTC antihistamine. If rash has not sub-
sided in two days, return to office. Otherwise, prn.

Karen Larsen

Karen Larsen, MD/ls

Problem-Oriented Medical Records (POMR)

Another form of record keeping revolves around a list of the patient's problems. A record organized in this way is referred to as a **problem-oriented medical record** (**POMR**). In a problem-oriented medical record, there are three essential components: a database, an initial plan, and a problem list

Database. The database consists of the patient's complete history, including the problem, history of present illness, past medical history, family history, social history, and review of systems, followed by information derived from a complete examination and routine diagnostic tests.

Initial Plan. Based on the database and the initial problems of the patient, the physician begins a course of treatment, detailed in this section.

Problem List. The problem list is a running account of the patient's problems. It is referred to and updated at each clinic visit. This procedure helps assure that all problems are considered during a visit. Using the list, the physician can, at a glance, learn what problems the patient has had, how often they have appeared, and the treatment prescribed. This list saves time in that the physician does not have to study the patient's entire chart before obtaining relevant information.

Generally, the SOAP format is used for organizing entries within the problem list. The SOAP format may also be used to outline the history and physical for the database section. Figure 4.12 is an example of a problem-oriented medical record. Notice how each entry begins with the date of the patient visit, followed by a reference to the problem being treated—*PROBLEM 1*, *PROBLEM 2*, and so on.

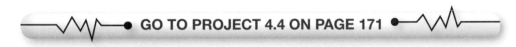

GO TO PROJECT 4.4 ON PAGE 171

4.4 OWNERSHIP, QUALITY ASSURANCE, AND RECORD RETENTION

Every medical practice has a variety of files that need to be preserved. Patient medical records, in particular, require special attention because of their importance to the practice and their value as legal documents. All medical records should be kept until the possibility of a malpractice suit has passed. This time period is determined by each state's statute of limitations. Although most medical records are, in fact, kept permanently, they are generally removed from an active file (pertaining to current patients) to an inactive file or closed storage (for patients who have died, moved away, or terminated their relationship with the physician).

Every provider should have guidelines for transferring patient medical records from one classification to another. These guidelines should specify the information that is to be kept and, if possible, the type of storage medium to be used. It is important for an administrative medical assistant to be familiar with these guidelines, since their application will help protect the physician and the practice from potential legal complications.

Ownership

The ownership of medical records is addressed by the American Medical Association Council on Ethical and Judicial Affairs. According to the Council, medical notes made by a physician—the actual chart notes, reports, and other materials—are the physician's property. The notes are for the physician's use in the treatment of the patient.

Figure 4.12

Chart Note for a
Problem-Oriented
Medical Record (POMR)

CHART NOTE

Pander, Ian
DOB: 08/02/19--   Age: 22

March 7, 20--
PROBLEM 1: Tonsillitis.

CHIEF COMPLAINT: Sore throat times two days.

S: Sore throat, difficulty swallowing.

O: Temperature 101°. Pharyngitis with exudative tonsillitis.

PLAN: 1. Throat culture.
         2. 1.2 units CR Bicillin.
         3. Recheck in 10 days.

Karen Larsen

Karen Larsen, MD/ls

March 14, 20--
PROBLEM 1:

S: Recheck. Patient feels better.

O: Temperature, normal. No problem with swallowing.

A: Problem 1 resolved.

P: Gargle with warm salt water if necessary. Pharyngitis with exudative
   tonsillitis resolved.

Karen Larsen

Karen Larsen, MD/ls

June 11, 20--
PROBLEM 2: Chip fracture lunate, left.

S: Pain in instep and tarsal bones.

O: Swelling and ecchymosis, left foot.

A: X-ray shows questionable undisplaced chip fracture of lunate.

P: 1. Continue supportive shoes.
        2. Referred to orthopedics for further evaluation.

Karen Larsen

Karen Larsen, MD/ls

However, the physician cannot use or withhold the information in the record according to his or her own wishes. For example, the physician is ethically obligated to furnish copies of office notes to any physician who is assuming responsibility for care of the patient. Even though, under the TPO portion of HIPAA, a signed release of information from the patient is no longer required, some practices still ask their patients to sign a release of information prior to releasing PHI to another physician for the continuity of the patient's care. It is understood that, even though the physician's notes are the physician's property, the information in the record—the nature of the patient's diagnosis and so on—belongs to the patient. For this reason, patients have the right to control the amount and type of information released from their medical record. Furthermore, patients alone hold the authority to release information to anyone not directly involved in their care, such as an attorney or a spouse. A fee may be charged for furnishing copies of complex medical reports; however, information should not be withheld because of an unpaid fee. State laws should be referenced when determining if a patient may be charged for copied medical documents and, if so, how much may be charged.

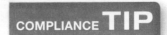

Credibility of the record is called into question when there is delayed filing of reports and physicians' notes, or when there are incomplete files, illegible records, or alterations in the record.

To ensure that files are complete, a standard office procedure should be used to follow up on pending reports for x-rays and other diagnostic procedures. A separate file marked "Pending Work" might be used, or a reminder might be placed in a tickler file.

Quality Assurance

The medical record probably is the best measure of the quality of care given a patient. The assistant helps the physician maintain high standards of care by paying attention to the data entered in the medical record.

If the assistant is unsure about a word written or dictated (for example, it may be unclear whether the physician means "15" or "50" milligrams), the item should be flagged for the physician's attention. The assistant should not interrupt the physician if he or she is attending to other tasks at that time.

The assistant should make sure that each record contains the following:

- Dated notations describing the service received by the patient
- Notations regarding every procedure performed
- Accurate notations; an addendum by the physician should be made if a discrepancy occurs (for example, a previous notation about a condition may have stated "left side," while the latest notation states "right side")
- Justification for hospitalization
- If necessary, a discharge summary regarding hospitalization before the patient arrives for a follow-up visit

Patients also have the right to inspect their medical documentation. If they feel an entry error has occurred, they should notify the provider, in writing, and ask that the correction be made. The provider must respond to the request. If the healthcare team reviews the documentation and, in fact, an error has occurred, a correction should be made in the chart and the patient notified of the correction. Correction should be made using the previously discussed method. If the corrective entry is longer than would fit either above or below the correction line, an addendum should be made in the medical record. However, if the physician does not feel an error has occurred he or she cannot be forced to make a corrective entry. In this situation, the patient should submit his or her own version of the encounter, which should then be included in the medical record.

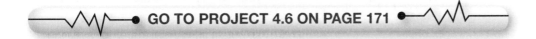

GO TO PROJECT 4.6 ON PAGE 171

Retention of Records

Every medical practice has files from previous years and all types of information. For example, patient medical records include files for patients who are currently being treated by the physician, those who have not seen the physician for some time, and those who are no longer patients.

For management purposes, these files are classified as

- **Active files**, pertaining to current patients.
- **Inactive files**, related to patients who have not seen the physician for 6 months or longer. Depending on the medical specialty, this time period may be longer. For example, a file may be considered inactive in a family medical practice after 6 months of

inactivity; however, a file in an OB-GYN practice may be considered inactive after 24 months of nonactivity.

- **Closed files**, those of patients who have died, moved away, or terminated their relationship with the physician.

Each office sets the criteria and time frames for placing files in one of the categories. This policy is part of a larger policy for record **retention**—the length of time records must be retained and the proper disposition of them when they should no longer be stored. Record retention policies protect physicians from exposure to legal problems.

Legal Requirements. Federal law does not regulate retention time frames for patients' medical records. Many states, however, have specific requirements for the length of time such records must be kept. Existing state laws and regulations must always be observed. Healthcare providers who receive payment under the federal Medicare program must also comply with Medicare's conditions for record retention.

In January 1997, the American Health Information Management Association (**AHIMA**) proposed this guideline in one of its practice briefs:

> Each healthcare provider should develop a retention schedule for patient health information that meets the demands of its patients, physicians, researchers, and other legitimate users while complying with all legal, regulatory, and accreditation requirements. Providers should also create guidelines that specify what information should be kept, the time period for which it will be kept, and the type of storage medium in which it shall be kept (paper, microfilm, optical disk, magnetic tape, or other).

Retention Time Frames. AHIMA has recommended the following time frames as retention schedules, subject to local laws and regulations:

- *Patient health records (adults):* Ten years after patient's most recent encounter
- *Patient health records (minors):* Age of majority (varies between 18 and 21 years of age) plus statute of limitations on malpractice; in most states, the time period ranges from one to four years
- *Diagnostic images (such as x-rays):* Indefinitely
- *Master patient index, register of births, register of deaths, register of surgical procedures:* Permanently

The office policy should include a variety of other records related to the physician's practice management:

- *Insurance policies:* Current policies are kept in safe storage in an accessible file. Professional liability policies are kept permanently.
- *Tax records:* Tax records for the three latest years are kept in a readily accessible file. The remaining records may be kept in a less accessible storage area.
- *Receipts for equipment:* Receipts for both medical and office equipment are kept until the various pieces of equipment are fully depreciated—that is, until the value of the equipment has completely diminished.
- *Personal records and licenses:* Professional licenses and certificates are kept permanently in safe storage. Banking records, such as statements and deposit slips, are kept in the file for three years. They may then be moved to a storage area. Other personal records, such as noncurrent partnership agreements, property records, or other business agreements, are also kept permanently in a storage area.

Paper Versus Electronic Records. To save space, paper records can be stored through a process called **micrographics**, in which miniaturized images of the records are created. These images are usually in a microfiche (sheet of film holding 90 images) or ultrafiche (compacted film holding up to 1,000 images) format and are viewed on readers that enlarge the images. Micrographic records may be stored in card files or binders. With the increased use of the large memory capacity afforded by computers, paper records may also be scanned and stored in a space-saving way on a hard disk, CD, or DVD. As electronic health records become the norm, traditional hardcopy patient records must be scanned into the practice program. This is a time-consuming task, and some practices have created employee positions for the sole purpose of scanning paper documents into the electronic health record program. Other medical practices have contracted with an outside agency to scan documents. Scanners may work during hours when patients and employees typically are away from the office. Using off-hours to scan documents makes patient medical data available to medical personnel as patients are being seen. All electronically stored records must be kept according to the same retention schedule as that for paper records.

Disposition of Records. Records that have been closed and those that must be kept permanently—patient records, personal records, and business records—may be transferred and are said to be in **dead storage**, a storage area separate from the area where active files are kept. Dead storage need not be easily accessible and can be in a location other than the office. The storage area should provide a secure, safe area for records.

There are financial and storage considerations for every practice. All records cannot be kept indefinitely. Some states have laws related to the destruction of records and even specify the method of destruction. General guidelines provided by AHIMA include the following:

- Appropriate ways to destroy records include burning, shredding, and pulping. Records must be destroyed so that there is no possibility of reconstructing them.
- When destroying computerized data, overwriting data or reformatting the disk should be done. Other methods delete file names but do not really destroy data. Microfilm, microfiche, and laser disks may be destroyed by pulverizing.

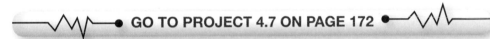

GO TO PROJECT 4.7 ON PAGE 172

4.5 FILING SYSTEMS

Filing Equipment and Supplies

Records management is the systematic control of records from their creation through maintenance to eventual storage or destruction. Records may be managed electronically or manually (paper records). To handle these tasks, administrative medical assistants have a source of helpful information in the Association of Records Managers and Administrators (**ARMA**). This international organization's members include information managers, archivists (those who specialize in control of records storage), librarians, and educators. One of the major purposes of the organization is to set standards for the filing and retention of records. Although ARMA standards are voluntary, rather than set by the government, following them makes it possible for medical offices to manage records more efficiently.

Medical offices may use the ARMA guidelines as a basis for the records management procedures and adapt the guidelines to fit individual office records management needs. For consistency, it is important to include written policy and procedures for records management in the office manual. A good question to ask is "Using the office records management policy, can the correct record be retrieved in a timely manner by an office employee and data given to the right individual to make informed medical decisions?"

ARMA
International
11880 College Blvd.
Suite 450
Overland Park,
KS 66210
Phone: 913-341-3808
or 800-422-2762
Web site:
www.arma.org
E-mail: hq@arma.org

Recorded information in any form—whether in an electronic file, in a paper document, or on external devices such as flash drives, disks, or digital image—is considered a record. In medical offices, the three main types of records are (1) patient medical records, (2) correspondence related to healthcare, and (3) practice management records.

1. *Patient medical records.* The central responsibility of the physician's practice is patient care. For this reason, the proper handling of the patient medical record is critical. This contains chart notes, all medical and laboratory reports, and all correspondence to, from, and about a patient.

2. *Correspondence related to healthcare.* General correspondence includes items about the operation of the office, such as orders for medical supplies. It also includes physicians' research reports; articles from medical journals related to new procedures or treatments; and correspondence, newsletters, and announcements from professional organizations.

3. *Practice management records.* Materials about the business and financial management of the practice must also be carefully kept. These documents include insurance policies, income and expense records, copies of tax returns for the practice, financial statements, and leases or contracts related to office space or the premises. Also kept are copies of managed care contracts and the office's compliance program and privacy policy. Personnel and payroll records are also part of practice management.

Two broad categories of files are centralized files and decentralized files. Centralized files—those kept in one place—must be used by many people in the medical office. Thus, ease of access is necessary. Information of use to only one staff member, such as a physician's correspondence, is stored in a decentralized file convenient to the user. The kinds of filing equipment and supplies that best suit a medical office depend on how records are used and who needs to use them.

Filing Equipment

Open-Shelf Files

Open-shelf files are bookcase-type shelves that hold files. These shelves may be adjustable or fixed and may extend from floor to ceiling. Folders are placed in the files sideways with identifying tabs protruding, as shown in Figure 4.13.

Figure 4.13

The assistant must understand the ways in which the office files are used, the organization of the files, and the principles and procedures for accurate filing. *How can an assistant get help in learning the filing procedures of a specific medical office?*

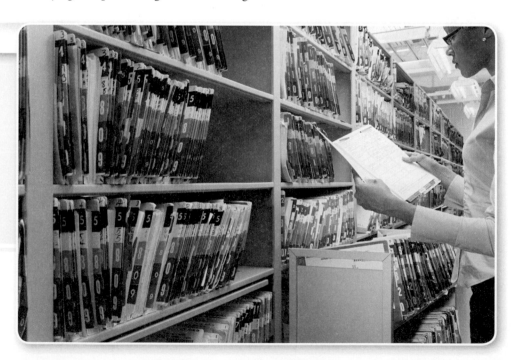

The need to conserve space in many offices has made open-shelf files popular. They take up less floor and aisle space and are less expensive to purchase than most other kinds of filing equipment. Because staff members do not need to open drawers, these files also save time and labor. However, open shelves do mean that records are less secure than if they were held in closed steel drawers. The records are also more vulnerable to accidents, including fire and water damage. Therefore, open-shelf filing equipment should have doors that can be closed and locked to protect medical records from theft and natural disasters, such as fire or flood.

Filing Cabinets

Many kinds of filing cabinets are available. The best choice for a particular office will be based on available space, the cost, and the level of security that is desirable.

Vertical Files. Drawer files, called **vertical files**, are contained in cabinets of various sizes. These letter-size cabinets, meant for documents that are $8\frac{1}{2}$ by 11 inches, are usually metal. They vary in capacity from one to five drawers; files are arranged from front to back in each drawer. Vertical files, shown in Figure 4.14, are popular because they provide a large amount of filing space. Vertical files can be moved fairly easily compared to open-shelf files. However, because these cabinets have drawers that must be opened and closed, using vertical files takes more of an assistant's time in filing and retrieving records. The space required to open the drawers is also a consideration in planning efficient use of storage and aisle space.

Lateral Files. In **lateral files**, the drawers or shelves open horizontally and files are arranged sideways, from left to right, instead of from front to back. Lateral files, as

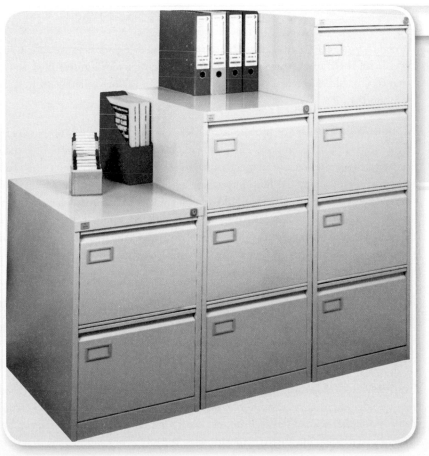

Figure 4.14

Vertical file cabinets are commonly used to store business documents and files. *Do business documents need to be more or less accessible to medical personnel than medical records do?*

Copyright © 2012 McGraw-Hill Higher Education

Figure 4.15

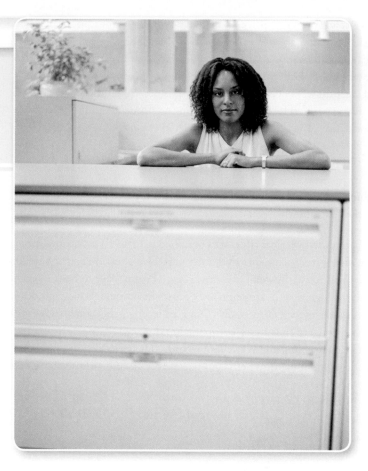

Drawers open horizontally in lateral file cabinets to provide easy access. *How important is it for the assistant to have easy access to files?*

shown in Figure 4.15, may have standard drawers or doors that are rolled down from the top of the shelf and retract when the shelf is being used. Lateral files do not project as far into an aisle as vertical files. Thus, if space is a major consideration, lateral files may be a good choice.

Mobile-Aisle Files. The **mobile-aisle files** contain open-shelf files that are moved manually or, more often, by a motor. The platform on which shelves are mounted may be specially constructed, or the tracks and mechanism may be on the floor. When these files are motorized, the person using the files may access a file quickly and easily. Mobile-aisle filing systems, shown in Figure 4.16, also hold a large volume of records. Because this system holds so many records and because the system is mechanized, safety features, such as an electronic eye to sense when someone is using another portion of the files and to prevent movement of the files, and the amount of weight the files will safely hold are important factors in the decision to install this system.

Filing Supplies

Folders, labels, tabs, and guides are all designed to make the location of and access to files efficient. Important considerations in choosing filing supplies are the durability of the material and the uses of color and positioning within a file to make the user's task easier.

Folders. File **folders**, which may be open on one, two, or three sides, hold the items that are filed. Folders may be purchased in various colors, styles, weights, and tab cuts. **Tabs** are the projections that extend beyond the rest of the folder, so that the folder can be labeled and easily viewed. **Tab cuts** are to the positions of the tabs. For example, the first cut creates a tab

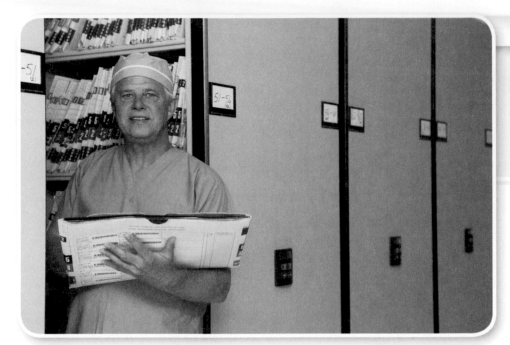

Figure 4.16

Mobile-aisle files save space and are easily accessible. *Which kinds of files seem most suitable for a single-physician office? A multi-physician office? A clinic? A hospital?*

at the left; a center cut, at the center. The most popular position of a tab for a patient chart is a third-cut tab, which places a tab at the right of the chart. Folders are filed in such a way that tab cuts, with the accompanying labels, are read in an orderly fashion from left to right.

Labels. Oblong pieces of paper, frequently self-adhesive, are called **labels**. Once the person establishing the file has keyed in a descriptive title or subject on the label, it is used to identify a file. (Handwritten labels are to be avoided, as they are hard to read.) Labels are available in perforated rolls or on self-adhesive strips. Many assistants use a computer and printer to key in file titles and print out the required labels. Labels with a color band on top for ease of identification are also available. Scanners and bar codes may be used to identify patient charts. Codified data, such as a patient name or number, are placed in a bar code and read by the programmed scanner, similar to purchasing items at a store and having them scanned for purchase.

Guides. **Guides** are rigid dividers placed at the end of a section of files to indicate where a new section or category of files begins. Because guides are made of rigid material, they support folders and are visual clues to the user of the file, showing exactly where in the file drawer new main subjects begin.

Out Guides. An **out guide** is a card or sheet that is placed as a substitute when a file or information from a file is removed. Out guides are particularly useful when there are many users of a particular set of files. Everyone always knows where information may be found. The front of the out guide has lines to record the name of the person who is taking the information, the date it was removed, the material which was removed, and the date it is to be returned. When the information is returned, these annotations are crossed out and the out guide is removed and may be reused. Out folders may be substituted for a patient chart when it is removed. They serve as a temporary storage unit until the original record is returned. Any accumulated documents in the temporary out folder will then be transferred into the original patient chart.

Cross-Reference Sheets. Many documents can be coded and filed under more than one heading. For example, a letter from the physician's insurance company verifying coverage may be placed in the physician's correspondence file. It may also belong with insurance policies kept in a different file. In cases such as this, a **cross-reference sheet** is prepared to indicate where the original material is filed and where in the files other copies may be found. The cross-reference sheet may be in a different color from the file folders to make identification simpler.

Steps in Filing

Following logical, consistent, systematic steps in preparing materials for filing enables the assistant to file accurately, to find materials quickly, and to refile documents efficiently.

The following are the steps in filing:

1. Inspecting documents
2. Indexing
3. Coding
4. Sorting
5. Storing

Inspecting Documents. The assistant is responsible for **inspecting documents** received for filing. Each document should be in good physical condition, and the information should be complete. For example, if an attachment is indicated, it should be present. If the document says that an action should be taken—such as a form letter should be sent to an insurance company—the item relating to the action should be present or there should be an indication, such as a check mark, that the action was taken. The document must also bear a release mark. **Releasing** is the indication, by initial or by some other agreed-upon mark, that the document has been inspected and acted upon and is ready for filing. Note that a release mark is different from a time-date stamp, which is documentation of the time and date a correspondence or document was received.

Indexing. Once a document has been released, it is ready to be indexed. **Indexing** is the mental process of selecting the name, title, or classification under which an item will be filed and arranging the units of the title or name in the proper order. For example, information about a patient named *José Gomez* would be filed under *G* for *Gomez*. Selecting the proper classification for an item is critical to finding the document when it is needed.

Coding. **Coding** is the placing of a number, a letter, or an underscore beneath a word to indicate where the document should be filed. For example, in the correspondence of José Gomez, the name *Gomez* would be underscored or coded in some way. Or the code might be written on the document, usually in the upper right-hand corner.

If the document should be coded and filed under more than one title or heading, cross-referencing the document is required. The cross-reference sheet is filed under the cross-reference location. For example, a cross-reference sheet for *José Gomez* might be found under "José."

Sorting. The assistant working with a number of items prepares them for the file by **sorting** them, or arranging them in the order in which they will be filed. Before they can be sorted, documents must be indexed and coded. When the assistant is indexing the item, the code should also be chosen.

Storing. **Storing**, or filing, is the actual placement of an item in its correct place in the file. When the item is placed in the folder, the top of the item should be to the left. Documents are placed in the folder with the most current document on top. The folder is then placed in the file cabinet with the tab side to the rear of the file.

Follow-Up Procedures. Many items that have been stored may require some further action to be taken. For example, even though the correspondence relating to José Gomez has

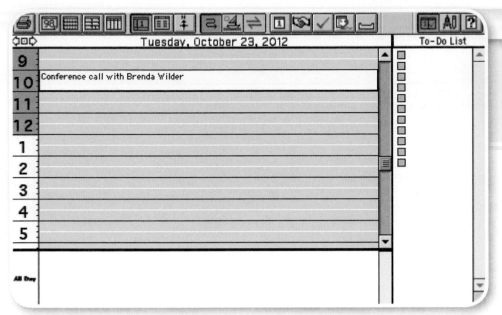

Figure 4.17

An automatic tickler serves as a reminder for follow-up tasks and appointments. *What kinds of items might be noted?*

been filed, Mr. Gomez may require a reminder to return for his annual checkup, which can be done with the use of a tickler file.

A useful tickler file should be consulted daily. An arrangement of index cards by months of the year and, within each month, by days of the month is practical. Notations of actions to be taken are placed on cards behind specific dates of the month. At the end of the current month, new cards are placed behind each date of the next month. There are also electronic monthly calendars available in most software application suites, as shown in Figure 4.17. If actions to be taken are entered on specific dates of the electronic calendar, the software will provide an automatic tickler—a message on the screen—on the appropriate date. The assistant may find this system more efficient and easier to use.

Another way to be reminded of a follow-up action is to use a colored index tab clipped to a patient's record. The colored tab indicates that action is required. Different colors may be assigned to stand for different kinds of actions.

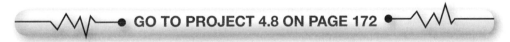

GO TO PROJECT 4.8 ON PAGE 172

Filing Methods

Effective records management requires records to be filed in the way they will be accessed. Most offices use more than one filing method to organize their different types of information. The major filing methods are alphabetic, numeric, and subject. Each method has advantages as well as disadvantages.

Alphabetic Filing.   The most popular filing method is **alphabetic filing**, the arrangement of names, titles, or classifications in alphabetic order. This method is popular because it is based on the familiar letters of the alphabet. It provides a direct reference—if the name is known, the record can be located. An alphabetic method enables a user to find a misfiled paper document easily and has low setup and maintenance costs. It is commonly used by word processing and database software to organize lists of files. Most programs include a sort feature, which automatically alphabetizes a list of entries (Figure 4.18).

COMPLIANCE **TIP**

To protect the confidentiality of medical records and patient PHI, medical charts should be placed backwards in holding areas-the label containing the patient's name will not be visible to anyone walking past the chart.

Figure 4.18

Alphabetized Patient List
in Medisoft®

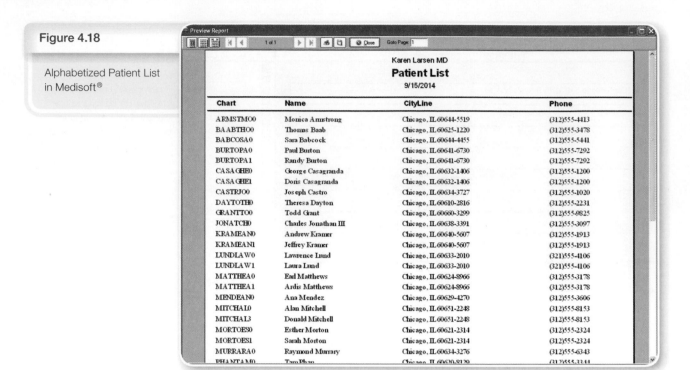

Karen Larsen MD
Patient List
9/15/2014

Chart	Name	CityLine	Phone
ARMSTMO0	Monica Amstrong	Chicago, IL 60644-5519	(312)555-4413
BAABTHO0	Thoms Baab	Chicago, IL 60625-1220	(312)555-3478
BABCOSA0	Sara Babcock	Chicago, IL 60644-4455	(312)555-5441
BURTOPA0	Paul Burton	Chicago, IL 60641-6730	(312)555-7292
BURTOPA1	Randy Burton	Chicago, IL 60641-6730	(312)555-7292
CASAGHE0	George Casagranda	Chicago, IL 60632-1406	(312)555-1200
CASAGHE1	Doris Casagranda	Chicago, IL 60632-1406	(312)555-1200
CASTRJO0	Joseph Castro	Chicago, IL 60634-3727	(312)555-1020
DAYTOTH0	Theresa Dayton	Chicago, IL 60610-2816	(312)555-2231
GRANTTO0	Todd Grant	Chicago, IL 60660-3299	(312)555-9825
JONATCH0	Charles Jonathan III	Chicago, IL 60638-3391	(312)555-3097
KRAMEAN0	Andrew Kramer	Chicago, IL 60640-5607	(312)555-1913
KRAMEAN1	Jeffrey Kramer	Chicago, IL 60640-5607	(312)555-1913
LUNDLAW0	Lawrence Lund	Chicago, IL 60633-2010	(321)555-4106
LUNDLAW1	Laura Lund	Chicago, IL 60633-2010	(321)555-4106
MATTHEA0	Earl Matthews	Chicago, IL 60624-8966	(312)555-3178
MATTHEA1	Ardis Matthews	Chicago, IL 60624-8966	(312)555-3178
MENDEAN0	Ana Mendez	Chicago, IL 60629-4270	(312)555-3606
MITCHAL0	Alan Mitchell	Chicago, IL 60651-2248	(312)555-8153
MITCHAL3	Donald Mitchell	Chicago, IL 60651-2248	(312)555-8153
MORTOES0	Esther Morton	Chicago, IL 60621-2314	(312)555-2324
MORTOES1	Sarah Morton	Chicago, IL 60621-2314	(312)555-2324
MURRARA0	Raymond Murray	Chicago, IL 60634-3276	(312)555-6343
PHANTAM0	Tam Phan	Chicago, IL 60630-8120	(312)555-3344

There are, however, several disadvantages to alphabetic filing. Because the method is so simple and so easily recognizable, there is much less confidentiality. File labels may be easily seen and read; computer files can be quickly searched. It is also possible that similar names will be confused or that a letter will be transposed and the document misfiled. A typing error can cause a patient's information to be filed incorrectly. An alphabetic method for paper records offers limited filing space and makes expanding the system difficult when folders labeled alphabetically are full.

The assistant must thoroughly understand the basic rules for alphabetizing and indexing in order to accurately manage records. ARMA's general rules for alphabetic filing, which are the standard for medical offices, are described in this section.

General Filing Rules

a. Each filing segment is considered a unit.
b. Alphabetize units by comparing letter-by-letter within that unit.
c. Ignore all punctuation marks.
d. File "nothing before something." In a letter-by-letter comparison of two terms, if one term has nothing and the other has an "a," the term with nothing is put first.
e. Arabic and roman numerals are filed sequentially before alphabetic files, with Arabic numerals coming before roman numerals.

Rule 1. Index individual names in the following order: surname (last name), given name (first name), and then middle name or initial.

Names	Indexing Order		
	1	2	3
Wade R. Benje	Benje	Wade	R
Wayne Benje	Benje	Wayne	
Wayne M. Benje	Benje	Wayne	M

Rule 2. Prefixes are considered part of the surname, not separate units. Some prefixes are *Aba, Abd, a la, D', Da, De, Del, De la, Den, Des, Di, Dos, Du, El, Fitz, ibn, La, Las, Le, Lo,*

Los, M, Mac, Mc, O', Saint, San, Santa, Santo, St., Te, Ten, Ter, Van, Van de, Van der, Von, and *Von der.*

Names	Indexing Order		
	1	**2**	**3**
Lorne Fitzgerald	Fitzgerald	Lorne	
Esther Ann O'Reilly	Oreilly	Esther	Ann
David R. Van de Wan	Vandewan	David	R

Rule 3. Index hyphenated names as one unit.

Names	Indexing Order	
	1	**2**
Karen Ames-Battle	Amesbattle	Karen
Ann-Marie Lesa	Lesa	Annmarie

Rule 4. Abbreviated and shortened forms of personal names are not spelled out. Use the abbreviation or shortened form. Make sure the patient states his or her legal name.

Names	Indexing Order		
	1	**2**	**3**
Bill J. Wicks	Wicks	Bill	J
Geo. Lester Wilson	Wilson	Geo	Lester

Rule 5. Professional or personal titles *(Dr., Mr., Mrs., Ms., Prof.)*, professional suffixes *(MD, DDS, Ph.D., CPA)*, and seniority designations are the last indexing unit. When a name has both a title and a suffix, the title is the last unit. If you have only a title and one name, index the name as it is written. In seniority terms, the sequence is numbers *(2nd, 3rd)*, roman numerals *(I, II)*, and then *junior (Jr.)* and *senior (Sr.)*.

Names	Indexing Order		
	1	**2**	**3**
Alan Berg MD	Berg	Alan	MD
Matthew Blue 2nd	Blue	Matthew	2
Charles Jonathan III	Jonathan	Charles	III
Charles Jonathan Jr.	Jonathan	Charles	Jr
Sister Mary-Margaret	Sister	Marymargaret	

Rule 6. When names are identical, index the names by city, state (spelled in full), street name, quadrant *(NE, NW, SE, SW)*, and house or building number in numeric order (lowest number first).

Names

Emily Beck
1055 Maple Lane
Chicago, IL 60623-9623

Emily Beck
8275 Maple Lane
Chicago, IL 60623-9627

Indexing Order

1	2	3	4	5	6	7
Beck	Emily	Chicago	Illinois	Maple	Lane	1055
Beck	Emily	Chicago	Illinois	Maple	Lane	8275

Rule 7. Index business and organizational names as written. When *The, A,* or *An* is the first word of the name, it is indexed as the last unit. Prepositions *(of, in, on, over)* are separate units. Compound expressions are treated as written—if there is a space between terms,

the terms are separate units. Single letters are indexed as written—if they are separated by a space, then they are separate units. Spell out symbols (&, #). Acronyms and call letters (for TV and radio) are single units.

Names	Indexing Order			
	1	2	3	4
A B C Clinic	A	B	C	Clinic
A&D Surgical Supplies	AandD	Surgical	Supplies	
A-B-C Clinic	ABC	Clinic		
Clinic On Main	Clinic	On	Main	
The Free Clinic	Free	Clinic	The	
John St. Claire Clinic	John	Stclaire	Clinic	
South West Clinic	South	West	Clinic	
Southwest Clinic	Southwest	Clinic		
Kare TV Station	Kare	TV	Station	

Rule 8. Arabic numerals and roman numerals are considered a single unit and are filed in numeric order before alphabetic characters (Arabic comes before roman). Ignore ordinal endings (*st, d, th*).

Names	Indexing Order		
	1	2	3
1-A Physical Therapy	1A	Physical	Therapy
5th Avenue Clinic	5	Avenue	Clinic
50+ Retirement Group	50plus	Retirement	Group
Sixty-Third Street Pharmacy	Sixtythird	Street	Pharmacy

Rule 9. Committees, hospitals, universities, hotels, motels, and churches are indexed as written. Cross-reference items to ensure finding them.

Names	Indexing Order			
	1	2	3	4
Alexander Hotel	Alexander	Hotel		
Committee for Academic Affairs (Could be cross-referenced under *Academic Affairs Committee for*)	Committee	for	Academic	Affairs
St. Paul's Medical Center	Stpauls	Medical	Center	
University of Illinois Hospital	University	of	Illinois	Hospital

Rule 10. Government names are indexed first by the governmental unit (country, state, county, or city). Next, index the name of the department, bureau, office, or board. Words such as *Office of* and *Department of* are separate indexing units and are transposed.

Federal Government
The first three units of all federal government names are *United States Government.*

Names	Indexing Order				
	1	2	3	4	5
U.S. Department of Health and Human Services	United	States	Government	Health	and
	6	7	8	9	
	Human	Services	Department	of	

State and Local Governments

Names	Indexing Order				
	1	2	3	4	5
City of Anoka Health Department	Anoka	City	Health	Department	of
Anoka County Health Department	Anoka	County	Health	Department	
Illinois Bureau of Health	Illinois	Health	Bureau	of	

Foreign Governments

Names	Indexing Order				
	1	2	3	4	5
Republic of Sweden Health Department	Sweden	Republic	Health	Department	of

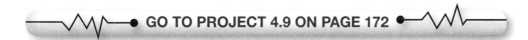

GO TO PROJECT 4.9 ON PAGE 172

Numeric Filing. Offices with a large volume of patient records may use a **numeric filing** system, that is, one in which each patient is assigned a number. The patient number is assigned from an **accession book**, which is a book of consecutive numbers indicating the next available number to be assigned. A cross-index is then prepared to match the numbers with the names. Many electronic medical database programs automatically assign the next available number from within the program's database. In order to access a patient's file, the assistant must first locate the patient's number and then, using the patient's number, access the patient's records. This is considered an indirect access method of locating records. Larger medical facilities maintain a master patient index (MPI), which identifies all patients who have received care at the facility. Patient information can be accessed only after retrieving the assigned patient number from the MPI.

There are several ways to assign numeric values. Two of the most frequently used ways are straight-numeric filing and terminal-digit filing.

1. *Straight-numeric filing*: The straight-numeric system uses ascending numbers in consecutive order. For example, File 125203 would be filed after File 125202 and before File 125204.
2. *Terminal-digit filing*: The terminal-digit system uses the terminal (last) digit, or set of digits, as the indexing unit. The file numbered 33-52-12 would be filed in Section 12 (the last digit) behind 52 (the guide number) and would be the 33rd item in sequence.

There is a filing method that is a combination of alphabetic and numeric filing. This alphanumeric system is used in software available for use in physicians' practices. Medisoft® uses both the alphabet and numbers to assign patient codes (Figure 4.19).

Numeric filing is a very accurate method of filing. It is more difficult to misfile or to lose files. Therefore, there is speedier storage and retrieval. It is a method that helps maintain confidentiality of files. In a numeric filing system, expansion is unlimited, depending only on the next unassigned number in the sequence.

Although numbers provide accuracy, there is still an opportunity to transpose numbers, especially if the sequence is a long one. More guides are required, and there is a need to consult and maintain an alphabetic cross-index. Using the system efficiently also requires a thorough training program for staff members.

Figure 4.19

Medisoft® Screen
Showing Patient Account
Numbers

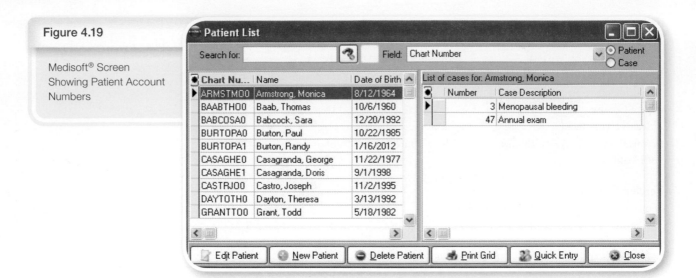

Subject Filing.

Subject filing is the placement of related material alphabetically by subject categories. It is a useful method for keeping nonpatient correspondence, research articles, practice management files, and other material of a general nature. A computer database is also organized by subject. For example, in the Medisoft® program, databases are set up for patients, insurance companies, physicians, and guarantors. (A guarantor is the person who is responsible for payment to the physician.) In each database, the entries are listed alphabetically.

Subject categories depend on the specific needs of the physician and on the amount of material to be filed under each heading. Manuscripts are filed alphabetically under the title of the article or book. Reviews of, and references to, the physician's own writing are also filed under the title of the article or book. Abstracts of research articles, excerpts, and other reviews may be clippings from magazines or newspapers. Whether these are filed by the author's name or by the subject depends on how the physician plans to use the items. Figure 4.20 illustrates a relative subject index with a sample of headings that might be used in subject filing.

When all items pertaining to the same subject may be found in one location, as they are with subject filing, valuable time is saved. Statistics and other types of information are easily accessible. The relative subject index is easy to expand. However, when there is a great amount of material, subject categories may overlap or extensive cross-referencing may be required for complex topics. It can become time-consuming, even for those who are experienced in filing, to file and retrieve materials.

Color-coding.

Color-coding is used in many medical offices. In a color-coded system, typically, the first two or three letters of the surname are placed on the tab. Each letter of the alphabet is a different color; for instance, A is green, B is blue, and so on. All folders within the A section of the files should have a green first label. Therefore, a folder containing a yellow label in the first position would be a misfiled chart. Using this system, it is easy to locate misfiled charts.

Multi-physician practices may use color-coded patient charts. Each physician's patients' charts are identified by color. Differentiating between charts becomes more efficient using this method.

Another use of color-coding indicates different functions. Different colored files are used for various documents, such as lab reports, signature files, or imaging results. Special-colored folders may also be used to forward information for insurance specialists, nurses, office managers, and so on.

Figure 4.20 Relative Subject Index

Advertisements
Drugs
Medical
Office

Automobile
Insurance
Maintenance

Clinic Property
Building
Inventory
Maintenance
Medical Equipment
Office Equipment

Collections
Accounts Receivable
Agency Contracts
Form Letters

Education
Doctor's Continuing
Employee
Patient

Entertainment

Financial Information
Annual Financial
Banking
Monthly Financial

Forms
Applications
Consent
Release from Work
Release of Information

Hospital
Policy
Reports
Staff Meetings

Insurance
Clinic
Fire
Liability—Doctor's

Patients
Index Control File
Patient Billing List

Personnel
Applications—Inactive
Benefits and Policies
Current Employees
Doctor's Personal File—Diplomas,
    Licenses, Publications

Referral Information

Society Information
American Medical Association
Seminars
State Medical Society

Subscriptions and Publications
Drug Companies
Lobby Magazines
Medical Magazines
Newspapers
Professional Library

Supplies
Inventory
Medical
Office
Order Forms

Taxes
Payroll
Personal (Doctor's)
Property

Travel
Expenses
Pending

Utilities
Electricity
Gas
Telephone
Water

Locating Missing Files. Even in a well-organized office, paper documents will occasionally be lost or misfiled. Here are a number of suggestions for locating a missing file:

- Look directly behind and in front of where the item should be filed.
- Look between other files in the area.
- Look in the bottom of the file drawer and under the file folders if they are suspended.
- Check for the transposition of first and last names—for example, *Wheng, Hart* instead of *Hart, Wheng*.
- Check alternate spellings of the name—for example, *Thomasen* and *Thomason*.
- In a numeric filing system, check for transposed numbers—for example, *19-63-01* instead of *19-01-63*.
- In a subject filing system, check related subject files or the Miscellaneous file.
- With the permission of those who have used the file recently, search the desk or work area of previous users of the file.
- Check with other office personnel.

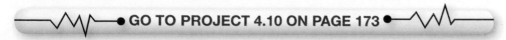
GO TO PROJECT 4.10 ON PAGE 173

The need to store large amounts of medical data and to protect that data efficiently is a primary concern of the medical and governmental communities. Laws have been passed and large sums of money have been and are being invested in the implementation of healthcare reform. Mandatory implementation of **electronic health records (EHRs)** is part of national healthcare reform. Billions of dollars have been directed to be used as incentives for implementing the use of EHRs. Advances in technology and their subsequent affordability make EHRs accessible to healthcare facilities and physicians' practices. It is estimated that 80 percent of healthcare facilities and 50 percent of physicians' practices have already voluntarily implemented EHRs.

Electronic health records are the assimilation and interoperability (electronic systems working together) of various healthcare databases compiled over the course of different patient encounters. Patient demographics, clinical assessment data, lab and other reports, medication lists, progress notes, and other medical data are entered into a software program and then stored electronically. The medical database of the patient is retrieved and updated at each patient encounter. The encounter may be face to face, such as when a child comes to the office for an immunization. It may also be a nonvisit update of the patient's database, as when a patient calls to have a prescription refilled. Figure 4.21 shows an example of a chart summary screen within an EHR, and Figure 4.22 is an example of patient progress note.

Laptops may be in each exam room and/or working area, or the medical team members may carry a TabletPC with them from station to station. Templates and drop-down menus are used to input data into the EHR, with menus providing other selections for the personnel. Space is provided for additional notes and comments. As an example, "blurred vision and headache" may be entered into the chief complaint screen and a drop-down menu of related symptoms may appear. From that point, a screen for review of systems for the cardiovascular system may be provided.

Advantages of Electronic Health Records

EHRs have many advantages over paper-based systems, including accessibility for both medical care personnel and patients. More than one medical team member may use the stored data at the same time. Paper-based records can create a backlog of work when the

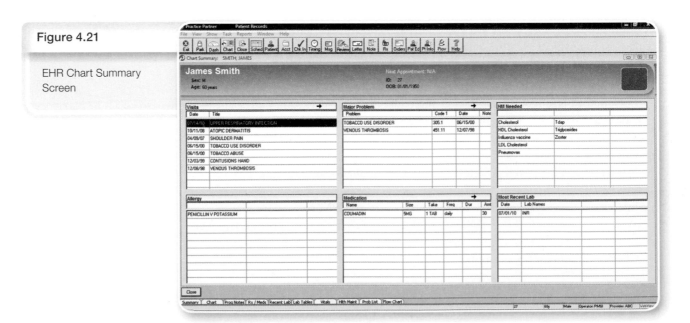

Figure 4.21

EHR Chart Summary Screen

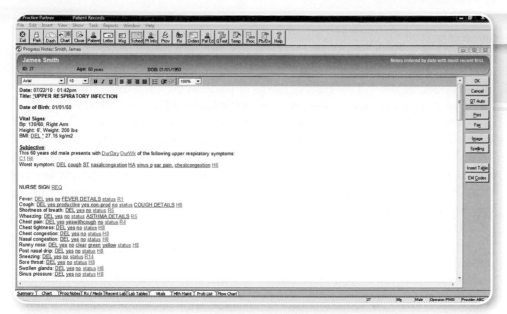

Figure 4.22

EHR Patient
Progress Note

same patient chart is needed to complete a task for different medical team members. Each medical team member has access to electronic data using an individually assigned password. The password allows the medical personnel access to all, or a limited amount, of the medical database. For example, nurses may have access to all areas of patient assessment but not have authorization to view insurance claim information. Using passwords will also create a usage log and an audit trail of individuals accessing medical data, which will increase record security. As more medical records become accessible through the Internet, patients will have access to areas of their EHR. The following are additional advantages offered by EHRs:

1. Easy and quick updating of medical records
2. Automatic verification of medications
3. Fewer medical misinterpretations due to poor handwriting
4. Higher level of data security by use of passwords, encryption, and frequent backup of medical data; minimum backup requirements are to perform a daily backup, with some practices conducting backups throughout the work shift
5. Greater amount of time spent in patient care as a result of less time spent updating medical records
6. Faster questions and answers related to patient medical information
7. Electronic input and submission of orders and prescriptions
8. Electronic reminders sent either directly to patients or to office personnel for follow-up

Challenges of Electronic Health Records

The advantages of converting from paper-based medical records to electronic health records are many, but it is not without challenges. For many facilities and private practices, the cost of EHRs is still prohibitive. Initial cost and contract fees can be too costly for healthcare providers. When evaluating EHR software, update of the system should be a consideration. As the field progresses, technologies advance, and government regulations change, it would be cost-effective for the medical practice to be contracted with a software vendor that will provide the mandatory updates to the system for a contracted amount or as part of the initial cost. Before investing in an electronic health records system, seek information from others who have used or are using the system.

Frequent and ongoing training for medical team members is imperative to ensure the integrity of the input data and the security of the system. New computer and other technology is introduced to society at a fast pace, and healthcare providers must look to cutting-edge technology for medical records storage. Policies and procedures for updating medical personnel and evidence of the training should be placed in the compliance manual.

Converting paper-based records to electronic health records requires the scanning of paper records into the electronic database. This task can be costly and time-consuming—many healthcare providers have chosen to create a position specifically for scanning documents. Even after all office medical documents have been scanned into the system, hardcopy lab reports, consultation letters, and so on may still be received and will need to be scanned into the patient's electronic record. Until electronic health records are fully implemented into the healthcare system, scanners will be needed.

As in a paper-based record, errors will occur, such as transposition of letters and numbers. After a patient encounter, the new electronic medical data should be reviewed and proofread for errors. Medical transcriptionists are skilled in grammar, punctuation, medical terminology, anatomy and physiology, and format. Their expertise provides a needed second look at the documentation. To correct an electronic medical record error, use the same method used to correct a paper-based record. Strike out the erroneous information with a single, straight line. Apply an electronic signature or initials to the correction and key in the correct information. If possible, date the correction. The original electronic data are not removed but may appear lighter than other data. Completely removing electronic data could give the appearance of fraud and is not permissible in many programs.

4.7 MEDICAL TERMINOLOGY AND ABBREVIATIONS

In medical documents, care must be taken with the use of medical terminology and abbreviations. It is important to use only standard, approved abbreviations. Figure 4.23 contains a list of abbreviations commonly used in medical records. The list includes the following types of abbreviations, grouped together and arranged in alphabetical order for ease of use:

- Weights and measures (mainly medication dosages and lab values)—for example, *mL* ("milliliter")
- Designations of times and methods—for example, *b.i.d.* ("twice a day")
- Terms typically found in chart notes—for example, *TPR* ("temperature, pulse, respirations")

It is also important to keep up to date on medical abbreviations that are obsolete or are targeted for nonuse, as shown in Figure 4.24.

4.8 TECHNOLOGIES FOR DATA INPUT

The one thing employees can count on to be consistent is that change will happen. Desktop computers are being replaced by laptops and TabletPCs, and physicians and other healthcare personnel are using smartphones, such as an iPhone, to enter patient data, research medical resources, and keep in contact with other team members. Newer technologies, when used effectively, can help improve productivity and efficiency. Traditional methods of inputting medical data are being integrated, updated, and, in some cases, replaced. As an administrative medical assistant, you must be open to learning new skills and technologies, such as voice recognition for data input, to enhance patient care and increase office productivity.

Figure 4.23 Abbreviations Commonly Used in Medical Records

a.c.	before meals	HEENT	head, eyes, ears, nose, throat	PERRLA	pupils equal, round, reactive to light and accommodation
AP	anteroposterio	HPI	history of present illness		
b.i.d.	twice a day	HS	hour of sleep	PMH	past medical history
BP	blood pressure	I&D	incision and drainage	PSA	prostate specific antigen
BUN	blood urea nitrogen	ICU	intensive care unit	R/O	rule out
C&S	culture and sensitivity	IM	intramuscular	ROS	review of systems
CBC	complete blood count	IV	intravenous	RTC	return to clinic
CC	chief complaint	kg	kilogram	RLQ	right lower quadrant
cc	cubic centimeter	L	liter	RUQ	right upper quadrant
cm	centimeter	LLQ	left lower quadrant	Rx	prescription
CNS	central nervous system	LMP	last menstrual period	SDA	same day appointment
CPE	complete physical exam	LUQ	left upper quadrant	SH	social history
D&C	dilation and curettage	m	meter	S/P	status post
DS	double strength	mcg	microgram	stat or	immediately
DTR	deep tendon reflexes	mEq	milliequivalent	STAT	
Dx	diagnosis	mg	milligram	STD	sexually transmitted disease
ECG	electrocardiogram	mL	milliliter		
EEG	electroencephalogram	mm	millimeter	T&A	tonsillectomy and adenoidectomy
EENT	eyes, ears, nose, throat	n.p.o.	nothing by mouth		
ENT	ears, nose, throat	OB	obstetrics	t.i.d.	three times a day
EOM	extraocular movements	OTC	over-the-counter (as in medications)	TM	tympanic membrane
ER	emergency room			TPR	temperature, pulse, respirations
FH	family history	P&A	percussion and auscultation		
F/U	follow-up			UA	urinalysis
FUO	fever unknown origin	p.c.	after meals	UC	urine culture
Fx	fracture	p.o.	per os (by mouth)	URI	upper respiratory infection
g or gm	gram	p.r.n.	as desired or as needed	UTI	urinary tract infection
GI	gastrointestinal	PE	physical exam	VD	venereal disease
gr	grain	PERLA	pupils equal, reactive to light and accommodation	VS	vital signs
GU	genitourinary			wbc	white blood cells
GYN	gynecology			WBC	white blood count
h	hour			WNL	within normal limits
H&P	history and physical				

Traditional Data Input

Electronic recording and storage of medical data is rapidly becoming the preferred method of documenting medical data. Prior to electronic storage, medical data were and, for some offices still are, maintained through verbal recordings and typed/keyed.

Transcription. Many offices today input medical data using the **transcription** method. The physician, or other provider of medical care, dictates the medical data into a recording device (tape recorder or phone recording system) to be transcribed by a keyboardist who specializes in medical data keyboarding. The transcriptionist will listen to the dictation, either from tapes or from other recorded media, and transcribe the verbal medical data into keyed format. Medical offices may employ their own transcriptionist or may use a transcription service.

A thorough knowledge of grammar and punctuation, medical terminology, and anatomy and physiology and accurate keyboarding skills are required. Medical transcriptionists must also be able to proofread medical documents with a high level of proficiency. Mistakes in medical documentation can lead to a vast array of consequences. Misdiagnoses can take place when medical decisions are made based on errors in transcribed documents. Consider

Figure 4.24 The Joint Commission

Official "Do Not Use" List[1]

Do Not Use	Potential Problem	Use Instead
U (unit)	Mistaken for "0" (zero), the number "4" (four), or "cc"	Write "unit"
IU (International Unit)	Mistaken for IV (intravenous) or the number 10 (ten)	Write "International Unit"
Q.D., QD, q.d., qd (daily)	Mistaken for each other	Write "daily"
Q.O.D., QOD, q.o.d, qod (every other day)	Period after the Q mistaken for "I" and the "O" mistaken for "I"	Write "every other day"
Trailing zero (X.0 mg)*	Decimal point is missed	Write X mg
Lack of leading zero (.X mg)		Write 0.X mg
MS	Can mean morphine sulfate or magnesium sulfate	Write "morphine sulfate" Write "magnesium sulfate"
MSO$_4$ and MgSO$_4$	Confused for one another	

[1] Applies to all orders and all medication-related documentation that is handwritten (including free-text computer entry) or on pre-printed forms.

*Exception: A "trailing zero" may be used only where required to demonstrate the level of precision of the value being reported, such as for laboratory results, imaging studies that report size of lesions, or catheter/tube sizes. It may not be used in medication orders or other medication-related documentation.

Additional Abbreviations, Acronyms, and Symbols
(For possible future inclusion in the Official "Do Not Use" List)

Do Not Use	Potential Problem	Use Instead
> (greater than)	Misinterpreted as the number "7" (seven) or the letter "L"	Write "greater than"
< (less than)	Confused for one another	Write "less than"
Abbreviations for drug names	Misinterpreted due to similar abbreviations for multiple drugs	Write drug names in full
Apothecary units	Unfamiliar to many practitioners Confused with metric units	Use metric units
@	Mistaken for the number "2" (two)	Write "at"
cc	Mistaken for U (units) when poorly written	Write "mL" or "ml" or "milliliters" ("mL" is preferred)
μg	Mistaken for mg (milligrams) resulting in one thousand-fold overdose	Write "mcg" or "micrograms"

© The Joint Commission, 2010. Reprinted with permission.

what would happen to a patient who was directed to take 5 mg of a prescribed medication when the amount should have been 0.5 mg.

Transcriptionists use templates to input medical data. Different formats include a history and physical format for general practitioners, radiologic reports for radiologists, and cardiovascular evaluations for thoracic surgeons. Although medical specialties may adjust formats to meet their documentation requirements, generalized rules for transcribing materials should be used. A sampling of these guidelines can be found at the Online Learning Center for this textbook.

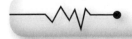 **GO TO PROJECT 4.5, IF ASSIGNED, ON PAGE 171**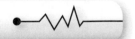

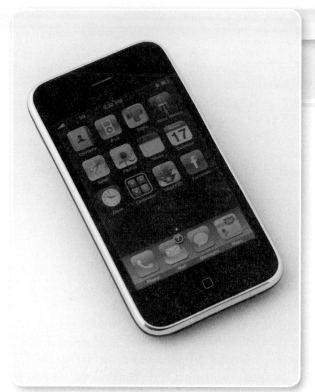

Figure 4.25

Wireless Smartphone Device

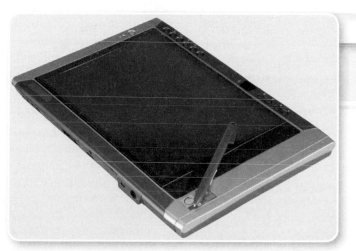

Figure 4.26

Portable Wireless Notepad

The future of transcription is changing. As electronic health records are implemented in the medical field, transcriptionists may proofread and edit documentation. Different input technologies, discussed in the next section, allow physicians to input data directly into medical records. However, proofreading and editing medical documentation for errors, such as punctuation, will still be a much-needed skill. The high cost of implementing electronic health records makes the highly skilled transcriptionist a valued medical team member.

Newer Input Technologies

Voice-Recognition Technology. A technology being used in medical and other offices for data input is **voice-recognition technology**. Using voice-recognition software, the dictator speaks into a headset that has been specifically trained for his or her voice. As the dictator speaks, data are input into the medical record. Some refer to this as "typing on the fly." Software efficiency varies. Some software requires the dictator to dictate all punctuation, while other software punctuations are based on the next given command, such as "new paragraph." Voice-recognition technology provides a hands-free input method that can reduce the possibility of keyed errors. With practice, data that are input with voice-recognition technology can be recorded at a faster rate than keyed words per minute, and individuals can multitask. This is not always an advantage, however, as errors can occur with dictation when attention is diverted to other tasks. Noise-filtering headsets should be used to filter out unwanted noise in the surrounding environment. Another disadvantage is that different lingual accents may "confuse" the software and produce flawed documentation.

Wireless Technology. Wireless technology, such as Smartphones, is used not only for social networking and communication but also for medical data input. Physicians may use these technologies to access and update patient and other medical office information. Wireless technologies allow medical team members to retrieve items such as e-mail and calendars through electronic devices. Patient information can be retrieved through Internet medical records, and medical decisions can be made without the need for the physician to return to the office. Current technologies for wireless devices require Internet accessibility through WiFi or an Internet service plan, which may be costly to a medical practice. Wireless iPods provide many of the same features as a wireless Smartphone device. However, a wireless iPod requires a WiFi connection instead of an Internet service plan; consequently, this device must be used in locations that have a WiFi connection. Wireless iPods are not phones—the physician must carry a separate phone. Physicians also use personal digital assistants (PDAs) and iPods for data input. Both are small and portable, making them convenient for mobile and remote data entry. Wireless devices are illustrated in Figures 4.25 and 4.26.

Remember, change will happen. As electronic health records are fully implemented in the medical environment, assistants must be flexible and willing to learn new technologies and to integrate the old with the new. It is an exciting time to be part of such a progressive environment.

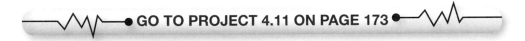

GO TO PROJECT 4.11 ON PAGE 173

Chapter Projects

Project 4.1 · **Internet Research: E-mail Features**

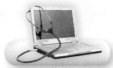

Using the Internet, research the features of an e-mail service. Create a list of five e-mail facts. Send this list as an attachment in an e-mail to your instructor.

Project 4.2 · **Computer Technology**

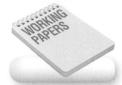

WP 39 contains statements that refer to computer technology in the medical office. Mark each statement with either "T" for true or "F" for false. For false statements, state why the statement is false. Be prepared to discuss your answers.

Project 4.3 · **Internet Research: Medical Records Institute**

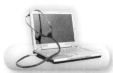

The Medical Records Institute promotes the development and acceptance of electronic health records systems nationally and internationally. The organization offers resources on electronic health records. It also is a network for exchanging knowledge, experiences, and solutions among healthcare professionals who are using or are interested in using electronic medical records systems. Visit the Web site at www.medrecinst.com, and check the current survey results regarding barriers to electronic records, possible solutions, and facilities that use electronic records.

Project 4.4 · **Chart Entries**

Dr. Larsen instructs you to make the following chart notations for her signature. Both should be dated October 13.

- Sara Babcock: Patient called for refill of Ortho Tri-Cyclen®. She has a physical scheduled for October 21, and we will deal with the prescription renewal at that time.
- Jeffrey Kramer: Father called for OTC help for Jeffrey for sore throat and earache. I advised the father to make an appointment as soon as possible. Patient to gargle with warm salt water q.3-4h. and be given children's Tylenol® for pain relief p.r.n.

Project 4.5 · **Chart Transcription—Optional Project**

Dr. Larsen has dictated her findings on the patients from October 14 and 15. Obtain the transcription source from your instructor. Use the formats presented in Figures 4.11 and 4.12 to transcribe the dictation onto each patient's medical record.

Project 4.6 · **Lab Message Entries**

The following lab results were received by telephone message. Dr. Larsen instructed you to make notations in the charts for her signature.

- October 16: Gary Robertson's urine culture results from October 14 show Enterobacter greater than 100,000 colonies, sensitive to sulfa. Left message for patient with results. Patient to continue Septra and follow up in two weeks, sooner p.r.n.
- October 16: Erin Mitchell's urine culture results from October 14 revealed bacterial count greater than 100,000/mL. Talked with patient today. Patient to continue ciprofloxacin as directed. RTC if symptoms do not clear.

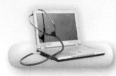

Project 4.7 | **Internet Research: Using AHIMA as a Resource**

AHIMA exists to serve health information management professionals. The organization offers credentials such as Registered Health Information Administrator. Like many professional groups, this organization also keeps those responsible for managing information current with the latest legislation and news and serves consumers of healthcare with topics of interest to them. Visit the AHIMA Web site at www.ahima.org. Follow the link from the home page to the page that allows you to search by key word. Key in the term *patient record* and read one of the articles related to this topic. Two other key words that will be of interest are *information security* and *patient confidentiality.* Read at least one article on each of these topics. Be prepared to share the results of your reading with the class. Contact information for AHIMA is shown below.

> American Health Information Management Association
> 233 North Michigan Avenue, Suite 2150
> Chicago, IL 60601
> Phone: 312-233-1100
> Web site: www.ahima.org
> E-mail: info@ahima.org

Project 4.8 | **Cross-Referencing**

Indicate the file and cross-reference entries for the following:

- Randolph Car Service (formerly Carl's Car Service)
- James Henry University
- File folders bought from Oliver Systems and Viking Office Supplies

Project 4.9 | **Preparing Patients' Files**

Dr. Larsen maintains a file folder for each patient. You will find the patient information forms on the CD-ROM that accompanies this text workbook. Print out each form and begin an alphabetic file for each patient. Note that each patient should have an individual chart or file. Material that pertains to each patient should be filed chronologically within that patient's folder. Prepare a chart note and new folder whenever a new patient arrives for an appointment.

Prepare the chart note in this way: Center the words *CHART NOTE* on the first line. Triple space; then key information about the patient as shown below. Save the document on your external storage device by the patient's last name, followed by the first initial: *Armstrong, M.*

Update information on the patient information form as necessary. You may update the form on the CD-ROM and print a new form if a patient changes a home address, for example. Place the alphabetized patient folders in your expandable portfolio.

medisoft

Print a list of all patients. Check this list against the patient information forms you printed from the CD-ROM. (*Hint:* The Patient List report is available on the Reports menu, under the Custom Report List option.)

Project 4.10 Using Subject Filing

On a plain sheet of paper, write the subject heading for each of the following items. Use Figure 4.20 as a guideline for your choices. Be prepared to discuss your answers in class.

- A copy of an article that Dr. Larsen had published in the *Journal of the American Medical Association (JAMA)*
- A new contract for employees' health insurance
- A bulletin about next month's continuing education seminar for the nursing staff
- The minutes from the hospital staff's last meeting
- A December itinerary for a symposium related to family practice physicians that Dr. Larsen will attend.

Project 4.11

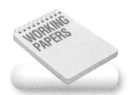

WP 40 contains statements that refer to electronic health records. Write "True" or False" in the blank to indicate whether you think the statement is true or false. If the answer is false, indicate what makes the statement false. Be prepared to discuss your answers.

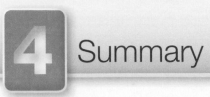
4.1 Classify various uses of computer technology. Pages 128–139	<ul><li>Computer usage in a medical environment has increased tremendously in recent years. Office tasks that traditionally were completed by hand are now done with a high degree of efficiency by using a computer<ul><li>Scheduling—Appointment availability can be quickly accessed and schedules can be completed. Past, current, and future appointments can be viewed, created, and changed within specific computer menus.</li><li>Medical data entry—Patients' medical records can be created electronically. Patient data can be input into the electronic health records, prescriptions may be electronically prepared and either given to the patient or sent directly to the pharmacy, and orders for lab tests and procedures can be automatically processed.</li><li>Communications—Information is transmitted via the Internet within the office or across the globe. The ease, cost-effectiveness, and speed of e-mail have made it the leading form of intraoffice and interoffice communications.</li><li>Research—Physicians can research medical conditions, search for drug interactions, conduct webinars, and perform other clinical tasks through the use of technology.</li></ul></li><li>Computers have integrated all phases of the medical community and will continue to be an asset to patient care.</li></ul>
4.2 Recall reasons for maintaining a medical chart and documents which compile the medical chart. Pages 139–142	<ul><li>Medical records are used as the main source of medical data for patients and they provide for continuity of care. They supply health information and protected health information such as diagnoses and treatments for patients. Medical charts are legal documents.</li><li>Examples of documents that may be found in a medical chart are<ul><li>Chart notes.</li><li>History and physicals.</li><li>Clinical forms.</li><li>Medical reports.</li><li>Communications with the patient or with other medical personnel concerning the patient.</li></ul></li></ul>

4.3 Identify components of a paper-based medical record and explain how the same components will be compiled in an electronic health record format. Pages 142–147	• Notes from the patient encounter, such as the chief complaint, history, examination, impression/diagnosis, and treatment plan, are documented in a patient medical chart using various formats, such as SOAP. Lab reports, nurses' assessment, dietician plans, and so on are placed into the chart either by encounter or by category—for instance, all nurses' assessments, would be placed in a section. • Electronic input of these and other medical chart components is completed through main screens and drop-down menus. As data are input into the electronic health record, other options may be presented or additional space will be provided for comments. • Electronic health records can be quickly searched for data, and information from encounters can be compared.
4.4 Distinguish among active, inactive, and closed files. Pages 147–151	• In a medical environment, a large number of medical records must be managed. Records are often classified by their activity. Three broad classifications are — Active files—medical records for current patients. — Inactive files—medical records for patients who have not seen the physician in a predetermined amount of time, such as six months to a year. — Closed files—medical records for patients who have moved away, have terminated their patient-physician relationship, or are deceased. As each medical specialty has its own requirements, a retention schedule should be developed by the practice based on its needs and state statutes.
4.5 Differentiate among the records management systems that may be used in a medical office. Pages 151–163	• Commonly used records management systems are alphabetic, numeric, and subject. — Alphabetic filing—traditionally, the most frequently used system. This system manages records based on the alphabet and is easy to train office personnel in its use. However, the lack of confidentiality (the patient's name is on the label) makes this system vulnerable to unintentional disclosure of PHI.

	— Numeric filing—uses a combination of numbers, not a Social Security number, to maintain patient information. Because the patient's name does not appear on the label, this system provides a higher level of protection for PHI. Numeric filing is widely used in medical environments. Indirect access and employee training are two disadvantages of numeric filing. — Subject filing—classifies records by subject titles, such as Invoices or Journals. This is useful when a group of similar data needs to be filed together. Indexes must be used for both the subject and numeric systems.
4.6 Discuss the advantages and challenges of electronic health records implementation. Pages 164–166	• As the mandatory use of EHRs quickly approaches, many advantages may be gained from implementation: — Multiple users at the same time — Data protection through passwords, encryption, and backup — Quick and easy update of records — Automatic verification of prescriptions — Fewer errors due to handwriting — More time spent with patients — Faster access to data — Electronic submission of orders and prescriptions — Electronic reminders to patients • Implementation also presents challenges: — Updating of system — Ongoing training — Scanning of hardcopy documents into the system — Inputting typographical errors
4.7 List three medical abbreviations that have been targeted by JACHO as not to be used. Page 166	• Similar medical abbreviations may contribute to a misdiagnosis or misinterpretation. JACHO has distributed a listing of "Do Not Use" abbreviations. The following are three examples: — U for unit — IU for international unit — Q. or q. for every — MS for either morphine sulfate or magnesium sulfate

4.8 Discuss the various input technologies used to create medical documentation. Pages 166–170	• Newer input technologies, such as voice-recognition software, wireless devices, and PDAs, allow the input of data with greater speed and mobility. This, in turn, allows more time for patient care.
	— Voice-recognition software enables the dictator to train the program to his or her voice, and data are input by speaking into the trained device.
	— Wireless technology, such as Smartphones, allow the input of medical data into extremely small, portable devices. WiFi connection is now available at many locations, allowing data to be input directly into a patient's electronic health record. A physician visiting a patient in the hospital can research medical contraindications from his or her wireless device without the need to leave the patient's room or the facility.
	— Traditionally, transcription has been used for medical data input. Physicians dictate data into recording devices and transcriptionists key in transcribed documents for the physician's verification and signature. The field of transcription is evolving, just as technology continues to evolve. Transcriptionists will be needed to edit medical data entered through electronic devices, such as voice recognition. Opportunities for "scribes"—individuals who input patient medical data into electronic storage as the physician dictates or provides data—exist for individuals with transcription training and/or experience.

Soft Skills Success

Teamwork

Effective teamwork can produce incredible results, but teamwork does not just happen. It takes a great deal of work and compromise. Knowing how to work on or with a team will be crucial to your success. Before we can reward teamwork and collaboration that integrates care, we need applications that let clinicians communicate patient information instantly and securely. **How can teamwork be beneficial to EHR and the medical office?**

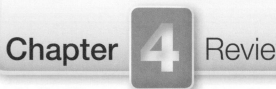 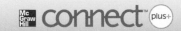
USING TERMINOLOGY

Match the term or phrase on the left with the correct answer on the right.

_____ 1. (LO 4.1) Word processing

_____ 2. (LO 4.3) SOAP

_____ 3. (LO 4.4) Active record

_____ 4. (LO 4.1) File server

_____ 5. (LO 4.5) Out indicator

_____ 6. (LO 4.6) Electronic health record

_____ 7. (LO 4.2) Medicolegal

_____ 8. (LO 4.3) ROS

_____ 9. (LO 4.8) Wireless communication

_____ 10. (LO 4.8) Voice-recognition technology

a. The use of radio waves to transmit data

b. A record of removed information

c. Records that provide proof of legal medical care

d. Software program used to enter, edit, format, and print documents

e. Technology used to input data using speech training

f. Heath care databases that work together to compile complete patient healthcare records

g. Medical documentation format that includes subjective and objective data, assessment of data, and course of treatment

h. A subjective assessment of pertinent body systems

i. Records of current patients

j. Centralized storage of shared network electronic data

CHECK YOUR UNDERSTANDING

Select the most correct answer.

1. (LO 4.1) Maria works exclusively inputting data into medical records. She seldom takes a break from inputting and works 4 days per week, 10 hours each day. While driving, she noticed a change in her distance vision. Which of the following should she do to help ease eye strain while working?

   a. Place her hands and wrists in horizontal alignment

   b. Regularly focus on a distant object

   c. Place source documents flat beside her computer

   d. Frequently rotate her neck and shoulders

2. (LO 4.2) Lori works for a medical practice that uses the first three letters of the patient's last name and the date of birth as patient numbers. When Lori was filing medical insurance claims, she noticed that a chart note had been made in the wrong chart. The physician sees twin females, and the chart for the wrong twin had been noted. To correct the error, she should

   a. Eliminate the chart note with correction fluid.

   b. Use a wide, permanent black marker to cross out the chart note.

   c. Place a straight line through the entry, making sure it is still legible; mark it "error"; date her correction; and initial the correction.

   d. Place a wavy line through the entry, making sure it is still legible; mark it "error"; date her correction; and initial the correction.

3. (LO 4.3) When Dr. Lee opened the EHR for his next patient, he was able to quickly view a listing of all the patient's current and previously treated medical conditions. Which documentation format does Dr. Lee use?

   a. SOAP
   b. CHEDDAR
   c. DATABASE
   d. POMR

4. (LO 4.4) After 10 years of practice, the administrative medical assistant observed that the medical charts container was full and hardcopy records were hard to retrieve and return due to overcrowding. No retention schedule had yet been developed. Which of the following strategies could be used efficiently to ease the overcrowding?

   a. Shred all records for patients who have not been seen in three years or more
   b. Retrieve all the inactive folders and place them in a corner
   c. Remove and shred all files for deceased patients
   d. Remove folders for inactive and closed files and move them to a secure, secondary location

5. (LO 4.5) Medical records in the office are marked with the patient number in the upper right-hand corner of the documents. This is known as

   a. Inspecting a document.
   b. Indexing a document.
   c. Coding a document.
   d. Storing a document.

6. (LO 4.6) Because of the high cost of EHR implementation and anticipated software updates, which of the following should not be considered when purchasing a program?

   a. A software program package that does not include future updates as part of the initial cost or at a stated cost
   b. Availability of ongoing software training by the manufacturer
   c. Ease of use
   d. Information from others who use the software

7. (LO 4.7) Which of the following is an acceptable chart notation for "as needed"?

   a. q.4h
   b. p.r.n.
   c. a.n.
   d. as ndd

8. (LO 4.8) Jamie does transcription for a local multi-physician practice. She has heard about the implementation of EHRs and is concerned about the future of her position. Which of the following would be beneficial for Jamie?

   a. Immediately resign from her position and return to school for training in a different field
   b. Become involved in the selection process of an EHR program and contribute observations on the documentation template
   c. Continue to update herself on grammar, punctuation, and format
   d. Both b and c are beneficial options for Jamie.

MEDICAL VOCABULARY USED WITH OPTIONAL TRANSCRIPTION

Be sure that you are familiar with the following terms:

adnexa   accessory parts to the main structure
amoxicillin   an antibiotic
anginal   relating to constricting chest pain
bronchitis   inflammation in the bronchi
bruit   murmur
colonoscopy   visualization of the colon with a scope
costochondritis   inflammation of the cartilage between the ribs
dysmenorrhea   menstrual cramps
dysuria   painful or difficult urination
ecchymosis   black and blue or purple skin discoloration; bruise
exudative   relating to tissue material deposited as a result of infection
gallop   an abnormal heart sound
hepatosplenomegaly   liver and spleen enlargement
injection   inserting a solution under the skin (subcutaneously, intravenously, or intra-muscularly) using a syringe or a needle
lymphadenopathy   enlargement of lymph nodes
malaise   feeling of uneasiness
normocephalic   relating to a normal-size head
ophthalmic   relating to the eye
otitis media   inflammation of the ear
PE tubes   polyethylene tubes
pharyngitis   inflammation of the throat
rhonchi   musical pitch heard on chest auscultation
sclera   the white of the eye
Sitz bath   a type of bath that consists of soaking the area from the tailbone to the lower abdomen in a tub of warm water
supple   easily moveable
tinea cruris   a fungal infection in the male perineal or groin area
tonsillitis   inflammation of the tonsils

THINKING IT THROUGH

These questions cover the most important points in this chapter. Using your critical-thinking skills, play the role of an administrative medical assistant as you answer each question. Be prepared to present your responses in class.

1. You are going through a patient's medical record to find information on a specific lab report, and you notice that several chart notes are not dated. What should you do?
2. How does the use of the SOAP format for record keeping minimize a provider's exposure to legal risk?

3. You retrieve a patient's medical record and notice that the abbreviation *WDWNWF* is used several times in the chart notes. You know that this is not an approved abbreviation, though you eventually figure out that it stands for "well-developed, well-nourished white female." What do you do with this information?

4. You are asked to retrieve information regarding a patient's family history of intestinal cancer. The physician generally uses the POMR format. Where in the file should you look?

5. A former patient calls, hoping to locate x-rays taken more than five years ago. What should you say?

6. A patient calls and is moving out of town. She is concerned about her medical record. What would you suggest?

7. You are transcribing the physician's dictation and cannot understand several words in a chart note. What do you do?

Simulation 1

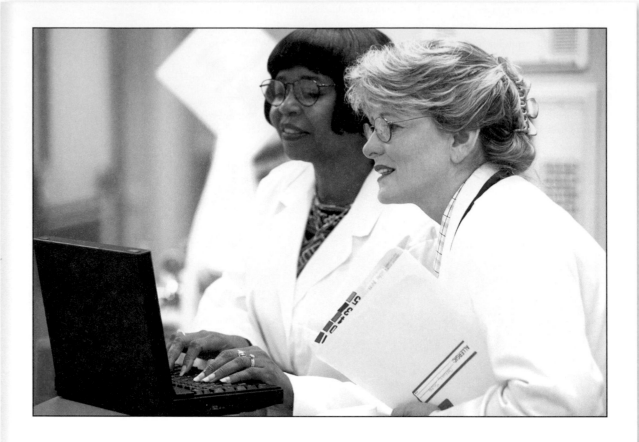

YOUR ROLE

Welcome to the practice of Dr. Karen Larsen! Today, you begin to apply the skills you have learned in this text as you assume the role of Linda Schwartz, Dr. Larsen's administrative medical assistant.

Simulation 1 is the first of three simulations in the text. These simulations provide practical experience in working in a physician's office. You will discover how various tasks relate to each other. The daily events in the office are narrated on the Simulation Recordings that accompany the text. As you listen to the recordings, you will handle various assignments as the assistant. Your simulation work will include making and canceling appointments, preparing messages, creating communications, preparing various medical forms, and following through on daily tasks.

Simulation 1

BEFORE YOU START

The following suggestions apply to all the simulations:

1. Review the content of the previous chapters to ensure familiarity with procedures.
2. Prepare three file folders:
   a. Label as *Day 1 and your name.*
   b. Label as *Day 2 and your name.*
   c. Label as *Day 3 and your name.*
3. Assemble and organize necessary materials as listed under *Materials* on the next page.
4. Set priorities each day by organizing your work in order of importance and completing the work in that sequence. Any work left over from Day 1 should be carried over into Day 2, and so forth. The work left over from any previous day should be taken into account in setting the priorities for that day. It is also possible that you may have work left over from the final day. It is important to remember to complete major tasks each day.
5. Be prepared for interruptions. These occur frequently as they would in a physician's office. Do not let interruptions upset you—learn to rearrange priorities.
6. Develop shortcuts, easier procedures, and better ways of doing tasks.

PROCEDURES

Day 1, Tuesday, October 14

1. Check today's appointments. Pull chart folders for today's appointments. Keep them together.
2. Organize any other materials you will need. Arrange your desk in an orderly fashion, leaving room for you to work.
3. Use your *To-Do List* (WP 55), checking off tasks as you complete them.

4. Use the *Telephone Log* form (WP 54) to list the answering service and all incoming calls. Make only brief notations on this form, checking off items as you follow through on them.
5. The simulation begins with the call to the answering service. You will hear conversations between the assistant and the answering service, the patients, and other callers. (Remember, you are assuming the role of Linda Schwartz, administrative medical assistant for Karen Larsen, MD.) You will hear Dr. Larsen giving you directions and dictation. You will *not* hear the voices of all patients—only those who ask you to do something.
6. Dr. Larsen may give new directions. There may be additional telephone calls. Listen to the conversations continuously, stopping to obtain information, to have information repeated, and to obtain the appointment calendar, message blanks, and other items. Make appropriate notes as you listen.
7. As you complete tasks, place them in your *Day 1* folder, organizing them as directed by your instructor. Place any incomplete work in your *Day 2* folder.

Day 2, Wednesday, October 15

1. Follow the same procedures as in Day 1. Remember that some of Day 2's new items may be more important than work left over from Day 1. Again, listen to conversations continuously, stopping as necessary.
2. At the end of Day 2, put all your completed work in the Day 2 folder, following your instructor's directions. Follow your instructor's advice with what to do with incomplete work.

Simulation 1

MATERIALS

You will need the following materials to complete Simulation 1. If these materials are not already in the proper folders, obtain them from the sources indicated.

Materials	Source
Appointment calendar	
Supplies folder:	
Appointment cards	WP 35
Letterhead	CD-ROM
Notepad	You provide.
Plain paper	You provide.
Patient information forms	WP 51 & 52
Records release form	WP 53
Telephone log	WP 54
Telephone message blanks	WP 9–16
To-do list	WP 55

To-Do Items

Note: If you have completed all the projects and do not have the following listed items, discuss the missing items with your instructor.

Day 1 folder:
Place patients' charts for October 14.

Day 2 folder:
Place patients' charts for October 15.

Miscellaneous folder:
Wanda Norberg, MD—message (Project 3.5) and interoffice memo (Project 3.2)

Patients' folders:

The following patients' folders (charts) should contain the chart note, patient information form, and any other items listed.

Armstrong, Monica
Baab, Thomas
Babcock, Sara—message   (Project 3.5)
Burton, Randy
Casagranda, Doris
Castro, Joseph
Dayton, Theresa
Grant, Todd
Jonathan, Charles III
Kramer, Jeffrey—message   (Project 3.5)
Matthews, Ardis
Mendez, Ana
Morton, Sarah
Murrary, Raymond
Phan, Marc
Richards, Warren
Roberts, Suzanne
Robertson, Gary
Sherman, Florence—referral letter,   (Project 3.1)
  chart note, and envelope
Sinclair, Gene
Sun, Cheng
Villano, Stephen

EVALUATION

You will be evaluated as follows:

1. Good judgment in establishing priorities—did you use good judgment? Did you accomplish the most important tasks?
2. Work of good quality—are tasks accurate and neat?
3. Quantity—did you complete a reasonable amount of work? Would a physician be satisfied with your rate of accomplishment?

medisoft MEDISOFT® INSTRUCTIONS

If your instructor has assigned the use of Medisoft®, you will complete certain parts of Simulation 1 using the software program.

To complete this simulation in Medisoft®, you must be able to:

- Schedule appointments
- Print a physician's schedule
- Enter new patients
- Update patient information

Specific instructions are in Appendix A.

Enter the new appointments in Office Hours. Then print Dr. Larsen's schedule for October 14 and 15. Remember that Office Hours uses the Windows System Date as the default date, so you will need to change the date that appears in the Office Hours calendar.

Enter the two new patients. Information about new patients is entered in the Patient/Guarantor dialog box and the Case dialog box. In the Patient/Guarantor dialog box, complete the following boxes:

Name, Address Tab
Chart Number
Last Name
First Name
Middle Name
Street
City
State
ZIP Code
Home Phone
Birthdate
Sex
Social Security Number

Other Information Tab
Type
Assigned Provider
Signature on File
Emergency Contact: Name, Home Phone

In the Case dialog box, data should be entered in the following boxes:

Personal Tab
Description
Guarantor
Marital Status

Policy 1
Insurance 1
Policy Holder 1
Relationship to Insured
Policy Number
Group Number
Assignment of Benefits/Accept Assignment (yes)
Insurance Coverage Percents:
  Box A: 80
  Boxes B–H: 0

Edit the record for the patient whose phone number has changed. Edit the record for the patient whose phone number and address have changed.

Office Management

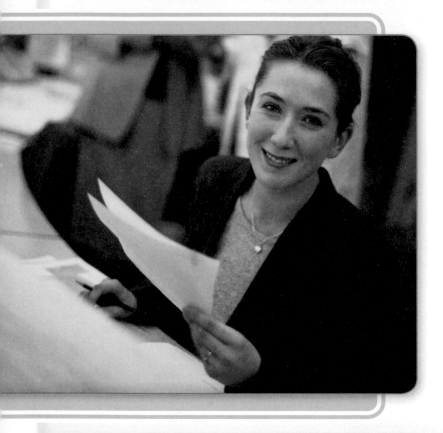

Copyright © 2012 McGraw-Hill Higher Education

LEARNING OUTCOMES
After studying this chapter, you will be able to:

5.1 Design a medical office waiting area that exhibits the priority of patient comfort.

5.2 Identify three stress triggers in your own life and define at least one method of reducing the associated negative stress.

5.3 Differentiate among three common leadership/management styles.

5.4 Explain why an administrative medical assistant needs to know how to collect and assimilate research data.

5.5 Classify items into major categories of needed information when making traveling arrangements.

5.6 Justify why a policies and procedures manual should be developed and used in a medical office.

KEY TERMS
Study these important words, which are defined in this chapter, to build your professional vocabulary:

agenda

authoritarian/autocratic

delegative/laissez-faire

ergonomics

itinerary

management qualifications

meeting minutes

outside services file

participative/democratic

patient education materials

patient information brochure

perfectionism

policies and procedures manual

reprints

stress

travel agent

Chapter 5

ABHES

- Adapt to change.
- Maintain confidentiality at all times.
- Use appropriate guidelines when releasing records or information.
- Project a positive attitude.
- Be cognizant of ethical boundaries.
- Evidence a responsible attitude.
- Conduct work within scope of education, training, and ability.
- Professional components.
- Maintain licenses and accreditation.
- Maintain liability coverage.
- Monitor legislation related to current healthcare issues and practices.
- Locate resources and information for patients and employers.
- Manage physician's professional schedule.
- Use proper telephone techniques.
- Apply electronic technology.
- Apply computer concepts for office procedures.
- Follow established policy in initiating or terminating medical treatment.

➡ Cognitive
➡ Psychomotor
➡ Affective

- Exercise efficient time management.
- Receive, organize, prioritize, and transmit information efficiently.
- Fundamental writing skills.
- Orient and train personnel.

CAAHEP

➡ Identify nonverbal communication.
➡ Recognize communication barriers.
➡ Identify techniques for overcoming communication barriers.
➡ Discuss the role of assertiveness in effective professional communication.
➡ Identify time management principles.
➡ List and discuss legal and illegal interview questions.
➡ Identify how the Americans with Disabilities Act (ADA) applies to the medical assisting profession.
➡ Discuss all levels of governmental legislation and regulation as they apply to the medical assisting practice, including FDA and DEA regulations.
➡ Describe the process to follow if an error is made in patient care.
➡ Respond to issues of confidentiality.
➡ Complete an incident report.
➡ Demonstrate sensitivity to patients' rights.
➡ Recognize the importance of local, state, and federal legislation and regulations in a practice setting.

INTRODUCTION

The word *administrative* in the administrative medical assistant's job title refers to more than clerical or office tasks that contribute to the care of patients. The word also describes the management functions that assistants fulfill on a daily basis. In many practices, career advancement to office management may be an outgrowth of skills and abilities used every day on the job.

This chapter deals with management of the physical medical office environment; the types of management, such as stress and conflict management; and **management qualifications**—the skills, abilities, and responsibilities of the medical assistant in the role of office manager, including

- Helping with editorial research projects.
- Making travel and meeting arrangements.
- Evaluating, updating, and distributing patient information and instruction handouts.
- Creating and maintaining office policies and procedures manuals.

5.1 PHYSICAL ENVIRONMENT

Analyzing the needs of the medical office and matching the overall medical office layout and design to those needs will contribute to a smoothly running office. An office design that is attractive, functional, and professional can assist personnel with meeting the healthcare needs of patients in a more productive manner. Patients, in turn, will be more satisfied with their care and the medical office team will be positively motivated.

Patient Waiting Area

With the exception of the building exterior, the waiting area will give patients their first physical impression of the medical office team. On their arrival, patients may evaluate the professionalism of the staff based on the overall appearance and comfort of the waiting area. Reading material in disarray, trash on the floor, and tattered furnishings provide the impression that the office staff does not consider the comfort of patients to be a priority. Many patients are apprehensive when arriving for medical services, and the waiting area should provide a comfortable, clean environment. An already nervous patient should be made to feel as comfortable as possible while waiting for their medical encounter.

A waiting area should not be oversized. A smaller area that is well lit and clean and has drinking water and current applicable reading material will help a patient feel more at ease such as the patient seen in Figure 5.1. If children will be waiting in the area, provide a larger space and an area with quiet toys for them to use while they wait. Do not provide items that children can place into their mouth or that pose other hazards. An area for sick patients should be separate from the waiting area for healthy patients. Remote controls for viewing media, such as a television, should be kept by the office staff. Maintain a station that has comfortable

Figure 5.1

Patient's waiting area should help patients feel at ease. *Why is it important for a successful medical practice to have a well-designed and equipped waiting area?*

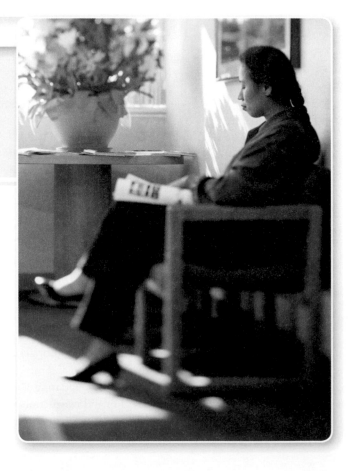

Why is there a problem with patients being able to see the patient sign-in sheet?

content, such as a travel or cooking station, and avoid viewing content that may contain questionable content (such as soap operas). DVDs for patient education are a good viewing choice.

Seats should be without tears and arranged to provide adequate walking space for patients. Leave enough room to allow for those using assistance devices, such as a walker or a wheelchair. Provide wall décor that is professional and will not create anxiety for patients. Calming scenes, such as a shoreline or mountains, are appropriate options, and soft, cool wall colors (neutrals, light pastels) are psychologically soothing. Live foliage helps purify the air and, when properly maintained, contributes to a comfortable waiting area. Beware of plants which may cause allergies for waiting patients or for office personnel. All decisions about the design of the waiting area should be made with the health and comfort of patients as the main goals. If necessary, consult an interior design professional.

Reception Area

Patient confidentially should be the primary focus of the reception area. Patient information on the log should be visible only to the receptionist. Information is frequently displayed on walls close to the reception area. However, this can clutter up the reception area, and patient information on the log may be viewed by others. Consider placing office information in a patient brochure or, if it needs to be displayed, place it on walls farther from the reception area. Placing items in the examination room for patients to read as they wait can help eliminate clutter at the reception area. If clear partitions are used between the reception area and the staff, unless they are soundproof material, conversations can still be heard, risking a breach of patient confidentiality.

Work Area

Fewer steps taken means more time spent on patient care. Workflow of individuals should be analyzed when designing work areas. Consider areas used by different components of the medical office team. Physicians and other clinical personnel use examination rooms, laboratories, and medication areas. Medical administrative personnel use reception and checkout areas, records storage facilities, and a generalized administrative work area. Work areas used by similar team members should be grouped in close proximity and provide little to no backtracking when completing patient care.

The design of furniture and equipment can help prevent occupational injuries and conditions, such as carpal tunnel syndrome. Individual body needs of those using the furniture and equipment are factors to consider when purchasing furniture and equipment: size, height, left- or right-handedness, and gender are primary considerations. **Ergonomics** attempts to match the individual's physiological factors to the equipment and furniture needed to complete tasks while reducing the risk of injury and hazards without decreasing output. Increased levels of stress may result when furniture and office equipment do not ergonomically meet the needs of the medical office team members. The next section discusses various items that can cause stress and how to manage them.

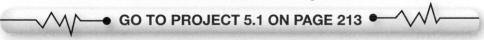

GO TO PROJECT 5.1 ON PAGE 213

Many things in life require individuals to be effective and efficient managers—stress, time, anger or conflict, and health, just to mention a few. As technology continues to change and provide faster methods of completing tasks, employees are expected to produce more in shorter amounts of time and with fewer resources. Effective management of self and other resources will allow an administrative medical assistant to be a valuable asset to the medical office team and its patients.

Stress

The word **stress** typically has a negative connotation. However, not all stress is negative. Stress can be a positive motivator for individuals. Why do students take this course or read this passage? For various reasons, individuals are learning new information to be applied in the medical office setting. This is a positive emotional or physiological response to an external requirement (achieving an educational goal, improving job performance, etc.). Good stress (eustress) is our body's nudge to maintain its function. For example, when you are feeling hungry, your body is experiencing eustress—go eat. However, when speaking of stress, the reference is normally to bad stress (distress), often referred to as the body's emotional and/or physiological reactions to external motivators. It can produce fatigue, sickness, and confusion which negatively affects the medical office environment.

Everything in life is a choice, and an individual's reactions to external requirements are also a choice. Some may disagree with this statement, but please read on. Getting out of bed today—that is a choice. Taking a shower—that is a choice. Completing homework for class—again, that is a choice. Consider all the things individuals do or do not do each day. Many will say they did not have a choice, but there are choices.

Now, let's apply this to the medical office environment.

- As patients begin to come into the office, a member of the medical office team can either choose to greet them in a comfortable, professional manner or not.
- One of the medical team members may be in a particularly unpleasant mood—fellow team members can make the choice to respond in a similar demeanor or can choose a different, positive response. Sometimes that response is simply not to say what is truly being thought at that instance. Always consider what is best for the medical office team as a whole.

Before effectively choosing how to respond to stress, an individual must first learn to recognize possible stress triggers. The following are a few of the stress triggers. There are many other external motivators for stress, and it is up to each person to learn what those are in his or her own personal and professional environment.

- Workplace expectations. Employees are expected to produce at a high level of efficiency, regardless of the position. This is a positive motivator, but emotional and physiological responses to work expectations can either propel employees forward in a positive manner, such as learning a new EHR program; hold an employee static; or even push an employee professionally backwards. When was the last time you heard someone complain or perhaps you complained about an anticipated change? In the medical office environment, change is constant, and being adaptable to change will contribute to a positive work environment.
- Single-parent provider. Many employees are the sole family caregiver. This creates a tremendous amount of pressure on an employee. Often, a single-parent provider does not have others to help care for a sick child or children. In turn, a single parent may have a higher rate of absenteeism simply because he or she does not have help.

- Caregiver to an aging family member. As the aging population increases, many in the workforce are also caring for aging family members, such as parents, other relatives, and friends. This is a time-consuming responsibility, which takes an emotional toll on the caregiver. Employees who are also caring for aging individuals often deal with painful medical processes, such as dementia and Alzheimer's disease, and financial responsibilities and decisions. Many must make the decision whether to place a loved one in a long-term care facility. Many caregivers must miss work in order to take care of needed medical and financial business.
- Multi-career family units. When both individuals in a relationship have career and job responsibilities outside the home, balancing work and home responsibilities can be a stress trigger if individual, specific responsibilities are not clearly defined. Consider this—one individual may assume the other is responsible for dinner on Tuesday when, in fact, the other individual thinks just the opposite. The bottom line is that no one plans for dinner on Tuesday evening.
- Financial pressures. It is a fact; today's money buys less than it bought just a few years ago. Individuals earn an income but it just seems not to go as far. Whether this is due to a lack of sufficient income, poor financial choices, or just the inability to say no, financial pressures are a trigger stress for many, if not most, Americans.

As employees begin to recognize stress triggers, some of the following stress-reducing suggestions can be used to benefit from positive stress and reduce the emotional and physiological effects of chronic stress.

- Get organized. Make a to-do list of items to be completed. Make a daily, a weekly, and even a monthly list. Lists can be maintained in paper format or electronically such as in electronic organizers and calendars as seen in Figure 5.2. Set reasonable

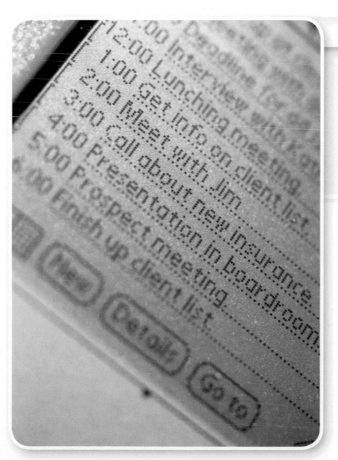

Figure 5.2

Electronic organizers through smartphones and e-mail options can be used to maintain schedules. *What are the pros and cons of electronic and paper-based organizers?*

and achievable goals and allow for flexibility and interruptions. Check off items as they are completed—this provides a visual sense of accomplishment.

- Set priorities. What must be complete today? Which task(s) must be completed prior to the arrival of patients? Recognize your own limitations. Being a team member in a medical office environment means that many times administrative medical assistants say yes to extra tasks. But when your resources (time, energy, knowledge, etc.) are limited and not sufficient to complete the tasks, ask for help or, if appropriate, respectfully ask for another solution.

- Develop a "whatever" category. Know the items that create negative stress. If the situation can be changed effectively and constructively, then do so. If not, then let it fall into a positive, not negative, "whatever" category and choose to react positively. Focus attention on other needed tasks. Also, practice taking a deep breath before reacting. Remember, change will happen, interruptions will occur, and plans will be revised. Adaptable employees will contribute to the smooth flow of the medical office environment.

- Be an achiever, not a perfectionist. **Perfectionism** is setting unrealistic expectations and goals and being dissatisfied with anything less. Perfectionists are often displeased with the end result. Achieving is accomplishing a goal or finishing a task.

- Maintain your health. Eat properly and exercise regularly. This will be discussed later in this chapter.

- Balance both work and play. Work hard while at work, but allow for the opportunity to play or relax. Watch a movie, read something just for fun, sing in the shower, or do any other activity that helps you reduce stress. If a medical team member does not take care of his or her physical and emotional needs, that member will find it difficult to be an effective, efficient part of the medical office team.

Time Management

Throughout the day, many people say, "I wish I had more time in the day," but is that what they really need? Everyone's day has 24 hours. If there were 28 hours in a day, individuals would simply fill all 28 hours and say, "I wish I had more time in the day." Time is a resource to be managed. Setting priorities and goals and creating to-do lists are two ways to manage time. Following are other time management tips:

- Identify time wasters. Keep a time log for a certain period, such as one full week (seven days). Record what you do, the time you started, and how long it took to complete the task. Nothing is too trivial for the log. Record when you wake up, take a shower, eat breakfast, watch the news, and so on. It is important to account for all your time in the log. Prioritize tasks using a rating system, such as 1, 2, 3 or A, B, C. Evaluate the log for each day and determine when the most productive and least productive times were to identify which tasks were time wasters.

- Delegate tasks. Everything cannot be accomplished by one employee. Sometimes it is necessary to ask others for help.

- Use technology. Technologies, such as computers and the Internet, allow tasks that traditionally needed to be completed using a greater amount of time, such as searching for the most efficient office furniture, to be completed by using search engines and Web sites. Using the telephone to call first before using time and other resources to physically go to a location is good not only for time management but also for the environment.

- Defeat procrastination. "When is the last day I can send in the lab work and still receive the results prior to the patient's appointment?" Procrastination is unnecessarily delaying the completion of a task. Employees delay completing a task for different reasons. Perhaps they are afraid of failing, overwhelmed (where do I start?), or upset at being asked to do the task. Or maybe it just isn't high on the employees' priority list. Also, technology failures may cause delays and, if an individual has already procrastinated and is almost at the deadline, this can disrupt the flow of the medical environment.

- Use a calendar. Many electronic calendars are available in various formats. Individuals also use traditional, printed calendars. Whatever format is preferred, choose one and use it consistently to record appointments, deadlines, and so on.

Anger and Conflict Management

Mismanagement of anger and conflict is one of the top triggers for producing negative stress. Consider the last time someone pulled out in front of you while you were driving. Did you consider why they pulled out without regard to you or did you just get mad? Choosing how to respond to internal anger motivated by external causes will help you avoid possible explosive situations and will reduce your negative emotional and physiological responses. Consider applying the following strategies when confronted with a possible conflict:

- Distinguish between perceived and realistic situations. How a situation is perceived may not be the reality of the situation. Determine facts and separate those from feelings.
- Breathe. When reacting to anger, bodies begin to exhibit physiological signs, such as tension in muscles, increased blood pressure, and/or a dry mouth. Deep breathing can help reduce the physiological effects of anger and allow an individual time to reconsider a different response. Rolling the neck and shoulders can reduce built-up tension in those areas.
- Save the e-mail. If responding to a communication such as an e-mail, do not click the Send button. Key in a response and either minimize it or save it—do not send the e-mail when angry. Allow time to gather more data and reevaluate your first response.
- Leave/walk away. Sometimes it is in the best interest of all involved to physically walk away from the conflict, allowing everyone time and space to calm down and/or rethink the situation. If physically leaving the area is not an option, emotionally take a walk. Count to 3 or 10, or imagine a comforting scene (mountains, beach, etc.) when the signs of anger begin to manifest themselves.

Health Management

Like a vehicle, when a body is not maintained and fueled properly, it does not function as it should. When the Check Engine light comes on, it is an indication that something is wrong and needs to be checked. A body has indicator lights as well. Some examples are chronic fatigue; changes in diet, sleep pattern, skin, or other physiological systems or loss of interest. Many medical conditions cannot be avoided; however, choosing to maintain your body with a healthy lifestyle can contribute to your effectiveness as an administrative medical assistant.

- Exercise regularly. To exercise regularly does not mean joining a gym and spending two hours, five days per week exercising, although that is one option. Decide on an activity and do it. Walking, canoeing, biking, yoga, hiking, strength training, dancing—the list is as varied as there are individuals. The key is to be consistent with exercising and vary the activity (to avoid boredom). If you like to exercise with other people, find someone who shares your interest and hold each other accountable. Little changes can make a difference; park at the end of the parking lot instead of in the closest space to the door or take the stairs instead of the elevator—there are many options.
- Eat regularly and correctly. The standard of three meal per day is still good. However, many health professionals recommend three main meals with small snacks—one snack between breakfast and lunch/dinner and another snack between lunch and dinner/supper. Still other health professionals recommend six smaller meals each day. But all agree, eat. When the body is not fueled on a regular basis, it begins to conserve fuel (calories) instead of using those calories. Foods high in fat

content can contribute to cardiovascular disease, one of the fastest-growing categories of disease in America.

- Manage stress. As discussed previously in this chapter, bodies can and do react to stress in physiological ways. Physiological reactions lead to decreased work efficiency and high absenteeism.

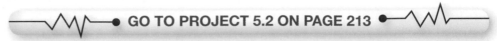

GO TO PROJECT 5.2 ON PAGE 213

5.3 THE OFFICE MANAGER'S ROLE

Advancing from the position of administrative medical assistant to office manager requires experience and specific skills and abilities. The experience ensures a broad and deep understanding of the many ways in which the medical practice is a business uniquely designed to serve people's most important and intimate needs. A high level of skill ensures a readiness to exercise initiative and to direct others.

Moving into an office management position sometimes requires a change of duties. It always requires a change of emphasis in job responsibilities. While the employee working as an assistant must have certain planning and management skills, the emphasis is most often on carefully following instructions, implementing plans made by the physician or other managers, and responding skillfully to a variety of situations. Office management requires the exercise of initiative that lets assistants act confidently because they grasp the goals and purposes of the practice.

Office management responsibilities involve the following managerial skills and abilities:

- *Being a team player:* It is important to understand the social fabric of the relationships in the office and to be recognized as someone who helps generously; freely gives credit to other employees for their work; contributes to a pleasant atmosphere; and relates well to colleagues as well as to managers.
- *Increasing productivity:* Understanding how to complete tasks more efficiently, actually increasing output, is the mark of a good manager. Directing others so that they are able

Figure 5.3

Medical office staff meetings provide an opportunity to share ideas. *What do you think are the most important aspects of effective meetings?*

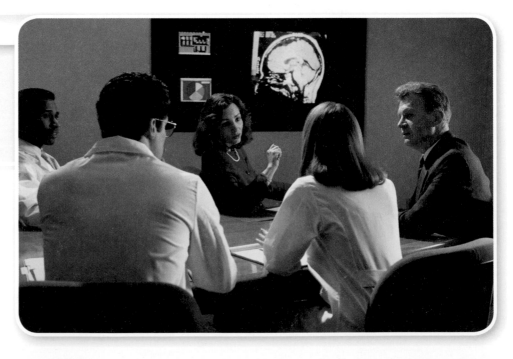

to get more tasks done more efficiently may be part of the office manager's responsibility. In addition to overseeing tasks performed by others, an effective manager delegates tasks. Thus, the manager's own development of time management skills and efficient ways of doing tasks is critical.

- *Planning strategically:* The office manager is expected to see beyond an immediate assignment, to view the whole business of the practice so as to contribute in ways that improve the daily operations of the office. This may involve anything from selecting a new electronic health records system to recommending the choice of a new supplier because of quality or price.

- *Using problem-solving skills:* The employer counts on the office manager to be able to analyze situations, determine the critical factors, apply knowledge gained in past working experience, and propose and implement solutions. Disputes and disagreements will develop between office team members, and the office manager must be able to remain impartial and to listen to all parties objectively. Critical-thinking and problem-solving skills can then be applied to reach a successful resolution.

- *Using available resources:* When physicians delegate the day-to-day management of the office, they may expect the office manager to get help from experts: an accountant, a lawyer, an insurance representative, even a time management expert. Companies specializing in office management, known as medical management consultants, are available to assist the office manager. The consultant will spend time analyzing the accounting system, the appointment scheduling and flow of patients, the filing methods, and the work habits of everyone on staff, including the physicians. The consultant will then make recommendations for changes. Perhaps the appointment scheduling system will need to be changed to accommodate physicians or patients better. There may be ways that office expenses can be reduced. A consultant may also provide comprehensive training for office personnel. If the practice can afford the use of such a resource, the help may be very valuable, especially to a newly appointed office manager. Managers should use Internet search engines to research topics and gain information related to decisions they need to make.

The ability to manage the office on a daily basis demands, above all, the quality of leadership. This quality enables the office manager to choose what to achieve, to plan for complex tasks, to prioritize time and tasks, and to motivate other employees to work effectively and efficiently.

Leadership Styles

A manager leads and motivates by example, either good or bad. Coaches motivate players, parents motivate children, and managers motivate employees. Before office managers can effectively manage situations, they must first know which management/leadership style is needed. Leadership styles fall broadly into three categories, with varying degrees of styles within each category.

Authoritarian/autocractic. An authoritarian/autocratic leader provides clear and definitive expectations to his or her team members. Each member knows how and when a task is to be completed and who is responsible for each part of the project. The manager makes decisions with little or no input from others. This style works best when there is minimal time to make decisions, such as in emergency situations.

Participative/democratic. A participative/democratic leader offers advice but is also a participant in the team dynamics and seeks input from other team members. An atmosphere of "your input is important" makes this a positively motivating style of leadership. However, the office manager retains authority to make final decisions.

Delegative/laissez-faire. A delegative/laissez-faire leader employs a "hands-off" policy and tends to allow other office team members to make their own decisions. Little guidance is given, and the manager becomes involved only when the situation makes it necessary.

Good managers must be able to analyze the dynamics of each situation and implement the most appropriate leadership style. Using one style in all situations can lead to employee dissatisfaction and poor work efficiency.

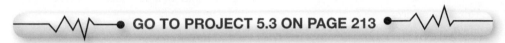

GO TO PROJECT 5.3 ON PAGE 213

5.4 EDITORIAL RESEARCH PROJECTS

The physician may be involved with research in a wide variety of areas, including investigating clinical procedures, instruments, or drugs and conducting experiments. Perhaps the physician needs to prepare a medical case history of particular interest or an article summarizing findings to the scientific community. Whether it is for a lecture, an article, or a book, the assistant may become involved in initial stages of research through obtaining material for the physician's reports at the library. The assistant will also keep copies of medical journals and will obtain and file reprints of articles in the physician's areas of interest or articles the physician has written.

Using the Library

In specialized medical libraries, such as those found in large medical centers or universities, librarians have educational qualifications in medical research and are prepared to be helpful to those who need to use the library. Public libraries have large computerized databases of materials in various medical specialties. These databases are quite simple to use because most of them include tips on how to search and are searchable by topic. If the document is located in another library, that information is also usually given. If the physician has given you only a topic and brief description, it may be efficient to print out those entries pertaining to the topic and ask the physician to check off those entries that seem most pertinent to the research. This will give direction to your search and will ensure that the most useful books or articles are provided.

Online databases are available in medical libraries and on the Internet, and information sites such as the Health Libraries or Health Sciences Resource List are also useful. Other helpful resources are listed here.

- Dedicated Web sites—such as MEDLINE (www.medline.cos.com), developed by the National Library of Medicine, and PubMed (www.ncbi.nlm.nih.gov/pubmed)—provide MEDLINE software, which gives immediate access to abstracts and journals and allows the full text of journal articles to be retrieved online.
- Compact disks for use at home or in an office may contain whole medical books, periodicals, journals, or even interactive training (for example, on how to perform a particular surgery, complete with pictures, animations, photographs, and videos).
- Specialized e-mail bulletin boards provide an opportunity for physicians to communicate publicly or privately with other physicians through e-mail messages.

Medical Journals

Most medical societies publish their own journals. The American Medical Association (AMA) publishes about a dozen periodicals on special subjects. In addition, the AMA publishes the official publication of the society, the *Journal of the American Medical Association* (*JAMA*).

JAMA contains articles on all aspects of the field of medicine. Most medical specialties have their own journals. Physicians who receive hardcopy journals will find it useful to have them bound and stored. Many physicians find it more time- and cost-efficient to retrieve and read journals online. *JAMA* articles, archived and current, can be retrieved at http://jama.ama-assn.org. In addition to viewing articles, physicians can participate in forum discussions and listen to podcasts of guests presenting research and other information. These contain much valuable information for reference and research. It is useful for you to know that each journal publishes a topical index at the end of a publishing cycle, although this cycle may not correlate exactly to a calendar year. Some research material that you may need may be found in the office storage area where these journals are kept.

Reprints

Physicians may inform their colleagues about their work by writing, lecturing, and publishing articles and papers on researched topics. If a physician presents a paper at a meeting of medical colleagues, the paper is usually published in the proceedings of the conference, in the organization's own publication, or in another medical journal. However, the physician may have submitted the article to a journal without having first presented it at a meeting.

Once the article is published, the author may receive a certain number of free copies of the article, called **reprints**. Additional copies are usually available at cost. The physician sends these reprints to colleagues interested in the same field or allied fields. You should keep a record of the names and addresses of those who receive copies of the article and of those who have acknowledged receiving the article.

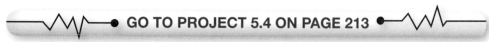

GO TO PROJECT 5.4 ON PAGE 213

5.5 TRAVEL AND MEETING ARRANGEMENTS

When the physician travels for professional or personal reasons, you will be involved in preparing for the trip. You need to know and understand the physician's preferences well in order to handle travel arrangements satisfactorily.

There are three general guidelines for handling travel:

1. Always consult with the physician in advance to be sure that the physician's preferences will be honored. Consider preferences in airline and airplane seating. First-class seating offers amenities such as larger seats, which are not available in coach-class seating. A traveler who is tall may prefer first class or, if traveling in coach class, an aisle seat. Other items to make notations of preferred choices are dietary needs or preferences in airplane meals; lodging requirements and the geographic relationship of the hotel to the meeting or conference site; car size, make, and model; car rental company of choice or limousine service or other ground transportation; preferred times of travel; airport, if there is more than one in the departure or destination city; and any need for information about the city—places of interest or restaurants, for example.

   The assistant should maintain a travel folder containing the physician's preferences, as well as other items relating to travel. This includes applicable discounts, such as membership discounts; financial items used to make reservations; and past itineraries for reference. When you are making travel arrangements, refer to this folder to save time.

2. Since the tragic events of September 11, 2001, travel requirements, especially when using airlines, have changed. Prior to traveling, the physician should be made aware of any changes made by the Transportation Security Administration (TSA) in traveling regulations. For example, as of the publication date of this text, the 3-1-1 rules for

carry-on liquids are applied. Liquid containers of 3.4 ounces or less may be placed in one 1-quart plastic ziplock bag, with one bag per traveler. Consult the TSA's Web site (www.tsa.gov/travelers) for up-to-date travel regulations.

3. Be sure to use the services of a skilled **travel agent** at a reputable agency or Web site. The travel agent does not charge the customer or may charge a small fee, and it is the agent's job to make all transportation, car rental, and lodging arrangements requested by the traveler. Sightseeing and pleasure arrangements can also be made through the travel agent. Communicate the physician's preferences to the agent. Many agents require the completion of a written travel profile that states the traveler's needs and preferences. This is a valuable tool because the physician does not have to take time to answer these questions every time a trip is planned.

Web sites for travel companies, airlines, and airports are also a valuable time-saving tool for making travel arrangements. Using the Web sites allows for price comparison. Features such as room amenities and airline seat location can also be verified without making a reservation.

Reservations

A request to a travel agent should be made as early as possible, so that the agent can research and obtain the best fare. Because many airlines use electronic tickets, called "e-tickets," the airline provides a confirmation of the reservation and purchase, rather than a printed ticket. This confirmation may be used at curbside to check luggage and/or at the ticket counter to obtain a boarding pass. Boarding passes may also be printed by the travel agent or assistant within 24 hours of the scheduled flight. Airlines will provide a printed ticket if there is a specific request for one. Having a printed ticket makes changing airlines easier, should that be necessary during the trip.

Most travelers prefer to stay either at the meeting site or very close to it. A delay in making the needed hotel reservations could mean that the physician will not be able to stay at the meeting site. This could lead to increased transportation costs and require additional travel time to and from the site. Provide maps of the area with the travel documents to facilitate travel time and help provide directions. Internet services, such as Mapquest and other online direction services, can provide valuable and time-saving information. If it is anticipated or possible that the physician will arrive late, be sure the hotel has been notified. Hotels have a stated "late arrival time," such as 6 P.M.

Once you have given the agent all relevant information on arrangements, request written or e-mail confirmation, if there is time. In any case, the agent provides multiple copies of an **itinerary**, or daily schedule of events, including flight times listed in the local departing and arrival destinations' times, flight numbers, hotel and car arrangements, and all pertinent addresses and phone numbers. Direct flights do not require the traveler to change planes but do have at least one stop before reaching their destination, and a nonstop flight is a direct flight with no stops. A sample of an itinerary is shown in Figure 5.4. As soon as you receive the itinerary, check to be sure that every arrangement is the same as what was originally requested or agreed upon. This itinerary, along with the confirmation ticket or airline ticket, should then be placed in a folder until the physician needs the information. However, you should notify the physician as soon as the itinerary arrives, so that copies can be sent to the physician's family members and any others whom the physician specifies. One copy for reference should be kept in a convenient place in the office.

Changes in Travel Plans

Changes and delays sometimes occur in the physician's travel plans. Ordinarily, the physician will share with you information on how likely it is that the trip will occur. This is important because airplane tickets that are refundable or that may be used at another time are more

Figure 5.4

Travel Itinerary. *Why are travel itineraries important?*

ITINERARY

For Karen Larsen, MD

March 10-14, 20—

Friday, March 10

5:00 p.m.   <u>Depart Chicago</u>, O'Hare International Airport, American Airlines 104, nonstop, 737

8:00 p.m.   <u>Arrive New York City</u>, JFK International Airport

Hotel: Mariott Marquis
1535 Broadway, Manhattan
212-555-5000
Conf. No.: GX476T02; nonsmoking room requested

Sunday, March 12

7:00 p.m.   <u>Depart New York</u>, LaGuardia Airport, American Airlines 526, nonstop, 737

8:01 p.m.   <u>Arrive Boston</u>, Logan International Airport

Hotel: Sheraton-Boston Hotel
Prudential Center, Boston
613-555-6789
Conf. No.: TZE32145, nonsmoking room requested

Monday, March 13

<u>Reminder:</u>   Make restaurant reservations.

7:30 p.m.   Dinner with Dr. and Mrs. Lawrence Carley

Tuesday, March 14

6:45 p.m.   <u>Depart Boston</u>, Logan International Airport, American Airlines 175, nonstop, 737

8:12 p.m.   <u>Arrive Chicago</u>, O'Hare International Airport

Travel and accommodations arranged by Linda Solomon, Chicago Travel, 312-555-6777.

expensive than nonrefundable tickets. However, it may be cost-effective to purchase a more expensive ticket or purchase travel insurance to allow for some flexibility in the physician's plans.

Because most hotel reservations are secured with a credit or debit card, it is also important to cancel a room reservation as soon as the travel plan changes. Each hotel has its own rules about cancellation without a financial penalty. The travel agent should be notified immediately, or you should call the hotel yourself to cancel the reservation. Request confirmation from the hotel that the reservation has been cancelled. Confirmation is usually in the form of an e-mail or a cancellation confirmation number. If a charge is made mistakenly to the credit card, it will be easier to deal with the credit card company if there is a verification of cancellation.

Duties Related to the Physician's Absence

Be certain that you have instructions about how to handle phone calls, correspondence, and appointments in the physician's absence. Mark the days on the calendar when the physician will be away, so that no patients are scheduled. Notify those patients who are already scheduled that the physician will be away and either make new appointments or refer the patients to the physician who will be substituting in the physician's absence. It is also useful to keep a running daily summary of phone calls, incidents, and patient inquiries, specifying the action that was taken while the physician was away. While away from the office, most business travelers check e-mail and call the office on a regular or predetermined time schedule. Keep a log of important information to be discussed with the physician during calls, and organize your phone discussion beforehand to make this valuable time more productive.

Meeting Arrangements

Many physicians belong to the AMA. In addition, there are organizations related to all of the medical specialties. Most national organizations also have state and local levels, and physicians belong to the association at all three levels. These organizations provide a valuable way for physicians to exchange information, learn about new developments, continue their education, and contribute to their profession.

Participation in organizations may involve simply attending meetings or may consist of working on or chairing committees. Your responsibilities will vary, depending on the physician's responsibilities.

National and state societies hold meetings once or twice a year. The dates, times, and places of a national or state meeting are usually determined a year in advance. This information is printed several months in advance in the state or national journal and on the organization's Web page. Notices of the meeting are sent to organization members well in advance of the meeting. The notice should contain pertinent information about the meeting: who is to attend, what the meeting is about, when the meeting begins and ends (including dates and times); where the meeting is being held (including directions, if needed), what will be discussed, and information for guests to RSVP. Enter meeting information on the physician's appointment calendar as soon as notice of the meeting arrives. It is helpful to put a reminder in the tickler file, so that you can meet with the physician to find out about preferences in travel schedules and arrangements.

Local meetings are usually held on the same day of each month—for example, on the second Tuesday. Meeting dates and programs are published in the journal or newsletter. Mark the dates on the physician's appointment calendar, and send a memo or an e-mail to the physician several days before the meeting each month as a reminder.

Special meetings may be called to discuss important business matters pertaining to the organization. In these cases, an announcement of the meeting is sent to each member. A sample of such an announcement is shown in Figure 5.5.

Figure 5.5

Meeting Announcement

THE CHICAGO MEDICAL SOCIETY
ELECTION OF OFFICERS MEETING

Tuesday, October 7, 20--
8:00 p.m.

UNIVERSITY HOSPITAL
5500 North Ridgeway Avenue
Room 254C

Preparing for Meetings

A physician who is the chair of a committee or an officer of the organization may be responsible for making the arrangements for the meeting. In many cases, the physician will delegate that responsibility to the assistant. If the meeting is to be held locally, arranging for the meeting is simpler. However, contracting for a meeting room, food or other refreshments, and equipment will still be necessary.

The following arrangements need to be made:

- Once you know how many people are expected, contact several conference centers or hotels to price the arrangements. Most conference centers and hotels have catering managers or conference planners available to help you. Know whether or not meals or other refreshments will be required; what type of media support—computers and projectors, flip charts and pens, microphones, recording equipment, and so on—will be required; the length of time the room will be needed; whether or not a lectern or table should be at the front of the room; and whether chairs alone or chairs and tables will be needed for the audience. If the group is to take notes, the hotel will ordinarily provide pads and pens. The hotel will also supply complimentary pitchers of ice water and glasses for the speaker and guests. Many facilities will fax you a worksheet for specifying all requirements, so that you can obtain the total cost.

- If there is to be a speaker, the physician will usually invite the person. However, you may need to confirm the person's attendance and the topic of the presentation. You may also need to make travel and hotel arrangements. The speaker should provide you with a brief *vitae* (biographical and credentialing information), so that the physician can make a proper introduction. The *vitae* should be placed in the physician's travel folder. You may also volunteer to prepare copies of handouts and to mail these to the meeting place. However, many handouts are presented in a more "eco-friendly" format. Presenters e-mail their presentation handouts in the form of an electronic file to the meeting facilitator. Attendees are then sent notification of the location of the handout. They may view it electronically or make a hardcopy for reference. Laptops may be used during the meeting to view the handouts and take notes.

- The physician may ask you to prepare an **agenda**, an outline of the meeting, that specifies the location, time, and major topics to be covered. A sample of an agenda is shown in Figure 5.6. Notice the large amount of white space, which enables attendees to make notes. Agendas are ordinarily sent out well ahead of the meeting to allow members to prepare for the business of the meeting.

- You will need to prepare and send, either by postal mail or e-mail, an invitation to each person who is expected to attend the meeting. Those invited must also be told how and when to return their acceptance of the invitation. Frequently, travel directions to the meeting site are included as a courtesy. If the meeting is local, invitations should be sent at least one week, but not more than two weeks, prior to the meeting date. If the meeting is to be held in another city, invitations must be sent approximately eight weeks before the meeting.

- Keep a record of the names, addresses, and telephone numbers of all those to whom you have sent invitations. It is also wise to keep a copy of the invitation and agenda in a convenient place. You will need to make copies of the agenda to hand out on the day of the meeting.

Last-Minute Meeting Preparations. There may be times when you must personally visit the meeting room just before the meeting to ensure that everything has been provided and that the attendees will be comfortable. You may want to call the representative of the facility with whom you have dealt and ask that person to be available when you visit the meeting room. If food or other refreshments will be served, it is also a good idea to confirm

Figure 5.6

Meeting Agenda

THE CHICAGO MEDICAL SOCIETY

Agenda

Monthly Meeting

Tuesday, October 7, 20-- — 8:00 p.m.

University Hospital, Room 254C

1. Call to order

2. Reading of minutes of previous meeting (approved or changed)

3. Reading of correspondence

4. Reading of treasurer's report

5. Old business

    a. Choice of dates for state-level meeting for next year

    b. Arrangements for meeting room for monthly meetings

6. New business

    a. Reviewing plan for increasing membership

    b. Voting on increase of membership dues

7. Program: Thang Huai, MD, Urban Hospital Medical Center, Department of Oncology, "The Patient's Informed Decision About Radiation and/or Chemotherapy Treatment"

8. Announcements

9. Adjournment

the times of service and what is to be served. Be sure to check the meeting room for the following:

- Appropriate temperature
- Correct number of chairs
- Audiovisual and electronic equipment requested and in working order; many presenters prefer to use a pointing device to help them call attention to electronically displayed data, and the device is frequently combined with the ability to advance and reverse audiovisual slides during the presentation
- Lectern or table at the front of the room to accommodate the speaker and chairperson, along with a microphone if necessary
- Notepads and pens for note taking
- Pitchers of ice water and glasses
- Name tags if required
- Copies of the agenda for the attendees

You may also be called upon to greet the guests when they arrive and the physician may have requested that you remain, so that you can record the minutes of the meeting.

Recording Minutes. The official record of the proceedings of a meeting is called the **meeting minutes.** Many meetings are conducted according to parliamentary procedure, and the minutes are then formatted in a formal way. Other meetings may proceed less formally. Minutes, therefore, may be formatted formally or informally, as shown in Figures 5.7a and 5.7b. Whatever the appropriate format, certain information is always included:

- Name of the organization or society holding the meeting
- Date, time, and location of the meeting
- Purpose of the meeting or indication that it is a monthly (quarterly, and so on) meeting
- Name of the presiding officer
- Names of the members in attendance and absent
- Order of business as it is taken up and any departures from the order as shown in the agenda
- Motions made and whether these were approved or rejected. (some organizations state the names of the people who motioned and who seconded)
- Summaries of discussions

Figure 5.7(a)

Example of Formal Minutes

THE CHICAGO MEDICAL SOCIETY

Minutes

Monthly Meeting

Tuesday, October 7, 20--

The monthly meeting of the Chicago Medical Society was held on October 7, 20--, in Room 254C of the University Hospital. The meeting was called to order at 8:00 p.m. by Dr. Lee Wentworth.

The following members were present: Drs. Brian Cleary, Ernest Dodson, Jane Gunderson, Michael Pope, Yan Tuo, Lisa Twelvetrees, and Lee Wentworth.

The following members were absent: Drs. Roger Ahmed and Gloria Mahibir.

The reading of the minutes from the last meeting was waived.

The Treasurer reported that the Society's balance, as of October 1, 20--, was $1257.72. There is one outstanding bill of $175.43 payable to the University Hospital Catering Service. A motion was made, seconded, and unanimously passed to pay this bill.

The next matter of business was the announcement of dates during which the state-level meeting will be held. Dr. Wentworth reported that the meeting was scheduled for December 4, 20—.

Dr. Gunderson reported that the University Hospital had renewed its agreement with the Society to allow the Society to use Room 254C for two more years.

A committee was formed to study ways to increase membership and will meet on November 1, 20--. Dr. Twelvetrees volunteered to chair the committee, and Drs. Cleary and Dodson agreed to serve as committee members.

For this month's program, Dr. Thang Huai, Urban Hospital Medical Center, Department of Oncology, gave a talk entitled "The Patient's Informed Decision About Radiation and/or Chemotherapy Treatment." A copy of the presentation is attached.

A motion was made to increase membership dues by $100 for the next year. It was seconded and unanimously carried.

The meeting was adjourned at 9:45 p.m.

_____   _____
Recorder   President

Figure 5.7(b)

MEMO TO: Membership Committee of the
          Chicago Medical Society

FROM: Lisa Twelvetrees, MD
             Committee Chair

DATE: November 2, 20--

SUBJECT: Minutes of the Membership Committee
             Meeting of November 1, 20--

Present: Drs. Brian Cleary and Ernest Dodson

Absent: None

1. **Discussion of the Committee's objectives.** The Committee will explore
   ways to increase membership in the Chicago Medical Society. The
   Committee set a goal of attracting ten new members for the next year.

2. **Discussion of courses of action.** The Committee discussed acquiring
   hospital mailing lists, sending an informational mailer to potential
   members, advertising in hospital bulletins, holding a hospitality
   evening for potential members, and offering incentives to current
   members who recruit new members.

3. **Actions to be taken.** Dr. Cleary agreed to research the cost of acquiring mailing lists and producing an informational mailer. Dr. Dodson
   agreed to get information on advertising and holding a hospitality
   evening. Dr. Twelvetrees agreed to speak with the Treasurer of the
   Society about incentives to current members for recruitment of new
   members. Committee members will report their findings at the next
   meeting of the Committee.

The next meeting of the Membership Committee will be held at 7:30 p.m.,
on December 6, 20--, at the office of Dr. Twelvetrees, University Hospital.

Lisa Twelvetrees, MD

rp

Distribution:

Dr. Brian Cleary
Dr. Ernest Dodson
Dr. Lee Wentworth

At certain meetings, portions of the minutes may need to be verbatim—that is, exactly as spoken. When this is necessary, the meeting is often taped and later transcribed.

It is usual for most organizations to have an assistant, sometimes called the "recorder." It is this person's responsibility to record the minutes of every meeting. The recorder may request that you transcribe the minutes after the meeting. The minutes are signed by the recorder. Minutes are kept in an official book of minutes and are taken to every meeting.

In the absence of an official recorder, you may be requested to take the minutes. Be sure to familiarize yourself with the agenda, review the names of the attendees, and concentrate on the meeting. Sit next to the presiding officer if possible. Review and refer to the minutes of previous meetings. Do not hesitate to ask for clarification or the repetition of a point if you are unclear about what was said.

A laptop or notebook computer may be used to record meeting minutes. Tape recorders may also be used. If these are used, the assistant should consult the office policies and procedures manual to determine how and how long the tapes should be maintained. Minutes may also be taken by hand using a pen and notebook and transcribing them after the meeting.

5.6 PATIENT AND EMPLOYEE EDUCATION

Information intended to educate patients about the practice and about their own healthcare is offered in many formats, including brochures, fact sheets, and newsletters. Videotapes, CD-ROMs, and in-person seminars are also used. Most practices display information on a Web page. You should work with the Web designer (Webmaster) to include and update pages for patient education.

Information important to employees is often gathered in an office policies and procedures manual. It contains key procedures about office operation.

Patient Information Brochure

A **patient information brochure**, or booklet, provides the patient with vital information that is particularly useful because it is in writing and can be kept in a convenient place in the patient's home or, if an electronic brochure is used, in an electronic file on the patient's electronic device. However, the brochure does not take the place of a personal orientation for new patients.

A patient information brochure can be used as a marketing tool for the medical practice, as well as a way to inform patients about the practice. Current and future patients should be well informed of the practice's policies and procedures.

Deciding on the contents of the brochure is the first step that must be taken. Topics to be considered include

- A description of the services offered by the practice, including classes and medical testing programs.
- A list of physicians' names, specialties, and qualifications.
- The names, functions, and office telephone numbers of the members of the office staff.
- Instructions for scheduling appointments. Be sure to list office hours and provide patients with instructions for emergencies, such as "Use 911 in life-threatening emergencies." Inform patients if the office has a 24-hour telephone service for emergency situations.
- Policies and procedures related to physicians' fees and payment, prescription refills, and medical insurance and other forms.
- A statement of any other policies that are relevant and that you may be directed to include, such as the practice's Notice of Privacy Agreement.
- A brief section expressing gratitude to patients for choosing the practice and for taking the time to read about the services it provides. Include a statement such as "If you have any questions about our clinic, please telephone us at [phone number] or e-mail us at [address]."

Patient Education Materials

In some practices, depending on the size, specialties, and resources available, there may be an opportunity to provide other **patient education materials**: for example, descriptions of frequently ordered testing and surgical procedures along with an account of the restrictions on diet or activity that the procedures impose. A list of resources—agencies, DVDs, Internet sites, specialized libraries in the area—may also be useful to patients. A list of preventive actions or "tips," intended to promote good health, may also be provided: getting regular checkups; limiting alcohol consumption; exercising regularly; avoiding tobacco; reducing stress, for example. A list of safety tips for avoiding injury at home and at work may also be appreciated.

Design Considerations

In many offices, the brochure is developed using a desktop publishing program. In others, this job is given to an outside resource.

There are many local businesses that specialize in designing and printing brochures, information sheets, and booklets. You will need to make clear to the professional who is assisting you the basic specifications of the piece you wish to create: length, quality of paper, and two-color (black ink and one other color for contrast) or full color. In addition, you will want to give the designer a sense of how you want the piece to look: visual appeal, use of photographs, and white (blank) space to make it easy to read. If you have friends who work in other practices, it would help you to evaluate the patient information brochures developed in their offices. This assessment will clarify the features you find effective. If this is not possible, you may cut out visually appealing magazine articles to show the designer and search the Internet for design and layout suggestions.

In addition to design considerations, there are issues of ease of understanding. Whether you or a professional writer creates the text, it must be easy to understand. The use of technical words should be minimal. You should also consider the cultural population in your service area and have the brochure written both in English and in other languages.

Policies and Procedures Manual

The **policies and procedures manual**, or employee handbook, is the reference that provides all employees with information about the work environment. Because employees are likely to refer to the manual often, it needs to be kept current and complete. The manual serves as a reminder of tasks to be done (referred to as policies) and how to complete the tasks (procedures). During the office manager's temporary absence due to illness or vacation, the manual helps keep the office running smoothly. It is a great help in training new employees, substitutes, and successors.

Format. A looseleaf binder with tab divisions is an ideal holder for a policies and procedures manual. Pages may easily be added or taken out. New topics only require additional tabs, inserted in a logical place. The only other format that offers as much flexibility is the computer. An electronic format, using a word processing program, would be easy to establish. Copies could be e-mailed to each employee. Updates, or instructions about deletions, could be sent the same way. It is important that every page be dated, so that the most recent update is easily identifiable.

Contents. Prepare an outline of topics that must be covered. The following suggestions for topics and the order of presentation will not address every situation. However, certain topics are common to almost all practices.

- *Office personnel directory:* This directory should contain the names, positions, physical locations, telephone or extension numbers, cell phone numbers, and pager numbers of everyone in the office, along with the numbers for building services, such as maintenance and security. E-mail addresses should also be included for each individual and department.
- *Job descriptions:* This section lists the major responsibilities and duties of all employees other than the physicians—for example, administrative medical assistants, clerks, receptionist, technicians, and billing specialists. A list of the names of the people currently holding the positions is often included, along with the name, e-mail address, and telephone number of a person to be contacted in case of emergency for each employee. Either in this section or in a separate section dealing with procedures, descriptions of how to perform the duties of the position are given. If job duties overlap, or if employees are expected to substitute for each other in case of absence or illness, that should be stated in this section of the manual.

- *Procedures:* Once the duties of the positions have been stated, a section on specific procedures may follow. Appropriate forms may be included with the procedures for which they are used. Figures 5.8a and 5.8b show pages designed to describe procedures. The following are examples of entries for the procedures section of the manual:

Daily Routine

1. List the duties to be performed to prepare the office each morning before patients arrive. These include checking the neatness and cleanliness of the office; calling the answering service or checking the answering machine for messages; checking e-mails; processing incoming and/or outgoing mail; pulling charts for the day's appointments; preparing the appointment schedule; and checking to see that the examination rooms are ready to be used. Throughout the day, canceled and/or missed appointments should be recorded in the patient's record.

Section 4: HANDLING RECORDS

PATIENTS WHO HAVE MOVED

Procedure:

DECEASED PATIENTS

Procedure:

TRANSFER OF RECORDS

Procedure:

SUPERVISION OF FILING SYSTEM

Procedure:

Figure 5.8(a)

Page from a Procedures Manual Showing Form for Describing Administrative Procedures

Figure 5.8(*b*)

Page from a Procedures
Manual Showing Form for
Describing Medical
Procedures

COMMONLY PERFORMED PROCEDURES

NAME OF PROCEDURE _____

USUAL TIME REQUIREMENT _____

SUPPLIES AND INSTRUMENTS:

PATIENT PREPARATION:

SPECIAL INSTRUCTIONS:

2. List other routine duties, including preparing correspondence and patient records, maintaining financial records, and completing insurance forms.
3. List the duties that must be done at the end of the day: locking desks and files, turning off and covering certain equipment, verifying that all computers have been either logged off or shut down, and programming the answering machine for after-hours calls.

Filing
1. Describe the filing method used, and provide a diagram, if necessary, of the locations of sections—active, inactive, closed, transient.
2. Indicate the length of time for keeping records in active files (retention schedule).
3. If colors are used as a filing aid, explain what each color designates.
4. Describe the preferred order of documents in the patients' medical records, including medication sheets, progress notes, laboratory reports, x-ray reports, special procedures notes, correspondence, and hospital summaries. This also includes the section and order in which electronic medical data are placed into EHRs.

5. List the types of medical reports that must be attached to a patient's chart or present in the electronic chart before a physician reviews it.
6. Describe follow-up procedures for test results.

Transferring Patients' Records
1. State which staff member is responsible for handling the transfer.
2. List the rules for what can and cannot be transferred.
3. Describe the procedures for copying records to be transferred.
4. Describe the procedures for faxing records to be transferred.
5. Describe the procedure for recording when and what information was transferred.
6. Describe the procedure for filing the release-of-information form.

Scheduling Appointments
1. List the schedule commitments for each physician, including office hours, hospital hours, and teaching or research schedule.
2. Note which physicians have special scheduling requests, such as limiting the number of physical examinations to no more than two in the morning or scheduling no physical examinations on Monday mornings or Friday afternoons.
3. List the procedure for canceling and rescheduling appointments, including whether or not patients are called or notified electronically on the day before the appointment for confirmation.
4. List the information required from patients for scheduling an appointment.
5. List the standard length of time required for various procedures, such as one hour for a complete physical examination, one-half hour for school physicals, and so forth.

Orientation for New Patients
1. Describe the information to be provided to new patients and how it will be provided, including office hours and emergency care procedures.
2. List the hospitals affiliated with the practice and their addresses, telephone numbers, and visiting hours.
3. Describe the procedures for obtaining medication refills.

Telephone Procedures
1. Give the preferred greeting for answering the telephone.
2. Explain the triage procedure, covering what calls should be put through to the physician. Include a flowchart listing the questions to ask patients when they are being triaged.
3. List the ways in which questions should be phrased when obtaining information about patients over the phone.
4. Provide suggestions for referring a patient to a physician on call, to the hospital emergency room, to another facility, or to sources of financial assistance.

Patient Care
This section may be the most significant portion of the manual, covering everything from the level of the interpersonal skills expected of the office staff to the specific ways to perform a variety of procedures.

Billing
1. Provide a sample patient statement, and explain the method of billing.
2. Note the name, address, and telephone number of any accounting service that is used.
3. If there is a billing specialist in the practice, state the procedures for disclosing and/or using information.

Collections

1. State and explain the steps established by the practice in the standard collection process.
2. Show sample collection letters, and provide a sample of the form used to track the collection process.

Processing Insurance Forms

1. Provide detailed instructions for handling each insurance account, for completing each type of form, for using and disclosing patient information to obtain third-party payment, and for billing patients who have insurance.
2. For each insurance carrier, provide the name of a contact person and the company's address, phone number, and e-mail address.
3. List the approximate turnaround time for processing claims for each insurance carrier.

Forms and Supplies

If samples of forms, with instructions for completing them, have not been included in topical sections, a separate section should familiarize employees with all the forms used in the practice. Even if the forms are in an electronic format, a hardcopy should be included in the manual for reference and training.

Equipment

Include an inventory of all office equipment. It is also useful to list equipment model and registration numbers. List the names, addresses, e-mail addresses, and phone numbers of equipment manufacturers, dealers, and local repair services.

Inventory and Ordering Procedures

1. Describe the rules for taking inventory and reporting on inventory levels. Include the required schedule for taking inventory—for example, every week.
2. State who is responsible for certain kinds of inventory. Nursing personnel may be responsible for medications, drugs, surgical gloves, and examination supplies. Administrative medical assistants may be responsible for desk, stationery, and maintenance supplies. Certain items, such as linens—laboratory coats, examination gowns, and towels—may be the property of the practice or may be rented from a linen supply company. Be sure to address how the linen supply is handled.
3. Provide the forms for ordering supplies and directions for completing them.

Employee Hiring Policies

1. Include a statement of nondiscrimination in hiring.
2. Describe hiring procedures, and indicate whose responsibility it is to interview and to recommend hiring for specific positions. If committees are used, indicate the positions that are to be on the committee—physician, office manager, administrative medical assistant. Positions on hiring committees will vary, depending on the vacancy being filled.

Employee Evaluation Policies

1. Indicate how often employees are evaluated, and explain the process.
2. Define the rating system, if one is used, and the relationship of ratings to the amount of salary increase.
3. Include a copy of the blank appraisal form.
4. Describe the procedures related to unsatisfactory performance and the steps leading to job probation and/or termination of employment.
5. Describe the grievance or arbitration procedure in place that employees may use if they have a serious complaint.

Employee Benefits Policies

1. State the rules regarding vacations, sick days, personal leaves, and the reporting of sickness or absence. The Family Medical Leave Act should be included in this section.
2. Describe the insurance benefits and the options employees may choose.
3. Describe any savings plans , 401k plans, and other retirement investment opportunities that are in place for employees.

Office Dress Code

State the rules related to professional dress established in the practice.

Meeting Schedule

1. List the established dates or days of staff meetings and committee meetings.
2. For each committee, list the members and the purposes of the committee.
3. Describe the role and responsibilities or degree of involvement of the physician with each committee.

Maintenance, Safety, and Office Security

1. Describe the schedule of building maintenance along with the names, e-mail addresses, and telephone numbers of the building maintenance staff or of the custodial service with which the practice has a contract.
2. If the office staff has specific duties to help keep the office clean and tidy, describe the duties and who is to handle them.
3. List the guidelines for office safety. Employee safety training schedules and how this training is to be documented should also be included in this section. Policies and procedures for maintaining Occupational Safety and Health Administration (OSHA) compliance are included. How to handle, process, and dispose of medical waste and contaminates should be clearly outlined.
4. Describe how building security works: requirements for identification badges and the security system itself—locks, alarms, and so forth. Include the rules for keeping doors locked or using buzzers for admittance. Provide the names of the security staff and their work telephone numbers and e-mail addresses. Include in this section reminders about securing personal property and demanding proper identification of strangers in the building.

Outside Services File

In addition to referring patients to other physicians, every physician must at times refer patients to agencies or businesses for help of various kinds, including health services and medical supplies. The policies and procedures manual should include an **outside services file** containing the names, addresses, e-mail addresses, and phone numbers of those to whom the physician may refer patients for services, such as

- Convalescent and nursing homes.
- Dentists and dental specialists.
- Health insurance organizations.
- Home healthcare agencies and hospices.
- Laboratories.
- Medical specialists for referrals.
- Pharmacies.
- Medical supply companies.
- Social services agencies.
- Human services agencies.
- Temporary agencies for staffing of medical personnel.
- Web site addresses of services and sites in your city that provide additional information and/or services.

Responsibility for Records

As office manager, the assistant may be responsible for supervising other staff members and keeping records relating to their employment. Each employee will have a separate file containing information such as an application form and a cover letter, a résumé, a letter of employment agreement, performance evaluations, and an attendance record. These are confidential records and are stored in a locked drawer or secure electronic files.

Each physician will want to keep a personal file containing additional information regarding licenses—state license, narcotics license, workers' compensation registration, for example. Social Security information and insurance identification numbers should also be kept in this file. A file listing the physician's affiliations with medical societies, organizations, and hospitals is kept along with a list of continuing education requirements. A list should be kept, related to these files, that contains license and membership renewal dates, fees, and any necessary identifying numbers.

Office Manager's Resources

It can easily be seen by the extensive list of topics to be covered in the office policies and procedures manual that the assistant serving as office manager has an enormous amount of responsibility. Even though it is difficult to keep the manual current, the manual can be an extraordinarily useful tool. It makes the task of managing both daily routines and personnel less problematic. The routines are made explicit and directions are given for handling daily tasks. Staff members are able to understand thoroughly their job responsibilities. This knowledge, in turn, helps them understand the expectations that managers have of them.

Another extremely useful tool is the computer. The information available on the Internet is a great help. There are a number of search engines designed to assist in locating services, articles and books required for physicians' research, travel directions, medical organizations and societies, and contact information for companies and professionals.

Also, standard printed references and resources should be available in every office, including dictionaries (standard and medical); a thesaurus; English language usage references to provide formatting instructions, grammar rules, and writing style guidelines; drug references to provide information on medications, such as brand and generic names, manufacturers, and dosages; state and local medical directories to provide credential information about medical personnel—correct spelling of names, office addresses, and telephone numbers.

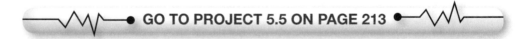

GO TO PROJECT 5.5 ON PAGE 213

Project 5.1 ## Designing a Waiting Area

The goal of waiting room design is to create a place where patients can relax—to allow them to collect their thoughts before seeing the physician and to calm their nerves to prepare them for their appointment. Patients will form their first impression of your office when they enter the waiting room. The look of the office could influence how likely they are to return for future care. Design a waiting room for a local physician's practice. Be sure to focus on the mechanics of patient flow and office efficiency.

Project 5.2 ## Analyze Usage of Time

Keep a time log for seven consecutive days. Document all 24 hours of the day—for example, 6:30 A.M. to 7:30 A.M.: got out of bed and got ready for school. 7:30 A.M. to 8:20 A.M.: drove to school. Determine the most and least productive times of the day and time wasters. Annotate the less productive time periods with ways to improve your time management skills.

Project 5.3 ## Internet Research: Improving Office Management Skills

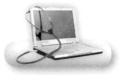

It is important to have some good resources for informational and motivational articles. Using your favorite Web browser, find articles on time management, prioritizing, problem-solving, initiative, strategic planning, and leadership. Choose at least three articles, and summarize the content. Submit this document to your instructor. Also be prepared to discuss your research in class.

Project 5.4 ## Internet Research: Journal Articles

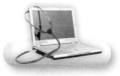

Dr. Larsen has asked you to search the Internet for recent articles (within the last year) on chickenpox (varicella) or mumps (parotiditis). Write a short summary of the articles you locate, including bibliographical data.

Project 5.5 ## Internet Research: Qualifications for Office Management

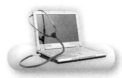

At the Web site for the American Association of Medical Assistants (AAMA), www.aama-ntl.org, there is a feature on the home page under "Medical Assisting & CMAs" called "Profiles of CMAs" (Certified Medical Assistants). Click this feature and read one or two profiles. Make a list of the qualifications, qualities, and experience required for the position of a Certified Medical Assistant based on the profiles you have read. Submit this list to your instructor and be prepared to discuss your list in class. Determine the specific skills needed to convey practice policies and procedures to patients and employees.

5.1 Design a medical office waiting area that exhibits the priority of patient comfort. Pages 188–189	• When considering the design of patient waiting areas in a medical office, consider each of the following: — Size of the area — Arrangements of chairs and walkways — Wall color, décor, and lighting, — Available reading material and comforts (such as drinking water) — Separate areas for healthy patients, sick patients, and children — Visual, kinesthetic, auditory, or other forms of entertainment Patient confidentially when registering on arrival is the primary focus of design.
5.2 Identify three stress triggers in your own life and define at least one method of reducing the associated negative stress. Pages 190–194	• Stress triggers are as varied as there are individuals. Some of the most common stress triggers are associated with expected work productivity levels. Others include financial pressures and family-unit pressure (single parent, multi-career, caregiver of an aging family member). Health issues also cause stress. • Certain strategies will help reduce the negative effects of stress: — Analyzing how we use time and applying time management techniques — Managing our anger and reactions to conflict — Getting organized and setting priorities — Staying physically and mentally healthy — Taking time to relax
5.3 Differentiate among three common leadership/management styles. Pages 194–196	• Managers lead and manage using different styles. The manager must choose the style best suited to meet the current situation. — Authoritarian/autocratic leaders make decisions with little or no input from others. — Leaders who prefer to seek advice and input from those involved are using the participative/democratic style of leadership. — A common leadership style is used by the manager who encourages team members to make their own decisions with little input or direction from the manager. This is known as delegative/laissez-faire management. An effective manager is able to analyze the situation and match it with the correct leadership style.

5.4 Explain why an administrative medical assistant needs to know how to collect and assimilate research data. Pages 196–197	• Physicians often research medical cases and data to gather treatment protocol for a condition or disease, to keep up to date on medical trends, and to prepare articles for professional medical journals and presentations. The physician will often rely on the administrative medical assistant to collect data from medical libraries and other sources. Collating and preparing the information in proper, keyed format are also skills needed by an AMA.
5.5 Classify items into major categories of needed information when making traveling arrangements. Pages 197–205	• When making travel arrangements for yourself or for others, maintain a reference folder with the following preferences: — *Method of travel*—air or ground • *Air travel*—airline, seat, meal, travel time, type of flight • *Ground travel*—rental company, size/make/model, smoking or nonsmoking — *Lodging*—smoking or nonsmoking accommodations, room and bed size, proximity to event, room/resort amenities — *Membership discounts*—professional social affiliations — *Past itineraries*—use for reference
5.6 Justify why a policies and procedures manual should be developed and used in a medical office. Pages 205–212	• Employees frequently need to be instructed in office policies and how to implement or complete tasks. A thorough and up-to-date manual provides a reference for current and new employees on topics related to all areas of the medical office. • When someone is absent, reference can be made to the manual for the completion of tasks; lost productivity because of someone's absence is reduced or does not occur. • When an employee has a question concerning office policy or procedure, reference can be made to the manual, thus reducing lost income due to errors. • Proof of compliance and employee training documentation can be maintained within the manual, reducing the possibilities of financial penalties. • Time and money spent preparing and maintaining a policies and procedures manual are justified when compared with the cost of lost income due to errors, absence of employees, and noncompliance.

Soft Skills Success

Adaptability

In today's business world, change is coming faster than ever before. Even minor change can be unsettling and intimidating. Stress and resistance will follow. This is especially true of the healthcare industry, where the only thing that remains the same is change. Change is important, and so is the way you react to it. During times of change, adaptability is required to foster progress and to help you remain effective and productive. **How well do you adapt to change? Describe a situation in the medical practice that would require you to make a change.**

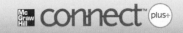
USING TERMINOLOGY

Match the term or phrase on the left with the correct answer on the right.

_____ 1. (LO 5.5) Travel agent

_____ 2. (LO 5.5) Itinerary

_____ 3. (LO 5.1) Ergonomics

_____ 4. (LO 5.3) Participative

_____ 5. (LO 5.2) Perfectionism

_____ 6. (LO 5.2) Stress

_____ 7. (LO 5.6) Patient information brochure

_____ 8. (LO 5.3) Delegative

a. "Hand-off" management style

b. Setting unrealistic goals; being dissatisfied with anything less

c. Management style in which a manager gives advice and participates in the decision process

d. Emotional and/or physiological reactions to external stimuli

e. Matching equipment/furniture and physical needs in order to complete tasks without decreasing productivity

f. Provides patient-related details of a medical practice

g. Daily schedule of travel events

h. Individual or agency used to assist with travel arrangements

CHECK YOUR UNDERSTANDING

Select the most correct answer.

1. (LO 5.1) Which of the following is a HIPAA-compliant method for patient registration in the waiting area?

   a. Have patients sign their first and last names on a sign-in log.
   b. Ask patients to verbally state their full name to the AMA.
   c. Ask patients to sign a detachable label log, which is immediately removed prior to the next patient's signing the log.
   d. Have patients sign their names on a log and mark it out with a highlighter.

2. (LO 5.2) During the monthly office meeting, Carrie became defensive and angry when she received the news that all office staff would need to attend a two-day training workshop on the new EHR software. She is behind on her work and being out of the office will just put her more behind. How might Carrie control her anger during the meeting without becoming a disruption?

   a. She can take a quiet, deep breath and reevaluate her perception of the news.
   b. She can walk out of the meeting.
   c. She can key in a quick comment on a social network.
   d. None of the above are appropriate responses.

3. (LO 5.3) An effective office manager is one who has which of the following attributes?

   a. Understands the different roles of the office team members
   b. Delegates tasks and resources needed to accomplish
   c. Manages available time
   d. All of the above

4. (LO 5.4) Felicia, Dr. Gomez's AMA, needs to locate current information on fibromyalgia for a presentation Dr. Gomez will give at the next state medical conference. Which of the following would not be a credible source of information?

   a. Online medical journals
   b. Case studies
   c. Reprints from colleagues who published articles on fibromyalgia during the last three years
   d. Verbal information gathered during lunch break

5. (LO 5.5) Caitlin, AMA, will continue to work in the medical office while Dr. Smith attends the American Medical Association National Conference. Dr. Smith will use her Smartphone to receive and send information and to correspond through e-mail. In addition, Dr. Smith would like to talk to Caitlin on Tuesday and Thursday at 12:30 P.M. during a conference break. To prepare for the phone calls, Caitlin should

   a. Wait to see what Dr. Smith wants to discuss and then retrieve the information.
   b. Keep a log of important phone calls, mail, and messages, along with the related patient information, such as a chart or flagged EHR for quick reference.
   c. Call other office staff and let them know when the doctor is going to call.
   d. Take a nap prior to the call, so that she is refreshed.

6. (LO 5.6) When asked to design and construct a method to convey practice information to patients, Natalie was unsure of how to begin. She works for a new pediatrician and the general parent population of their patients is below the age of 30. Which of the following would be a productive first step?

   a. Compile all the procedures and policies of the practice in a brochure format.
   b. Research local printing cost.
   c. Take a class on Web design.
   d. Conduct a survey of the patients' parents to determine their desired mode of delivery, such as electronic, written, or both.

THINKING IT THROUGH

These questions cover the most important points in this chapter. Using your critical-thinking skills, play the role of an administrative medical assistant as you answer each question. Be prepared to present your responses in class.

1. In the following situation, show how you use these three qualifications for office management—being a team player, planning strategically, and increasing productivity: There are three physicians in the practice where you are employed. Each physician has an administrative medical assistant and a technician, and there is an office receptionist. As office manager, you have just received approval to present a proposal for purchasing new waiting room furniture. How will you use your office management skills to handle this task?

2. Of the four main office management tasks discussed in this chapter, which one appeals to you most? Which task has the least appeal? Discuss reasons for your answers.

3. What are several things you can do to ensure that the physician's travel is as pleasant as possible?

4. The physician who is your employer is responsible for the next meeting of the local chapter of a professional association. What are three major tasks you must accomplish in making the arrangements for this meeting?

5. Prepare a rough draft outline—major points only—for a patient information brochure.

6. Design an office brochure to educate patients about your practice. This will be provided to new patients, and it should be functional for a physician's waiting room area. This brochure will represent the practice and the services provided. Patients retain only 20 percent of what they hear, so written information from a healthcare professional is very important. Keep in mind what you would want to know about a medical practice.

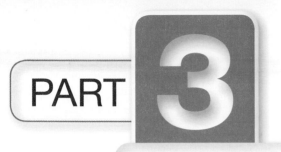

PART 3

Practice Financials

CHAPTER 6
Insurance and Coding

CHAPTER 7
Billing, Reimbursement, and Collections

CHAPTER 8
Practice Finances

Part 3 discusses the important duties of the administrative medical assistant in managing the financial aspects of a practice. Presented are insurance and coding, billing, payments, and accounting tasks.

CONSIDER THIS: Financial duties are very important to a successful practice, and computers are primarily used to help handle this task. *How can you improve your computer-related skills?*

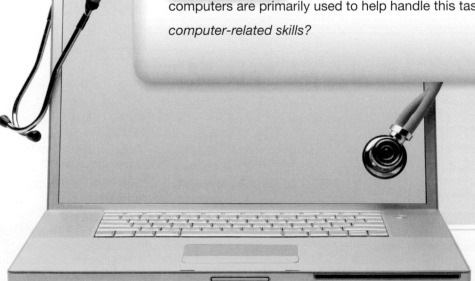

Insurance and Coding

LEARNING OUTCOMES
After studying this chapter, you will be able to:

6.1. Define *medical insurance* and *coding terminology*.

6.2. Explain the differences among the types of insurance plans.

6.3. Compare and contrast PAR and nonPAR and the methods insurance companies use to determine how much a provider is paid.

6.4. Explain diagnostic coding, procedural coding, and coding compliance.

6.5. Identify structural changes in coding with the implementation of *ICD-10* and explain the advantages of the changes.

KEY TERMS
Study these important words, which are defined in this chapter, to build your professional vocabulary:

accepting assignment

allowed charge

assignment of benefits

balance billing

birthday rule

Blue Cross and Blue Shield Association (BCBS)

capitation

carrier

Centers for Medicare and Medicaid Services (CMS)

CHAMPVA

code linkage

coinsurance

coordination of benefits (COB)

copayment (copay)

CPT

customary fee

deductible

Defense Enrollment Eligibility Reporting System (DEERS)

diagnosis-related groups (DRGs)

fee-for-service

HCPCS

HMO (health maintenance organization)

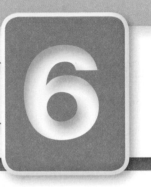

Chapter 6

ABHES

- Maintain confidentiality at all times.
- Be cognizant of ethical boundaries.
- Apply computer concepts for office procedures.
- Serve as a liaison between the physicians and others.
- Receive, organize, prioritize, and transmit information expediently.
- Monitor legislation related to current healthcare issues and practices.
- Exercise efficient time management.
- Use manual and computerized bookkeeping systems.
- Analyze and use current third-party guidelines for reimbursement.
- Perform billing and collecting procedures.
- Complete insurance claim forms.
- Implement current procedural terminology and *ICD-9-CM* coding.
- Use physician fee schedule.

CAAHEP

➡ Identify types of insurance plans.
➡ Identify models of managed care.
➡ Discuss workers' compensation as it applies to patients.

➡ Cognitive
➡ Psychomotor
➡ Affective

➡ Describe procedures for implementing both managed care and insurance plans.
➡ Discuss utilization review principles.
➡ Discuss the referral process for patients in a managed care program.
➡ Describe how guidelines are used in processing an insurance claim.
➡ Compare process for filing insurance claims both manually and electronically.
➡ Describe guidelines for third-party claims.
➡ Discuss types of physician fee schedules.
➡ Describe the concepts of RBRVS.
➡ Define diagnosis-related groups (DRGs).
➡ Describe liability, professional, personal injury, and third-party insurance.
➡ Apply both managed care policies and procedures.
➡ Apply third-party guidelines.
➡ Complete insurance claim forms.
➡ Obtain precertification, including documentation.
➡ Obtain preauthorization, including documentation.
➡ Verify eligibility for managed care services.
➡ Incorporate the Patient's Bill of Rights into personal practice and medical office policies and procedures.
➡ Respond to issues of confidentiality.
➡ Demonstrate assertive communication with managed care and/or insurance providers.
➡ Demonstrate sensitivity in communicating with both providers and patients.
➡ Communicate in language the patient can understand regarding managed care and insurance plans.

ICD-9-CM	participating (PAR) provider	primary care provider (PCP)	sponsor
indemnity plan	patient encounter form	provider	third-party payer
insured	PPO (preferred provider organization)	reasonable fee	TRICARE
managed care	preauthorization	referral	usual fee
Medicaid	premium	relative value scale (RVS)	workers' compensation
Medicare		resource-based relative value scale (RBRVS)	

INTRODUCTION

Medical insurance, also known as "health insurance," refers to insurance protection against medical care expenses. Administrative medical assistants must under-stand insurance in order to answer patients' questions about their health insurance policies and to process insurance claim forms properly, so that the physician receives compensation for services.

6.1 INSURANCE TERMINOLOGY

The administrative medical assistant must be familiar with basic insurance terminology in order to be helpful to patients and to process insurance claims.

The Medical Insurance Contract

Medical insurance is a policy, or certificate of coverage, between a person, called the "policyholder," and an insurance company, or **carrier**. The policyholder pays a certain amount of money to the insurance company in return for benefits. The benefits are in the form of payments from the insurance company for the medical services received.

In the medical insurance contract, the insurance company agrees to carry the risk of paying for services required by the policyholder. The patient agrees to make regular payments to the insurance company to keep the policy intact. As with other types of insurance companies, medical insurance companies manage the risk that some individuals they insure will require very expensive services by spreading that risk among many policyholders.

Insured. The person who takes out the insurance policy is referred to as the **insured**. Since a medical insurance policy often covers the insured and the insured's dependents, in the strict sense of the term, *policyholder* refers to the person in whose name the policy is written (the person who is responsible for making payments) and the term *insured* refers to anyone, such as the policyholder or a spouse, covered by the medical policy.

Premium. The rate charged to the policyholder for the insurance policy is the **premium**. Premiums are usually paid by the policyholder on a regular basis—for example, monthly or quarterly.

Third-Party Payer. According to contract law, when a physician agrees to treat a patient who is seeking medical services, there is an unwritten contract between the two. The physician or other healthcare professional—the **provider** (the "first party")—agrees to treat the patient, and the patient (the "second party") assumes the legal responsibility of paying for the services received. If the patient has a policy with an insurance company, in which the insurance company agrees to carry the risk of paying for those services, the insurance company is referred to as the "third party" and is therefore called a **third-party payer.**

A patient who does not have insurance is referred to as a "self-pay." A self-pay patient is responsible for paying the physician directly for all services received.

Coordination of Benefits. The clause relating to **coordination of benefits (COB)** in an insurance policy provides that a patient who has two or more insurance policies can have only a maximum benefit of 100 percent of the health costs. If the insurance companies do not communicate with each other, there is the possibility that more than 100 percent of the cost of the covered services will be reimbursed.

Under the terms of the coordination-of-benefits clause, one insurance carrier is named the primary carrier. The clause explains how the policy will pay—whether as a primary or secondary carrier—if more than one insurance policy applies to the claim. For example, the primary carrier may pay up to 80 percent and the secondary carrier 20 percent, not to exceed a maximum benefit of 100 percent.

The Birthday Rule. The **birthday rule** is used as a guideline for determining which of two parents with medical coverage has the primary insurance for a child. The rule states that the policy of the insured with the earlier birthday in the calendar year is the primary policy. The policy of the other parent, the secondary policy, may cover costs that are not covered by the primary policy. This ensures that the maximum benefit will not exceed 100 percent of the charge for covered services.

Types of Medical Insurance Coverage

Medical insurance coverage can be purchased in a variety of forms for different levels of coverage. The greater the coverage, the more expensive the plan. It can also be purchased for a group or for an individual.

Under group insurance, one master policy is issued to an organization or employer and it covers the eligible members or employees and their dependents. Thus, all the members or employees have the same healthcare coverage. Group insurance provides better benefits with lower premiums than does individual insurance.

Individual insurance is usually purchased by people who are not eligible for group insurance, such as by those who are self-employed. Because it is not obtained at a group rate, the cost is higher than for group insurance.

The following are examples of the types of health insurance coverage that are available:

- *Basic:* A basic insurance plan generally includes coverage of hospitalization, lab tests, surgery, and x-rays.
- *Medical:* Medical insurance covers benefits for outpatient medical care. An outpatient is a person who receives medical care at a hospital or other medical facility but is generally admitted for less than 23 hours. The term *medical* refers to the physician's costs for nonsurgical services, whether in the office or in a hospital. Special provisions are made for pathology, x-ray, and diagnostic lab fees.

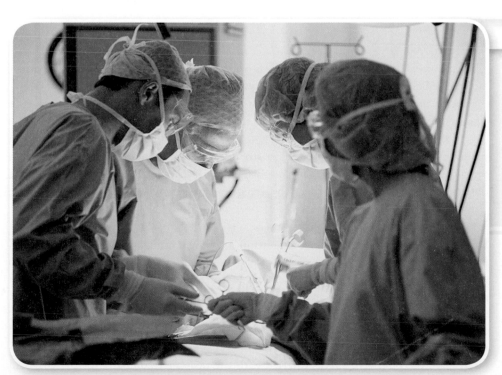

Figure 6.1

Medical insurance helps people pay for medical, surgical, and hospital costs. *Why is it important to both the patient and the provider for the administrative medical assistant to file insurance claims accurately and promptly?*

- *Hospital:* Hospital insurance provides protection against the costs of inpatient hospital care. It generally provides a room allowance (a stated amount per day for a semiprivate room) with a maximum number of days per year. Special provisions are made for operating room charges, x-rays, laboratory work, drugs, and other medically necessary items while the insured person is an inpatient. An inpatient is a person who is admitted to the hospital for more than 23 hours.
- *Surgical:* Surgical insurance provides protection for the cost of a physician's fee for surgery, whether it is performed in a hospital, in a physician's office, or elsewhere (such as in a surgical center). Charges for anesthesia generally are covered by surgical insurance.
- *Major medical:* Major medical insurance offers protection from large medical expenses, such as extensive injuries from a car accident or those associated with a prolonged illness, that go above and beyond the maximum established by a regular health insurance policy.
- *Disability:* Disability insurance provides reimbursement for income lost because of the insured person's inability to work as a result of an illness or injury, which may or may not be work-related.
- *Dental insurance:* Dental insurance can be obtained, often under a separate policy, to cover all or part of the costs of dental care.
- *Vision care:* Vision insurance can be obtained, often under a separate policy, to cover all or part of eye care cost, such as eye exams and prescriptions for glasses and contact lenses.

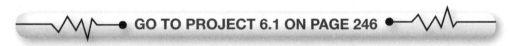

GO TO PROJECT 6.1 ON PAGE 246

6.2 INSURANCE PLANS: IDENTIFYING PLANS AND PAYERS

There are many medical insurance plans from which people can choose and many different insurance companies that offer them. Most insurance plans use one of two payment methods: fee-for-service or capitation.

Fee-for-Service

The first type of payment, **fee-for-service**, is made by the insurance carrier *after* the patient has received medical services. The insured pays for the medical services at the time of receiving them, and the insurance carrier reimburses the insured after receiving an insurance claim. Alternatively, the insured may instruct the carrier to pay the physician directly.

In a fee-for-service plan, fees are usually set by the physician. An insurance carrier and a physician may negotiate a *discounted fee-for-service* payment schedule. Under this schedule, a physician agrees to provide services for less than the usual charge. The physician makes up the difference in payment, at least in theory, by seeing more patients who have that insurance plan.

Capitation

Under the second type of payment, **capitation**, a payment is made in advance. Capitation is the *prepayment* by the insurance carrier of a fixed (per capita, or per head) amount to a physician to cover the healthcare services for each member of one of its plans for a specified period of time, such as for a month. It is common for the payment to be based on categories such as patient gender and age. For the per member per month (PMPM) payment, the physician must provide all the care needed according to a predetermined set of services to each patient for which a capitation PMPM payment is made. In a capitated plan, the physician shares the risk with the insurance company for the cost and frequency of the services provided. For example, a physician may receive $30 per month for each assigned patient, regardless of the number of times the patient visits the physician during the month, or even if the patient receives no care that month.

Types of Plans

Most medical insurance plans fall into one of two categories, depending on their payment arrangements. Plans that use a fee-for-service payment arrangement are mostly indemnity plans. Those that use capitation are generally managed care plans.

Indemnity Plans. Under most **indemnity plans**, the insurance company reimburses medical costs on a fee-for-service basis. This type of plan pays for a percentage of the allowable cost, and the patient is responsible for the remaining portion. Patients receive medical services from the providers they choose, who usually file the required claims for payment on behalf of patients.

For each claim, three conditions must be met before reimbursement is made:

1. The policy's premium payment must be up to date.
2. A deductible has been paid. A **deductible** is a certain amount of allowable or covered medical expense the insured must incur before the insurance carrier will begin paying benefits. Deductibles usually range from $200 to $500 annually.
3. Any coinsurance has been taken into account. **Coinsurance** is the percentage of each covered claim that the insured must pay, according to the terms of the insurance policy. The coinsurance rate is expressed in terms of percentages, with the percentage the insurance company is to pay listed first. For example, a coinsurance rate of 80-20 means that the insurance company will pay 80 percent of the physician's allowable fee and the insured must pay the remaining 20 percent.

Managed Care Plans. **Managed care** plans generally use capitation as the basis for making payments to physicians. These plans are the predominant type of medical insurance in the United States. There are two main types of managed care plans—HMOs and PPOs.

HMOs

The oldest form of managed care, an **HMO (health maintenance organization)** is a medical center or a designated group of physicians that provides medical services to insured persons for a monthly or an annual premium. The insured is able to obtain health care on a regular basis with unlimited medical attention and minimal coinsurance payments. Thus, HMOs encourage insured persons to take advantage of preventive healthcare services in an attempt to make healthcare coverage more cost-efficient.

HMOs attempt to control costs by using a number of methods:

- *Restricting patients' choice of providers*: After enrolling in an HMO, members must receive services from the network of physicians, hospitals, pharmacies, and other healthcare providers connected with that HMO. The insurance will not cover visits to out-of-network providers, except for emergency care or in urgent situations when the member is away from home.
- *Requiring cost sharing*: Every time HMO members visit their physician, they pay a set charge called a **copayment (copay)**—$10 to $20. Higher copayments, such as $50 to $100, are required when patients go to an emergency room or visit the office of a specialist.
- *Requiring preauthorization/precertification for services*: Often HMOs require **preauthorization**, also known as precertification, before the physician will deliver certain types of service. This enables the HMO to verify ahead of time that the service is medically necessary and is covered under the patient's policy. The HMO may also require a second opinion, from a different physician, about whether a planned procedure is necessary before granting authorization. Figure 6.2 shows an example of a precertification form.

Figure 6.2

Precertification Form

PRECERTIFICATION FORM

Certification for [ ] admission and/or [ ] surgery and/or [ ] _____

Insurance carrier _____

Patient name _____

Street address _____

City/state/ZIP _____

Date of birth _____ Telephone _____

Subscriber name _____

Employer _____

Member no. _____ Group no. _____

Admitting physician _____

Provider no. _____

Hospital/facility _____

Planned admission/procedure date _____

Diagnosis/symptoms code _____

Treatment/procedure _____

Estimated length of stay _____

Complicating factors _____

Second opinion required [ ] Yes [ ] No If yes, [ ] Obtained

Corroborating physician _____

Insurance carrier representative _____

Approval [ ] Yes [ ] No If yes, certification no. _____

If no, reason(s) for denial _____

- *Controlling access to services:* In most HMOs, patients are required to select a **primary care provider (PCP)** from the HMO's list of general or family practitioners, internists, and pediatricians. The PCP's role is to act as a gatekeeper, coordinating patients' overall care and ensuring that all services provided are, in the PCP's judgment, necessary. For example, HMOs require members to obtain a medical **referral** from the PCP before seeing a specialist or for hospital admission. The referral document names the provider the patient is to use and specifies the services the patient can receive. If a member visits a provider without a referral, the member is directly responsible for the full cost of the service.

Preferred Provider Organizations

Another type of managed care plan, more popular now than HMOs, are PPOs. The **PPO (preferred provider organization)** contracts to perform services for PPO members at specified rates. These rates, or fees, are generally lower than the fees charged to regular patients. The PPO gives the insured a list of PPO providers from which to receive healthcare at PPO rates. If a patient chooses to receive treatment from a provider who is not in the PPO network, the patient has to pay more—usually a higher copayment or deductible or any difference between the PPO's rate and the outside provider's rate.

PPOs, like HMOs, are managed care systems. This means PPOs use many of the same types of practices as HMOs to control the cost of healthcare. For example, they encourage members to use providers in their own PPO network, they usually require preauthorization for some procedures, and they require members to share in the cost of care by making co-payments each time they have an encounter with a provider.

Unlike HMOs, PPOs do not generally require patients to choose a primary care physician to oversee their care. Nor are referrals to specialists required. As a result, however, premiums and copayments tend to be higher than those for HMO members.

Medical Insurance Payers

Medical insurance plans, whether indemnity plans or managed care plans, are available through commercial insurance companies in the private sector, such as Aetna or WellPoint, Inc., or, for eligible individuals, through government-sponsored programs, such as Medicare and Medicaid.

Private-Sector Payers. The private-sector market is made up chiefly of a few very large national firms that offer all the leading types of insurance plans. Although most of these payers are for-profit, some are nonprofit, such as Kaiser Permanente, which is the largest nonprofit HMO.

The **Blue Cross and Blue Shield Association (BCBS)**, one of the largest private-sector payers in the United States, has both for-profit and nonprofit components. As with many of the private-sector payers, BCBS offers both indemnity and managed care plans, with many individual policy variations in each category. Its HMO network, HMO Blue USA, is the largest managed care network in the country, providing coverage to more than 14 million members in 47 states and the District of Columbia. BCBS member plans offer many types of managed care programs, including an HMO, a PPO, and others. There are also BCBS plans that make it easy for patients to receive treatment outside their local service area (the BlueCard program); nationwide BCBS plans for corporations with offices in more than one state; and a BCBS Federal Employee Program (FEP), which has been part of the Federal Employee Health Benefit Program (FEHBP) since its inception in 1960.

Medicare. **Medicare** is a federal health plan that provides insurance to citizens and permanent residents aged 65 and older; people with disabilities, including kidney failure; and spouses of entitled individuals. Medicare is divided into two parts—Part A, hospitalization insurance, and Part B, medical insurance.

Medicare Part A, also known as hospital insurance, covers hospital, nursing facility, home health, hospice, and inpatient care. Those who are eligible for Social Security benefits are automatically enrolled in Medicare Part A. Medicare Part B, also known as supplementary insurance, covers outpatient services, services by physicians, durable medical equipment, and other services and supplies. Medicare Part B coverage is optional. Everyone eligible for Part A can choose to enroll in Part B by paying monthly premiums.

Medicare Part C (originally called Medicare + Choice) is available for individuals enrolled in Parts A and B. Under Part C, CMS (Centers for Medicare and Medicaid Services) contracts with private insurance carriers to offer Medicare beneficiaries Medicare Advantage plans, which are competitive with the original Medicare plan, which includes Medicare Parts A and B. Medicare Advantage Plans, another name for Medicare Part C, must offer all the benefits covered in Medicare A and B but does not have to offer them at the same rate. In addition, Medicare Advantage Plans (Medicare Part C) offer other coverage, such as hearing, vision, and prescription.

Medicare Part D, known as the prescription plan, provides voluntary Medicare prescription drug coverage for Medicare-eligible individuals. Part D plans are offered through private insurance plans, and most beneficiaries pay a monthly premium. Individuals who subscribe to a Medicare Advantage Plan including prescription coverage do not need Part D. Beneficiaries enrolled in the original Medicare plan and desiring prescription coverage may enroll in a Medicare Part D plan.

All deductibles must be met before payment benefits begin, such as the first $155 for services covered in Part B. In a traditional fee-for-service program (Part B), after the deductible has been met, Medicare pays 80 percent of approved charges and the patient is responsible for the remaining 20 percent. In a Medicare managed care program, the terms are different: most managed care plans charge a monthly premium and a small copayment for each office visit but do not charge a deductible.

Medicaid. **Medicaid** is a health benefit program, jointly funded by federal and state governments, that is designed for people with low incomes who cannot afford medical care. Each state formulates its own Medicaid program under broad federal guidelines. As a result, programs vary in coverage and benefits from state to state. In some states, the program is known by a different name. For example, in California, Medicaid is called MediCal.

The State Children's Health Insurance Program (SCHIP) was enacted by federal legislation in 1997. It offers states the opportunity to develop and implement plans that offer health insurance coverage for uninsured children. Children covered through SCHIP come from low-income families whose income is too high to qualify for Medicaid. Children up to 19 years of age may be covered.

TRICARE. **TRICARE** (formerly *CHAMPUS*) is the Department of Defense's health insurance plan for military personnel (referred to as **sponsors**) and their families. Those eligible include active or retired members of the following uniformed services and their families: the U.S. Army, Navy, Marines, Air Force, Coast Guard, Public Health Service, and National Oceanic and Atmospheric Administration. Coverage also applies to the dependents of military personnel killed while on active duty.

All military treatment facilities (MTFs), including hospitals and clinics, are part of the TRICARE system, which also contracts with civilian facilities and physicians to provide more extensive services to beneficiaries. TRICARE offers three healthcare plans: TRICARE Standard, TRICARE Prime, and TRICARE Extra. TRICARE Standard, a fee-for-service program, is the most expensive of the plans. TRICARE Prime is a managed care plan, similar to an HMO, and TRICARE Extra is an alternative managed care plan for individuals who want to receive services primarily from civilian facilities and physicians rather than from military facilities. To be certain a patient is eligible, the administrative medical assistant checks the individual's military ID card and ensures that coverage is still valid by examining the expiration date.

If the eligible individual is not certain if he or she has coverage, the sponsor (the uniformed service member) may contact the **Defense Enrollment Eligibility Reporting System (DEERS)** to verify eligibility; the provider may not contact DEERS directly because the information is protected by the Privacy Act.

CHAMPVA. **CHAMPVA**, which stands for Civilian Health and Medical Program of the Veterans Administration, is a government health insurance program that covers the expenses of the families of veterans with total, permanent, service-connected disabilities. It also covers surviving spouses and dependent children of veterans who died in the line of duty. Each eligible beneficiary possesses a CHAMPVA authorization card. Most CHAMPVA enrollees pay an annual deductible and a portion of their healthcare charges.

Workers' Compensation. Each state has its own **workers' compensation** laws to guarantee that an employee who is injured or who becomes ill in the course of employment will have adequate medical care and an adequate means of support while unable to work. The employer must obtain insurance against workers' compensation liability and is liable whether or not the employee is at fault for an accident or injury. Workers' compensation insurance operates under the jurisdiction of the state department of labor or an industrial commission.

The administrative medical assistant must verify with the employer that a patient who claims workers' compensation was indeed injured or became ill in the course of employment. The physician must submit a report, usually within 48 hours, to the workers' compensation insurance carrier, which notifies the Workers' Compensation Board. (The time period during which the physician must file the report varies by state and ranges from 24 hours to 10 days.) The report must include the patient's case history, symptoms, complete medical findings, tentative diagnosis, prescribed treatment, and length and extent of disability or injury. Work-related injuries are grouped into five categories, which are defined by the state and administered by its department of labor:

- Injury without disability
- Injury with temporary disability
- Injury with permanent disability
- Injury requiring vocational rehabilitation
- Injury resulting in death

Progress reports on the case must be filed regularly until the physician releases the patient from care. The final report must be designated as such, indicating that the patient has recovered to the maximum capacity from the work-related disability.

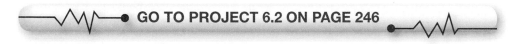
GO TO PROJECT 6.2 ON PAGE 246

6.3 PARTICIPATION AND PAYMENT METHODS

Physicians must decide with which insurance plans they want to participate. They judge which plans to join based on the types of patients they serve and the financial arrangements the plans offer them. Because more people are members of managed care plans than any other type of plan today, most physicians have contracts with a number of managed care plans in their area. Often, to avoid confusion, a medical practice displays a list of plans it participates in, so that patients know what to expect, given the insurance they have. Figure 6.3 is an example of such a list.

Figure 6.3

Example of an Insurance Plan Participation List

Welcome to our practice.

In order to make your visit as pleasant as possible, we have compiled a list of the most commonly asked questions regarding insurance and billing in this office.

With which insurance plans does the physician participate?

Aetna/US Healthcare Plans	Medicaid
CIGNA	MedSpan
Blue Choice PPO: POS, PPO, Prestige, Select	MD Health Plan
Focus Workers Compensation PPO	Oxford Health Plan
Health Care Value Management, Inc.	Physician Health Services
Health Choice	Prudential Healthcare
Health Direct	POS Plan
Kaiser Permanente	Wellcare
Medicare	

What can I expect if the physician participates with my insurance?

We will file a claim with your insurance company for any charges. Your insurance may require you to pay a copay at the time of services. You are responsible for any deductibles and non-covered services. You may need to obtain a referral from your primary care physician. Failure to obtain a referral may result in rescheduling of your appointment until you can obtain one.

What can I expect if the physician does not participate with my insurance?

Payment is expected at the time of service. You will receive a statement within two weeks. Use it to file a claim. As a courtesy, we will submit any surgery claims to your insurance carrier, but you are responsible for payment.

Plan Participation

A physician who joins an insurance plan is a **participating (PAR) provider** in that plan. As a participating provider, the physician agrees to provide medical services to the insurance plan members according to the plan's rules and payment schedules. The insurance carrier offers various incentives, such as faster payment, to participating providers.

A nonparticipating provider, or nonPAR, chooses not to join a particular insurance plan. A nonPAR physician who treats members of a plan does not have to obey the rules or follow the payment schedule of that plan. At the same time, a nonPAR physician will not receive any of the benefits of participation.

HIPAATIPS   Some physicians' offices outsource billing services. Offices using outside billing services must sign a business associates agreement because the information needed to process insurance claims is confidential. The agreement verifies that the services are HIPAA compliant and will keep the patient information confidential.

What private health information would be shared with an outside billing agency?

Fee Schedules

In a private managed care plan, contracts that set fees are often negotiated between the insurance company and the physician. In Medicare, the **Centers for Medicare and Medicaid Services (CMS)** is responsible for setting up the terms of the plan, referred to as the Medicare Fee Schedule (MFS). This agency was called the Health Care Financing Administration, commonly known as "HCFA" (pronounced "hic-fuh"), before 2001. An agency of the Department of Health and Human Services (HHS), CMS administers the Medicare and Medicaid programs to millions of Americans. Part of its role is to review managed care plans that want to become Medicare coverage providers.

Payment Concepts

Every health insurance plan has its own payment methods, rules, and regulations. An administrative medical assistant must keep up with the different options available in each plan in order to be sure a patient has coverage for a given service and to process insurance claims for patients properly. Following is a list of the basic concepts used in insurance contracts regarding methods of making payments to providers.

Allowed Charge. When insurance companies set up the payment terms for an insurance contract, many set an **allowed charge** for each procedure or service a provider performs. This amount is the most the insurance company will pay any provider for that work and may not be the same as the charged amount. Insurance carriers may refer to their allowed charge as the allowed amount or allowable fee.

Balance Billing. When the amount the physician charges is more than the insurance company's allowed charge, the difference in cost must be absorbed by either the patient or the physician. If the physician decides the patient should absorb the cost, the physician bills the patient for the unclaimed amount, a practice referred to as **balance billing**.

Many insurance plans specify that a participating provider may *not* bill patients for balances. This means a PAR provider must accept the allowable charge of the insurance carrier and payment from the insurance carrier and patient up to that amount as payment in full for the procedure and not collect ("write off") the difference between the physician's usual fee and the allowed charge. In other words, the physician subtracts the unpaid amount from the patient's bill.

Accepting Assignment. A PAR provider who agrees to accept the allowed charge set forth by the insurance company as payment in full for a service and not bill the patient for the balance is **accepting assignment**. PAR providers must always accept assignment.

For some plans, such as Medicare, a nonPAR provider may decide whether to accept assignments on a claim-by-claim basis. A nonPAR provider who decides to accept assignment on a given claim does not bill the patient for the balance. Conversely, if the nonPAR provider decides not to accept assignment, the patient is billed for the unclaimed amount.

Assignment of Benefits. A physician who accepts an **assignment of benefits** agrees to receive payment directly from the patient's insurance carrier. In this case, the patient signs an assignment of benefits statement, usually on the patient information form, and a notation is made on an insurance claim form that the patient has a signature on file (SOF) for the assignment of benefits. If the provider is participating with the patient's insurance carrier and a direct payment of benefits is part of the participation agreement, the patient's signature for assignment of benefits is not needed.

When a nonPAR physician does not accept assignment on a claim, the patient is usually asked to pay for the service in full at the time of the visit, so that the medical office can avoid having to collect payment later. Some practices ask the patient to assign benefits for

COMPLIANCE TIP

In a private plan, a nonparticipating provider can usually bill the patient for any unpaid balance after the insurance company has paid its responsibility. In the case of government-sponsored programs, however, other rules protect the patient. In a Medicare plan, for example, nonPAR providers are subject to a limiting charge for each procedure. The limiting charge is a way of preventing Medicare patients from having to pay the unclaimed portion of a bill.

the claim at the time of the visit, then bill the patient later for any amount the insurance company does not pay.

Examples of PAR and NonPAR Provider Fees for a Medicare Patient. Suppose a patient whose primary insurance carrier is Medicare visits a physician for a procedure. Normally, the physician charges $120 for the procedure; the Medicare allowed charge for the procedure, however, is only $60. How much can the physician charge for the procedure, and how much will Medicare reimburse? Depending on whether the physician participates in the Medicare program (physicians decide each year whether to participate), the amount the physician can charge will vary. PAR providers are reimbursed more than nonPAR providers. As part of its standard policy, Medicare sets the fees for nonPAR providers 5 percent less than those for PAR providers for the same services.

Furthermore, depending on whether a nonparticipating physician decides to accept assignment or not, and the limiting charge imposed on a nonPAR provider who does not accept assignment, the amount Medicare pays varies. If a nonPAR provider decides not to accept the Medicare assigned amount as payment in full, and decides rather to bill the patient for the balance, Medicare subjects the assigned amount to a limiting charge, thus limiting the amount of unpaid balance the physician can bill the patient. The limiting charge is 115 percent of the fee listed in the nonPAR Medicare fee schedule (MFS). For example, if the nonPAR amount for a covered service was $115.26, the limiting charge amount would be $132.55 ($115.26 × 115%). In effect, the limiting charge prevents the physician from balance billing the patient for the full unclaimed amount.

The following three fee structures illustrate the three possible scenarios:

Participating Provider

Physician's standard fee	$120.00
Medicare fee	60.00
Medicare pays 80% ($60.00 × 80%)	48.00
Patient or supplemental plan pays 20% ($60.00 × 20%)	12.00
Provider adjustment ($120.00 − $60.00)	60.00

Nonparticipating Provider Who Accepts Assignment

Physician's standard fee	$120.00
Medicare nonPAR fee ($60.00 × 95%)	57.00
Medicare pays 80% ($57.00 × 80%)	45.60
Patient or supplemental plan pays 20% ($57.00 × 20%)	11.40
Provider adjustment ($120.00 − $57.00)	63.00

Nonparticipating Provider Who Does Not Accept Assignment

Physician's standard fee	$120.00
Medicare nonPAR fee	57.00
Limiting charge ($57.00 × 115%)	65.55
Patient billed	65.55
Medicare pays patient ($57.00 × 80%)	45.60
Total provider can collect	65.55
Patient pays balance ($65.55 − $45.60)	19.95
Provider adjustment ($120.00 − $65.55)	54.45

These examples can also be used to illustrate the different options for assigning benefits on Medicare claims. In the first and second scenarios, since the physician has agreed to accept the assigned Medicare amounts ($60 and $57, respectively) as reimbursement in full for the procedure, the physician would also accept an assignment of benefits, authorizing Medicare to pay the physician directly.

In the third scenario, since the provider has decided not to accept the Medicare assigned amount of $57 as payment in full for the procedure, the provider will also not accept an assignment of benefits for the claim. Instead, Medicare will send the payment directly to the patient, and the patient will be responsible for paying the bill in full, including the balance.

Setting Fees

Third-party payers use different formulas and systems for setting up fee schedules for the procedures and services they will reimburse. The most common types of payment systems are

- A list of usual, customary, and reasonable (UCR) fees.
- A relative value scale (RVS).
- A resource-based relative value scale (RBRVS).
- Diagnosis-related groups (DRGs).

UCR Fees. To set fees for their services, providers establish a list of their usual fees for the procedures and services they frequently perform. In every geographic area, there is a normal range of fees for each procedure. Different practices set their fees at some point along this range. Third-party payers, to set the rates they pay providers, analyze providers' usual fees and establish a schedule of UCR (for usual, customary, and reasonable) fees for each procedure.

- A **usual fee** is an individual provider's average charge for a certain procedure.
- A **customary fee** is determined by what physicians with similar training and experience in a certain geographic location typically charge for a procedure.
- A **reasonable fee** is one that meets the two previous criteria, or a fee allowed or approved by the insurance carrier for a difficult or complicated service.

Relative Value Scale (RVS). Another payment system is the **relative value scale (RVS)**. A relative value scale sets fees for medical services based on an analysis of the skill and time required to provide them.

Resource-Based Relative Value Scale (RBRVS). The payment system used by Medicare is the **resource-based relative value scale (RBRVS)**. The RBRVS, like the RVS on which it is based, is a scale that establishes relative prices for services. It is based on three factors: (1) the national relative value unit (RVU) which represents the amount of resources required (time, skill, overhead) to complete a service, (2) an adjustment factor for the geographic location, and (3) a national conversion factor.

Also, many private insurance companies use resource-based fee structures to establish what to pay for each procedure when company managers believe a resource-based fee structure more fairly reflects the real costs involved in providing medical services than the historical fees.

Diagnosis-Related Groups (DRGs). Another payment system, used by Medicare for establishing payment for hospital stays, is **diagnosis-related groups (DRGs)**. Diagnostic groupings are based on the resources that physicians and hospitals have used nationally for patients with similar conditions, taking into account factors such as age, gender, and medical complications.

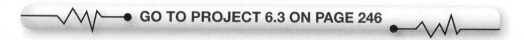

GO TO PROJECT 6.3 ON PAGE 246

To keep track of the many thousands of possible diagnoses and of procedures and services rendered by physicians, and to simplify the process of verifying the medical necessity of each procedure, two coding systems are used:

- *Diagnostic coding:* Codes for reporting what is wrong with the patient, or what brought the patient to see the physician
- *Procedural coding:* Codes for reporting each procedure and service the physician performed in treating the patient

These systems are used to convert the physician's medical terminology into numeric (or alphanumeric) codes. In some medical practices, the physicians assign these codes; in others, a medical coder or a medical insurance specialist handles this task. In either case, an administrative medical assistant must be familiar with coding systems to work effectively with encounter forms and insurance claims. A **patient encounter form** is the form used in the medical office to record the diagnosis (or diagnoses) and the procedures performed during a patient's visit.

Diagnostic Coding

Accurate diagnostic coding gives insurance carriers clearly defined diagnoses to help them process claims efficiently. An error in coding conveys to an insurance carrier the wrong reason a patient received medical services. This causes confusion, a delay in processing, and possibly a reduced payment or denial of a claim. An incorrect code may also raise the question of fraudulent billing if the insurance company decides that, based on the diagnosis, the services provided were not medically necessary. Active diagnostic code databases can also provide statistics for medical researchers, physicians, and third-party payers about costs, trends, and future healthcare needs.

The *ICD-9-CM.* The diagnosis codes are found in the **ICD-9-CM**, the *International Classification of Diseases*. The *ICD* lists codes according to a system assigned by the World Health Organization of the United Nations. *ICD* codes are used by government healthcare programs, professional standards review organizations, medical researchers, hospitals, physicians, and other healthcare providers. Private and public medical insurance carriers also use the codes.

The *ICD* has been revised a number of times. In the title, *ICD-9-CM*, the initials *CM* indicate that the edition is a clinical modification. For example, the *ICD-9-CM* is the clinical modification of the ninth revision of the *ICD*. Codes in this modification describe various conditions and illnesses with more precision than did earlier codes. Since 1988, *ICD-9-CM* coding has been required on all Medicare claims. HIPAA mandates the use of current *ICD-9-CM* codes on insurance claim forms. Updates of the *ICD-9-CM* are published every year. Medical offices should have a copy of the most recent publication.

The *ICD-9-CM* uses three-digit codes for broad categories of diseases, injuries, and symptoms. Fourth- and fifth-level codes are created by the addition of a decimal point followed by a one- or two-digit subclassification suffix (for example, *380.01* [2010 edition] represents a fifth-level diagnostic code). Such subclassification permits the specification of a diagnosis as exactly as possible.

In addition to the categories for diseases, there are two sections of *ICD-9-CM* codes that begin with the letters *V* and *E*. These letters are followed by up to four digits. The codes that begin with a *V* are used for visits for reasons other than illness or injury. In these situations, patients often do not have a complaint or an active diagnosis. For example, a routine annual physical examination is a reason for an office visit without a complaint. Visits for treatments for already diagnosed conditions, such as for chemotherapy for cancer, also receive codes beginning with a *V*. Codes beginning with an *E* indicate the external cause of an injury or a poisoning. For example, a patient's harmful reaction to the proper dosage of a drug is assigned an E code. V codes and E codes are described in more detail later in this section.

An insurance claim for a patient must show the diagnosis that represents the patient's major health problem for *that encounter's* claim. This condition is known as the "primary diagnosis." The primary diagnosis must provide the reason for medical services listed on that claim. At times, there is more than one diagnosis because many patients are treated by a healthcare provider for more than one illness. The primary diagnosis—the underlying condition—is listed first on the insurance claim. After that, as many as three other coexisting conditions may be listed. Coexisting conditions occur at the same time as the primary diagnosis and affect the treatment or recovery from the primary condition. For example, a patient sustained a severe laceration on the right forearm and also has Type 1 diabetes. The laceration is the primary condition and Type 1 diabetes does affect the treatment and recovery of the laceration. Consequently, the patient's Type 1 diabetes is a coexisting condition.

The information for identifying a patient's diagnosis and any coexisting conditions is found in the patient's medical record. Notes about the patient's chief complaint may be entered in the patient's medical record by an administrative medical assistant, a nurse, or a physician. However, *only* the physician determines the diagnosis. A good rule-of-thumb to remember is "if it is not documented, it was not done" and, therefore, may not be coded. Thorough documentation by the provider is a must for accurate coding. All medical office team members who enter encounter data in the patient's chart should make clear and complete medical entries. Ongoing training for all personnel is a key element in keeping the medical office team up to date on documentation guidelines and maintaining accurate medical documentation.

When the diagnosis is reported on the patient encounter form after the patient's visit, the physician or coder converts the physician's written diagnosis statement to the correct code. In many medical offices, the encounter form lists the most frequently used diagnoses together with their codes for that medical practice. The physician can then simply check off the appropriate diagnosis from the list on the form, without having to look up the code in the *ICD-9-CM*.

When a diagnosis code is not provided by the physician, the coder must know how to use the *ICD-9-CM* to look up and correctly code the physician's written statement about the diagnosis. Similarly, an administrative medical assistant may need to use the *ICD-9-CM* to verify a diagnosis code or to ensure that the codes listed on the office's current encounter form are consistent with the annual updates of the *ICD-9-CM*.

Using the *ICD-9-CM*

Whether the *ICD-9-CM* is bound as a single book or a set of two or three books, three sections are available:

Volume 1—Diseases: Tabular List
Volume 2—Diseases: Alphabetic Index
Volume 3—Procedures: Tabular List and Alphabetic Index

Notice that the *ICD-9-CM* covers two major areas—diseases and procedures. The procedures (Volume 3) are used only for hospital tests and treatments. Codes from Volume 3 are used by hospital coders. An administrative medical assistant in a medical office would generally need to refer only to the diagnosis codes (Volumes 1 and 2).

In the *ICD-9-CM* diagnoses are listed two ways, as illustrated in Figures 6.4 and 6.5. One is the Alphabetic Index, which lists diagnoses in alphabetic order with their corresponding diagnosis codes. The other is the Tabular List, which provides diagnosis codes in numeric order with additional instructions. Since the Alphabetic Index (Volume 2) is referenced first when locating a diagnostic code, many publishers now place Volume 2 in front of Volume 1 in coding references.

COMPLIANCE **TIP**

Using fourth- and fifth-level *ICD* codes is not optional. When coding, always use the highest code digit available. Use a three-digit code only if there are no four-digit codes within the category. Likewise, use a four-digit code only if there is no five-digit code for that subcategory. Use the five-digit subclassification code wherever possible. Most *ICD-9-CM* books use a symbol, such as ⑤, next to a subcategory to indicate that a five-digit code is required.

Figure 6.4

Example of the *ICD-9-CM* Alphabetic Index

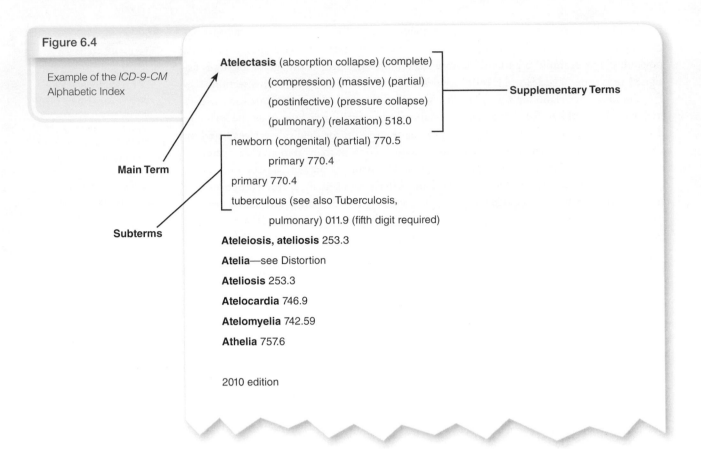

Both the Alphabetic Index and the Tabular List are used to find the right code. The Alphabetic Index is never used alone, because it does not contain all the necessary information. After a code is located in the Alphabetic Index, it is looked up in the Tabular List. Notes in this list may suggest or require the use of additional codes. Alternatively, notes may indicate that conditions should be coded differently because of exclusion from a category.

The Alphabetic Index is organized by main terms in boldface type according to condition, as shown in Figure 6.4. A main term may be followed by a series of terms in parentheses, called "supplementary terms." These supplementary terms help define the main term but have no effect on the selection of the code. Because of this fact, they are referred to as "nonessential" supplementary terms. Another type of term, a "subterm," is indented underneath the main term in regular type. Subterms do affect the selection of appropriate diagnosis codes. They describe essential differences in body sites, etiology (the cause of disease), or clinical type.

In contrast to the Alphabetic Index, the Tabular List, as shown in Figure 6.5, in the *ICD-9-CM* presents diagnosis codes in numeric order. It also organizes the codes according to body system, site, or type of procedure, rather than according to medical condition, as in the Alphabetic Index.

V codes and E codes are found in numeric order following the Tabular List. V codes classify factors that influence health status or give reasons that a patient may seek medical services when there is no clear diagnosis or disease process. Examples of V codes include routine care during pregnancy and immunizations.

Some insurance companies accept V codes for primary diagnoses. In these cases, the V code is listed first, followed by the code for the condition that requires medication or treatment. Other insurance companies require that the condition being treated be listed first, followed by a V code. Medical insurance specialists verify the requirement of each plan.

④ **362 Other retinal disorders**

> **Excludes** *chorioretinal scars (363.30–363.35)*
>
> *chorioretinitis (363.0–363.2)*

⑤ ***362.0*** *Diabetic retinopathy*

Code first diabetes (249.5, 250.5)

+362.01 **Background diabetic retinopathy**

Diabetic retinal microaneurysms

Diabetic retinopathy NOS

+362.02 **Proliferative diabetic retinopathy**

+362.03 **Nonproliferative diabetic retinopathy, NOS**

+362.04 **Nonproliferative diabetic retinopathy**

+362.05 **Moderate nonproliferative diabetic retinopathy**

+362.06 **Severe nonproliferative diabetic retinopathy**

+362.07 **Diabetic macular edema**

Diabetic retinal edema

Note: Code 362.07 must be used with a code for

diabetic retinopathy (362.01-362.06)

⑤ **362.1** **Other background retinopathy and retinal**

vascular changes

362.10 **Background retinopathy, unspecified**

362.11 **Hypertensive retinopathy**

362.12 **Exudative retinopathy**

Coats' syndrome

362.13 **Changes in vascular appearance**

Vascular sheathing of retina

Use additional code for any associated

atherosclerosis (440.8)

2010 edition

Figure 6.5

Example of the *ICD-9-CM* Tabular List

It is appropriate to use V codes

- When a patient is not sick but receives a service for a purpose, such as an ultrasound during pregnancy.
- When a patient with a current or recurring condition receives treatments, such as physical therapy.
- When a patient has a past condition that affects current health status or has a family history of disease.

E codes are diagnosis codes for external causes of poisonings and injuries. E codes are used *in addition to* the main code that describes the injury or poisoning itself; they are never used as primary codes. For example, if a person had a concussion from the impact sustained in a car accident, an E code would be used to indicate the external cause of the diagnosis. E codes are required for workers' compensation and liability insurance, since they are used to define what happened and where it happened.

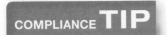
Basic Steps in Diagnostic Coding

Diagnostic coding follows a five-step process:

Step 1 *Locate the statement of the diagnosis in the patient's medical record.* If necessary, decide which is the main term or condition of the diagnosis. For example, in the diagnosis *peptic ulcer*, the main condition is *ulcer*, and peptic describes what type of ulcer it is.

Step 2 *Find the diagnosis in the ICD-9-CM's Alphabetic Index.* Look for the condition first. Then find descriptive words that make the condition more specific. Read all cross-references to check all the possibilities for a term and its synonyms. Examine all subterms under the main term in the Alphabetic Index to be sure the correct term is found. Do not stop at the first one that "sounds right." When you find the correct term, make a note of the code that follows it.

Step 3 *Locate the code from the Alphabetic Index in the ICD-9-CM's Tabular List.* The Tabular List gives codes in numeric order. Look for the number in boldface type.

Step 4 *Read all information and subclassifications to get the code that corresponds to the patient's specific disease or condition. Note fourth- or fifth-digit code requirements and exclusions.* Observe all notes for help in locating the exact code. For example, the *ICD-9-CM* may indicate "fifth code required." This note means that the correct code for the diagnosis must have five digits. The *ICD-9-CM* may also use the boxed and italicized word *Excludes* under a main term to indicate that a certain entry is not to be included as part of the preceding code. The note may also give the correct location of the excluded condition.

Fourth- and fifth-digit code requirements and exclusions are generally used in the *ICD-9-CM* to accommodate the changes in diagnoses that occur over time. Where, in the past, a single code was used for a condition, now multiple codes might be used to specify the various types and complications of the condition. This requires adding more digits to a code or grouping related codes differently.

Step 5 *Record the diagnosis code on the insurance claim, and proofread the numbers.* As part of the proofreading process, a coder should always ask: Have all the numbers been entered in the right order? Are the codes complete? Has the highest code level been used?

Coding becomes easier with practice, but do not be tempted to take shortcuts. Every case is different, and additional terms or digits may be necessary to make a diagnosis code as specific as possible. If a step is skipped, important information may be missed. If more than one diagnosis is listed in a patient's medical record, work on only one diagnosis at a time to avoid coding errors.

Procedural Coding

The procedural coding system classifies services rendered by physicians. Each procedure code represents a medical, surgical, or diagnostic service performed by a provider. A coding specialist in an insurance company compares the procedure codes with the stated diagnoses on every insurance claim to determine whether the procedures were medically necessary. An administrative medical assistant should be very meticulous in working with codes on encounter forms and insurance claims, since accurate diagnostic and procedural coding is the only way to ensure that providers receive the allowable maximum reimbursement for services.

CPT-4. The most commonly used system of procedure codes is found in the *Current Procedural Terminology*, fourth edition, a book published by the American Medical Association and known as the **CPT**. An updated edition of the *CPT* is published every year to reflect changes in medical practice. Newly developed procedures are added, and old ones that have become obsolete are deleted. These changes are also available in a computer file, because some medical offices use a computer-based version of the *CPT*.

CPT codes are five-digit numbers, organized into six sections as follows:

Section	Range of Codes
Evaluation and Management	99201–99499
Anesthesiology	00100–01999, 99100–99140
Surgery	10021–69990
Radiology	70010–79999
Pathology and Laboratory	80047–89398
Medicine (except Anesthesiology)	90281–99607

Note: 2010 Edition

With the exception of the first two sections, the *CPT* is arranged in numeric order. Codes for evaluation and management are listed first, out of numeric order, because they are used most often. Each section opens with important guidelines that apply to its procedures. This material should be checked carefully before a procedure code is chosen.

Procedure codes are located by referring to the *CPT*'s index, an alphabetic list of procedures, organs, and conditions in the back of the book. Boldface main terms may be followed by descriptions and groups of indented terms. The coder selects the correct code by reviewing each description and indented term under the main term.

CPT Organization

The six primary sections of the *CPT* are divided into categories. These in turn are further divided into headings according to the type of test, service, or body system. Code number ranges included on each page are found in the upper-right corner. This helps the coder locate a code quickly after using the index.

In the *CPT* sections, four symbols are used to highlight changes or special points. A bullet, which looks like a black circle (●), indicates a new procedure code. A triangle (▲) indicates a change in the code's description. The triangle appears in only the year the descriptor (the description of the numeric code) is revised. Facing triangles (▶ ◀) enclose other new or revised information with the exception of the code's descriptor. A plus sign (+) is used for add-on codes, indicating procedures that are usually carried out in addition to another procedure. For example, Code 90471 covers one immunization administration, and Code +90472 covers administering an additional shot. Add-on codes are never reported alone. They are used together with the primary code. A bullet inside a circle (⊙) beside a code means conscious sedation is part of the procedure. When conscious sedation is used, the patient is in a moderate, drug-induced depression of consciousness and can still respond to verbal commands. When a product, such as a vaccine, is pending FDA approval, a thunderbolt symbol (⚡) is used. Once the product is approved, the symbol is removed and the code may be used. New to the 2010 edition is the "#" symbol, which precedes a code that has been resequenced or is an out-of-order code. Also, a new appendix, Appendix N, has been added to list all resequenced and out-of-order codes.

The *CPT* uses a special format to show codes and their descriptions. The "parent code" description begins with a capital letter and may be followed by indented descriptive codes. The indented codes include the description of the parent code up to the semicolon, plus the indented information. See Figure 6.6 for an example of *CPT-4* code listings.

Notes and Modifiers

CPT listings may also contain notes, which are explanations for categories and individual codes. Notes often appear in parentheses after a code. Many notes suggest other codes that should be considered before a final code is selected.

COMPLIANCE **TIP**

Medical offices should have the current year's *ICD-9-CM* and *CPT* available for reference. Previous years' books should also be kept, in case there is a question about already submitted insurance claims.

Figure 6.6

Example of the *CPT-4*
Code Listings

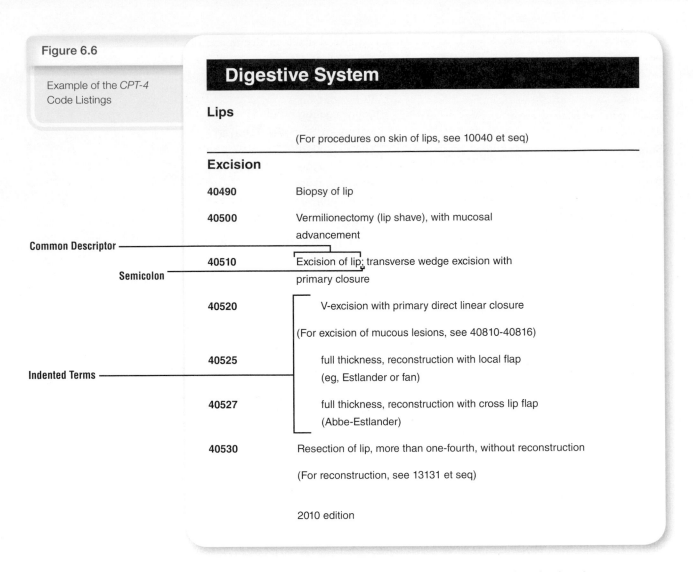

Common Descriptor

Semicolon

Indented Terms

Digestive System

Lips

(For procedures on skin of lips, see 10040 et seq)

Excision

40490	Biopsy of lip
40500	Vermilionectomy (lip shave), with mucosal advancement
40510	Excision of lip; transverse wedge excision with primary closure
40520	V-excision with primary direct linear closure
	(For excision of mucous lesions, see 40810-40816)
40525	full thickness, reconstruction with local flap (eg, Estlander or fan)
40527	full thickness, reconstruction with cross lip flap (Abbe-Estlander)
40530	Resection of lip, more than one-fourth, without reconstruction
	(For reconstruction, see 13131 et seq)

2010 edition

One or more two-digit modifiers may need to be assigned to the five-digit main number. Modifiers are written with a hyphen before the two-digit number. Modifiers show that some special circumstance applies to the service or procedure the physician performed. Appendix A of the *CPT* explains the proper use of each modifier.

Some services or procedures occur so infrequently that they are not listed in the *CPT*. Others are too new to be included. Unlisted procedures codes are provided for these situations. When a code for an unlisted procedure is used, a report must be attached to the insurance claim. It describes the procedure, its extent, and the reason it was performed.

Coding Evaluation and Management Services

To diagnose conditions and plan treatments, physicians use different amounts of time and effort, as well as different kinds of skill, depending on the patient and the circumstance. In the guidelines to the Evaluation and Management (E/M) section, the *CPT* explains how to code different levels of these services. Three key factors documented in the patient's medical record help determine the level of service:

- The extent of the patient history taken
- The extent of the examination conducted
- The complexity of the medical decision making

In addition to level of service, insurance carriers want to know whether the physician treated a *new patient* or an *established patient*. Physicians often spend more time during new patients' visits than during visits from established patients, so the E/M codes for the two types of patients are separate. For reporting purposes, the CPT considers a patient "new" if that person has not received professional services from the physician or a physician of the same specialty practicing within the same group in the past three years. Medical offices commonly use the abbreviation *NP* for a new patient. An established patient is one who has seen the physician or a physician of the same specialty within the same group in the past three years. (Note that the current visit need not be for a problem treated previously.) Medical offices commonly use the abbreviation *EP* for an established patient. Emergency patients are not classified as either new or established patients.

The CPT has a range of codes for new-patient or established-patient encounters. The lowest-level code is often called a Level I code; the codes continue to go higher, such as a Level V code. Annual physical examinations are located under the heading *Preventive Medicine Services* in the E/M section and are coded based on the age of new or established patients. For example, the procedure code 99395 (2010 edition), in the "established patient" category, covers the routine examination, with tests and counseling, of a patient between the ages of 18 and 39.

Location of the service is also important, because different E/M codes apply to services performed in a physician's office, a hospital inpatient room, a hospital emergency department, a nursing facility, an extended-care facility, or a patient's home.

Coders should also be familiar with the difference between a referral and a consultation, since codes connected with these services are different. Sometimes one physician sends a patient to another physician for examination and treatment. This transferring of the responsibility for the patient's care for that condition is called a "referral." Standard E/M codes are used by the physician who assumes the responsibility. In contrast, a consultation occurs when an attending physician requests advice from another physician but retains responsibility for the care of the patient. The CPT E/M section lists several codes for consultations, depending on the level and location of the service.

As of January 1, 2010, physicians providing consultation services to Medicare patients and billing the services to Medicare can no longer use any of the consultation codes. CMS no longer makes a differentiation between consultation codes and nonconsultation codes. Higher monies previously paid for the consultation codes will be redistributed among the office and hospital E/M service codes. For example, a physician who sees a patient and conducts a comprehensive history and examination using high-complexity medical decision making would have used code 99245 prior to January 1, 2010. Currently, however, the physician must use code 99205 if the patient was a new patient to the physician or code 99215 if the patient is considered established. Currently, consultation codes may be used for other insurance carriers.

Coding Surgical Procedures

In the Surgery section, a "separate procedure" is a surgical procedure usually performed as an integral part of a full surgical package (multiple services combined into one code). When the procedure is done independently, it may be reported by itself or with another procedure or service by adding the modifier -59 to the separate procedure code. In contrast to these procedures, most codes listed in the Surgery section include all routine elements.

Coding Laboratory Procedures

Organ or disease-oriented panels listed in the Pathology and Laboratory section of the CPT include tests frequently ordered together. An acute hepatitis panel, for example, includes tests for hepatitis A antibody, IgM antibody; hepatitis B core antibody, IgM antibody; hepatitis B surface antigen; and hepatitis C antibody (2010 edition). Each element of the panel has its own procedure code. However, when the tests are performed together, the coder must use the code for the panel, rather than list each test separately.

COMPLIANCE TIP

If each test in a panel or procedure in a surgical package is listed separately, it will "unbundle" the panel or package. The review performed by the insurance carrier's claims department will rebundle the services under the appropriate code, which could delay payment. Note that when unbundling is done intentionally to receive more payment than is correct, the claim is likely to be considered fraudulent.

Coding Immunizations

Injections and infusions of immune globulins, vaccines, toxoids, and other substances require two codes—one for giving the injection and one for the particular vaccine or toxoid that is given. For example, for an influenza shot, the administration code 90471 is used for the injection, along with one of the codes for the specific vaccine, such as 90281, 96360, or 96365 (2010 edition). If a significant, separately identifiable E/M service was provided, the appropriate E/M code should also be reported in addition to the vaccine and toxoid administration codes.

HCPCS Codes. The Health Care Financing Administration's Common Procedure Coding System, commonly referred to as **HCPCS**, was developed by the CMS, and in 1996 HIPAA mandated the use of not only the *CPT* codes for billing and coding but also HCPCS codes. The *CPT* Level II codes, HCPCS (pronounced "hic-picks") are a coding system that uses both all the codes in the *CPT* (considered *CPT* Level I codes) and additional codes that cover many supplies, such as sterile trays, drugs, and durable medical equipment (DME). The additional codes have five characters—numbers, letters, or both—and a different set of modifiers. Examples of these codes follow.

Code Number	Description
G0104	Colorectal cancer screening; flexible sigmoidoscopy
V5299	Hearing service, miscellaneous

In medical offices where the HCPCS system is used, regulations issued by the CMS are reviewed to determine the correct code and modifier for claims.

Basic Steps in Procedural Coding. Five steps are used for finding procedure codes in the *CPT*, as follows.

Step 1 *Become familiar with the* CPT. Read the introduction and main section guidelines and notes. For example, look at the guidelines for the Evaluation and Management section. They include definitions of key terms, such as *new patient, established patient, chief complaint, concurrent care,* and *counseling.* They also explain the way E/M codes should be selected.

Step 2 *Find the services that were provided.* The next step is to check the patient's encounter form to see which services were performed. For E/M procedures, look for clues as to the extent of history, examination, and decision making that were involved and the amount of time the physician spent with the patient.

Step 3 *Look up the procedure code.* First, pick out a specific procedure or service, organ, or condition. Find the procedure code in the *CPT*'s index. For example, to find the code for "burns, dressing," first look alphabetically in the index for the procedure. Then, turn to the procedure code in the body of the *CPT* to be sure the code accurately reflects the service performed. Although it may seem tempting to record the procedure code directly from the index, resist the shortcut. Critical information is placed at the beginning of each chapter and sections within the chapter. Read all information prior to using a code. Explanations and notes in the guidelines and main sections more accurately lead to finding main numbers and modifiers that reflect the services performed. That is the only way to ensure reimbursement at the highest allowed level.

Step 4 *Determine appropriate modifiers.* Check section guidelines and Appendix A to find modifiers that elaborate on details of the procedure being coded. For example, a bilateral breast reconstruction requires the modifier –50. Find the code for "breast reconstruction with free flap": 19364. To show the insurance carrier that the procedure was performed on both breasts, attach –50: 19364–50.

Step 5 *Record the procedure code.* After the procedure code is verified, it is posted to the insurance claim form (see Chapter 7). If the patient has more than one diagnosis for a single claim, the primary diagnosis is listed first. Likewise, the corresponding primary procedure is listed first. The *primary procedure* is the main service performed for the condition listed as the primary diagnosis.

The physician may perform additional procedures at the same time or in the same session as the primary procedure. If additional procedures are performed, match each procedure with its corresponding diagnosis. If this is not done, the procedures will not be considered medically necessary and the claim will be denied.

For example, Ms. Silvers, who saw Dr. Rucker for chest pain and shortness of breath, also has asthma. While the patient was in the office, Dr. Rucker renewed her prescription for asthma medication along with performing the ECG. If the ECG is mistakenly shown as a procedure for asthma, the claim will be denied, because that procedure is not medically necessary for that diagnosis.

Coding procedures become easier as the coder becomes more familiar with *CPT* codes. In fact, most medical offices use only a limited number of procedure codes.

Coding Compliance

On correct claims, each reported service is connected to a diagnosis that supports the procedure as necessary to investigate or treat the patient's condition. Insurance company representatives analyze this connection between the diagnostic and the procedural information, called **code linkage**, to evaluate the medical necessity of the reported charges. Correct claims also comply with many other regulations from government agencies and private payers.

Diagnostic and procedure codes are updated quarterly and annually. Current codes must be used to identify the diagnoses and procedures that are performed. Code numbers may be added or deleted and code descriptions may be modified. Current-year coding books are available in October and January. Updates are also published quarterly on the CMS Web site. To not use the current year's code is considered noncompliant coding. When new codes go into effect, all office resources, such as charge slips, must be updated to reflect the new codes. Many offices use coding software programs, which have to be updated to include the current codes.

Claims are denied because of lack of medical necessity when the reported services are not consistent with the symptoms or the diagnosis and when they are not in keeping with generally accepted professional medical standards. Correctly linked codes that support medical necessity meet these conditions:

- The *CPT-4* procedure codes match the *ICD-9-CM* diagnosis codes.
- The procedures are not elective, experimental, or nonessential.
- The procedures are furnished at an appropriate level.

Medical necessity rules are established by each third-party payer. For example, each Medicare carrier has its own guidelines for particular procedures and the diagnoses that must be linked for payment. Private payers may impose a different set of rules, and contradictions are not uncommon.

Common Coding Errors. There are many factors that contribute to coding errors. Some of the more common coding errors are

- Reporting diagnosis codes that are not at the highest level of specificity available.
- Using out-of-date codes.
- Altering documentation after the services are reported.

- Coding without proper documentation to back up the codes selected.
- Reporting services provided by unlicensed or unqualified clinical personnel.
- Reporting services that are not covered or that have limited coverage.
- Using modifiers incorrectly, or not at all.
- Upcoding—using a procedure code that provides a higher reimbursement rate than the code that actually reflects the service provided.
- Unbundling—billing the parts of a bundled procedure as separate procedures.

Most medical practices have a system, formal or informal, for evaluating coding errors in an effort to achieve better coding compliance. Some examples of efforts that can be made include the appointment of a compliance officer and committee, regular training plans, and ongoing monitoring and auditing of claim preparation.

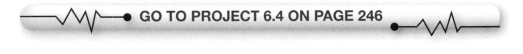

GO TO PROJECT 6.4 ON PAGE 246

6.5 ICD-10

The tenth edition of the *ICD* was published by the World Health Organization (WHO) in 1990. In the United States, the new *ICD-10* is being field tested and reviewed by healthcare professionals. *ICD-10-CM* is expected to be adopted by the United States as the mandatory code set for diagnostic coding. *ICD-10-PCS* (the current Volume 3 of *ICD-9-CM*) will be used for inpatient procedures. The Department of Health and Human Services has mandated implementation of the new *ICD-10* code set by October 1, 2013.

Some of the major changes include

- More categories and codes than *ICD-9-CM*. Currently, *ICD-10-CM* contains more than 187,000 codes, which is a substantial change from the available codes in the *ICD-9-CM* set (13,500). *ICD-10-PCS* will increase from 4,000 codes in *ICD-9-CM* Volume 3 to approximately 200,000 codes. The creation of more codes allows a higher level of specificity when reporting diseases and newly recognized conditions. It will also allow for expansion within categories.
- Alphanumeric codes, containing a letter followed by up to five numbers will be used.
- A sixth digit is added to capture clinical details. For example, all codes that relate to pregnancy, labor, and childbirth include a digit that indicates the patient's trimester.
- New codes are added to show bilateralness (which side of the body is affected) for a disease or condition that can be involved with the right side, the left side, or both sides. For example, separate codes are listed for a malignant neoplasm of right upper-inner quadrant of the female breast and for a malignant neoplasm of the left upper-quadrant of the female breast.

A crosswalk, a resource that connects the two sets of codes, will be available to assist medical office personnel with the transition. The crosswalk, referred to as a General Equivalency Mapping (GEM), connecting *ICD-10-CM* to *ICD-9-CM* will be used by medical office personnel to relate the two coding systems. Figure 6.7 shows an example of a crosswalk. Although the code numbers look different, the basic systems are very similar. Individuals who are familiar with the current codes will find their training quickly applied to the new *ICD-10* system.

EXAMPLE 1

ICD-9-CM 896.2 Traumatic amputation of foot (complete) (partial) Bilateral, without mention of complication

ICD-10-CM Choose one of the following:

• S98.911A Complete traumatic amputation of right foot, level unspecified, initial encounter OR S98.921A Partial Traumatic Amputation of right foot, level unspecified, initial encounter   AND
• Choose one of the following:
• S98.912A Complete, traumatic amputation of left foot, level unspecified, initial encounter OR   S98.922A Partial traumatic amputation of left foot, level unspecified, initial encounter

Two *ICD-10-CM* codes are required for coding the bilateral amputation. The two codes specify both the bilateral amputation and whether the amputation was complete or partial. The *ICD-9-CM* code of 896.2 does not specify if the amputation was complete or partial.

EXAMPLE 2

ICD-9-CM
428.1 Left heart failure

ICD-10-CM
I50.1 Left ventricular failure

Notice that the new *ICD-10-CM* code provides the specific location of the failure—the left ventricle.

EXAMPLE 3

ICD-9-CM
728.86 Necrotizing fasciitis

ICD-10-CM
M72.6 Necrotizing fasciitis

Notice that the *ICD-9-CM* and the *ICD-10-CM* code descriptions are the same.

Chapter Projects

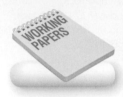

Project 6.1 **Insurance Terminology**

On WP 41, match each insurance term in Column 2 with its definition in Column 1. Be prepared to discuss your answers in class.

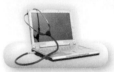

Project 6.2 **Internet Research: The Medicare Web Site**

The official U.S. government Web site for Medicare information provides information about Medicare basics, Medicare plan choices, publications, nursing homes, a participating physician directory for your area, the top 20 questions from the Medicare helpline, and more. Visit www.medicare.gov and look up information about the different Medicare plan choices available nationally, as well as what plans are available in your area. Be prepared to share the results of your reading with the class.

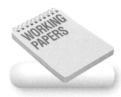

Project 6.3 **Insurance Plans, Payers, and Payment Methods**

WP 42 contains statements that refer to the obligations of the physician and/or medical law. Mark each statement with either "T" for *true* or "F" for *false*. For each *false* answer, document on a separate sheet of paper what makes the statement *false.* Also be prepared to share your answers in class.

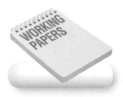

Project 6.4 **Identifying Diagnostic and Procedure Codes**

Refer to WP 43 *(ICD-9-CM* diagnostic codes) and WP 44 (patient encounter form for Janet Provost's annual exam) to answer the following questions regarding diagnostic and procedure codes.

1. What is the *ICD-9-CM* diagnostic code for each of the following conditions?
   a. Migraine headache   _____
   b. Chest pain   _____
   c. Lightheadedness   _____
   d. Annual physical exam, age 39   _____
   e. Family history of heart disease   _____
   f. Test for pregnancy   _____
   g. Osteoarthritis   _____

2. Review Janet Provost's patient encounter form.
   a. What is the diagnostic code for Janet Provost's visit? _____
   b. What is the description given in the *ICD-9-CM* for this code? _____
   c. What procedures did Dr. Larsen perform? List the *CPT-4* procedure codes for each: _____
   d. How much did Dr. Larsen charge for the complete blood count (CBC)? _____

3. Do you think the *CPT-4* procedure codes marked off on the encounter form are in compliance with the *ICD-9-CM* diagnosis code given? _____

Chapter 6 Summary

6.1 Define *medical insurance* and *coding terminology*. Pages 222–224	• Administrative medical assistants should be familiar with basic terms and concepts of medical insurance, including coding and compliance. Insurance carriers may use different terminology, and medical office personnel need to know current terminology.
6.2 Explain differences among types of insurance plans. Pages 224–229	• Indemnity plans are usually fee-for-service plans that pay after services are provided. They offer benefits in exchange for regular payments of a fixed premium by the insured. In addition, the insured must also pay deductibles and coinsurance. • Managed care plans, in contrast, often use capitation payments, which are fixed, prospective payments made for services to be provided during a specified period of time. It is common to base capitation rates on gender and age. Managed care organizations contract with both patients and providers. • In an HMO, patients agree to receive services from providers who have contracts with the HMO; usually, a PCP coordinates the patient's care and makes referrals. • In a PPO, patients are offered lower fees in exchange for receiving services from plan providers but are usually not required to choose a PCP.
6.3 Compare and contrast PAR and nonPAR and the methods used by insurance companies to determine how much a provider is paid. Pages 229–233	• PAR providers agree to render medical services to plan members according to the plan's rules and payment schedules; a nonPAR provider is not contractually obligated to abide by the rules or the payment schedule when treating members. • PAR providers receive a direct benefit payment from the insurance carrier through an agreed-upon assignment of benefits; a nonPAR provider collects payment from the patient at the time of service and the patient receives payment from the insurance carrier. • Common types of payment systems used by third-party payers for reimbursing physicians are based on (a) usual, customary, and reasonable (UCR) fees; (b) a relative value scale (RVS); (c) a resource-based relative value scale (RBRVS); or (d) diagnosis-related groups (DRGs).

| 6.4 Explain diagnostic coding, procedural coding, and coding compliance. Pages 234–244 | • The *ICD-9-CM* is used to report patients' conditions (diagnoses) on insurance claims. Codes consist of three, four, or five numbers and a description. The Alphabetic Index is used first to approximate the correct code for a diagnosis. Next, the Tabular List is used to verify and refine the final code selection. All notations and coding guidelines should be followed.
| | • *CPT-4*, a publication of the AMA, contains the most widely used system for physicians' medical services and procedures. There are two levels of procedural codes: *CPT-4* and HCPCS, which include temporary codes. *CPT-4* codes are required for reporting physician services on insurance claim forms. Codes consist of five digits and a description. Modifiers may be used to indicate a change to the code description. *CPT-4* contains six sections of codes:
| | — Evaluation and Management
| | — Anesthesia
| | — Surgery
| | — Radiology
| | — Pathology and Laboratory
| | — Medicine
| | These are followed by appendices and an index. The Alphabetic Index is used first in the process of selecting a code; then the code number is referenced in the Tabular List. Notes, exclusions, inclusions, and other critical information are contained within the Tabular List. Therefore, *never* code directly from the Alphabetic Index without verifying the code selection in the Tabular List.
| | • HCPCS codes are used to code supplies, equipment, and procedures not listed in the *CPT-4*. HCPCS codes are selected the same way as *CPT-4* codes. Refer to the Alphabetic Index first and then verify the code selection in the Tabular List. Within HCPCS, codes are alphanumeric.
| | • Coding compliance is the process of coding using actions that satisfy federal official requirements and guidelines. Individual carrier guidelines must also be followed in order to be considered compliant.

6.5 Identify the structural changes in coding with the implementation of *ICD-10* and explain the advantages of these changes. Pages 244–245	• *ICD-10* is scheduled for mandated implementation October 1, 2013. It will replace the *ICD-9-CM* coding system. *ICD-10-CM* will replace the current *ICD-9-CM* Volumes 1 and 2 used by physicians' offices and other outpatient facilities. *ICD-10-PCS* will replace the current *ICD-9-CM* Volume 3 used to code inpatient hospital procedures. • *ICD-10* will contain substantially more codes from which to choose and the codes will be alphanumeric, containing a letter followed by up to five digits. Clinical details will be noted using a sixth digit. Also, *ICD-10* codes will be added to show laterality or bilaterality. • Increasing the number of available codes permits a higher level of specificity when reporting disease and will incorporate newly recognized conditions.

Soft Skills Success

Time Management

How often do you find yourself running out of time? Many feel that there is just never enough time in the day to get everything done. When you know how to manage your time, you gain control. Effective time management helps you choose what to work on and when. This is important if you want to achieve anything of any real worth. To start managing time effectively, you need to set goals. Consider setting a goal of producing clean claims (an error-free claim) at a rate of 98 percent or above for a given submission period (such as one work day). Without proper goal setting, your time will be wasted on the confusion of conflicting priorities. People tend to neglect goal setting because it requires time and effort. A little time and effort put in now saves an enormous amount of time, effort, and frustration in the future. **Are your time management skills strong? Describe how your skills could be improved, or share how your skills have helped you become successful.**

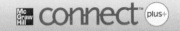
USING TERMINOLOGY

Match the term or phrase on the left with the correct answer on the right.

_____ 1. (LO 6.2) Capitation

_____ 2. (LO 6.3) PAR

_____ 3. (LO 6.1) Premium

_____ 4. (LO 6.3) CMS

_____ 5. (LO 6.4) Patient encounter form

_____ 6. (LO 6.1) Third-party payer

_____ 7. (LO 6.2) Managed care

_____ 8. (LO 6.1) Provider

_____ 9. (LO 6.4) HCPCS

_____ 10. (LO 6.2) Coinsurance

a. Stated amount an insured must pay for an insurance policy

b. Physician or other provider who agrees to treat the patient

c. Insurance payment that pays a prepaid, stated amount to the provider for covered services within a stated period of time

d. Percentage of a covered claim that the insured must pay

e. Provider who agrees to offer covered services per a plan's contract rules and regulations

f. Organization that administers Medicare and Medicaid

g. Used to record patient encounter diagnoses and procedures

h. Alphanumeric coding system used to record supplies and procedures

i. Insurance carrier

j. Most popular insurance plan in the United States

CHECK YOUR UNDERSTANDING

Select the most correct answer.

1. (LO 6.1) Patient A had a CBC and a PFT performed. Which type of insurance will cover the services?

    a. Major medical
    b. Surgical
    c. Basic
    d. Disability

2. (LO 6.2) Noelle's insurance policy states she has a coinsurance of 90/10 of covered services. When she received her notice from the insurance carrier, it stated that the charges for her last office visit were not allowed. How much of the charges is Noelle responsible for?

    a. 90 percent
    b. 10 percent
    c. 0 percent
    d. 100 percent

3. (LO 6.2) Under his insurance plan, Tyler is required to have prior approval for his upcoming knee replacement. Before the surgery, the surgeon must have which approval document from the insurance plan for the surgery?

   a. Informed consent
   b. Expressed consent
   c. Patient encounter form
   d. Preauthorization/precertification approval

4. (LO 6.2) Michelle and her husband, Drew, just had a baby. Michelle is laid off from her job and Drew works part-time at a gas station. They are without insurance coverage. The administrative medical assistant should supply Michelle and Drew with the contact information for

   a. Medicare.
   b. Medicaid.
   c. TRICARE.
   d. CHAMPVA.

5. (LO 6.3) Dr. Abrams receives payment from BCBS for services rendered to patients covered by the plan. This is known as

   a. Assignment of benefits.
   b. Accepting assignment.
   c. Balance billing.
   d. Preauthorization of services.

6. (LO 6.3) If the standard fee for a Medicare covered service is $150 and the Medicare nonPAR fee schedule for the service is $80, what is the limiting charge for the service?

   a. $120
   b. $92
   c. $30
   d. $50

7. (LO 6.4) The insurance carrier has requested codes to indicate where its insured's injury took place. Which of the following code categories will be used?

   a. V codes
   b. HCPCS codes
   c. Evaluation and management codes
   d. E codes

8. (LO 6.4) Luke last visited his physician, who has a single-physician practice, in September 2006. He is at the office today for a sore throat and chest congestion. Since he was already a patient, the medical insurance coder submitted an established patient E/M code to Luke's insurance carrier for payment. The insurance carrier requested additional documentation on the visit. Which of the following may have been the reason?

   a. Luke's visit should have been coded from the HCPCS code selections.
   b. The medical insurance coder did not submit the claim to the insurance carrier on the actual day of Luke's visit.
   c. Luke's visit should have been coded from the new patient E/M category.
   d. There was no reason for the insurance carrier to request additional documentation.

9. (LO 6.4) During Luke's visit mentioned in Question 8, a CBC was performed. Which type of code(s) should be used for the service?

    a. Unbundled codes

    b. E codes

    c. Bundled code

    d. Medicine code

10. (LO 6.5) Which of the following is not an advantage of *ICD-10*?

    a. Higher level of specificity

    b. Expansion of and within categories

    c. Increased number of bilateral codes

    d. Fewer and more concise categories

THINKING IT THROUGH

These questions cover the most important points in this chapter. Using your critical-thinking skills, play the role of an administrative medical assistant as you answer each question. Be prepared to present your responses in class.

1. How would you explain to a patient who is unfamiliar with insurance terminology what is meant by the term *third-party payer*? How was the term derived?

2. Ellen Gold, a Medicare patient, does not understand her last month's medical statement. She already paid her deductible, yet the bill states that she owes $20 on a total bill of $100. How would you explain the bill to her?

3. Joe Cantinori inquires about his unpaid bill and asks whether the physician received payment from his insurance company. When you check his record, you find that your office submitted the insurance form on his behalf. However, the physician did not accept assignment on the claim, since he is not a PAR provider in that program. This means that the insurance company will send the payment directly to Joe. How would you explain this to Joe?

4. A patient complained of symptoms usually associated with arthritis. The physician ordered the following tests: rheumatoid factor, uric acid, sedimentation rate, and fluorescent noninfectious agent screening. The insurance claim submitted contained procedure codes for each test. You have not received any response from the insurance carrier, even though payments for other claims sent to the same carrier on that day have been received. What do you think accounts for the delay?

Billing, Reimbursement, and Collections

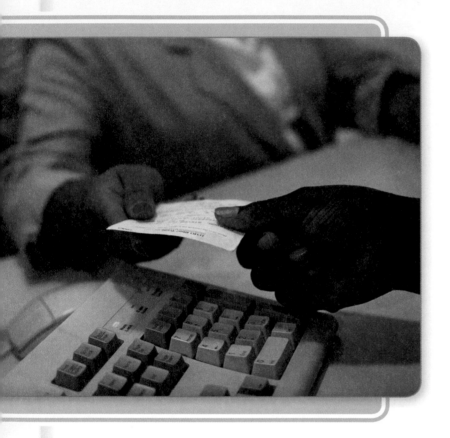

LEARNING OUTCOMES

After studying this chapter, you will be able to:

7.1 Recognize and calculate charges for medical services and process patient statements based on the patient encounter form and the physician's fee schedule.

7.2 Compare and contrast the process of completing and transmitting insurance claims using both hardcopy and electronic methods.

7.3 Describe the different types of billing options used by medical practices for billing patients.

7.4 Paraphrase the procedures and options available for collecting delinquent accounts.

KEY TERMS

Study these important words, which are defined in this chapter, to build your professional vocabulary:

clearinghouse	collection ratio	fee adjustment	scrubber program
clean claim	cycle billing	fee schedule	terminated account
CMS-1500 claim form	dependent	guarantor	third-party liability
collection agency	electronic claims	monthly billing	write-off
collection at the time of service	EOB	patient information form	
	ERA	patient statement	

Chapter 7

ABHES

- Adapt to change.
- Maintain confidentiality at all times.
- Use appropriate guidelines when releasing records or information.
- Project a positive attitude.
- Be cognizant of ethical boundaries.
- Evidence a responsible attitude.
- Conduct work within scope of education, training, and ability.
- Professional components.
- Monitor legislation related to current healthcare issues and practices.
- Locate resources and information for patients and employers.
- Use proper telephone techniques.
- Apply electronic technology.
- Apply computer concepts for office procedures.
- Orient patients to office policies and procedures.
- Adapt what is said to the recipient's level of comprehension.
- Adapt for individualized needs.
- Apply managed care policies and procedures.
- Obtain managed care referrals and precertification.
- Follow established policy in initiating or terminating medical treatment.
- Establish and maintain a petty cash fund.
- Perform basic secretarial skills.
- Prepare a bank statement.
- Reconcile a bank statement.

- ➡ Cognitive
- ➡ Psychomotor
- ➡ Affective

- Maintain records for accounting and banking purposes.
- Post entries on a day sheet.
- Prepare a check.
- Post collection agency payments.
- Prepare a check.
- Post collection agency payments.
- Use manual and computerized bookkeeping systems.
- Manage accounts payable and receivable.
- Be courteous and diplomatic.

CAAHEP

- ➡ Compare manual and computerized bookkeeping systems used in ambulatory healthcare.
- ➡ Explain both billing and payment options.
- ➡ Identify procedures for preparing patient accounts.
- ➡ Discuss procedures for collecting outstanding accounts.
- ➡ Discuss precautions for accepting checks.
- ➡ Compare types of endorsements.
- ➡ Differentiate between accounts payable and accounts receivable.
- ➡ Describe the impact of both the Fair Debt Collection Act and the Federal Truth in Lending Act of 1968 as they apply to collections.
- ➡ Perform accounts receivable procedures: (a) post entries on a day sheet; (b) perform billing procedures; (c) perform collection procedures; (d) post adjustments; (e) process a credit balance; (f) process refunds; (g) post nonsufficient fund (NSF) checks; (h) post collective agency payments.
- ➡ Utilize computerized office billing systems.
- ➡ Demonstrate sensitivity and professionalism in handling accounts receivable activities with clients.

INTRODUCTION

Administrative medical assistants help maintain physicians' financial records. This includes billing patients, filing insurance claims, and collecting the appropriate fees. Billing, reimbursement, and collections are extremely important because the office depends on the cash flow generated by these functions. All the expenses of running the office, such as supplies, payroll, and liability insurance, depend on the revenue from patients' and insurance companies' payments. General rules for filing healthcare claim forms, billing patients, and implementing collection procedures are discussed in this chapter.

7.1 RECORDING TRANSACTIONS

Administrative medical assistants keep track of the services rendered and any payments made during a visit to the physician. After the patient completes the office visit, the administrative medical assistant updates the patient ledger to show the financial information for the encounter.

Patient Encounter Form

To facilitate the process of billing patients for physicians' services, medical offices use a patient encounter form. A blank patient encounter form (also called a charge slip, superbill, routing slip, or patient service form) is attached to the patient's medical record for completion. It is used to record the details of patients' encounters for billing and insurance purposes. In particular, it is designed to record each procedure the physician performs, the fee charged for each, and the diagnosis connected with the treatment.

Most encounter forms contain sections for recording the following information (see Figure 7.1 for an example):

- Patient's name, address, phone information, and type of insurance, as well as patient return information, such as two weeks, prn
- Date of service
- Diagnosis for the current visit
- Procedure information—a checklist of the most commonly administered examinations, lab tests, injections, and other procedures in that office and the physician's fee for each
- Financial information—the total fees for the day, payments made—and amount due for that visit
- Physician identifying information—address, fax and phone numbers, national provider identification (NPI), employer identification number (EIN), and individual insurance provider numbers

Preprinted forms should be numbered to provide a higher level of audit control over the forms, thereby reducing the possibility of fraudulent claims. All numbered forms must be accounted for and any missing forms found. The word "VOID" should be written in large red letters across encounter forms that are not to be used (i.e., error on the form such as wrong patient name) and should be included with other daily encounter forms.

Forms should be updated annually and the codes verified with the current year's diagnostic and procedural codes. Documentation of the update is usually placed in the right lower corner, indicating when the form was last updated, such as "January 1, 2011."

The procedures listed on a patient encounter form are customized to represent the most commonly administered examinations, lab tests, injections, and other procedures for that practice. On some encounter forms, the fee for each procedure is printed beside the procedure code. In most cases, however, because the physician's fees may change from year to year, and because they are sometimes adjusted or discounted for different patients and insurance

Figure 7.1

Completed Patient
Encounter Form

No.	Date	Description	Charge	Credit		Current Balance
				Payment	Adjustment	
	05/15/2008	Annual exam, HGB, UA	173.00	34.60	-------	138.40

Patient Information

7911 Riverview Lane N.
Address

Chicago, IL 60632-1979
City, State, Zip

312-555-6685   312-555-3385
Home phone   **Work phone**

Alison Becker   self
Responsible Person   **Relationship**

Real Insurance   470-55-8533
Insurance   **Contract numbers**

Patient _____ Becker, Alison _____

Date: 05/15/2008   **Chart #** 1324

Karen Larsen, MD
2235 S. Ridgeway Avenue
Chicago, IL 60623-2240

312-555-6022

FAX: 213-555-0025
NPI: 1234567

Diagnoses:

1. ___ V70.0 ___

2. _____

3. _____

4. _____

OFFICE VISITS

New Patient			Established Patient	
		Preventive Medicine		
	___ 99381	under 1 year	___ 99391	
___ 99201	___ 99382	1–4	___ 99392	___ 99211
___ 99202	___ 99383	5–11	___ 99393	___ 99212
___ 99203	___ 99384	12–17	___ 99394	___ 99213
___ 99204	___ 99385	18–39	136.00 99395	___ 99214
___ 99205	___ 99386	40–64	___ 99396	___ 99215
	___ 99387	65+	___ 99397	

Hospital Visits
Initial:
___ 99221
___ 99222
___ 99223
Subsequent:
___ 99231
___ 99232
___ 99233
Nursing Facility
Initial:
___ 99304
___ 99305
___ 99306

Subsequent:
___ 99307
___ 99308
___ 99309
___ 99310
Discharge
___ 99315
___ 99316

Other
___ 99318

Return visit: Two weeks

Lab:
___ 80048 Basic
    metabolic panel
    (SMA-8)
___ 87110 Chlamydia
    culture
___ 85651 ESR;
    nonautomated
___ 83001 FSH
___ 82947 Glucose,
    blood
___ 85025 Hemogram
    (CBC) with
    differential
___ 80076 Hepatic
    function panel
13.00 85018 HGB
___ 86701 HIV-1
___ 83002 LH
___ 80061 Lipid panel
___ 86617 Lyme
    antibody

___ 86308 Monospot
    test
___ 88150 Pap
___ 85610 Prothrombin
    time
___ 84152 PSA
___ 86430 Rheumatoid
    factor
___ 82270 Stool
    hemoccult x 3
___ 87430 Strep screen
___ 84478 Triglycerides
___ 84443 TSH
24.00 81001 UA with
    microscopy
___ 87088 UC
___ 84550 Uric acid,
    blood
___ 81025 Urine
    pregnancy test
_____
_____

Injections:
___ 90471 admin 1 vac
___ 90472 each add'l
    vac
___ 90716 Chickenpox
___ 90702 DT
___ 90701 DTP
___ 90657 Influenza
    6-35 months
___ 90658 Influenza
    3 years +
___ 90665 Lyme disease
___ 90707 MMR
___ 90704 Mumps
___ 90713 Polio vac
    inactivated (IPV)
___ 90703 Tetanus Tox
ECG: ___ 93000 ECG

Other
_____
_____

Updated January 1, 2011

plans, a space is provided before each code (as in Figure 7.1) for the administrative medical assistant to enter the appropriate fee at the time of the visit

Procedural and diagnostic codes listed on the encounter form should be updated to reflect current year codes. Placing on the form the date it was updated—for example, in the bottom right-hand corner—will show which year's codes are on the form.

The following is the procedure for using a patient encounter form:

1. An encounter form is attached to the patient's file when the patient registers for the visit.

2. As the physician performs various procedures during the visit, check marks are made in the appropriate boxes on the encounter form (or the appropriate items on the form are circled). The diagnoses and corresponding codes are also recorded on the form.

3. At the end of the visit, the form is taken to the checkout area for the administrative medical assistant to record, or post, the necessary transactions in the office's billing system.

Practices using electronic health records (EHRs) will input data traditionally documented on an encounter form into the patient's EHR. Codes and charges will be linked to the documentation and the patient's electronic account will be automatically updated and charged. A hardcopy encounter form may still be given to the patient to use during checkout.

Fee Schedule

Each physician or medical practice has a **fee schedule**, which lists the usual procedures the office performs and the corresponding charges. The administrative medical assistant should always refer to the practice's fee schedule in determining the total cost for each patient's visit.

Some medical practices have more than one fee schedule. For example, if a physician is a participating provider in a preferred provider organization (PPO), the procedures may be discounted for PPO members according to an agreed-upon amount between the physician and the plan.

While dealing with the office's fee schedule, the assistant should also be familiar with the policy of the office regarding financial arrangements: the charges when a reduction of the fee is possible, the acceptable minimal payment, and any other facts needed to deal efficiently with problems concerning patients' payments.

Patients who call to make a first appointment may inquire about the charges. Patients should be told that it is difficult to discuss exact charges prior to a visit because the charges will depend on the extent of the examination, the tests, and the type of treatment provided. Ideally, the patient should be told the approximate cost of the procedures before treatment begins. Many insurance carriers require that patients be given written notification of noncovered and/or excluded charges. The form must contain specific information, such as a description of the noncovered services, amount, acknowledgment of patient payment responsibility, and the patient's dated signature. Without the completed document on file prior to services being rendered, neither the patient nor the insurance carrier may be charged for the service. Medicare refers to this form as an advanced beneficiary notice. Other insurance carrier contracts should be referenced for the proper procedure regarding noncovered services. Providing this information in advance will help avoid misunderstandings and will make collection of payments easier.

It may be necessary to explain the fee by calling attention to the time involved; the cost of medications or supplies; and the skill, knowledge, and experience of the physician. Either the physician or the administrative medical assistant can discuss the fee with patients. If the physician discusses the fee with a patient, the assistant needs to know what has been discussed.

It is a fair assumption that a patient who inquires about charges before a visit is concerned about the price and should be shown every consideration. If a definite amount is quoted and this amount seems to worry the patient, the administrative medical assistant can reassure the patient by saying that arrangements can be made to ease payment.

Patient Statements

The administrative medical assistant records all transactions—that is, charges incurred by the patient for office visits, x-rays, laboratory tests, and so on and all adjustments and payments made by the patient or the patient's insurance company—in the patient ledger. The patient's copy of the information stored in the patient ledger (hardcopy or electronic) is referred to as the **patient statement**, or patient bill.

The patient statement shows the professional services rendered to the patient, the charge for each service, payments made, and the balance owed. Figure 7.2 shows an example of a patient statement. Notice that the statement contains transactions for two people— Alison and Mike Becker—since both are members of the same family and are under the same account.

Figure 7.2

Patient Statement

STATEMENT

Statement Date: 03/11/20--

Account Number: 1324

Any change or payments made after the statement date will appear on the next statement.

Amount Enclosed _____

Please remit all payments to:

Karen Larsen, MD
2235 South Ridgeway Avenue
Chicago, IL 60623-2240
312-555-6022   Fax: 312-555-0025

Responsible Person's Name

Alison C. Becker
7911 Riverview Lane N.
Chicago, IL 60632-1979

Service Date	Patient's Name	Procedure Code	Diagnosis Code	Service Description	Charge	Insurance Paid	Adj.	Patient Paid	Amount Due
03-11-09	Alison	99201	786.2	NP problem focused	54.00	-0-	-0-	54.00	-0-
03-15-11	Mike	99202	729.1	NP expanded visit	73.00	-0-	-0-	-0-	73.00
04-01-11								73.00	-0-
05-15-11	Alison	99395	V70.0	Annual exam	136.00			34.60	101.40
		85018		HGB	13.00				114.40
		81001		UA	24.00				138.40
05-31-11				Real Insurance		138.40			-0-

ANY AMOUNT NOT PAID BY INSURANCE IS NOW THE PATIENT'S RESPONSIBILITY

ACCOUNT NUMBER	SSN	CURRENT	OVER 30 DAYS	OVER 60 DAYS	OVER 90 DAYS	OVER 120 DAYS	INSURANCE PENDING	AMOUNT DUE
1324	470-55-8533	-0-	-0-	-0-	-0-	-0-	-0-	-0-

Abbreviations:

CBC (complete blood count)	HV (hospital visit)	UA (urinalysis)
ECG (electrocardiogram)	LAB (laboratory work)	UC (urine culture)
EP (established patient)	NP (new patient)	

Listing, or itemizing, the procedures on the statement reminds patients when they visited the physician and what services were performed. To save space on the statement, some common procedures are listed using procedure codes only, with no descriptions.

The statement is generally sent to the patient who received treatment, although in some cases another person may be designated as the one responsible for receiving and paying the bill. A copy of legal documents, such as a durable power of attorney and/or medical power of attorney, should be maintained in the patient's medical documentation and notation made of the authorized individual(s). Careful attention must be used to prevent the unauthorized disclosure of PHI. In general, parents are responsible for the medical bills of minor children living in their home.

Computerized Billing

Most medical practices, even though they may not be using a complete EHR system, use a computerized billing program to generate patient statements. Many software programs, such as Medisoft®, are available to handle patients' billing. Figure 7.3 shows an example of a Medisoft®

Figure 7.3

Computerized Patient
Statement from the
Medisoft® Program

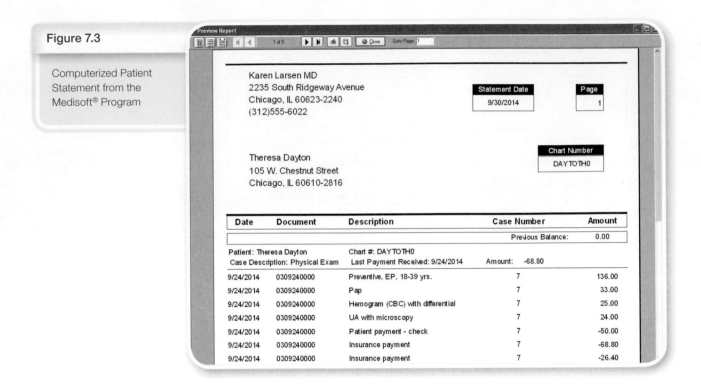

patient statement. In addition to generating itemized patient statements, a computerized billing system is usually used to produce the following reports for accounting purposes:

- A daily report, called a "day sheet," listing all charges, payments, and adjustments entered during that day
- Monthly reports summarizing the operation of the practice
- Aging reports, which list the outstanding balances owed to the practice by insurance companies or patients
- Lists of the amounts of money generated by various departments, such as laboratory, x-ray, and physical therapy
- Lists of the amounts generated by individual physicians in the practice
- Reports on the frequency of procedure codes reported by each physician in the practice

A patient billing program can also be used to print out blank patient encounter forms each day for patients who have appointments on that day. Medical billing programs are a valuable accounting tool for the physician, and the administrative medical assistant should be familiar with their use.

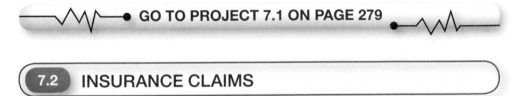

GO TO PROJECT 7.1 ON PAGE 279

7.2 INSURANCE CLAIMS

Overview of the Process

When patients receive services from a medical practice, either they pay for services themselves or the charges are submitted to their insurance company or government agency for payment. Most medical practices complete an insurance claim form on behalf of the patient. The insurance claim form contains both clinical and financial information and is transmitted to the patient's insurance carrier for partial or full reimbursement of the services rendered.

Using the CMS-1500 Paper Claim Form. The most commonly used paper claim form is the **CMS-1500 claim form** (formerly known as the HCFA-1500 claim form). See Figure 7.4 for an example. Accepted by private as well as government-sponsored programs, it is also called the "universal claim form." Two medical office forms are used to complete the CMS-1500 claim form: the **patient information form**, which is filled out or updated by the patient, and the patient encounter form. The patient information form may also include release-of-information and assignment-of-benefits statements. Prior to HIPAA, if a provider submitted a claim for a patient, a release-of-information statement had to be completed by the patient. Since HIPAA, the payment portion of TPO gives providers the authority to release claim-pertinent PHI to obtain third-party payment. If the patient decides to authorize a nonPAR provider to receive payments for medical services directly from third-party payers, an assignment-of-benefits statement must be signed by the patient and filed in the patient's medical record. For participating physicians, an assigned (direct) payment is one of the incentives for participation, and the patient's signature authorizing assignment of benefits is not needed. For convenience, some medical practices

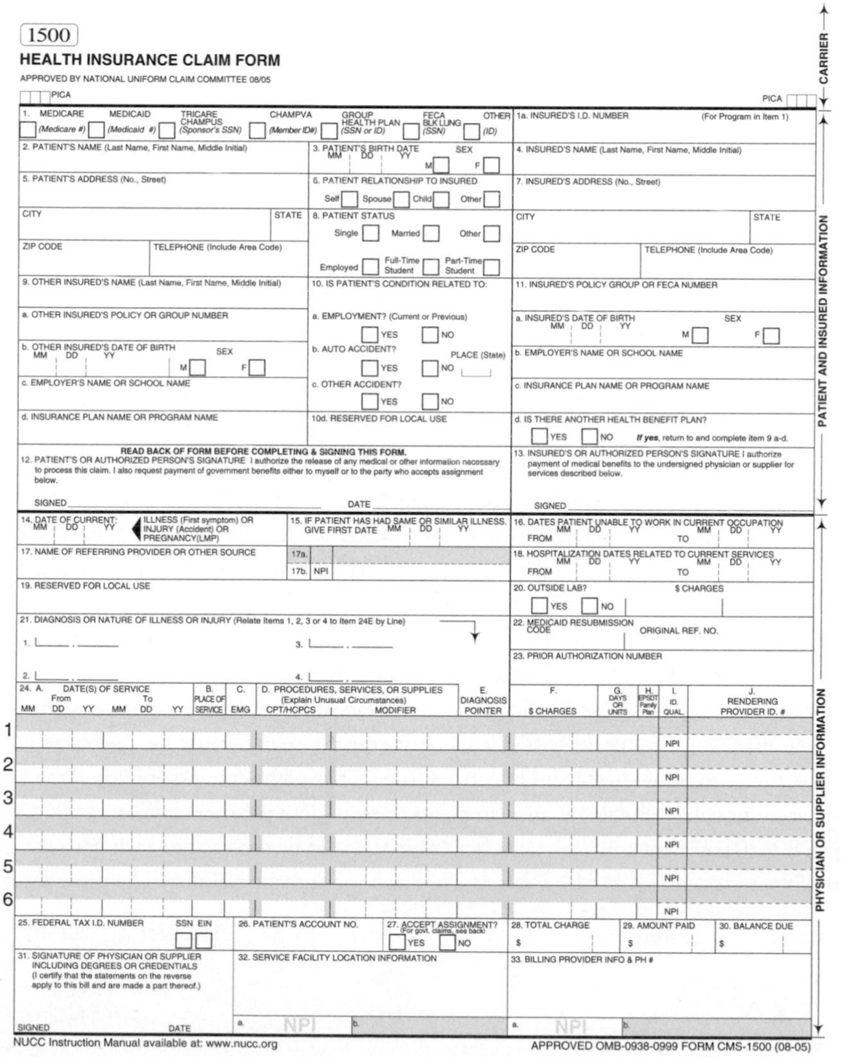
1500
HEALTH INSURANCE CLAIM FORM
APPROVED BY NATIONAL UNIFORM CLAIM COMMITTEE 08/05

PICA | PICA

1. MEDICARE (Medicare #) MEDICAID (Medicaid #) TRICARE CHAMPUS (Sponsor's SSN) CHAMPVA (Member ID#) GROUP HEALTH PLAN (SSN or ID) FECA BLK LUNG (SSN) OTHER (ID)
1a. INSURED'S I.D. NUMBER (For Program in Item 1)
2. PATIENT'S NAME (Last Name, First Name, Middle Initial)
3. PATIENT'S BIRTH DATE MM DD YY SEX M F
4. INSURED'S NAME (Last Name, First Name, Middle Initial)
5. PATIENT'S ADDRESS (No., Street)
6. PATIENT RELATIONSHIP TO INSURED Self Spouse Child Other
7. INSURED'S ADDRESS (No., Street)
CITY STATE
8. PATIENT STATUS Single Married Other
CITY STATE
ZIP CODE TELEPHONE (Include Area Code)
Employed Full-Time Student Part-Time Student
ZIP CODE TELEPHONE (Include Area Code)
9. OTHER INSURED'S NAME (Last Name, First Name, Middle Initial)
10. IS PATIENT'S CONDITION RELATED TO:
11. INSURED'S POLICY GROUP OR FECA NUMBER
a. OTHER INSURED'S POLICY OR GROUP NUMBER
a. EMPLOYMENT? (Current or Previous) YES NO
a. INSURED'S DATE OF BIRTH MM DD YY SEX M F
b. OTHER INSURED'S DATE OF BIRTH MM DD YY SEX M F
b. AUTO ACCIDENT? YES NO PLACE (State)
b. EMPLOYER'S NAME OR SCHOOL NAME
c. EMPLOYER'S NAME OR SCHOOL NAME
c. OTHER ACCIDENT? YES NO
c. INSURANCE PLAN NAME OR PROGRAM NAME
d. INSURANCE PLAN NAME OR PROGRAM NAME
10d. RESERVED FOR LOCAL USE
d. IS THERE ANOTHER HEALTH BENEFIT PLAN? YES NO *If yes,* return to and complete item 9 a-d.
READ BACK OF FORM BEFORE COMPLETING & SIGNING THIS FORM.
12. PATIENT'S OR AUTHORIZED PERSON'S SIGNATURE I authorize the release of any medical or other information necessary to process this claim. I also request payment of government benefits either to myself or to the party who accepts assignment below.
SIGNED DATE
13. INSURED'S OR AUTHORIZED PERSON'S SIGNATURE I authorize payment of medical benefits to the undersigned physician or supplier for services described below.
SIGNED
14. DATE OF CURRENT: MM DD YY ILLNESS (First symptom) OR INJURY (Accident) OR PREGNANCY(LMP)
15. IF PATIENT HAS HAD SAME OR SIMILAR ILLNESS. GIVE FIRST DATE MM DD YY
16. DATES PATIENT UNABLE TO WORK IN CURRENT OCCUPATION MM DD YY FROM TO
17. NAME OF REFERRING PROVIDER OR OTHER SOURCE 17a. 17b. NPI
18. HOSPITALIZATION DATES RELATED TO CURRENT SERVICES MM DD YY FROM TO
19. RESERVED FOR LOCAL USE
20. OUTSIDE LAB? YES NO $ CHARGES
21. DIAGNOSIS OR NATURE OF ILLNESS OR INJURY (Relate Items 1, 2, 3 or 4 to Item 24E by Line)
1. 2. 3. 4.
22. MEDICAID RESUBMISSION CODE ORIGINAL REF. NO.
23. PRIOR AUTHORIZATION NUMBER
24. A. DATE(S) OF SERVICE From MM DD YY To MM DD YY | B. PLACE OF SERVICE | C. EMG | D. PROCEDURES, SERVICES, OR SUPPLIES (Explain Unusual Circumstances) CPT/HCPCS MODIFIER | E. DIAGNOSIS POINTER | F. $ CHARGES | G. DAYS OR UNITS | H. EPSDT Family Plan | I. ID. QUAL. | J. RENDERING PROVIDER ID. #
1 NPI
2 NPI
3 NPI
4 NPI
5 NPI
6 NPI
25. FEDERAL TAX I.D. NUMBER SSN EIN
26. PATIENT'S ACCOUNT NO.
27. ACCEPT ASSIGNMENT? (For govt. claims, see back) YES NO
28. TOTAL CHARGE $
29. AMOUNT PAID $
30. BALANCE DUE $
31. SIGNATURE OF PHYSICIAN OR SUPPLIER INCLUDING DEGREES OR CREDENTIALS (I certify that the statements on the reverse apply to this bill and are made a part thereof.)
SIGNED DATE
32. SERVICE FACILITY LOCATION INFORMATION a. NPI b.
33. BILLING PROVIDER INFO & PH # a. NPI b.
NUCC Instruction Manual available at: www.nucc.org
APPROVED OMB-0938-0999 FORM CMS-1500 (08-05)

Figure 7.4

Blank CMS-1500 Form

include these statements on the patient information form. Other practices prefer to use separate forms for each of them.

Submitting Paper or Electronic Claims. Increasingly, medical offices are using computerized insurance claim forms, known as **electronic claims**, in place of paper claims. Electronic claims are prepared on a computer and transmitted electronically (from one computer to another) to an insurance carrier for processing. If necessary, an electronically prepared claim may be printed and and a hardcopy claim sent to the carrier by postal service or other non-electronic methods. The HIPAA 837 claim is the standard format for electronic claims. Currently, HIPAA 837 claim submissions are to be used by offices with 10 or more full-time employees or the equivalent of 10 full-time employees, such as 20 employees whose combined work status equals 10 full-time employees. Advantages of using electronic claims include immediate transmission, faster payment (Medicare claims are paid within 14 days versus 29 days), and easier tracking of claim status.

Processing by a Third-Party Payer. When the claim form arrives at the office of the insurance carrier, either on paper or as a computer file, the insurance carrier processes the claim. This entails reviewing the information for accuracy and completeness, verifying that the patient's policy is current, evaluating the treatment received, and deciding what benefits are due to the insured. The insurance company may determine to pay the fee, deny the claim, or pay less for some or all of the procedures.

Receiving an EOB or ERA. After the insurance carrier reviews the claim and makes a final reimbursement determination, it sends remittance advice to the patient and the provider with an explanation of its decision. The remittance advice also takes into account any deductibles or coinsurance the insured may owe. If the insurance company determines that there are benefits to be paid, a check for the appropriate amount is attached to the provider's report. In cases in which the benefits have not been assigned to the provider, the remittance is sent directly to the patient.

In the case of paper claims, the remittance advice sent by the insurance company in response to the claim is transmitted through the mail and is referred to as an **EOB** (explanation of benefits). Figure 7.5 shows an example of an EOB for an office visit. In the case of electronic claims, the report is transferred from one computer to another and is therefore referred to as an **ERA** (electronic remittance advice). As with an electronic claim, an ERA is never printed. Although the formats used for the EOB and the ERA differ, the information conveyed in both types of reports is the same—both explain the amount of benefits to be paid to, or on behalf of, the insured and how that amount was determined.

Frequently, providers receive bulk payments—a single benefit payment that covers more than one submitted claim. For example, the insurance carrier submits one payment covering benefits for 15 Blue Cross Blue Shield patients instead of processing a single payment for each claim. Administrative medical assistants who process payments must be able to separate the bulk payments into individual claim benefits and post the payment and /or adjustments to the patient's account. The following is an example of three patient payments on one bulk statement. Using an 80/20 payment split, calculate how much should be credited to each patient's account from the insurance carrier and how much is left as patient responsibility. The provider is PAR.

Pt Name & Number	Submitted	Plan Allowance	Ins Pay	Deduct	Coins/Copay
PATIENT A 0012BA					
09/16/20–	$ 80.00	$ 60.00	_____	$0.00	_____
09/23/20–	160.00	100.00	_____	0.00	_____

Figure 7.5

An Example of an EOB

Cross and Shield National Government Program
1290 Cimmons Road
Cincinnati, OH 45555

#FEI12398095643567#
Lena T. Crac
2520 Arizona Lane
Floyd, KY 4II99-2520

			EXPLANATION OF BENEFITS

Check sent to:	Karen Larsen, MD
Provider:	Karen Larsen, MD
Type:	PAR
Patient Name:	LENA CRAC
DOS:	03/23/20— to 03/23/20—
You Owe the Provider:	$20.00

EXPLANATION OF BENEFITS
This Is Not a Bill

ID Number:	R55559990
Claim Number:	R213213892308
Claim Paid On:	03/30/20--
Claim Received On:	03/25/20—
Claim Process On:	03/30/20—
Claim Processed By:	Annie B.

Service Rendered	Submitted Charge(s)	Allowance	Codes	Deductible Amount	COB	Coinsurance or Copayment	Plan Payment	Patient Owes
OFFICE VISIT	100.00	61.15	160			20.00	41.15	20.00
TOTALS:	100.00	61.15		0.00		20.00	41.15	20.00

160-The charge submitted by the provider exceeds the allowable amount for this service. You are not responsible for the difference between the submitted charge and the plan allowance.

On this claim your out-of-pocket expenses are:	
Yearly Deductible:	0.00
Admission Copay:	0.00
Coinsurance Amount:	0.00
Copayment Amount:	20.00
Preauthorization Penalty Charge:	0.00
YOUR TOTAL:	20.00

	Yearly Ded	PAR	NonPAR
What You Have Paid:	34.91	0.00	0.00
Family:	34.91	301.00	301.00
Your Annual Max	400.00	0.00	0.00
Family:	800.00	5,000.00	7,000.00

If you have a question concerning this claim, please call a customer service assistant. Refer to the Claims Section of your Service Booklet for disputed claims inf claims procedures.

1-800-555-5555

Pt Name & Number	Submitted	Plan Allowance	Ins Pay	Deduct	Coins/Copay
PATIENT B 0106SM					
09/02/20–	80.00	60.00	_____	0.00	_____
PATIENT C 0219LS					
09/15/20–	120.00	120.00	_____	0.00	_____
TOTALS	$440.00	$340.00	$272.00	$0.00	$68.00

Calculating the insurance payment and balance due from the patient using an 80/20 payment split:

Patient A
09/16/20–   Insurance payment of $48.00 and patient balance of $12.00
09/23/20–   Insurance payment of $80.00 and patient balance of $20.00

Patient B
09/02/20–   Insurance payment of $48.00 and patient balance of $12.00

Patient C
09/15/20–   Insurance payment of $96.00 and patient balance of $24.00

Patient A will require two entries—one for each date of service. Also, since the provider is PAR, an adjustment will need to be made to each patient's account for the difference between the submitted amount and the plan allowance amount. What is the amount to be adjusted off each patient's date of service?

Patient A
09/16/20–   Adjustment amount   _____
09/23/20–   Adjustment amount   _____

Patient B
09/02/20–   Adjustment amount   _____

Patient C
09/15/20–   Adjustment amount   _____

Patient A adjustments are $20.00 and $60.00, respectively. Patient B will have an adjustment of $20.00, and Patient C will have no adjustment to the account.

Checking the Reimbursement Details. After the medical office receives the remittance advice (the EOB or ERA), the administrative medical assistant reviews it and checks it against the original claim. If all is in order, the assistant files the report with the patient's financial records. If a check from the insurance company is attached to the EOB, the assistant posts the payment received to the appropriate patient's account and marks the check for deposit in the practice's bank account. Generally, if a claim is processed electronically, the method of payment is also electronic. In such cases, the payment attached to the ERA is deposited into the practice's bank account through an electronic funds transfer (EFT), rather than mailed in the form of a check to the medical practice.

Billing the Patient. If the patient still owes money to the medical practice after the EOB or ERA has been received—usually for charges that were not fully reimbursed by the insurance company or for noncovered services—the assistant bills the patient for the amount due. If the patient is confused or has any questions about payments, the assistant can try to help by going over the terms of the insurance plan with the patient. The assistant may also need to call the insurance carrier and act as a go-between for patients. The assistant can build goodwill for the physician's office by using problem-solving and communication skills to fulfill this role. Patients understandably get upset when they receive unexpectedly large bills or an incorrect payment. The assistant is the patient's advocate with the insurance carrier. Sometimes explaining the solution again to the patient in different terms after speaking with the insurance carrier will help clear up the problem.

Patients may also accuse the medical office of billing incorrectly when they are unhappy with the benefits received. The assistant should remember to use respect and care in solving any miscommunications or misunderstandings in such circumstances. It is important to separate the patient's feelings from the facts. When documented facts, such as EOB or ERA information, is professionally yet empathetically discussed with angry patients, they may be more accepting of the information. Be careful to avoid insurance and medical jargon; this will only add to patients' frustration.

Once the patient understands the terms of the payment due, the assistant follows up with the patient to see that the amount due is collected in a timely manner. When the patient pays the balance due, the account is listed as a zero balance and the insurance claim process is complete.

Appealing Claims. If the physician thinks that the reimbursement decision is incorrect or unfair, the medical office may initiate an appeal. Appeals must be filed within a stated period after the determination of claim benefits or denial. Most insurance carriers have an upward structure for appeals, beginning at the lowest level and progressing upward. For example, the first step may be to submit a formal complaint. If the provider is not satisfied with the outcome, the second step may be to file an appeal. A grievance would be filed if the appeal did not produce the desired results. When making an appeal of an electronic claim, include the electronic claim number. Each insurance company has its own appeal process. A representative from the insurance company can instruct the assistant on the appeal process the insurer uses, if necessary. This information may also be available on the Internet by initiating a search from the insurance carrier's Web site.

Completing and Transmitting the Claim Form

Completing and transmitting the claim form accurately for a patient is one of the most important steps in successful claim reimbursement. Therefore, the administrative medical assistant should be familiar with the details of the process.

Verifying Insurance Information. The first step in processing a claim is to verify the patient's insurance information. With new patients, most practices routinely check insurance coverage before the patient's first appointment. Basic information about the patient and the patient's insurance is obtained over the phone when the first appointment is scheduled. The assistant then contacts the insurer by telephone, fax, Internet, or other electronic methods specified by the insurance carrier to verify that the patient is currently enrolled in the plan as specified and has paid all required premiums or other charges.

Checking the Accuracy of Essential Claim Information. Claim forms must be completed accurately. The following basic information is required on most claim forms:

- Contract numbers—that is, the group number and the insured's identification number from the insured's current insurance card
- The patient's complete name, date of birth, gender, and relationship to the insured
- The insured's complete name, address, date of birth, and employer
- Information on a secondary carrier—subscriber's name, date of birth, and employer
- Information about whether the condition is job-related or accident-related and whether it is an illness or an injury
- The patient's account number (if the facility assigns numbers to patients)
- Complete and current diagnostic codes for the submitted claim
- Information about the provider—name, address, identifying codes, NPI and other required identifiers, and signatures
- A statement of services rendered, which should include dates, procedure codes, charges, and total charges

The following is information presented on an insured's insurance card submitted to the provider through the registration process.

```
CROSS AND SHIELD          PPO

INSURED
DAYS CATALINA S
ID NUMBER
R123456789XX
GROUP CODE           DOC
555                  04-19-20—
```

A claim was submitted with the following information and the claim was denied. What is wrong with the submitted claim information?

Patient name: Catalina S. Dayes   ID Number: R123456798XX   Group Code 555

Before submitting claims, the assistant must carefully check every bit of information for accuracy. Typographical errors and transposition of numbers are two of the most common claim submission errors. This example contains two errors—a misspelled name and transposition of the numbers in the ID number.

Completing the CMS-1500 Claim Form.

Most insurance companies accept the CMS-1500 for processing claims. However, the assistant may need to complete a specifically designed claim form for a carrier. Although the form may be different, the information required on most insurance claim forms is the same. If the assistant is familiar with the various fields on the CMS-1500 form, the same knowledge can be applied to other claim forms for successful completion.

Figure 7.6 shows a completed CMS-1500 claim form. Note that the form is divided horizontally into two parts: The top half contains patient and insured information (Items 1–13), while the bottom half contains physician or supplier information (Items 14–33). Figure 7.7 presents the information that should be entered in each numbered blank (called a "form locator").

After a claim has been completed and sent to the insurance company, make a notation in the patient ledger by entering the date and the phrase "Submitted to insurance" after the last entry. When insurance claims are submitted using an electronic submission program, the program places the submission date into the patient's electronic ledger account. An updated patient statement is then sent to the patient for billing purposes on the next billing date. The patient or another designated person is still responsible for the complete charge, even if insurance is involved.

Using Computer Billing Programs.

Generating claim forms (whether paper or electronic) on the computer is one of the major uses of computer technology in the medical office today. The computer automatically processes the information required to create a completed claim by transferring the patient's and the insured's information, the charges, the procedure and diagnostic codes, and so forth from the various databases set up in the computer onto the insurance claim form.

The computer stores facts about the medical practice in the practice database; information about the carriers that most patients use in the insurance carrier database; information about payments made by patients, as well as benefits received from insurance companies, in the transaction database; and information about each patient—personal as well as clinical data—in the patient database. Careful attention must be given when keying information and updating system data. Errors in keying will be transferred to the claim form.

When all new data and transaction information have been entered and checked regarding a patient's visit to the physician, the administrative medical assistant creates the electronic claim. The format for the claim—either the CMS-1500, HIPAA 837, or a specialized claim form—is also designated. The software program then organizes the necessary databases and selects the data from each one as needed to produce a completed claim form. When this is completed, the administrative medical assistant will electronically transmit the claim to the insurance carrier for processing.

Electronic Claims Versus Paper Claims.

The main difference between electronic claims and paper claims is the means by which they are transmitted to the insurance carrier. The use of electronic claims not only speeds up transmission and payments but also ensures a greater degree of accuracy and costs less.

Figure 7.6

Completed CMS-1500 Form

1500

HEALTH INSURANCE CLAIM FORM

APPROVED BY NATIONAL UNIFORM CLAIM COMMITTEE 08/05

CROSS AND SHIELD
1234 ANY STREET
ANYWHERE, USA 55555-5555

CARRIER

PICA

1. MEDICARE (Medicare #) MEDICAID (Medicaid #) TRICARE CHAMPUS (Sponsor's SSN) CHAMPVA (Member ID#) GROUP HEALTH PLAN (SSN or ID) [X] FECA BLK LUNG (SSN) OTHER (ID)

1a. INSURED'S I.D. NUMBER (For Program in Item 1): R123456789

2. PATIENT'S NAME (Last Name, First Name, Middle Initial): RICHARDS WARREN L

3. PATIENT'S BIRTH DATE MM DD YY: 04 09 1980 SEX M [X] F

4. INSURED'S NAME (Last Name, First Name, Middle Initial): RICHARDS NANCY J

5. PATIENT'S ADDRESS (No., Street): 7952 SPRINGFIELD AVENUE

6. PATIENT RELATIONSHIP TO INSURED: Self Spouse [X] Child Other

7. INSURED'S ADDRESS (No., Street): SAME

CITY: CHICAGO STATE: IL

8. PATIENT STATUS: Single Married [X] Other

CITY STATE

ZIP CODE: 60623-2579 TELEPHONE (Include Area Code): (312) 5553391

Employed [X] Full-Time Student Part-Time Student

ZIP CODE TELEPHONE (Include Area Code) ( )

9. OTHER INSURED'S NAME (Last Name, First Name, Middle Initial)

10. IS PATIENT'S CONDITION RELATED TO:

11. INSURED'S POLICY GROUP OR FECA NUMBER: FEP222

a. OTHER INSURED'S POLICY OR GROUP NUMBER

a. EMPLOYMENT? (Current or Previous) YES [X] NO

a. INSURED'S DATE OF BIRTH MM DD YY: 10 19 1979 SEX M F [X]

b. OTHER INSURED'S DATE OF BIRTH MM DD YY SEX M F

b. AUTO ACCIDENT? YES [X] NO PLACE (State)

b. EMPLOYER'S NAME OR SCHOOL NAME: DEPARTMENT OF JUSTICE

c. EMPLOYER'S NAME OR SCHOOL NAME

c. OTHER ACCIDENT? YES [X] NO

c. INSURANCE PLAN NAME OR PROGRAM NAME: CROSS AND SHIELD

d. INSURANCE PLAN NAME OR PROGRAM NAME

10d. RESERVED FOR LOCAL USE

d. IS THERE ANOTHER HEALTH BENEFIT PLAN? YES [X] NO *If yes, return to and complete item 9 a-d.*

READ BACK OF FORM BEFORE COMPLETING & SIGNING THIS FORM.

12. PATIENT'S OR AUTHORIZED PERSON'S SIGNATURE I authorize the release of any medical or other information necessary to process this claim. I also request payment of government benefits either to myself or to the party who accepts assignment below.

SIGNED SOF DATE 06 01 2010

13. INSURED'S OR AUTHORIZED PERSON'S SIGNATURE I authorize payment of medical benefits to the undersigned physician or supplier for services described below.

SIGNED SOF

PATIENT AND INSURED INFORMATION

14. DATE OF CURRENT: ILLNESS (First symptom) OR INJURY (Accident) OR PREGNANCY(LMP) MM DD YY: 03 07 2011

15. IF PATIENT HAS HAD SAME OR SIMILAR ILLNESS. GIVE FIRST DATE MM DD YY

16. DATES PATIENT UNABLE TO WORK IN CURRENT OCCUPATION FROM TO

17. NAME OF REFERRING PROVIDER OR OTHER SOURCE

17a. 17b. NPI

18. HOSPITALIZATION DATES RELATED TO CURRENT SERVICES FROM TO

19. RESERVED FOR LOCAL USE

20. OUTSIDE LAB? YES [X] NO $ CHARGES

21. DIAGNOSIS OR NATURE OF ILLNESS OR INJURY (Relate Items 1, 2, 3 or 4 to Item 24E by Line)

1. 726 10
2.
3.
4.

22. MEDICAID RESUBMISSION CODE ORIGINAL REF. NO.

23. PRIOR AUTHORIZATION NUMBER

	24. A. DATE(S) OF SERVICE From MM DD YY	To MM DD YY	B. PLACE OF SERVICE	C. EMG	D. PROCEDURES, SERVICES, OR SUPPLIES (Explain Unusual Circumstances) CPT/HCPCS	MODIFIER	E. DIAGNOSIS POINTER	F. $ CHARGES	G. DAYS OR UNITS	H. EPSDT Family Plan	I. ID. QUAL.	J. RENDERING PROVIDER ID. #
1	03 07 11		11		99212		1	55 00	1		NPI	0123456789
2											NPI	
3											NPI	
4											NPI	
5											NPI	
6											NPI	

PHYSICIAN OR SUPPLIER INFORMATION

25. FEDERAL TAX I.D. NUMBER: 16-55555555 SSN EIN [X]

26. PATIENT'S ACCOUNT NO.: RICHARDSW1

27. ACCEPT ASSIGNMENT? (For govt. claims, see back) [X] YES NO

28. TOTAL CHARGE: $ 55 00

29. AMOUNT PAID: $ 20 00

30. BALANCE DUE: $ 35 00

31. SIGNATURE OF PHYSICIAN OR SUPPLIER INCLUDING DEGREES OR CREDENTIALS (I certify that the statements on the reverse apply to this bill and are made a part thereof.)

SIGNED SOF 01 01 2011 DATE

32. SERVICE FACILITY LOCATION INFORMATION

a. NPI b.

33. BILLING PROVIDER INFO & PH # (555) 9670303
KAREN LARSEN MD
2235 SOUTH RIDGEWAY AVE
CHICAGO IL 60623-2240

a. 0123456789 b.

NUCC Instruction Manual available at: www.nucc.org

APPROVED OMB-0938-0999 FORM CMS-1500 (08-05)

Paper claims, whether printed from a computer billing program or typed, are usually transmitted to insurance carriers through the mail. When they reach the insurance carrier, the information on the form must be keyed into the insurance company's computer by data-entry personnel. Alternatively, the information may be scanned using an optical character reader (OCR). In either case, a certain percentage of error is introduced. If a claim form is to be scanned, it is a good idea for the administrative medical assistant to complete the form using all capital letters and avoid the use of symbols or punctuation. This will lead to fewer errors while scanning.

The following are more tips for preparing claims that will be scanned:

1. Use an eight-digit format for dates (01/02/2014).
2. Send reports and other supporting documentation unattached from the claim form.
3. Start over when a mistake is made on claim forms prepared by hand, and correct individual errors when prepared on the computer. Refrain from erasing, striking out errors, or applying white-out products.

Figure 7.7 CMS–1500 Guidelines Chart

CMS-1500 FORM GUIDELINES

ITEM NO.	DESCRIPTION	RESOURCE
1, 1a	Type of insurance and insured's ID number	ID card
2, 3, 5, 6	Patient's name, DOB, address, telephone number, and relationship to insured	Chart, patient's registration form
4, 7	Insured's name and address	Chart
8	Patient's marital and employment status	Chart
9, 9a–d	Other insured's name and information—policies that supplement the primary carrier	Chart
10a–c	Patient's condition related to a work injury, an automobile accident, or other type of accident	Chart
11, 11a–d	Primary carrier information	Chart
12	Release of information may have signature on *Authorization for Release of Medical Information Statement*—"patient's signature on file/SOF"	Patient's and/or insured's signature; may have signature on file in chart
13	Authorization of payment of benefits to provider ("patient's signature on file/SOF" if have signed authorization on file)	Patient's and/or insured's signature; may have signature on file in chart
14	Date of current illness (first-symptom date), injury (accident date), or pregnancy (LMP)	Chart
15	First date of same or similar illness	Chart
16	Dates patient unable to work	Chart
17, 17a, b	Referring physician and ID number (NPI and or PIN–provider individual number)	Chart, insurance manual
18	Hospitalization dates	Chart
19	Reserved for local carriers' specified information	Insurance manual
20	Usage of outside lab—complete if services from an outside lab were used	Ledger/chart
21	*ICD-9-CM* diagnostic codes with primary diagnosis listed first	Chart and code books
22	Only used on Medicaid claims	Medicaid procedures
23	Prior authorization number, if required by payer	Contact carrier
24A–G	Services rendered—one procedure per line, maximum of six lines on one claim	Chart, patient encounter form, ledger, coding books
24A	Dates of procedures	
24B	Place of service code: 11 Office 31 Skilled nursing facility 54 Intermediate care facility/mentally retarded 12 Patient's home 32 Nursing facility 55 Residential substance abuse treatment 21 Inpatient hospital 33 Custodial care facility 56 Psychiatric residential treatment center 22 Outpatient hospital 34 Hospice 61 Comprehensive inpatient rehabilitation 23 Hospital emergency room 42 Air or water ambulance 62 Comprehensive outpatient rehabilitation 24 Ambulatory surgical center 51 Inpatient psychiatric facility 65 End-stage renal disease treatment 25 Birthing center 52 Federally qualified health center 26 Military treatment center 53 Community mental-health center	
24C	EMG: Payer-specific code	
24D	*CPT* and/or HCPCS codes	
24E	Diagnosis code—relate the procedure codes to the appropriate diagnosis (i.e., 1, 2, 3)	
24F	Charges for each service	
24G	Number of days of units the procedure/services was given	
24H	Medicaid EPSDT Family Plan	Patient Medicaid ID Card
24I	ID qualifier type, such as NPI	Practice Records
24J	Rendering Provider ID #	
25	Employer's federal tax ID number (EIN)	Doctor's information
26	Patient's account number—if patient known as a number	Chart/ledger
27	Accept assignment	Doctor's information
28, 29, 30	Total, amount paid on services specific to the claim form, and balance due	Ledger
31	Signature of physician, including credentials, and date	Typed signature, signature stamp, electronic signature on file
32	Name and address of outside facility used other than home or office	Chart/ledger
33 a, b	Provider's billing name, complete address, telephone number, and ID numbers (NPI and other identifying numbers)	

Electronic claims, on the other hand, are transmitted from one computer to another over the telephone, Internet, or other electronic transmission method. Because claim information is entered once, not twice, chances of error or omission are greatly reduced. It also costs less to file claims electronically; fewer personnel are involved, and neither paper forms, envelopes, nor postage is required.

An advantage to transmitting claims electronically is that the medical office receives immediate feedback whenever claims are transmitted. Medical offices generally transmit claims in batches, grouped by insurer. Tracking numbers are used to follow the progress of claims. When an insurance carrier receives electronic claims, it sends a transmittal report back to the sender, acknowledging receipt of the claims. The administrative medical assistant should compare the acknowledgment of claims against the reports of sent claims. If a claim is not listed on the transmittal receipt, the claim should be retransmitted.

Each office has its own schedule for sending claims. The usual practice is to transmit claims every day or every other day. Larger practices may transmit claims multiple times a day, such as late morning and afternoon. Individual carriers will have time guidelines for providers to submit claims. Guidelines may be as little as 30 days from the date of service or as long as December 31 of the year after the year in which the service was provided. For example, a patient had a colonoscopy performed on March 18, 2014. Under the latter guidelines, the last date to submit this claim to the carrier would be December 31, 2015. Provider schedules for submitting claims to carriers should be based on the carrier's guidelines and any negotiated contract time guidelines.

When claims are transmitted electronically, the medical office receives a file acknowledgment—immediate feedback that tells the medical office the file has arrived at the insurance carrier's claims department. If the file is missing details (for example, if a required field is left blank) or if the claim form contains incorrect information, such as an invalid patient identification number, the computer will immediately notify the sender that the file has been rejected. The medical office that sent the claim can then fix the error and resubmit the claim.

Whether the claim is paper or electronic, it is often the overlooked, seemingly simple errors that prevent the provider from producing a **clean claim**—a claim that is accepted by the insurance payer for adjudication. The following are some common errors:

- Service facility names and associated information, such as address or phone number, are missing, incomplete, or incorrect.
- Referring provider information is missing.
- Patient birth date is invalid.
- Procedure and diagnostic codes are not current or are invalid.
- There are typographical errors and transposition of numbers.

Clean claims are processed in a more timely manner and, in turn, benefit payments are received faster by the provider. Software programs, known as **scrubber programs**, are used to check for errors on insurance claim forms before they are submitted.

Using Clearinghouses. A **clearinghouse** is a service bureau that collects electronic claims from many different medical practices and forwards the claims to the appropriate insurance carriers. Some insurance carriers who receive insurance claims electronically require information to be formatted in a particular way. Part of the service a clearinghouse provides is to translate claim data to fit the setup of each carrier's claims processing department. Because of this factor, many medical practices choose to use a clearinghouse instead of transmitting claims directly to insurance carriers themselves. Usually, a fee is negotiated with the clearinghouse for its services. With or without the use of a clearinghouse, electronic claims reach the insurance carrier almost immediately compared with paper claims.

COMPLIANCE **TIP**

Some physicians outsource their billing services. Because the information needed to process information claims is confidential, offices using outside billing services must sign a business associate agreement, which verifies that those services are HIPAA compliant. How else can you make sure that the patient's information stays confidential?

Following Up on Claims

When an EOB or ERA from a third-party payer arrives, the assistant checks that

- All the procedures listed on the claim also appear on the EOB/ERA.
- Any unpaid charges are explained.
- The codes on the EOB/ERA match those on the claim.
- The payment listed for each procedure is correct.

The assistant must routinely follow up on all submitted claims. Many medical offices use the Internet to contact carriers to check claim status. For claims submitted using HIPAA transactions, HIPAA 276/277 are used to ask payers about the status of a claim. The number 276 refers to the provider's inquiry, and 277 refers to the payer's response. The time line for the follow-up varies according to the insurance carrier, the insurance program, and, if participating, their written contract. Most medical offices follow up on claim status 7 to 14 days after the claims are submitted. Experience with insurance will enable you to know when follow-up on a claim is necessary.

Some physicians automatically rebill in 30 days if they have not heard from an insurance company. Most medical offices, however, send a tracer as the first contact about overdue claims. A tracer, whether sent in print or by e-mail, contains the basic billing information and asks the carrier about its status. Using an electronic program, an aging report can be produced and used to determine how long a claim has been submitted yet not paid or denied. Outstanding claims are aged, usually by a certain number of days, such as 1–30 days or 31–60 days.

In addition to regular claim follow-up, the administrative medical assistant will need to follow up claims that have been denied for unclear reasons or are late because of special situations. Examples include the following:

- An unclear denial of payment or an incorrect payment is received on an EOB or ERA; follow-up should be done to determine the cause of the problem and to rectify it.
- The carrier asks for more information to process the claim—namely, a report on a new procedure for which there is no *CPT* code; the assistant should follow up with a report from the physician, describing the procedure and the situation in which it was used.
- The carrier notifies the medical office that a claim is being investigated with regard to preexisting conditions; after a period of 30 days from receiving such a notice, if nothing further has been received, follow-up should be done.

In some situations, the administrative medical assistant will need to resubmit a claim. Examples include the following:

- A mistake has been made in billing: the physician forgot to check off a procedure on the patient encounter form.
- A claim was overlooked by the physician's office: a patient had a series of visits for allergy injections, and one of the visits was not included.

Similarly, there are situations in which the insurance carrier rejects a claim and asks for resubmission:

- The wrong diagnosis or procedure codes are submitted.
- Information is incomplete or missing (for example, no accident date is given).
- The charges, units, and costs do not total properly.

In short, the administrative medical assistant should study the ERA/EOB carefully to understand any uncovered benefits, deductibles, copayment responsibilities, and other reasons for any noncoverage in the claim. If any of the explanations on a claim seem unfair or unclear, the insurance carrier should be contacted for help. Most insurance carriers have staff members whose primary job is to answer questions about claims. If necessary, an appeal should be initiated by the medical office. It is the responsibility of the assistant to take the time and care necessary to process and complete clean insurance claims accurately and to follow up in whatever way is required, so that prompt and precise compensation is received.

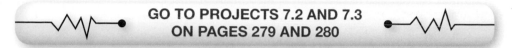

GO TO PROJECTS 7.2 AND 7.3
ON PAGES 279 AND 280

7.3 PAYMENTS FROM PATIENTS

Just as it is important for the medical office's cash flow to have claims approved and paid promptly by insurance carriers, it is also important to help ensure prompt payments from patients. The administrative medical assistant can facilitate the prompt receipt of payments from patients by keeping all transactions in each patient's account current and by being alert to the status of each account, such as 30 days past due.

The method of payment is arranged at the time of the patient's first visit. In most offices, a combination of methods is used and may include the following:

- Patients pay at the time of the visit by cash, check, debit card, or credit card. This type of collection is referred to as **collection at the time of service**. Copayments, as required by HMOs and other managed care plans, are always collected at the time of service.
- Bills are mailed to patients as designated by office policy, such as weekly or monthly or at the end of a procedure or hospital stay.
- Patients pay a fixed amount weekly or monthly until the bill is paid in full.
- Bills are sent to health insurance carriers.
- Some physicians work on a cash-only basis.
- A patient with a poor credit rating or whose checks have been returned for nonsufficient funds may be on a cash-only basis.

Methods of Payments

The assistant must be careful to enter each cash payment in the patient's ledger and in the daily summary record. The patient's name, the services rendered, the charges, the payment received on the account, and any balances should be included.

Payments should be given to the administrative medical assistant, not the physician. A receipt must be given to the patient who pays cash. An example of a receipt is shown in Figure 7.8. Copies of receipts are kept as permanent records. The patient should be advised

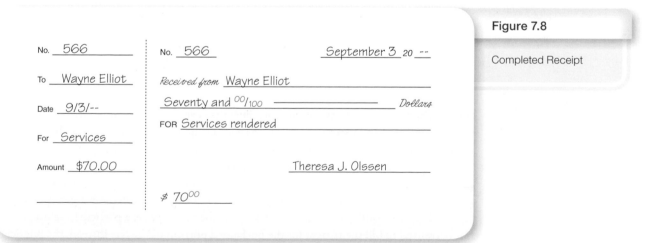

Figure 7.8

Completed Receipt

No. _566_

To _Wayne Elliot_

Date _9/3/--_

For _Services_

Amount _$70.00_

No. _566_   September 3 20 _--_

Received from _Wayne Elliot_

Seventy and ⁰⁰/₁₀₀ ———————— *Dollars*

FOR _Services rendered_

Theresa J. Olssen

$ 70⁰⁰

to keep the receipt and a copy of the patient encounter form for income tax purposes in claiming medical deductions. If the patient pays by check, the canceled check is the receipt. Credit and debit card charges appear on the patient's statement from his or her financial institution. Patients also receive a copy of the authorization. However, for smaller amounts (for example, $25 or less), patients may not need to sign an authorization form.

Certain rules must be observed to safeguard money received. Cash, checks, and money orders should be kept in a secure location, such as a locked drawer. Currency should be separated by denomination. Checks should be immediately stamped on the back with a restrictive endorsement, which specifies "Pay to the order of . . ." or "For deposit only." To minimize the danger of theft, money should be deposited in the bank daily.

Sending Statements

Although most bills are sent out once a month, a statement may be sent at the end of a procedure or upon discharge from the hospital. Practices decide to do either monthly billing or cycle billing. With **monthly billing**, bills are sent out once a month and are timed to reach the patient no later than the last day of the month, but preferably by the 25th of each month. Such a billing schedule enables patients to pay physicians' bills along with other monthly bills.

Traditionally, medical offices have used monthly billing. However, another system of billing, called **cycle billing**, is becoming more popular with medical offices. Cycle billing is designed to avoid once-a-month peak workloads and to stabilize the cash flow. It has been used by department stores, oil companies, and other large businesses for some time. With cycle billing, all accounts are divided into fairly equal groups, the number of groups depending on how many times you wish to do billing during a month. If you decide to do billing four times a month (once a week), for example, you would divide the accounts into four groups, usually alphabetically, with each group billed on a different date. If cycle billing is used, the patient should be informed on the first visit approximately when the bill will be mailed.

There are two advantages of using cycle billing: (1) the workload is apportioned throughout the entire month and (2) a consistent monetary flow occurs throughout the month versus an influx of payments during only a specific period during the month. Billing is a major task for the administrative medical assistant. If bills are prepared once a month, entire days are usually sacrificed from other routine duties during that period in order to get statements in the mail. Cycle billing allows the assistant to factor in billing as part of a daily or weekly routine. An additional benefit is that the possibility of error is reduced, because more time and consideration can be given to each account.

Payment Plans

For the patient who is unable to pay a medical bill in one lump sum, a schedule of payments, or contract, can be agreed upon. The agreement should be in writing, and a copy of the plan should be given to the patient as a reminder of the commitment to pay the physician. The amount to be paid weekly or monthly is stated in the agreement, and it is used as a reference when corresponding with the patient about unpaid bills.

Fee Adjustment

Should the need arise, the physician can adjust the cost of any procedure; the physician will then inform the administrative medical assistant of the **fee adjustment**. Fees should not be reduced as a way to receive payment quickly and avoid collection procedures.

One type of fee adjustment a medical office makes regularly with certain health plans is called a **write-off**. As explained in Chapter 6, according to the rules of many insurance plans—for example, with most HMOs—when the physician's fee for a given service is higher than the insurance company's allowed fee for that service, a participating provider is not permitted to bill the patient for the unclaimed portion of the fee. Instead, the physician must write off this amount by subtracting it from the patient's bill and accept the payment from the insurance company and the patient as payment in full—up to the allowable charge—for the procedure. Write-offs are entered into the patient ledger as fee adjustments. A nonparticipating physician who does not accept the allowable charge may be permitted to bill the patient up to the physician's normal fee and not write off the difference. As discussed in Chapter 6, this is called balance billing.

If a physician chooses to reduce or cancel a fee, the decision must be in writing for the protection of the physician, since it is possible for such a reduction or canceling of a fee to be misinterpreted and even lead to a malpractice suit. For the same reasons, in computerized billing programs, it is important not to delete any transactions. Rather, corrections, changes, and write-offs are made with adjustments to the existing transactions. Most billing programs contain a column in the patient ledger that displays such entries. The adjusting entries give both the medical office and the patient a history of events in case there is a billing inquiry or an audit.

In cases that involve a considerable sum, the patient may not be able to pay the fee and may have to seek financial assistance. The assistant should be acquainted with the local agencies to which a patient can be referred when financial assistance is needed.

In the past, physicians have chosen to waive—not collect—charges for services rendered to other medical personnel, such as another physician or nurse, and their family members. However, many federal and state laws now prohibit the practice of professional courtesy. Filing an insurance claim and collecting benefits while waiving deductibles and other required payments are unlawful and violate antikickback rules.

At times, it may be in the best interest of the practice to render services for lesser or no fees. Patients are asked to sign and date documentation of the financial agreement, known as a hardship agreement, which becomes a permanent part of the medical record.

Health Insurance

Many patients carry health insurance that provides payment for a portion of their medical expenses. Depending on whether or not the physician accepts the health insurance the patient has, the payment arrangement varies. Essentially, there are two options: patients are billed at the time of service or after the insurance claim has been processed.

After an office visit, the new charges are entered into the patient's account. If the physician has not accepted assignment and is not going to file a claim for a patient, patients are usually required to pay in full at the end of the visit. The administrative assistant gives the patient a receipt for the payment. In some cases, patients in this situation arrange to be billed later for payments due, depending on the office's policy. A written agreement containing the payment amount, the due date, and other pertinent payment information should be signed by the patient, and he or she should be given a copy of the contract.

In contrast, when the physician accepts assignment and is going to file a claim, the patient usually pays only the required deductible and any coshare (required percent or stated dollar amount) at the time of service. The amount of the patient's coshare payment is entered and subtracted from the balance due. Then the insurance claim for the service is created and transmitted to the insurance carrier. When insurance payment is received, it is entered in the patient's account. Ideally, the total paid by the patient and all carriers should equal the charges for the service provided.

If there are procedures for which the insurance company did not pay or paid less than expected, the administrative medical assistant must sort out the various charges and benefits. The assistant determines which charges the patient should be billed for, if any are to be written off by the medical office, and which, if any, should be resubmitted, or even appealed, by studying the EOB or ERA. The patient's account is then updated accordingly, and a patient statement is sent on the appropriate billing date.

Third-Party Liability

Sometimes a person other than the patient assumes liability, or responsibility, for the charges. Such responsibility is called **third-party liability**. The assistant must contact this third party for verification of financial obligation. Relatives, particularly children of aged parents, may say they will be responsible for payment of the bill, but this promise must be in writing. Oral promises are not legally binding. A third party is not obligated by law unless he or she has signed an agreement to pay the charges. Therefore, a signed promise obtained prior to treatment will greatly reduce the credit risk. Others examples of third-party liability are workers' compensation claims and auto accidents. Claim numbers are needed to submit claims and prior authorization, in most cases, is needed before treatment is rendered.

By contrast, a **guarantor** is an individual who is a policyholder for a patient of a medical practice. Essentially, the guarantor guarantees payment of the account charges. For example, a parent who is a policyholder may be the guarantor for his or her **dependent** children. As part of the Health Care Reform Legislation of 2010 and effective September 23, 2010, adult children covered under a parent's insurance policy may continue being covered under the parent's medical insurance policy up to the age of 26, regardless of whether the adult child is a student or married.

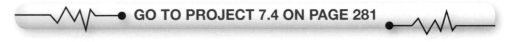 **GO TO PROJECT 7.4 ON PAGE 281**

7.4 DELINQUENT ACCOUNTS

A medical practice, like any business, has outstanding accounts. It is regrettable that patients are often slow and even delinquent in paying physicians. There are various reasons a patient might not pay a bill. For example, the patient may unintentionally or intentionally ignore the bill, the patient may not have the money to pay the bill, or the patient may be unwilling to pay the bill for a reason such as disagreeing with the amount of the bill. Other reasons for non-payment of medical bills include a patient's excessive debt, unemployment, illness, disability, family problems, and marital problems. The administrative medical assistant must know how to handle patients' accounts properly to reduce the physician's losses from unpaid bills.

Communicating with Patients

In a sense, the collection process actually begins with effective communications with patients about their responsibility to pay for services. When patients understand the charges and agree to pay them in advance, collecting the payments is not usually a problem. Most patients pay their bills on time. However, every practice has some patients who do not pay their bills when they receive their monthly statements.

One way to minimize problems with payments is to notify patients in advance of the probable cost of procedures that are not going to be covered by their plan. For example, many private plans, as well as Medicare, do not pay for most routine services, such as annual physical examinations. Many patients, however, consider preventive services a good idea and are willing to pay for them. For these noncovered services, patients should be asked to agree to pay in writing. A letter of agreement signed by the patient prior to service should also specify why the service will not be covered and the cost of the procedure. As mentioned previously, for Medicare patients, this form is called an advance beneficiary notice for noncovered services (ABN), a form that providers should have patients sign. It explains the service, the reason it will not be covered by Medicare, and the estimated charge. This form is also used when Medicare declares a service not reasonable and necessary and, therefore, does not cover it. Patients are asked to sign the ABN in advance of services being rendered.

A patient should also be informed about fees before a complicated set of procedures begins. Or a physician—in particular, a nonPAR physician—may need to clarify the payment arrangements with a patient before services are performed.

Guidelines for Payment

Management or the accounting department in every office must determine the **collection ratio** (total collections divided by net charges of the practice). The percentage will show the effectiveness of the collections (the higher the percentage, the more effective the collections). Management would then set the guidelines for payments—how much is to be collected daily, how much should be collected on each account, and so forth. As a general rule, at least one-third of the outstanding accounts should be collected each day.

Using the following figures, calculate the collection ratio and whether or not the collection methods are effective based on the guideline stated above.

	Total Collections	Net Charges	Collection Ratio	Effective Y/N
Day 1	$2,450.25	$6,320.00	_____	_____
Day 2	$1,425.50	$5,226.75	_____	_____

Collection methods are considered effective for Day 1—the collection ratio is 38.77 percent. However, the collection strategies for Day 2 are not effective. The collection ratio for Day 2 is only 27.27 percent.

The Office Collection Policy

It is often the duty of the administrative medical assistant to collect payments on overdue accounts. Each month delinquent accounts (any unpaid accounts with a balance that is 30 days past due) should be aged to show their status in the collection process (that is, 30, 60, or 90 days past due). If a computerized billing program is used, a patient aging report is generated to show which patients' payments are due or overdue. For this reason, payments must always be entered promptly, so that at billing time there is no question about any balance due. For example, if payments received by the office totaled $5,000 for the month of January and the net outstanding accounts (accounts receivable) was $25,000, the collection ratio is 20 percent ($5,000 divided by $25,000).

Laws Governing Collections

Collections from payers are considered business collections. Collections from patients, however, are consumer collections and are regulated by federal and state law. The Fair Debt Collection Practices Act of 1977 and the Telephone Consumer Protection Act of 1991 regulate debt collections, forbidding unfair practices, such as making threats, and the use of any form of deception or violence to collect a debt.

Course of Action

Every office needs to establish a written course of action to be taken on overdue accounts. The physician will need to establish the office policy regarding collection procedures, including when to send statements, reminders, and letters and when to take final action.

Usually, an automatic reminder notice and a second statement are mailed when a bill has not been paid 30 days after it was issued. Some medical offices phone a patient with a 30-day overdue account. If the bill is not then paid, a series of collection letters is generated at intervals, each more stringent in its tone and more direct in its approach. Collections letters should be sent using certified mail. Some medical offices use an outside **collection agency** to pursue large unpaid bills.

Federal laws regulate credit and collections for businesses. Also, individual states may have laws that guide the collection process. Usually as a last resort, payment for outstanding accounts may be pursued in small claims or civil claims court. The material in this chapter discusses only basic collection procedures.

Collection by Telephone

A common method of collection is to phone the patient personally. A phone call can be effective in reminding a person who has unintentionally forgotten to pay. Tact and experience are necessary in order to be effective in phone collections.

The following are some techniques of phone collection:

- Identify yourself, the practice, and the purpose of the call
- Be sure you are talking to the person who is responsible for payment of the account. Avoid disclosure of PHI by following HIPAA regulations.
- Make the collection call in the evening, especially if the person who is responsible for payment is out during the day, but no later than 9 P.M. Collection calls may be placed after 8 A.M. but no later than 9 P.M. and not on Sunday or another day the patient recognizes as a Sabbath day.
- Never call a patient at a place of employment to inquire about an unpaid bill.
- Always use a pleasant manner and positive wording (such as "May I process your payment today using your credit or debit card?"). In other words, speak with an expectation of payment. to reflect your confidence that the problem can be resolved.
- Ask to discuss the bill to determine whether the patient has any questions. This query should elicit some response, which is your cue to continue the rest of the conversation.
- Listen carefully.
- Do not show irritation in your voice or appear to be scolding the patient.
- Inform the person that you need to know why the bill has not been paid or why inquiries about the unpaid bill have not been answered.
- If the patient promises to pay, ask when you can expect a payment, the method of payment (cash, debit card, etc.), and the amount. Then make a note about the conversation, saying, for example, "I am making a note in your account file that you promised to pay $100 on September 10. Is that correct?"
- If the patient would prefer that you call his or her attorney, do not contact the patient directly again, unless asked to do so by the attorney. If the patient requests that no more calls be made to him or her concerning the debt, continue correspondence through the mail, with thorough documentation and evidence of delivery.

When collecting by phone, always keep complete, accurate records of who said what, who promised to pay, how much was promised, and when the payment was promised. Note any unusual circumstances. Ask the person responsible for the bill to write down the arrangement. An effective collection tool is to mail a confirmation of the phone details to the patient.

Collection by Letter

The longer a bill remains unpaid, the less likelihood there is of collecting it. A bill should be followed up most vigorously after being overdue for three months. An effective method of collection at this point is to write a letter to the patient. Writing collection letters that bring results is a skill. Collection letters should be personal letters, not form letters. The letter should show that you are sincerely interested in the patient's problem and want to work out a solution. Collection letters should be brief, with short sentences. The letters should appeal to the patient's sense of pride and fair play, as well as a desire for a good credit rating. The amount that is due should be stated clearly in each collection letter, and the patient should be asked to call the assistant to discuss the situation by a stated date. Figure 7.9 shows an example of an effective first collection letter.

It is common practice to send no more than three collection letters, each letter using a more assertive tone. The second letter should refer to the first sent letter, and the third letter often attempts to stress the importance of payment before the account is submitted to a collection agency.

Terminated Accounts

A physician who finds it impossible to extract payment from a patient may decide to terminate the physician-patient relationship. The account is then referred to as a **terminated account**.

If a patient comes to the office, requesting medical care after an account has been terminated, the physician should be consulted and may decide to see the patient on a cash-only basis. If a patient is dismissed, careful and thorough documentation should be made. A letter documenting the dismissal should be sent to the patient by certified mail, return receipt requested. An offer to continue providing care on a cash-only basis for a stated period of time is offered to the patient so the patient's current status of health is not endangered. It will also provide evidence that the physician has not medically abandoned nor refused care to the patient during the time when the patient is seeking another medical provider. Additionally, the physician may provide referrals and copies of the patient's records to other physicians for continuity of care.

Figure 7.9

Collection Letter

KAREN LARSEN, MD
2235 South Ridgeway Avenue   312-555-6022
Chicago, IL 60623-2240   Fax: 312-555-0025

July 1, 20--

Ms. Clair Munson
3492 Green Avenue South
Chicago, IL 60624-3422

Dear Ms. Munson:

In reviewing our accounts, I find that you have an overdue balance of $162.

As you are aware, all bills are due within 30 days of service. Is there some reason we have not heard from you?

Please send us your check for $162 by July 10, 20--, to clear your account or contact our office immediately.

Sincerely,

Theresa J. Olssen

Theresa J. Olssen
Medical Administrative Assistant

Collection by Agency

If the patient has not paid the bill after a reasonable time and routine collection procedures have failed, the physician has two ways of attempting collection. The physician can sue the patient and go to court, which is a time-consuming and costly procedure. The other method is to turn the account over to a collection agency. Once an account has been turned over for collection, the office will have no further contact with the patient concerning billing.

The use of a collection agency is not a very desirable option for collecting unpaid bills, as most agencies work on a contingency basis. Approximately 40 to 50 percent of the amount due is lost when the account is turned over to an agency, and the longer the bill goes unpaid, the less money the physician will receive when the account is finally settled.

There are various types of collection agencies, and a physician will want to investigate an agency thoroughly to determine its reputation.

Statute of Limitations

If the physician fails to collect a fee within a certain period of time, the collection becomes illegal under the statute of limitations and no further claim on the debt is possible. Each state sets its own time limitation, which varies from three to eight years. The physician should obtain legal counsel for advice concerning these statutes.

Credit Arrangements and the Truth in Lending Act

For large bills or special situations, some practices may elect to extend credit to patients. When credit agreements are made, patients and the practice agree to divide the bill into smaller payments over a period of months. If no finance charges are applied to unpaid balances, this type of arrangement is between the practice and the patient, and no legal regulations apply.

If, however, the practice adds finance or late charges and the number of payments is more than four installments, the arrangement is governed by the federal Truth in Lending Act, which became law on July 1, 1960, and is part of the Consumer Credit Card Protection Act. Regulation Z requires that a disclosure form be completed and signed. The disclosure form notifies the patient in writing about the total amount, the finance charges (stated as a percentage), when each payment is due and the amounts, and the date the last payment is due. The disclosure form must be signed by both the practice manager and the patient.

If a physician extends credit to one patient, under the Federal Equal Credit Opportunity Act (1975), the physician must extend the opportunity for credit arrangement to all patients who request it. Refusal can only be made based on ability or inability to pay and, if credit is refused, the physician must notify the patient of the refusal and reason for refusal. The patient has up to 60 days to request the reason for denial in writing.

Writing Off Uncollectible Accounts

If no payment has been made after the collection process, the administrative medical assistant follows the office policy on bills it does not expect to collect. Usually, if all collection attempts have been exhausted and it would cost more to continue than the amount to be collected, the process is ended. In this case, the amount is called an uncollectible account or bad debt and is written off from the expected revenues. Future services for patients who are responsible for uncollectible accounts are usually on a cash-only basis.

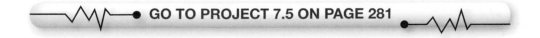

GO TO PROJECT 7.5 ON PAGE 281

Project 7.1   Updating Patient Statements

Dr. Larsen asks you to update the billing. Access the patients' ledgers in the Transaction Entry window in Medisoft®, and enter the charge transactions shown below for October 14 and 15. For the two new patients, David Kramer and Erin Mitchell, you will need to enter the diagnostic code listed below in the Diagnosis tab of the Case dialog box before you enter their charge transactions. The diagnostic codes for the remaining patients have already been entered.

    If a patient has more than one case—in this instance, Robertson, Lund, Baab, and Matthews—be sure to apply the transaction(s) to the correct case. (*Hint:* In the Transaction Entry window, click the triangle button inside the Case box to display a list of cases for the selected patient.) After entering the charge transactions, print patient statements for patients who have transactions on October 14 and 15.

Dr. Larsen asks you to update the billing. The established patients' statements are stored as files on the CD-ROM, labeled according to the patients' last names. Save the statements onto your own disk. These are the billing statements that you will work from. Use Dr. Larsen's fee schedule (WP 45) and the following information to update the patients' statements. After updating the statements, print all of them for your file.

October 14, 20–:

• David Kramer	NP preventive checkup, age 5; UA(81001); HGB	Diagnostic code: V20.2
• Erin Mitchell	99201; UA(81001); UC	Diagnostic code: 599.0
• Gary Robertson	99212; UA(81001); UC	Diagnostic code: 595.0
• Laura Lund	99213; Pap smear	Diagnostic code: 625.3
• Jeffrey Kramer	99212	Diagnostic code: 382.9
• Joseph Castro	99212	Diagnostic code: 930.8

October 15, 20–:

• Todd Grant	99212; ECG	Diagnostic code: 785.0
• Thomas Baab	EP preventive, age 54; UA(81001); CBC; SMA-8; PSA; fasting lipid panel	Diagnostic code: V70.0
• Ardis Matthews	99212	Diagnostic code: 008.8
• Marc Phan	99212	Diagnostic code 466.0

Project 7.2   Internet Research: Comparing Appeal Processes

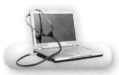

Every third-party payer has its own appeal process. Using your favorite search engine, visit the Web site of your health plan, a friend's plan, or a major plan you know about, and research the plan's appeal process. Then go to the Medicare Web site at www.medicare.gov and read about how to appeal a Medicare claim. How do the processes compare? Which process is more complicated? Why do you think this is the case? Answer these questions and submit them to your instructor.

Project 7.3   Completing Claim Forms

Using the information listed below, go to the Online Learning Center and use the online, electronic claim form to complete the following five insurance claims:

- The place of service is Code 11 (24B).
- The physician is Jack E. Smith, MD, Suite 101, 400 E. Elm Street, Anytown, US 12345-6789. His SS# is 111-22-3333. Phone (312) 555-0874. NPI# is 6374322.
- The patients all live in Anytown, US.
- Utilize the proper coding book to research diagnosis codes.

A. Edward Walker, 432 East High Street 12345
   Date of Birth: 3/18/31
   SS# 382277877
   Patient is insured person, Medicare
   Other insurance is BCBS# 3822778771
   Signature on file
   Abdominal pain and diabetes mellitus
   Seen in office

4/20/xx	Office visit, intermediate	$30.00
	Test feces for blood	$15.00
	Automated hemogram	$20.00
	Phlebotomy	$15.00

B. Amber Shemwell, 3456 Sweetberry Lane 12345
   Date of Birth: 11/27/82
   SS# 254893526
   Patient is insured person, Travelers Insurance Company
   No other insurance
   Not related to employment or accident
   Signature on file
   Arthritis, acute back pain
   Seen in office

4/21/xx	Office visit, intermediate	$30.00
	X-ray lumbar spine, AP & lateral	$129.00
	Phlebotomy	$15.00
	Automated hemogram	$20.00

C. Sherry Johnson, daughter. 2350 West Schaffer Road, 12345
   Date of Birth: 11/27/99
   SS# of insured 986236541
   Insured: Jeffrey Johnson   Date of Birth: 9/5/48
   Self-employed
   Phone # 312-555-4563
   BCBS Insurance   No other insurance
   Signature on file
   Impetigo
   Seen in office

4/22/xx	Office visit, limited	$25.00

D. Melissa Jones, wife. 286 South Roberts Road, 12345

Date of Birth: 12/3/73

Self-employed

Metropolitan Insurance

Insured: Brad Jones   Date of Birth: 10/15/68

SS# of insured: 459872124

No other insurance on file

Signature on file

Phone # 312-555-4845

Acute edema, cystitis, cervicitis

Seen in office

4/23/xx	Office visit, extended	$45.00
	Catheterization, urethra	$30.00
	Endometrial biopsy	$130.00
	Urinalysis	$20.00

E. Adam Westerfield, 2584 Bradford Road, 12345

Date of Birth: 8/13/25

Medicare and Aetna Insurance

SS# of insured: 414319911-A

Signature on file

Phone # 312-555-3635

Diabetes mellitus, coronary atherosclerosis

Seen in office

4/24/xx	Office visit, intermediate	$30.00
	Assay blood fluid, glucose	$30.00
	Phlebotomy	$15.00

Project 7.4 **Posting Payments**

The following patients stop in the office on October 15 with checks to update their accounts.

- Florence Sherman   Pays $35.20
- Theresa Dayton   Pays $33.60
- Thomas Baab   Pays $82.20

Enter and apply the patients' payments in Medisoft® using the Transaction Entry feature. If a patient has more than one open case, be sure to enter and apply the payment to the correct case. Print a walkout receipt for each patient who has made a payment.

Post the payments to their statements. Reprint these statements.

Project 7.5 **Preparing an Effective Collection Letter**

After updating the statements, you notice that Suzanne Roberts has not made a payment for three months. There are collection notations on her statement: September 30, reminder sent; October 10, a follow-up phone call. Compose a letter to Ms. Roberts, requesting payment. Date the letter October 20. This document should be typed and submitted to your instructor.

7.1 Recognize and calculate charges for medical services and process patient statements based on the patient encounter forms and the physician's fee schedule. Pages 256–260	• The administrative medical assistant handles patient transactions, including entering charges for medical services rendered and payments received from patients and third-party payers. • The assistant enters transactions in the appropriate patient's account by referring to information on the patient's encounter form for the visit and the physician's fee schedule. Other charges, such as hospital charges, should be entered from course documents, such as a hospital rounds report. • Determine any charges that are the patient's responsibility, such as an office visit copayment. • Update the patient's account.

7.2 Compare and contrast the process of completing and transmitting insurance claims using both hardcopy and electronic methods.
 	
Pages 260–271
	• Complete the insurance claim form, either electronic or paper. The most commonly used claim form format is the CMS-1500 claim format.
	• Verify patient demographic, encounter, and insurance information.
	• Transmit, electronically or by postal mail, the claim form to the insurance company, which decides to pay the fee, deny the claim, or pay a certain portion of the claim.
	• Verify the accuracy of the payment and post any payments received from the insurance company to the patient's account.
	• Bill patient for coshares.
	• Both paper and electronic claims
	  — Use patient information collected during the registration.
	  — Use diagnostic and procedural information from the patient's encounter.
	  — Gather needed information from either electronic or hardcopy records.
	• Electronic claims are entered only once, creating fewer opportunities for errors, whereas paper claims—even if produced electronically—may be scanned by the payer or physically reentered, creating greater opportunities for errors.
	• Payments resulting from electronic claims submission are faster and, most commonly, are electronic funds transfers. Payments from paper claims may be electronically deposited but may also be sent to the provider via a hardcopy check through the postal service creating a much slower process.

7.3 Describe the different types of billing options used by medical practices for billing patients. Pages 271–274	• The administrative medical assistant is responsible for receiving prompt payments from patients. The method of payment is arranged during the patient's first visit and may include a combination of the following: — Patients pay at the time of the visit by cash, check, debit/credit card (coshares are always collected at this time). — Bills are mailed to patients monthly or at the end of a procedure or hospital stay, using either monthly or cycle billing. — Patients may pay, if necessary, according to an agreed-upon payment plan. — Bills are sent to health insurance carriers, and after payment is received, depending on the terms of the plan, the patient is billed for any balance due. — Patients pay for all charges when physicians work on a cash-only basis. • The physician can adjust the cost of any procedure, should the need arise. However, the decision must be documented, in writing, to protect against a malpractice suit if the adjustment is ever misinterpreted. • Adjusting entries are used to make corrections to patient accounts within a computerized billing system. Transactions are never deleted—they are adjusted.
7.4 Paraphrase the procedures and options available for collecting delinquent accounts. Pages 274–278	• Guidelines are determined by each office in regard to payment—how much is to be collected daily, how much should be collected on each account, etc. • Communications with patients from the start about what is expected from them in terms of payment are the beginning of the collection process. • Patients should be notified in advance of all procedures that are not covered by insurance. • Policies and procedures for handling overdue accounts are determined by each office in conjunction with state and federal laws. • Collection processes may be ended and the amount written off as a bad debt when the amount to be collected is less than the cost of collecting the debt. • State statutes are used to determine the legal period of time to continue the collection of a debt.

Soft Skills Success

Listening Skills

Is listening the same as hearing? The answer is no. Hearing is a physical ability and listening is a skill. The ability to listen helps us make sense of what another person is saying. It greatly enhances our understanding and may even open doors that might not otherwise be open. If you are a good listener, you will be more productive in your career, and more opportunities will come your way. You should find it easy to establish positive working relationships with physicians, office managers, patients, and colleagues. Good listeners are well respected. As a healthcare professional, you will need to not only speak but also listen to the individuals whom you deal with on a daily basis. **Describe a situation in the physician's office that will require you to both listen and speak. What could occur if communication fails during this situation?**

Respond to Facts, Not Feelings

As a part of your responsibilities, you are answering the phones for the day. An angry patient calls and begins yelling at you about an EOB that she has received that denied her claim as being "not medically necessary." It will be important that you attempt to listen to the facts the patient is giving. **How would you handle this situation?**

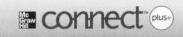
USING TERMINOLOGY

Match the term or phrase on the left with the correct answer on the right.

_____ 1. (LO 7.2) Electronic claim

_____ 2. (LO 7.2) CMS-1500 form

_____ 3. (LO 7.3) Cycle billing

_____ 4. (LO 7.4) Collection agency

_____ 5. (LO 7.1) Fee schedule

_____ 6. (LO 7.4) Collection ratio

_____ 7. (LO 7.3) Write-off

_____ 8. (LO 7.2) Clearinghouse

_____ 9. (LO 7.2) ERA

_____ 10. (LO 7.1) Patient statement

a. An accounting of patient services, charges, payments/adjustments, and balance

b. Payment determination report sent by insurance carrier

c. Percentage that shows the effectiveness of collection methods

d. Insurance claim prepared on and transmitted by computer

e. Service used to pursue payment for services

f. Listing of medical procedures/services and usual charges

g. Universal claim form

h. Billing method used to provide consistent cash flow

i. Service that collects, corrects, and transmits insurance claims

j. Financial adjustment for PAR providers of the difference between submitted and allowable charges

CHECK YOUR UNDERSTANDING

Select the most correct answer.

1. (LO 7.1) Dr. Alonzo has rendered a noncovered procedure to Mrs. Shepherd, who is covered by Medicare. She was not advised before the procedure that it is not covered. The medical office should

   a. Charge Mrs. Shepherd for the procedure.
   b. Obtain Mrs. Shepherd's signature on an ABN.
   c. Adjust the procedure charge off Mrs. Shepherd's account.
   d. Charge Mrs. Shepherd the Medicare allowable amount for the service.

2. (LO 7.1) An appointment was scheduled for a new patient, who asked how much the fee would be for the visit. The administrative medical assistant should

   a. Quote the highest new patient exam fee to the patient.
   b. Transfer the call to the office manager.
   c. Quote the mid-level new patient exam fee to the patient.
   d. Provide an estimate of the exam but explain that the estimate is prior to other services, such as blood work.

3. (LO 7.2) Hardcopy insurance claim forms will produce which of the following?

    a. ERA

    b. EHR

    c. PAR

    d. EOB

4. (LO 7.2) Which of the following is not necessary information on an insurance claim form?

    a. Patient's gender

    b. Patient's sexual orientation

    c. Insured's employment data

    d. Procedure codes

5. (LO 7.2) To complete the insurance form, the medical biller/coder needs the dates when Juan Gomez was unable to work. To find this information, the coder would refer to the

    a. Patient's chart.

    b. Patient registration form.

    c. Lab report.

    d. Patient's ledger.

6. (LO 7.2) Before mailing patient statements, which of the following reports should be reviewed for delinquent accounts?

    a. ERA

    b. Aging report

    c. Daily report

    d. EOB

7. (LO 7.3) At the end of her visit, Katie was asked to pay $20, which is her coshare cost for today's office visit through her managed care health plan. The $20 represents Katie's

    a. Prior account balance.

    b. Copayment.

    c. Payment toward a scheduled procedure.

    d. Monthly payment amount.

8. (LO 7.3) Listed on an account are the father, the mother, and two minor children. One insurance policy, held by the mother, covers all four family members. Who is the guarantor of the account?

    a. Mother

    b. Father

    c. Insurance carrier

    d. Mother and father

9. (LO 7.4) The administrative medical assistant must call patients whose accounts are 30 to 60 days past due. All of the following are recommended phone strategies except

    a. Call during evening hours prior to 9 P.M.

    b. Ask why the bill has not been paid.

    c. Discuss results of lab tests and/or procedures.

    d. Use effective listening techniques.

10. (LO 7.4) Statutes of limitations for collecting debt

    a. Are mandated by the federal government.

    b. May exceed 15 years.

    c. Are set state to state and may vary.

    d. Are not relevant to the office collection policy.

THINKING IT THROUGH

These questions cover the most important points in this chapter. Using your critical-thinking skills, play the role of an administrative medical assistant as you answer each question. Be prepared to present your responses in class.

1. Wayne Elliot asks you why he was charged for two office visits when his daughters, Emily and Rose, were seen at the same time in the same room for the same problem—an earache. Explain the reasoning behind the charges.

2. You receive an EOB for a patient who is covered by an HMO. The HMO did not pay for services received on May 5, which is when the patient visited Dr. Larsen for her annual Pap smear. You check your records and find that the same insurance carrier paid for previous Pap smears for the same patient in past years. What should you do?

3. You receive an ERA from Blue Cross Blue Shield for a Medicare patient. The amount received for the claim is $60, which is $20 less than the usual fee of $80. Since the doctor you work for accepts assignment for Medicare patients, the medical practice will need to write off this amount. You decide to delete the initial fee of $80 in the computerized patient ledger and key in $60, so that the account balances. Why is this a mistake?

4. You notice that an elderly patient is scheduled for a minor surgical procedure that will remove unsightly dark patches of skin, a procedure that is considered cosmetic by most insurance companies. Why is it a good idea to point this out to the patient before the procedure?

Simulation 2

SIMULATION 2

Today you will begin a second simulation in Dr. Larsen's office. The simulation dates are Monday, October 20; Tuesday, October 21; and Wednesday, October 22.

PROCEDURES

Review the section "Before You Start" in Simulation 1. Note that these procedures also apply to this simulation. Also review the "Procedures," because they apply to this simulation. Pull the patients' charts following the appointment calendar, and put them in the appropriate day folder.

MATERIALS

You will need the following materials to complete Simulation 2. If these materials are not already in the proper folder, obtain them from the sources indicated.

Materials	Source
Appointment calendar	
Diagnostic codes	**WP 43**
Fee schedule	**WP 45**
Supplies folder	

To-Do Items

Day 1 folder:

Place patients' charts for October 20.

Telephone log	WP 56
To-do list	WP 57
Letter from Dr. Tai	WP 58
Receipts	WP 59
Patient encounter forms	WP 60–64

Day 2 folder:

Place patients' charts for October 21.

Patient encounter forms	WP 65–67

Day 3 folder:

Place patients' charts for October 22.

Patient encounter forms	WP 68–73

Patients' folders:

The following items have been added to the patients' folders since Simulation 1.

Patient statements for all current patients	Project 7.1, 7.4

MEDICAL VOCABULARY

Before working through this simulation's assignments, review the following terms to be familiar with their spelling and meaning.

Ace wrap

bacitracin—anti-infective agent

chronicity—long duration of time

clindamycin—anti-infective agent

COPD—chronic obstructive pulmonary disease

DTP—diphtheria, tetanus, and pertussis vaccine

effusion—escape of fluid from blood vessels or lymphatics into tissues or a cavity

FSH—follicle-stimulating hormone

gravida—pregnant woman

HDL—high-density lipoprotein

hematuria—urine containing blood

hemoccult—test for hidden (occult) blood within stool

hidradenitis—inflammation of sweat glands

incontinence—inability to prevent discharge of excretions, such as urine or feces

IPV—inactivated polio vaccine

IVP—intravenous pyelogram

LDL—low-density liproprotein

lymphadenitis—inflammation of lymph node or nodes

mediocondylar—middle rounded prominence on a bone

MMR—measles-mumps-rubella vaccine

Naprosyn—analgesic, antipyretic

OTC—over-the-counter

proximal—nearest

purulent—containing pus

pustular—marked by pustules (small skin elevations containing pus)

pyelonephritis—inflammation of renal pelvis and kidney

Robaxin—skeletal muscle relaxant

suppurative—producing pus

tendonitis/tendinitis—inflammation of tendon

valgus—bent or twisted outward from midline of body

varus—bent or twisted inward toward the midline of body

Vicodin—analgesics

Z-pack—analgesics

medisoft MEDISOFT® INSTRUCTIONS

If your instructor has assigned the use of Medisoft®, you will complete certain parts of Simulation 2 using the software program. Follow these instructions:

To complete this simulation in Medisoft®, you must be able to:

- Schedule appointments
- Print a physician's schedule
- Enter charges
- Enter payments
- Print walkout receipts
- Print patient statements

Enter the new appointments in Office Hours. Then print Dr. Larsen's schedule for October 20, 21, and 22.

Enter all charge and payment transactions. Print walkout receipts for patients who made a payment.

Print statements for all patients who had transactions on October 20, 21, and 22.

Practice Finances

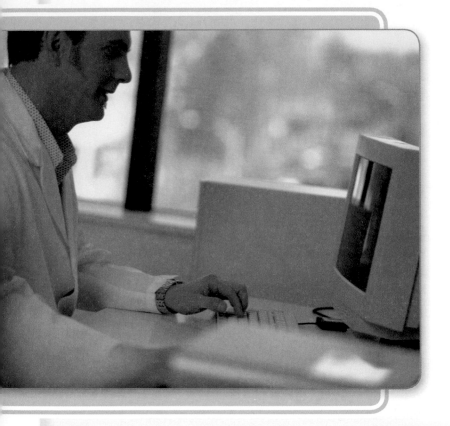

LEARNING OUTCOMES

After studying this chapter, you will be able to:

8.1 Explain, using accounting terminology, the procedures for maintaining two essential financial records.

8.2 Summarize the main focus of the Red Flag Requirements as they relate to the medical office as a business.

8.3 List three banking duties of the administrative medical assistant.

8.4 Explain how an employee's net salary is determined.

KEY TERMS

Study these important words, which are defined in this chapter, to build your professional vocabulary:

absolute accuracy	bank reconciliation	EFT	monthly summary
accounting	blank endorsement	employer identification number (EIN)	patient ledger cards
accounts payable (A/P)	bookkeeping	e-signature	payroll
accounts receivable (A/R)	cash basis	FICA	petty cash fund
accrual method	charge/receipt slips	full endorsement	posting
aging reports	daily journal	FUTA	practice analysis report
annual summary	deductions	income statement	procedure day sheet
audit	deposits	indirect earnings	Red Flag Requirements
balance sheet	direct earnings	interest	restrictive endorsement

Chapter 8

ABHES

- Adapt to change.
- Maintain confidentiality at all times.
- Use appropriate guidelines when releasing records or information.
- Project a positive attitude.
- Be cognizant of ethical boundaries.
- Evidence a responsible attitude.
- Conduct work within scope of education, training, and ability.
- Professional components.
- Apply electronic technology.
- Apply computer concepts for office procedures.
- Orient patients to office policies and procedures.
- Establish and maintain a petty cash fund.
- Perform basic secretarial skills.
- Prepare a bank statement.
- Reconcile a bank statement.
- Maintain records for accounting and banking purposes.
- Post entries on a day sheet.
- Prepare a check.
- Post collection agency payments.
- Use manual and computerized bookkeeping systems.
- Manage accounts payable and receivable.

CAAHEP

- ➡ Compare manual and computerized bookkeeping systems used in ambulatory healthcare.
- ➡ Explain both billing and payment options.
- ➡ Identify procedures for preparing patient accounts.
- ➡ Discuss procedures for collecting outstanding accounts.
- ➡ Discuss precautions for accepting checks.
- ➡ Compare types of endorsements.
- ➡ Differentiate between accounts payable and accounts receivable.
- ➡ Describe the impact of both the Fair Debt Collection Act and the Federal Truth in Lending Act of 1968 as they apply to collections.
- ➡ Perform accounts receivable procedures, including (a) post entries on a day sheet; (b) perform billing procedures; (c) perform collection procedures; (d) post nonsufficient fund (NSF) checks; (h) post collection agency payments.
- ➡ Utilize computerized office billing systems.
- ➡ Demonstrate sensitivity and professionalism in handling accounts receivable activities with clients.

- ➡ Cognitive
- ➡ Psychomotor
- ➡ Affective

INTRODUCTION

The physician's time and medical expertise are perhaps the most valuable assets in a medical practice. Because the practice is a business as well as a service, it is required to produce a profit. The administrative medical assistant protects and enhances the assets of the practice by handling many financial responsibilities on the business side. When assistants are working with patients' financial information, standards should be in place to protect patients from identity theft. Governmental Red Flag Requirements may extend to the physician's medical practice.

Administrative medical assistants help with **accounting**—the methodical recording, classifying, and summarizing of business transactions—in the medical office. The physician must have a record of all transactions and must be able to prepare tax records. Either an accountant employed by the practice or the Internal Revenue Service (IRS) may wish to perform an **audit**, or review of all financial data in order to ensure the accuracy and completeness of the data. The assistant also makes all records available to the IRS and keeps all source documents for tax purposes. These tasks require a working knowledge of tax regulations and of the accounting process. The part of the process that is the accurate recording of transactions is called **bookkeeping**.

Accounting for the practice may be done in one of two ways: on a cash basis or on an accrual basis. If the practice operates on a **cash basis**, charges for services are not recorded as income to the practice until payment is received and expenses are not recorded until they are paid. With the **accrual method**, income is recorded as soon as it is earned, whether or not the payment is received, and expenses are recorded when they are incurred. Whichever way the practice decides to keep its accounts, there are certain essential records that must be carefully kept and maintained. The assistant's task is to enter data accurately the first time on a record and to perform the tasks of **posting** to records, or transferring amounts from one record to another.

The financial records that are used daily in the practice include the following:

- *The daily journal:* The **daily journal** is a record of services rendered, daily fees charged, payments received, and adjustments. It is also called a "general journal," "day sheet," or "daily earnings record." Most medical providers now use computerized daily journals (day sheets), commonly referred to as a procedure day sheet (which will be discussed later in this chapter).
- *Charge/receipt slips:* **Charge/receipt slips** provide a record of the physician's services and the charges for these. These slips are also called patient encounter forms (discussed in Chapter 7).
- *Ledgers:* **Patient ledger cards** contain a patient's name, services rendered, charge, payment, and balance. Computerized patient ledgers are referred to as simply "patients' accounts." **Accounts payable (A/P)** ledgers record expense amounts owed to a supplier or creditor. Examples of accounts payable are rent, equipment rental, and office supplies. **Accounts receivable (A/R)** ledgers record the balance of payments due from patients or others (third-party payers) on current accounts.
- *Summaries:* The **monthly summary** shows the daily charges and payments for an entire month. The **annual summary** provides the monthly charges and payments for an entire year. In some practices, quarterly (a three-month period) summaries are prepared.

Each of these records may be maintained electronically, and most offices, even if they have not fully implemented EHRs, maintain their financial records with electronic software.

HIPAA TIPS A document containing any patient information is considered confidential; this includes personal checks. Documents such as this must be kept out of view from other patients and staff members who do not have permission to access any confidential patient information.

What type of staff member would not need to have access to confidential patient information?

The assistant is responsible for accurately entering the data and keeping these essential records current. Data input errors have a ripple effect. When a mistake is made on financial data, other financial areas are also affected. For example, a patient was evaluated at a 99213 level but the code 99214 was entered. The error affects not only the patient's account but also the daily accountability of how many procedures of each type have been rendered and their daily, weekly, and monthly totals. Accurate data input is a key skill for medical office personnel.

Financial records are the basis for ongoing decisions about collections and disbursements, and they provide a picture of the financial health of the practice. In all businesses, the managers speak of the importance of the **balance sheet**, the financial statement for a particular date that indicates the total assets (possessions of value, such as equipment), liabilities (debts), and capital (available dollars). Summaries are an important part of the balance sheet.

Another important financial "snapshot" of the practice is the **income statement**, which shows profit and loss for a stated period of time, such as a quarter or year. All income is categorized and reported as gross income (income prior to deductions). Expenses are also categorized and totals are listed. Taxes are included as a business expense. A net total (income after expenses are deducted) is calculated. Income statements are a critical analysis tool for determining the financial health of a business.

Accounting Software

Some offices still maintain financial records in a paper format. However, most practices use an accounting software package to perform all necessary accounting functions. Several software applications have been customized with vocabulary and features specific to medical practices. Software programs require some effort to learn and manipulate. However, they save time by automatically performing routine tasks and most mathematical calculations.

Daily Journal

The daily journal, manual and electronic, is used to record daily fees charged and payments received. It is, then, the financial source document (journal) used for accounts receivable (fees charged) and cash receipts (payments received). Fees charged, payments received, and adjustments must be recorded promptly in the daily journal.

It is necessary to have an accurate balance of accounts. The manual daily journal, used with older manual systems, in Figure 8.1 shows typical entries and balances entered onto a manual daily journal. Accuracy is obtained by using the section at the bottom of the journal page, in the center, labeled "Accounts Receivable Control." *Accounts Receivable* in the label refers to the balance due from patients on current accounts. By maintaining this section of the daily journal, the practice keeps a "control" on the amount of money it is owed. Every day, the charges are added and the payments are subtracted from the previous day's balance. The result is the current day's accounts receivable balance.

There is also a section, usually in the lower left corner of the page, labeled "Proof of Posting." In this case, *proof* does not mean that the correct amounts were charged. *Proof* means only that the columns balance.

The section labeled "Daily Cash" in the lower right corner is used to account for the daily cash flow, or the amount of cash received that day.

Computerized Daily Journal. Medical management software provides electronic daily journal forms. The example shown in Figure 8.2 is a feature of Medisoft®. It is called the **procedure day sheet** and lists numerically all procedures performed on a given day. It also provides patient names, document numbers, places of service (POS), and debits and credits.

Figure 8.1

Manual Daily Journal

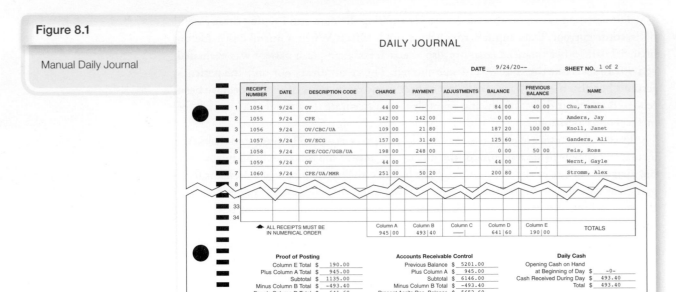

DAILY JOURNAL

DATE 9/24/20--   SHEET NO. 1 of 2

	RECEIPT NUMBER	DATE	DESCRIPTION CODE	CHARGE	PAYMENT	ADJUSTMENTS	BALANCE	PREVIOUS BALANCE	NAME
1	1054	9/24	OV	44 00	—	—	84 00	40 00	Chu, Tamara
2	1055	9/24	CPE	142 00	142 00	—	0 00		Amders, Jay
3	1056	9/24	OV/CBC/UA	109 00	21 80	—	187 20	100 00	Knoll, Janet
4	1057	9/24	OV/ECG	157 00	31 40	—	125 60		Ganders, Ali
5	1058	9/24	CPE/CGC/UGB/UA	198 00	248 00	—	0 00	50 00	Feis, Ross
6	1059	9/24	OV	44 00	—	—	44 00	—	Wernt, Gayle
7	1060	9/24	CPE/UA/MMR	251 00	50 20		200 80		Stromm, Alex
8									
33									
34									
▲ ALL RECEIPTS MUST BE IN NUMERICAL ORDER				Column A 945 00	Column B 493 40	Column C —	Column D 641 60	Column E 190 00	TOTALS

Proof of Posting		**Accounts Receivable Control**		**Daily Cash**	
Column E Total $	190.00	Previous Balance $	5201.00	Opening Cash on Hand	
Plus Column A Total $	945.00	Plus Column A $	945.00	at Beginning of Day $	-0-
Subtotal $	1135.00	Subtotal $	6146.00	Cash Received During Day $	493.40
Minus Column B Total $	-493.40	Minus Column B Total $	-493.40	Total $	493.40
Equals Column D Total $	641.60	Present Acc'ts Rec. Balance $	5652.60		

Figure 8.2

Medisoft® Procedure Day Sheet

Karen Larsen MD

Procedure Day Sheet

Show all data where the Date From is between 9/24/2014, 9/24/2014

Entry	Date	Chart	Name	Document	POS	Debits	Credits
80048							
146	9/24/2014	ROGERCL0	Rogers, Clarence	0309240000		51.00	
		Total of 80048			Quantity: 1	$51.00	$0.00
81001							
89	9/24/2014	DAYTOTH0	Dayton, Theresa	0309240000		24.00	
117	9/24/2014	MATTHEA1	Matthews, Ardis	0309240000		24.00	
		Total of 81001			Quantity: 2	$48.00	$0.00
85025							
88	9/24/2014	DAYTOTH0	Dayton, Theresa	0309240000	11	25.00	
116	9/24/2014	MATTHEA1	Matthews, Ardis	0309240000	11	25.00	
		Total of 85025			Quantity: 2	$50.00	$0.00
87088							
118	9/24/2014	MATTHEA1	Matthews, Ardis	0309240000		35.00	
		Total of 87088			Quantity: 1	$35.00	$0.00
88150							
87	9/24/2014	DAYTOTH0	Dayton, Theresa	0309240000		33.00	
125	9/24/2014	MENDEAN0	Mendez, Ana	0309240000		33.00	
		Total of 88150			Quantity: 2	$66.00	$0.00
93000							
145	9/24/2014	ROGERCL0	Rogers, Clarence	0309240000		70.00	
		Total of 93000			Quantity: 1	$70.00	$0.00

Methods of Bookkeeping

There are two main methods of bookkeeping: single-entry method and double-entry method. A third method, which is a manual accounting system referred to as a pegboard system, was used extensively by medical practices in the past, but most medical offices have transferred accounting functions to computerized systems. Debits and credits summarized in columns at the bottom of the day sheet are used to balance manual day sheets.

- *Single-entry method:* This system requires only one entry for each transaction and is the oldest system. It is, however, a difficult system to use because it is not a self-balancing method; therefore, users find it hard to recognize errors.
- *Double-entry method:* This system requires more knowledge of accounting principles than the other method does. It is a method based on the accounting equation: assets equal liabilities plus owner equity. In businesses where this method is used, one account must be debited and another account credited after each transaction. Thus, the system takes more time to use.

Summaries

In many practices, the physician will want to analyze charges, cash receipts, and disbursements at the end of the month, at the end of each quarter, and at the end of the year. The purpose of analyzing summaries is to compare the present financial performance of the practice with its performance last year, last quarter, or last month. The physician, and in some cases an accountant, will look at cash receipts from certain kinds of services (such as EP Level III E/M codes), the expenses involved in running the office, and other categories. The analysis will help the physician plan for the future of the practice by cutting back on expenses, for example, or by investing in equipment that will enable the practice to offer more patients a particularly profitable service.

Computer Summaries. The use of a software program to provide summaries is an efficient way to assemble information. The database can be manipulated to provide a summary by procedure code or by number of procedures within a certain time frame. It also can provide a comparative summary over time of payments used to make a deposit. Such software solutions are available in specialized medical accounting software programs.

In Medisoft®, for example, a **practice analysis report** may be generated monthly or for another specified period of time. The purpose of the report is, as its name shows, to analyze the revenue of the practice for a specified period of time. In the report, the description of and revenue for each procedure is shown first, as in Figure 8.3(*a*). A summary page at the end of the report then shows the total charges, patient payments, copayments, adjustments, and so on. The summary page is shown in Figure 8.3(*b*). This report may also be used to generate financial statements for the practice.

In addition, programs such as Medisoft® provide other useful summaries, such as **aging reports**. This analysis lists the amounts of money owed to the practice, and the report is organized according to the number of days due. In such a report, the "aging" begins on the date of the transaction and will report those debts that are current—or "0 to 30 days"—and several other time frames of past due debts. See the example of an aging report in Figure 8.4.

Software spreadsheet capabilities also enhance the physician's ability to analyze the performance of the practice. These spreadsheets may be designed to provide profit and loss reports, expense reports, and budget planning documents. To create a program to serve your practice, the designer customizes the spreadsheet by specifying the format and creating formulas that will provide the desired calculations.

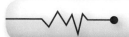 **IF ASSIGNED, GO TO OPTIONAL PROJECT 8.1 ON PAGE 308**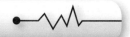

Figure 8.3

(a) Practice Analysis Report, Page 1
(b) Practice Analysis Report, Summary Page

Karen Larsen MD
Practice Analysis
Show all data where the Date From is between 9/1/2014, 9/30/2014

Code	Description	Amount	Units	Average	Cost	Net
80048	SMA-8 Basic metabolic panel	51.00	1	51.00	0.00	51.00
81001	UA with microscopy	48.00	2	24.00	0.00	48.00
85025	Hemogram (CBC) with differential	50.00	2	25.00	0.00	50.00
87088	UC	35.00	1	35.00	0.00	35.00
88150	Pap	66.00	2	33.00	0.00	66.00
93000	Electrocardiogram (ECG)	70.00	1	70.00	0.00	70.00
99212	OV, EP, Focused	44.00	1	44.00	0.00	44.00
99213	OV, EP, Expanded	60.00	1	60.00	0.00	60.00
99221	Initial hospital visit, detailed	121.00	1	121.00	0.00	121.00
99231	Subsequent hospital visit, focused	65.00	1	65.00	0.00	65.00
99395	Preventive, EP, 18-39 yrs.	272.00	2	136.00	0.00	272.00
INSPAY	Insurance payment	-543.20	12	-45.27	0.00	-543.20
PATPAY	Patient payment - check	-274.40	5	-54.88	0.00	-274.40

(a)

Karen Larsen MD
Practice Analysis
Show all data where the Date From is between 9/1/2014, 9/30/2014

Code	Description	Amount	Units	Average	Cost	Net
			Total Procedure Charges			$882.00
			Total Global Surgical Procedures			$0.00
			Total Product Charges			$0.00
			Total Inside Lab Charges			$0.00
			Total Outside Lab Charges			$0.00
			Total Billing Charges			$0.00
			Total Insurance Payments			-$543.20
			Total Cash Copayments			$0.00
			Total Check Copayments			$0.00
			Total Credit Card Copayments			$0.00
			Total Patient Cash Payments			$0.00
			Total Patient Check Payments			-$274.40
			Total Credit Card Payments			$0.00
			Total Debit Adjustments			$0.00
			Total Credit Adjustments			$0.00
			Total Insurance Debit Adjustments			$0.00
			Total Insurance Credit Adjustments			$0.00
			Total Insurance Withholds			$0.00
			Net Effect on Accounts Receivable			$64.40

(b)

Figure 8.4

Aging Report

Patient Aging by Date of Service
Karen Larsen MD
Show all data where the Charges/Payments/Adj is on or before 10/7/2014

Chart	Name	0-30	31-60	61-90	91-120	121+	Total
DAYTOTH0	Dayton, Theresa	33.60					33.60
MENDEAN0	Mendez, Ana	8.45					8.45
ROBERSU0	Roberts, Suzanne			156.00			156.00
ROGERCL0	Rogers, Clarence	86.20					86.20
Report Totals:		128.25	0.00	156.00	0.00	0.00	284.25

Just as HIPAA regulations were implemented to protect patients' nonpublic personal data, new regulations, known as **Red Flag Requirements**, focus on identifying and verifying individuals in relation to information presented to the practice. In other words, the medical practice must make sure that persons presenting for services are who they say they are. Using the criminal act of identity theft to acquire medical and other types of services illegally has become a growing challenge for society.

The following are some examples of possible identity theft:

- Checks with a different name other than the patient's
- Patient complaints about bills for services they did not receive
- Medical records showing treatment that is inconsistent with the physical exam and/or history as reported by the patient

As of 2010, the deadline for compliance with Red Flag Requirements has been extended five times. The current compliance deadline date is December 31, 2010.

Who Must Comply

Financial institutions (that is, banks, credit unions, and other lending institutions) and other "creditors" must comply with Red Flag Requirements. A "creditor" is any person or business that makes arrangements for extending, renewing, or continuing credit. This definition covers a large collection of businesses—auto dealerships, telecommunication companies, hospitals, collection agencies, and so on. There has been much discussion as to whether a medical practice fits the definition of a "creditor." The Federal Trade Commission says that any company/organization that provides services or other goods may qualify as a "creditor" if the company does not require the patient to pay in full at the time of service. Frequently, in a medical office, a patient receives services and is billed monthly and/or after the patient has received payment from the insurance carrier. According to the current definition, physicians' practices are considered "creditors." Additionally, if an individual obtains medical services by using another person's identity, there is a high risk that the victim's medical records will be intermixed with the criminal's records. This may lead to serious consequences when the victim seeks medical treatment. Therefore, medical practices must know with a reasonable amount of certainty that persons seeking and receiving treatment are actually who they say they are.

Covered Accounts

Accounts that must be protected are any personal accounts that allow multiple payments or transactions. This qualifies medical patients' accounts, as they usually are the primary source of financial transaction documents for the patient. Also, if there is a reasonable and predictable risk to the patient/customer or to the safety of the creditor, the account is considered a covered account because it is a transaction account. A transaction account is any account from which or into which the owner (patient) makes payments and/or transfers.

Red Flag Implementation

Each company/organization that fits the definition of a covered account must follow the Red Flag Requirements, also known as the Red Flag Rules. The following are the parts of the Red Flag Requirements as of the printing of this text:

1. *Recognize and list red flags (warning signs) pertinent to your practice.* Each practice should study and identify triggers that suggest identity fraud. Make a comprehensive list. Alerts and updates from a consumer reporting guide may be used to list red flags.

Other red flags may be in the form of suspicious documents, a change in PHI (such as an address change), and unusual account activity.

2. *Describe how your practice will discover/detect each red flag.*

   a. Put steps in place to obtain identifying information and to verify the identity of an individual who is seeking services.

   b. Implement effective methods of authenticating the identity of the patient requesting service or other transactions. Traditionally, a photo ID, such as a driver's license, was sufficient. However, more stringent methods may need to be used. Primary and secondary identifiers should be listed as acceptable forms of identification. Primary identifiers may include a valid driver's license or state I.D. card, valid passport, U.S. alien registration card, and military I.D. Fingerprint readers may be used to authenticate identity. Examples of secondary identifiers may include Social Security cards, firearm licenses, insurance cards, and voter registration cards. Patients should present either two primary identifiers or one primary and one secondary identifier—the policy of identifiers should be established, in writing, by the practice.

   c. Monitor the activity of your patients' accounts.

   d. Verify the authenticity of a change of address. Identity thieves will change the legitimate address on the account, so that all fraudulent activity is sent to the changed address.

3. *Prevent and diminish identity theft with appropriate responses.* The medical office should respond to identity theft triggers to an appropriate degree. For example, an account may only need to be monitored for identity abuse, or it may need to be closed.

4. *Update the Red Flag Requirements plan.* The effectiveness of policies and procedures need to be evaluated to ensure that they cover the current red flags.

A Red Flag Requirements plan should be overseen by individuals who are senior in the practice, such as the physician, office manager, and head nurse. Also, the plan must include steps for training medical team members in identity theft triggers and detection. Using guidelines from the federal government, medical offices should design and implement a plan that is appropriate for the size and nature of the practice. Many helpful Web sites contain information and suggestions for developing a Red Flag Requirements plan, including the Federal Trade Commission Web site, at http://ftc.gov.

8.3 • BANKING

It is clear that handling the banking functions of the practice accurately and promptly contributes to the financial health of the practice. The administrative medical assistant is responsible for many of these banking duties, including preparing deposits and reconciling bank statements. Banking tasks require **absolute accuracy**, correctness that is 100 percent, because the assistant acts as the physician's agent in these matters.

Checks and Checking Accounts

An order (written or electronic) to a bank to pay a specific amount of money to another party is referred to as a check. The practice may have at least two types of checking accounts—one regular business checking account and an account that pays interest. There may also be a savings account in the name of the practice. Money for taxes or expenses that are not immediate will be kept in a checking or savings account where it will earn **interest**, or money paid by the bank to depositors in return for the bank's use of the depositor's money. You will use the regular business account most frequently: to deposit patient payments and to draw checks for the payment of office expenses. Although this account may not pay interest, it allows for availability and flexibility.

Negotiable Checks. A check is an order to a bank to pay a specific amount of money. In order for the check to be negotiable—that is, to allow the legal transfer of money—it must meet several requirements. It is important for you to know what these are; you should examine all checks given to you before accepting them. To be negotiable, a check must

- State the specific amount to be paid.
- Be made out (made payable) to the payee. The payee may be the title of the practice rather than the physician's name, depending on the title of the account.
- Carry the name of the bank that is making the payment.
- Specify the date on which payment is to be made.
- Be signed by the payer, the person who writes the check and is promising to pay the money.

Be sure that you understand and follow office policies about accepting checks. For example, a patient visiting the office for the first time may be required to present identification before the check is accepted.

The following kinds of checks are usually not acceptable:

- *Postdated checks:* A check dated in the future (postdated) cannot be cashed until that future date.
- *Predated checks:* A check dated in the past (predated) is acceptable only if the date is *within* a six-month period before the date on which you receive it.
- *Third-party checks:* In this case, *third party* refers not to an insurer but to anyone other than the patient. A third-party check is a check written to the patient by a person unknown to the practice.
- *Checks annotated "Paid in Full":* When the amount of the check does not correspond to the total, or full, amount due for the services rendered, the office should not accept a check marked "Paid in Full."

Check Endorsements. All checks received should be endorsed as soon as they are accepted. This lessens the chance that they will be lost, stolen, or forgotten. Three types of endorsements may be used (Figure 8.5):

- *Blank endorsement:* In a **blank endorsement**, the signature of the person to whom the check is payable (the payee) is placed on the back of the check. Once a check is endorsed this way, the check may be cashed by anyone. Blank endorsements are not used in business.
- *Full endorsement:* A **full endorsement** indicates the person, company, account number, or bank to which the check is being transferred, followed by the payee's name.

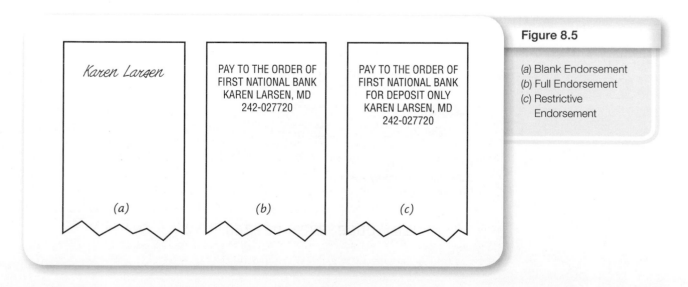

Figure 8.5

(a) Blank Endorsement
(b) Full Endorsement
(c) Restrictive Endorsement

- *Restrictive endorsement:* A **restrictive endorsement** is the safest and most commonly used endorsement in business. The check is "restricted" by being marked "For Deposit Only." The use of the check is thus limited because the party to whom the money should be paid and the purpose have been stated. The restrictive endorsement is convenient for business use. The assistant may use a "For Deposit Only" rubber stamp and may deposit the check without obtaining the physician's signature.

Deposits. The checks and cash placed into the account belonging to the practice are called **deposits**. Once the daily monetary intake from endorsed checks and cash has been verified using the procedure day sheet, a deposit slip is prepared. For a sizable practice, depositing checks daily is important because it improves the cash flow and ensures that checks sent by the practice will not bounce. If the practice is specialized or very small, deposits may be made less often during the week. The bank where the checking account is maintained provides deposit slips. These are preprinted with the title of the account and the account number. A sample deposit slip is shown in Figure 8.6. On the first line, marked "Cash," the amount of currency—bills and coins—is entered. Some deposit slips list "Cash" and "Coins" on separate lines. Beneath this entry, each check is listed separately. Some banks prefer to have the check identified by its number or bank name. The total amount, cash and checks, is entered on the appropriate line (usually the last line). The amount of the deposit is then entered on the first unused checkbook stub or in the check register. When manually preparing any banking document, only blue or black ink should be used. Other colors are difficult for electronic scanning equipment to read.

It is important to obtain a deposit receipt from the bank. All deposit slips, the checkbooks, and the check register should be kept in a secure and locked place in the office.

Returned Checks. The bank may return a check that has not been completed properly: the check may be missing a date or signature. The check will also be returned if there is not enough money in the account to cover the amount shown on the check. In this case, the check is stamped, or identified "NSF," or "nonsufficient funds." The bank may charge a fee for returned checks, and in turn the practice will charge the patient a fee for the returned check. After the returned check has been received, make a debit entry into the patient's account, recharging for the amount of the check. Include the returned check fee on the account. Notify the patient of the returned check and related fees. Usually, payment from the patient should be a cash or debit/credit card payment. Be sure to inform the patient of the due date and to document information discussed with the patient (if not in letter format). When this happens, you will need to contact the person who gave you the check.

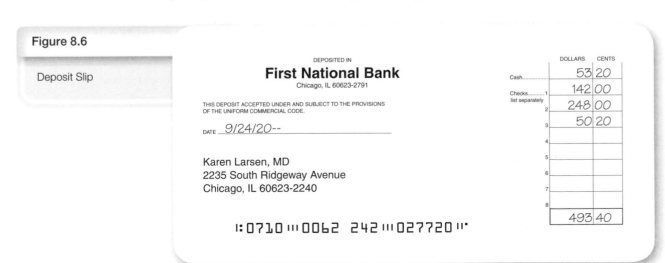

Figure 8.6

Deposit Slip

DEPOSITED IN
First National Bank
Chicago, IL 60623-2791

THIS DEPOSIT ACCEPTED UNDER AND SUBJECT TO THE PROVISIONS OF THE UNIFORM COMMERCIAL CODE.

DATE 9/24/20--

Karen Larsen, MD
2235 South Ridgeway Avenue
Chicago, IL 60623-2240

⑆0710⑆0062 242⑆027720⑆

	DOLLARS	CENTS
Cash	53	20
Checks 1 list separately	142	00
2	248	00
3	50	20
4		
5		
6		
7		
8		
	493	40

The Banking Policy of the Practice

The physician must indicate the persons in the practice authorized to sign all checks. One person may be authorized to write checks, and another may be authorized to sign. This is a good internal system to avoid mistakes and misappropriations. The physician may require two signatures for each check or may set limits on the amounts of money for which anyone other than the physician may write checks.

Bank Reconciliation

Each month the bank submits a statement of the checking account, such as the one shown in Figure 8.7. The monthly statement shows the beginning balance, total credits (deposits added to the account during the month), total debits (checks paid out of the account during the month), any service charges that apply, and the resulting new balance.

The new balance on the statement must be compared with the checkbook balance to determine whether there is a difference between the amounts. This process is known as reconciling

Figure 8.7

Bank Statement

First National Bank
Chicago, IL 60623-2791

STATEMENT OF
ACCOUNT NUMBER
242 027720

CLOSING DATE	ITEMS
6/25	12

KAREN LARSEN, MD
2235 SOUTH RIDGEWAY AVENUE
CHICAGO, IL 60623-2240

PERSONAL CHECKING ACCOUNT STATEMENT

BEGINNING BALANCE	(+) TOTAL CREDITS	(−) TOTAL DEBITS	(−) SERVICE CHARGE	(=) NEW BALANCE
2,592.74	1,030.00	919.06		2,703.68

CHECKS & OTHER DEBITS		DEPOSITS & OTHER CREDITS	DATE	BALANCE
	2.54	165.00	6/2	2,755.20
		100.00	6/4	2,855.20
	97.00		6/5	2,758.20
	450.00		6/6	2,308.20
		120.00	6/9	2,428.20
	29.37		6/11	
	13.00			2,385.83
		85.00	6/12	2,470.83
	7.00	210.00	6/16	2,673.83
	15.62		6/17	2,658.21
		90.00	6/18	2,748.21
	37.98	185.00	6/23	
	65.12			2,830.11
	145.00		6/24	
	15.00			2,670.11
	41.43	75.00	6/25	2,703.68

SYMBOLS

C = CORRECTION	DM = DEBIT MEMO	RI = RETURN ITEM	ST = SAVINGS TRANSFER
CM = CREDIT MEMO	OD = OVERDRAFT	SC = SERVICE CHARGE	

the bank statement, or **bank reconciliation.** Many banks provide a reconciliation form, such as the one shown in Figure 8.8, on one of the pages of the monthly statement.

The steps you should take in the reconciliation process are:

1. Compare the canceled checks returned by the bank with the items listed on the bank statement. When banks do not provide the actual canceled checks, miniaturized photostats of the checks are usually provided. These, in addition to the listing of the checks on the statement, may be used for reference.

2. Compare the checks listed on the bank statement with the checkbook stubs to verify that check numbers and amounts agree. Deductions, such as service charges, are explained on the bank statement. These must be recorded in the checkbook. Checks that were written during the last month but have not yet been paid by the bank are not

Figure 8.8

Reconciliation Section of a Bank Statement

CHANGE OF ADDRESS ORDER
TO CHANGE YOUR ADDRESS, PLEASE COMPLETE THIS FORM;
THEN CUT ALONG DOTTED LINE, AND MAIL OR BRING TO THE BANK.

NEW ADDRESS

NUMBER AND STREET

CITY   STATE AND ZIP CODE   NEW PHONE NUMBER

DATE   CUSTOMER'S SIGNATURE

OUTSTANDING CHECKS	
NUMBER	AMOUNT
	125 00
	18 65
	22 19
	48 90
TOTAL	214 74

TO RECONCILE YOUR STATEMENT AND CHECKBOOK

1. DEDUCT FROM YOUR CHECKBOOK BALANCE ANY SERVICE OR OTHER CHARGE ORIGINATED BY THE BANK. THESE CHARGES WILL BE IDENTIFIED BY SYMBOLS AS SHOWN ON FRONT.

2. ARRANGE ENDORSED CHECKS BY DATE OR NUMBER AND CHECK THEM OFF AGAINST THE STUBS IN YOUR CHECKBOOK.

3. LIST IN THE OUTSTANDING CHECKS SECTION AT THE LEFT ANY CHECKS ISSUED BY YOU AND NOT YET PAID BY US.

TO RECONCILE YOUR STATEMENT AND CHECKBOOK		
LAST BALANCE SHOWN ON STATEMENT	2,703	68
PLUS: DEPOSITS AND CREDITS MADE AFTER DATE OF LAST ENTRY ON STATEMENT	130	00
SUBTOTAL	2,833	68
MINUS: OUTSTANDING CHECKS	214	74
BALANCE: WHICH SHOULD AGREE WITH YOUR CHECKBOOK	2,618	94

included with the statement. These are called "outstanding checks" and should be listed on the reconciliation form as shown in Figure 8.8.

3. Compare the deposits recorded in the checkbook with the credits listed on the bank statement. A deposit listed in the checkbook but not recorded by the bank at the time the statement was issued is called a "deposit in transit."
4. If the checking account earns interest, record the interest as a credit, similar to a deposit, in the checkbook.
5. Complete the reconciliation form following the directions.

If the final amount on the reconciliation form does not agree with the amount in the checkbook, compare the monthly statement with the checkbook again.

- Recheck the deposits entered on the bank statement against those you have entered in the checkbook.
- Confirm that all service charges shown on the statement are entered in the checkbook and have been properly deducted.
- Make sure no check has been drawn that has not been recorded in the checkbook. Compare all checks with the stubs to make sure the amounts agree.
- Review the list of outstanding checks to see whether an old check is still outstanding.
- Recheck all addition and subtraction.

When the checkbook is reconciled, make a notation to that effect in the checkbook on the last-used stub or register line.

Banking Electronically

Banking by computer can contribute to both efficiency and accuracy. The tasks that you have when banking electronically are the same as those you perform when using paper procedures. You are still responsible for recording and physically depositing checks. You still need to reconcile statements but do not need to wait for a hardcopy statement to be mailed. Online banking is typically in real time and is up to date. However, the software makes all the calculations automatically. This not only saves time but also reduces the chances for error. You no longer need to worry about a secure storage place for the checkbook and deposit slips. The password you use to access the bank account is the only item you must protect.

Banks' software systems allow you to

- Check account balances.
- Receive electronic deposits.
- Find out which checks have cleared.
- Transfer money from one account to another.
- Pay certain bills.

Menus in banking software are user friendly. Main menus present broad topics, such as "Pay Bills," "Payment Center," and "Transfers." Reconciling monthly statements may also be done electronically with a computerized version of the reconciliation form. Technical support is available with most online banking software 24 hours a day, 7 days a week. The software is updated and maintained periodically, however, and during that time online banking transactions cannot be processed.

In June 2000, federal legislation was signed that granted electronic signatures, or e-signatures, the same legal standing as printed signatures. An **e-signature** is a unique identifier, or "signature," created for each person through computer code. It is not a computer image of a person's handwritten signature. Verifying the identities of those doing business in cyberspace is still an issue to be resolved. Many medical providers and other businesses are becoming technologically equipped to use e-signatures for processing financial and other documents. This practice will continue to grow as the technology becomes more efficient and economical.

The practice may also authorize a payer to transfer funds electronically. That is, a third-party payer, such as the federal government or an insurance company, deposits payment to the practice electronically directly into the practice's account.

Petty Cash

A **petty cash fund** contains small amounts of cash (such as $40–$100) to be used for small expenses. These expenses are usually so small that checks would not be written to pay for them: cab fares, postage stamps, payments to messengers, and delivery charges.

Each time you make a payment from the petty cash fund, make an entry in the petty cash register or complete a voucher if this is the system used in your office. The register or voucher provides a record of these small expenses and ensures that only authorized payments are made from this fund. Receipts for expenditures from petty cash should be placed with the petty cash register/voucher.

To obtain money for the petty cash fund, the minor expenses for the month are estimated. A check for the estimated amount is drawn, payable to "Cash" or "Petty Cash." The check is endorsed and cashed in an assortment of small bills and change. The money is kept in a secure place, such as a locked metal cash box in a drawer.

At the end of the month or when the amount of cash has been depleted to a predetermined amount, such as $25, the fund is replenished. First, from the record in the petty cash register and receipts, determine the total amount of disbursements made. Count the remaining cash in the fund. Be sure the two amounts add up to the original amount of the check that was last cashed. This procedure is called "proving the petty cash fund." A new check is then drawn to bring the fund back to its original amount.

> **EXAMPLE**
>
> The original amount of the petty cash fund was $100. According to the petty cash register, expenses added up to $89.75. Thus, there should be $10.25 in cash and $89.75 in receipts remaining in the fund. Count the cash to verify that the correct amount remains. Draw a check for $89.75 to bring the amount of petty cash back to $100 once the check has been cashed.
>
> The petty cash expenditures should be recorded in the correct columns on the monthly summary sheet. They may be entered as petty cash.

8.4 PAYROLL

The total earnings of all the employees in the practice is called the **payroll**. Services, such as ADP (Automatic Data Processing, Inc., at adp.com) will process payroll for companies. However, if you are responsible for handling the payroll in your office, you will be completing the following tasks:

- Calculating the earnings of employees
- Subtracting the correct amounts of taxes and other **deductions**, or amounts of money withheld from earnings
- Creating employee payroll records
- Preparing salary checks
- Submitting payroll taxes
- Keeping current with IRS formulas and regulations that affect payroll; many tax tables and other information can be found on the IRS Web site (www.irs.gov)

Creating Employee Payroll Records

Because accurate records are required and because the process is complex, you will want to create a payroll information record for each person employed in the practice. For each employee, list the following information:

* Name, address, Social Security number, marital status, and number of dependents
* Pay schedule; show how often the employee is paid—weekly or biweekly, for example
* Type of payment; show whether the employee is paid a straight salary or an hourly wage
* Employee-requested deductions; an employee may have payments to an employer-sponsored insurance plan, a flexible healthcare spending account, contributions to a savings plan sponsored by the practice, or additional tax contributions withheld

If any employees are not citizens of the United States, they must be authorized to work in the United States. A completed Employment Eligibility Verification Form (Form I-9) must be filed with the federal government within three business days of the date when employment begins and a copy of the I-9 form, along with supporting identification documents, should be kept with the payroll records. This document verifies that the person is a legally admitted alien or a person authorized to work in this country.

Employer and Employee Identification Numbers

All employers, whatever the size of the business, are required to have a tax identification number. This **employer identification number (EIN)** enables the IRS to track the financial activity of employers in meeting payroll and tax obligations. An example of an EIN is 12-3456789. The nine-digit number is obtained by requesting Form SS-4 from the IRS. Employees are required to be identified by Social Security numbers.

Taxes Deducted From Earnings

Direct earnings are salaries (fixed amounts paid regardless of hours worked) or wages (pay based on an hourly or daily specific rate) paid to employees. **Indirect earnings** are paid leaves or specific employer-paid benefit programs.

When employees are first hired, they must complete the Employee's Withholding Allowance Certification (Form W-4), on which they state the number of allowances or exemptions to be used when the employer is calculating how much money to withhold from their salaries as deductions. Employers should verify annually that the information on file is still current. A new W-4 should be completed when major life changes (marriage, divorce, births, or deaths) occur. Name changes should be made only when the change is verified by a new Social Security card. The amounts to be withheld from an employee's salary for federal and state taxes are determined from wage-bracket tables supplied by the IRS. The amount withheld depends on the amount of money earned, the number of exemptions claimed, and the current tax rate. The IRS also supplies wage-bracket tables that apply to various payroll cycles: daily, weekly biweekly, semimonthly, and monthly. Refer to the state and local tax tables to determine the additional amounts of money to be withheld.

FICA Tax

The Federal Insurance Contributions Act, or **FICA**, governs the Social Security system. This law requires that a certain amount of money be withheld for Social Security. The employee pays half the required contribution, and the employer pays the other half. This amount is deducted in two separate payroll taxes: one helps finance Medicare, and the other helps fund Social Security pension benefits. These amounts, dictated by the IRS, are a percentage of the employee's taxable earnings, considering payroll periods and allowances claimed. Since Congress can change this amount yearly, you must obtain information from the IRS or from the physician's accountant.

Calculating Payroll

Spreadsheet programs perform these complex calculations very quickly. It is important for you to understand the formulas used and the process involved. Web sites such as www.adp.com offer the opportunity to use free online payroll calculators.

- *Gross earnings:* Calculate gross earnings. For an employee on salary, the salary amount for the period is the employee's gross earnings, regardless of whether or not the employee worked more than 35 or 40 hours. For an hourly wage worker, the hourly rate multiplied by the number of hours worked yields the employee's gross earnings.

- *Exemptions; state and local tax deductions:* Find the number of exemptions the employee claimed on Form W-4. Refer to the IRS tax table (Circular E) for the amount to be deducted, based on the gross earnings and the exemptions. State and local taxes are often at a set rate—for example, 5 percent of gross earnings. Subtract this amount from gross earnings.

- *FICA taxes:* Withhold, and deduct, half the amount due for the pay period from the employee's gross earnings. The other half is paid by the practice. There is one rate for the Social Security deduction and another for the Medicare deduction Verify the current withholding rate prior to calculating the amounts.

- *Unemployment taxes:* These taxes vary from state to state. Some states tax only employers. Withhold these taxes as necessary.

- *Voluntary deductions:* Deduct any amounts the employee has requested for insurance, a savings plan, additional tax withholding, and so on.

- *Employer's obligation:* Post the employer's FICA contribution and taxes due to federal and state unemployment funds to the physician's account.

- *Net earnings:* When total deductions are taken from gross earnings, the result is the employee's net earnings.

- *Net pay statement:* Prepare an itemized statement, either hardcopy or electronic, of gross pay, deductions, and net pay, and include it with the employee's pay.

Employers' Tax Responsibilities

Employers are required to help fund a Federal Unemployment Tax Act, or **FUTA**, account, which is used to help those who have been without work for a specified time as they seek new employment. This dollar amount is a percentage of each employee's gross earnings but is not to be deducted from the employee's earnings. Usually, payments into a state unemployment fund are applied as credit against the amount of FUTA tax.

Unemployment laws in most states require only the employer to contribute to the unemployment insurance fund. There are states that make an exception, and both employers and employees contribute. There are also some states where an employer does not contribute if the company has very few employees.

Employers' Deposit and Tax Return Obligations. The practice must make federal tax withholding payments and FICA payments to a federal deposit account in a Federal Reserve Bank or in some authorized bank. The money must be deposited at least monthly. The IRS imposes a severe penalty for the failure to make these deposits.

The employer is required to file a quarterly tax return, Form 941, to report federal income and FICA taxes withheld from employee paychecks.

Employees' W-2 Forms. Employees need payroll information from the previous year to file their taxes with the federal and state governments. Employers prepare a W-2, showing wages and deductions, for each employee who received earnings during the previous year. Employer identification information is also listed on the W-2.

INDIVIDUAL EMPLOYEE'S EARNINGS RECORD

Name: Molly Benson Social Security No.: 301-48-7122 Position: M.A. (part-time)
Address: 5985 West Park Ave. Marital Status: Single Monthly Rate:
City: Chicago, IL 60650 No. of Allowances: 1 Weekly Rate: $528
Telephone: 555-4251 Birthdate: 5/29/1968 Overtime Rate: $25/hour

Period Ending	Hours Worked	Gross Earnings Regular	Overtime	Total	FICA	Federal Withholding	State Withholding	City Withholding	Insurance	Other	Total	Net Pay	Accumulated Earnings (Gross)
6-13	24	528 00		528 00	40 40	63 19	15 84				119 43	408 57	12,672 00
6-20	24	528 00		528 00	40 40	63 19	15 84				119 43	408 57	13,200 00
6-27	24	528 00		528 00	40 40	63 19	15 84				119 43	408 57	13,728 00
7-4	24	528 00		528 00	40 40	63 19	15 84				119 43	408 57	14,256 00
7-11	24	528 00		528 00	40 40	63 19	15 84				119 43	408 57	14,784 00
7-18	24	528 00		528 00	40 40	63 19	15 84				119 43	408 57	15,312 00
7-25	24	528 00		528 00	40 40	63 19	15 84				119 43	408 57	15,840 00
8-8	24	528 00		528 00	40 40	63 19	15 84				119 43	408 57	16,368 00
8-15	24	528 00		528 00	40 40	63 19	15 84				119 43	408 57	16,896 00

Figure 8.9

Individual Employee's Earnings Record

Payroll Records: Contents and Retention

The practice is required by law to retain payroll data for four years. A typical format for this record is shown in Figure 8.9.

Each employee's earnings record must contain the employee's name, Social Security number, address, number of exemptions claimed, gross salary earned, net salary paid, income taxes withheld, and FICA, state, and local taxes deducted. The column labeled "Other" is used to record certain other deductions required by law or voluntary deductions made under an agreement with the employer. For example, many employers deduct, at the employee's request, amounts for savings bonds, insurance, or union dues. All amounts deducted by the employer are held in trust. The employer must remit the monies to the proper authority in a timely manner.

Electronic Payroll: Direct Deposit

Through direct deposit, the employee's net pay is automatically withdrawn from the practice's account and deposited into the employee's account. The physician must contract with the bank for this procedure, known as **EFT** (electronic funds transfer), and employees must give employers their account numbers (banking routing number and employee's account number). The employee receives a deposit stub showing the gross pay, net pay, and specific deductions. This aspect of electronic banking has many advantages for both employers and employees:

1. The loss or theft of paychecks is eliminated. When an employee is on vacation or absent, the check is deposited.
2. Productivity and cost-saving are increased. Time and expense are saved because no paychecks need to be written.
3. Employees have the convenience of eliminating a trip to the bank to deposit a paycheck, and the money is available on the day of deposit.

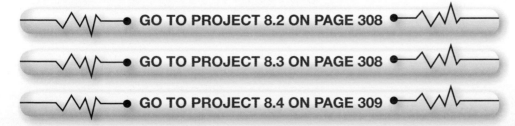

GO TO PROJECT 8.2 ON PAGE 308

GO TO PROJECT 8.3 ON PAGE 308

GO TO PROJECT 8.4 ON PAGE 309

Chapter Projects

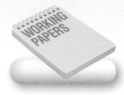

Optional Project 8.1 ## Updating Daily Journals

On October 23, you need to complete the daily journals started for October 20 (WP 46), October 21 (WP 47), and October 22 (WP 48).

Note that the patients have been listed for you. Use patient statements to obtain each previous balance. Post each day's transactions onto both the daily journal and the patient statement, computing the current balance. Information for charges has been obtained from each patient's encounter form or from payments received on account.

Total Columns A, B, C, D, and E. Complete the Proof of Posting, the Accounts Receivable Control, and Daily Cash sections. Post the daily ending accounts receivable balance onto the next daily journal.

Note that no deposits were yet made.

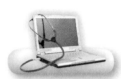

Project 8.2 ## Internet Research: Using the IRS as a Resource

Using a favorite search engine, key in "Internal Revenue Service." Go to the site for the IRS, and examine the information available. Look especially at the tax forms, the help for small businesses, and the section on payroll tax rules. Determine why this site is helpful to a medical practice. Write a "mini-paper" to be submitted to your instructor. Also be prepared to discuss with your peers the specific helpful information that you find.

Project 8.3 ## Updating Payments and Deposits

The following payments were received, in the form of checks, on October 24:

Joseph Castro	$44.00
Suzanne Roberts	$156.00
Gene Sinclair	$44.00

Enter and apply the payments. Print a walkout receipt for each patient who made a payment. Then complete a deposit slip (WP 50) for payments received October 20–24. In addition to the three checks received from Castro, Roberts, and Sinclair, a check for the Armstrong account in the amount of $48.20 was received on October 20. Cash payments in the amounts of $16.60 (October 20, Villano) and $8.80 (October 22, Mendez) were also received.

If the optional Project 8.1 was completed, then complete this portion of Project 8.3. Complete a daily journal (WP 49), and post transactions to patient statements. Complete a deposit slip (WP 50) for payments received October 20–24.

Project 8.4 Calculating an Employees' Payroll

Complete the following table by calculating the number of hours each employee worked during the payroll period. Then calculate the employee's gross wage by multiplying the number of hours worked in the payroll period by the employee's hourly wage. Round to the nearest cent.

Employee	M	T	W	TH	F	HOURS	Rate per Hour	Gross Pay
Connie Bradley	10	11	11	Off	10		12.00	
Dara Cecil	8	7	8	7	Off		12.00	
Misty Dark	Off	11	10	11	10		12.25	
Jennifer Eckel	5	Off	8	8	8		12.25	
Thomas Free	8	8	Off	7	6		12.50	
Anthony Gregson	Off	6	7	Off	8		13.50	
Tara Hughes	8	11	8	11	8		13.50	
Michael Ikard	9	9	9	9	9		15.25	
Leighanne Jones	7	8	Off	8	8		15.75	
Amanda Kat	11	8	11	10	9		14.25	

The following employees worked overtime hours. Using their rate per hour provided above, multiply that hourly rate by 1.5 and then multiply that amount by the employees' overtime hours. Round to the nearest cent.

Employee	Total Overtime Hours	Overtime Rate	Gross Earnings
Michael Ikard	5		
Misty Dark	2		
Connie Bradley	2		
Amanda Kat	9		
Tara Hughes	6		

8.1 Explain, using accounting terminology, the procedures for maintaining two essential financial records. Pages 292–296	<ul><li>Five accounting terms related to the assistant's responsibilities are<ul><li>*Accounts payable*—expense amounts owed to the supplier or creditors.</li><li>*Accounts receivable*—balance of payments due from patients or others on current accounts.</li><li>*Bookkeeping*—the part of accounting that is the accurate recording of transactions.</li><li>*Daily journal*—the record of services rendered, daily fees, charges, payments received, and adjustments.</li><li>*Audit*—an IRS review of all financial data to ensure the accuracy and completeness of the data.</li></ul></li><li>The procedures for maintaining two essential financial records (electronic or manual) are<ul><li>Daily journal:<ul><li>Daily record the fee charged.</li><li>Daily record the payments received.</li><li>Accurately maintain the Accounts Receivable Control section with the Record of Payments received from patients.</li><li>Daily balance the columns for Proof of Posting.</li><li>Accurately record the amount of cash received during the day in the Daily Cash section to account for cash flow.</li></ul></li><li>Monthly Summary:<ul><li>Accurately summarize the daily charges and payments on a monthly basis.</li></ul></li></ul></li></ul>
8.2 Summarize the main focus of the Red Flag Requirements as they relate to the medical office as a business. Pages 297–298	<ul><li>Medical practices must protect not only patients' protected health information under HIPAA but also patients' financial information under the Red Flag Requirements. Identity thieves have increasingly used criminal activities to gain medical services and benefits, such as insurance payments.</li><li>Medical practices must establish policies and procedures that enable them to form a reasonable belief that the individual requesting services is actually that person.</li></ul>

	• Policies and procedures should identify
	  — The primary and secondary types of identification required from patients.
	  — Account red flags.
	  — The courses of action to take when fraudulent activity is suspected.

8.3 List three banking duties of the assistant.
Pages 298–304
	• Three banking duties performed by the assistant are
	  — Accepting valid checks in payment for services rendered.
	  — Depositing cash, checks, and other forms of payment into the practice's account(s).
	  — Reconciling bank statements.

8.4 Explain how an employee's net salary is determined.
Pages 304–307
	• The assistant's duties related to the payroll process are as follows:
	  — Calculating gross earnings—determining the salary amount, or multiplying the number of hours worked by the hourly wage amount.
	  — Determining the proper exemptions, and state and local tax deductions—subtracting these from the gross earnings.
	  — Subtracting FICA tax—withholding half the specified amount from the employee's paycheck; the employer pays the other half.
	  — Subtracting voluntary deductions—if the employee has asked that amounts be withhold for insurance, savings, and so on, deducting these amounts.
	  — Subtracting the total deductions from the gross earning—the result is the employee's net salary.
	  — Posting the taxes that are the physician's obligation to the practice account.

Soft Skills Success

Integrity

As an administrative medical professional, it is your job to handle the payroll. You have worked with several of the employees for over five years, and you realize that a new hire is making more money hourly than the other employees in the same position. Somehow the employees have found out about this and they ask you if it is true. **How should you handle this situation?**

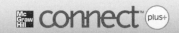
USING TERMINOLOGY

Match the term or phrase on the left with the correct answer on the right.

_____ 1. (LO 8.1) Procedure day sheet

_____ 2. (LO 8.1) Posting

_____ 3. (LO 8.3) Blank endorsement

_____ 4. (LO 8.4) Direct earnings

_____ 5. (LO 8.4) FICA

_____ 6. (LO 8.4) FUTA

_____ 7. (LO 8.1) Daily journal

_____ 8. (LO 8.3) Restrictive endorsement

_____ 9. (LO 8.2) Red Flag Requirements

_____ 10. (LO 8.1) Balance sheet

a. Record of provided services and their charges, payments received, and adjustments

b. Transferring accounts from one record to another

c. Period statement showing assets, liability, and capital

d. Numeric listing of all procedures and related information performed on a given day

e. Federal regulations requiring creditors to implement procedures to protect personal data pertaining to a covered account

f. Signature of the payee on the back of a check

g. States the payee and purpose of a check

h. Salaries/wages from an employer

i. Law requiring withholding from wages for Social Security

j. Law requiring employers to pay into an unemployment fund to be used by individuals unemployed for a specific amount of time but seeking new employment

CHECK YOUR UNDERSTANDING

Select the most correct answer.

1. (LO 8.1) Dr. Conna is considering purchasing her own EKG equipment to perform the procedure at the office instead of renting the equipment from a DME (durable medical equipment) distributor. She asked Evan (her administrative medical assistant) to give her the total number of EKGs performed and the revenue generated for the month of September. Which of the following reports should Evan reference for the information?

   a. Aging report

   b. Procedure day sheet

   c. Practice analysis report

   d. Income statement

2. (LO 8.1) To prepare for sending out patient statements for Dr. Conna's practice, Evan needs to know which accounts are more than 30 days past due. Which of the following reports should he reference for the information?

   a. Aging report
   b. Procedure day sheet
   c. Practice analysis report
   d. Income statement

3. (LO 8.2) Since Dr. Conna is a cardiologist, she performs many high-cost procedures, which require her patients to establish a monthly payment schedule. Her office extends credit in accordance with the Truth in Lending Act. Based on extending credit, the practice may be considered a

   a. FICA employer.
   b. FUTA employer.
   c. Red flag–covered account.
   d. Red flag creditor.

4. (LO 8.2) Evan has been asked by Dr. Conna to establish policies and procedures to protect patients from identity theft. Which of the following is an identity theft alert?

   a. A patient requests a change of address.
   b. A patient is billed for a service she did not receive.
   c. The name on a check is different from the patient's name.
   d. All of the above are identity theft alerts.

5. (LO 8.3) The monthly bank statement shows a balance of $5,060.13. Three checks in the amounts of $89.50, $310.92, and $25.00 are still outstanding. What is the actual available balance of the checking account?

   a. $5,485.55
   b. $5,060.13
   c. The available balance cannot be determined.
   d. $4,634.71

6. (LO 8.3) Using the same information from Question 5, calculate the monthly service charge of $10 into the actual available balance. What is the actual available balance after the service charge?

   a. $5,495.55
   b. $5,050.13
   c. The available balance still cannot be determined.
   d. $4,624.71

7. (LO 8.4) Evan's hourly wage is $18 and he works 7.5 hours per day, 5 days per week. Based on a tax withholding of 7.5 percent, how much should be withheld from his wages for taxes?

   a. $506.30
   b. $50.63
   c. $5.06
   d. $67.50

8. (LO 8.4) Using Evan's wage information from Question 7, if the state tax rate is 9 percent, what is his tax obligation?

   a. $6.08
   b. $607.50
   c. $60.75
   d. $61.00

THINKING IT THROUGH

These questions cover the most important points in this chapter. Using your critical-thinking skills, play the role of an administrative medical assistant as you answer each question. Be prepared to present your responses in class.

1. What are the major financial responsibilities that you have as an administrative medical assistant? What are the accounting terms used to describe these responsibilities?
2. You have been asked to help a colleague understand how to deal with the daily journal. How will you explain this?
3. Mr. Thompson is a patient whose insurance company has paid a portion of the fee for the physician's services; Mr. Thompson is responsible for the remaining amount. He is angry and determined to dispute the matter with the insurance company. For this reason, he has given you a postdated check for the amount owed to the doctor, $427.50. The check is dated three weeks from the current date. How will you handle this nonnegotiable check?
4. One of the staff members asks you to explain the difference between the terms *gross* and *net* on the paycheck. How do you respond?

SIMULATION 3

Today you will begin the third simulation in Dr. Larsen's office. The simulation dates are Monday, October 27; Tuesday, October 28; and Wednesday, October 29.

PROCEDURES

Review the section "Before You Start" in Simulation 1. Note that these procedures also apply to this simulation. Also review the "Procedures," because they apply to this simulation. Pull the patients' charts following the appointment calendar, and put them in the appropriate day folder.

MATERIALS

You will need the following materials to complete Simulation 3. If these materials are not already in the proper folder, obtain them from the sources indicated.

Materials	Source
Appointment calendar	
Diagnostic codes	WP 43
Fee schedule	WP 45
Supplies folder	

To-Do Items

Day 1 folder:

Place patients' charts for October 27.

Telephone log	WP 74
To-do list	WP 75
Patient encounter forms	WP 76–80
Checks received	WP 81
Daily journal #106	WP 82

Day 2 folder:

Place patients' charts for October 28.

Patient encounter forms	**WP 83–85**
Checks received	**WP 86**
Daily journal #107	**WP 87**

Day 3 folder:

Place patients' charts for October 29.

Patient encounter forms	**WP 88–93**
Checks received	**WP 94**
Daily journal #108	**WP 95**

Patients' folders:

The following items have been added to the patients' folders since the last simulation.

Patient statements for all current patients	(PROJECTS 8.1, 8.3)

Simulation 3

MEDICAL VOCABULARY

Before working through this simulation's assignments, review the following terms to be familiar with their spelling and meaning.

amoxicillin—antibiotic

ASCVD—arteriosclerotic cardiovascular disease

audiogram—graphic record of hearing results

Augmentin—anti-infective agent

cerumen—earwax

Cortisporin otic—ophthalmic anti-infective agent

costochondral—relating to costal cartilages

creatinine—lab test to diagnose impaired renal function

CVA—costovertebral angle

D&C—dilation (dilatation) and curettage

dentition—natural teeth

dorsalis pedis pulse—pulse in the foot

DTRs—deep tendon reflexes

dyspepsia—gastric indigestion

endocervical—within any cervix

fetor—offensive odor

gravida—number of pregnancies

hepatosplenomegaly—enlargement of liver and spleen

hyperlipidemia—abnormally large amount of lipids in blood

iliac—relating to ilium (broad portion of hip bone)

Lotrisone—antifungal

malaise—general discomfort or uneasiness

malar—relating to the cheek or cheekbone

malleolus—rounded bony prominence such as on side of ankle joint

menometrorrhagia—irregular or excessive bleeding during

menstruation and between menstrual periods

Midrin—antipyretic agent

osteoarthritis—degenerative joint disease

para—number of births

popliteal pulse—pulse behind the knee

retro-ocular—behind the eyeball

rhinorrhea—discharge from nose

RTC—return to clinic

scoliosis—lateral curvature of the spine

Septra DS—anti-infective agent

suboccipital—relating to below the back of head

thyromegaly—enlargement of thyroid gland

TIA—transient ischemic attack

TM—tympanic membrane

---

medisoft) MEDISOFT® INSTRUCTIONS

If your instructor has assigned the use of Medisoft®, you will complete certain parts of Simulation 3 using the software program. Follow these instructions:

To complete this simulation in Medisoft®, you must be able to:

- Schedule appointments
- Print a physician's schedule
- Enter charges
- Enter payments
- Print walkout receipts
- Print patient statements
- Print patient day sheets

Enter the new appointments in Office Hours. Then print Dr. Larsen's schedule for October 27, 28, and 29.

Enter all charge and payment transactions. Print walkout receipts for patients who made a payment.

Print patient statements for all patients who had transactions on October 27, 28, and 29.

Print patient day sheet reports for October 27, 28, and 29.

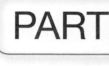

PART

Preparing for Employment

CHAPTER 9
Preparing for Employment in the Medical Office

Part 4 discusses the importance of preparation as the administrative medical assistant begins and progresses through the path to a medical career. Presented are steps and strategies to make the career search as successful as possible.

CONSIDER THIS: Self-analysis can help the administrative medical assistant match skills and attributes to a career choice. *What are your top five skills and personal attributes and how can they be used in a medical environment?*

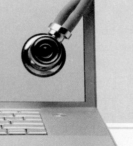

Preparing for Employment in the Medical Office

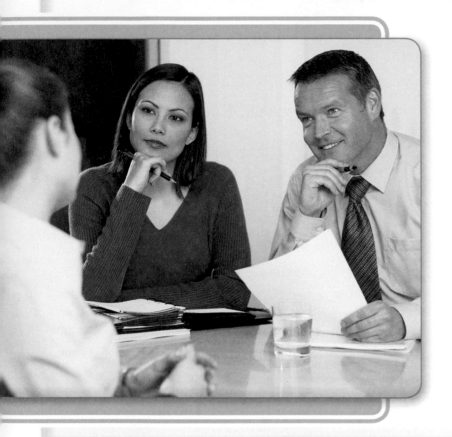

LEARNING OUTCOMES

After studying this chapter, you will be able to:

9.1 List and explore visible and hidden career-employment resources.

9.2 Assimilate information and prepare an employment application.

9.3 Compose a cover/application letter.

9.4 Assimilate data and compose résumés using different format styles.

9.5 Assemble personal and professional information and appropriate dress for the interview process and conduct a mock interview.

9.6 Compose a follow-up thank-you letter.

KEY TERMS

Study these important words, which are defined in this chapter, to build your professional vocabulary:

chronological résumé	hidden job markets	plain-text résumé	scannable résumé
cover letter	keywords	power words	visible job markets
functional résumé	personal reference	professional reference	

Chapter 9

ABHES

- Adapt to change.
- Project a positive attitude.
- Use proper telephone technique.
- Apply electronic technology.
- Be courteous and diplomatic.
- Fundamental writing skills.

CAAHEP

➡ Recognize elements of fundamental writing skills.
➡ List and discuss legal and illegal interview questions.
➡ Demonstrate awareness of how an individual's personal appearance affects anticipated responses.
➡ Analyze communications in providing appropriate responses/feedback.
➡ Compose professional/business letters.
➡ Apply active listening skills.

➡ Cognitive
➡ Psychomotor
➡ Affective

INTRODUCTION

Just a short time ago, employment opportunities were mostly confined to a local, state, or national job market. Many employees worked at and retired from first jobs with very little mobility. Times have changed and so have opportunities for employment. The workforce is very fluid and the Internet presents a global market.

Whether the job search is local or international, one key to being successful is being prepared. It begins with evaluating your skills and goals and matching them to various career opportunities. The search continues through exploring sources of career opportunities, composing a professional cover letter and accurately completing an application, preparing a résumé (or more than one), interviewing for a position, and conducting follow-up techniques.

Your Skills and Goals

As you begin your search for employment, first evaluate your skills (personal and professional) and your overall goal. Make a list of your personal traits and professional skills. Many individuals are not content in their current position for various reasons, one of which may be that their personal and professional skills are mismatched with their current job requirements. Following are some questions to ask yourself as you begin your list:

- Am I skilled in public communications?
- Do I enjoy searching for answers or solving problems (do I work puzzles/word searches, etc.)?
- Am I more productive working on my own or as a member of a team?
- Do I organize my personal and professional lives?
- Have I held or do I hold positions of leadership, such as club officer?
- What are my technical skills?
- Do I pursue above and beyond what is required of me?

As you begin to evaluate yourself through these and other questions, match your answers to general job requirements or environments. For example, someone who enjoys and is proficient at solving word searches may be suited to finding errors in submitted insurance claim forms and submitting corrected claims to carriers. An individual who frequently holds an office, such as president or treasurer, within an organization may not be content in a professional position that does not provide an opportunity to grow professionally and assume more responsibility. Listing and objectively evaluating personal and professional skills is the first step in seeking employment.

Sources of Employment Opportunities

After your have compiled an evaluation of your skills and traits, the next step is to begin searching for employment opportunities. Some sources are more visible and traditional, while others fall within the hidden job market of opportunities. At times, employers want a large number of responses for available positions; however, some position vacancies are complicated by a vast number of applicants. Traditional job markets, or **visible job markets** (job markets composed of resources that are traditional and the most obvious), produce a greater number of responses to positions, while nontraditional job markets, or **hidden job markets** (job markets that are less obvious and require more initiative by the job seekers to access) are more confined.

Visible Resources. Many resources are available to job seekers through easily accessible venues. Following is a sampling of some visible job markets:

- *Classified ads in national and local newspapers.* Ads may include desired information, such as the name and address of the organization, but many do not include specific data other than the position requirements. Résumés are frequently sent to a P.O. box and no company or individual name is listed. Most newspaper classified ads can also be found on the newspaper's Web page.
- *Professional publications.* Journals published by professional organizations contain position opportunities. Student memberships are available through most professional organizations, usually at a discounted rate. National organizations typically have local chapters, which can supply information about local career opportunities.
- *Career/job fairs.* Most schools will host an event that brings together prospective employers and employees. Local communities may also host a career fair. When attending a fair,

an applicant should be professionally dressed, have an application/cover letter (discussed later in this chapter), and résumés in various formats (also discussed later in this chapter).

- *Job boards.* Schools and businesses post available positions on accessible traditional and/or electronic bulletin boards. For businesses, positions may first be posted to provide currently employed individuals the opportunity to apply first (known as in-house posting). Beginning and ending dates are listed on the vacancy notice. For example, a volunteer within a medical facility will know when positions have been internally posted and the when external applicants may apply for the position. School career centers and/or placement offices also post the available positions that have been sent to them.

- *Internet.* Doing a topic search for job listings will produce a vast number of results. Several online employment services are available, such as www.Monster.com. Some sites collect résumés, which they forward to employers, while some sites list complete position information, including the employer. One advantage of using Internet employment Web sites is the number of choices they provide. However, corporations listed on these sites may receive a great number of résumés per day. Résumés that are not prepared in a computer-friendly format (discussed later in this chapter) may not convey the intended information, and therefore may not be reviewed.

- *Temporary employment agencies.* You can get short-term exposure to various positions through local temporary job services. Job seekers who have little or no experience may find it beneficial to use these services to gain documentable experience. There may be a fee for the services. The temporary position may change to a permanent opportunity; however, the goal of a temporary employment agency is to provide short-term coverage of job responsibilities.

- *Employment services.* Companies may fill positions through local and governmental employment services. Companies that have a vacancy contact the employment service and ask to review the files of individuals who meet the job requirements. Those selected are interviewed by the service or by the company. Individuals should keep the file with the employment service up to date. Privately owned employment services may charge a fee for their services.

This list is not inclusive of all career resources but gives job seekers some avenues to pursue for employment.

Hidden Resources. Many times, less obvious job markets are overlooked and opportunities are lost. Job seekers must have the initiative to seek out these markets and opportunities. Following are examples of hidden markets:

- *Face-to-face networking.* Everyone has a network of individuals, which frequently is overlooked in the job-seeking process. People in your network can provide up-to-date information on industry trends and changes, as well as current and upcoming vacancies. Teachers and classmates typically have the same or similar interests and goals. Relatives and friends, fellow club or organization members, and acquaintances from the community frequently know about upcoming vacancies before the positions are posted. If someone with whom you work is leaving, an opportunity could be provided for you to apply for the vacancy. A network also includes people from sporting events, health clubs and workout classes, physicians' offices—the list continues to include many, varied places where other individuals can be encountered.

- *Electronic networks.* These kinds of networks also are a vast source of employment opportunities However, you should be careful of seeking information electronically if you are currently employed and have not submitted a letter of resignation. Also, refrain from posting negative comments about your current employment and colleagues. Electronic information, once posted, spreads quickly.

Figure 9.1

Practicing Networking
Skills

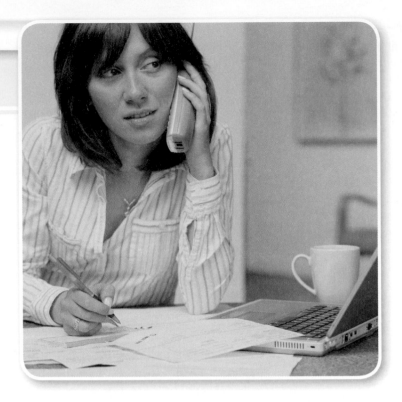

- *Telephone directories.* Yellow pages, traditional or electronic, are a valuable source of employers in a specific area. It is easy to locate all the physicians in a given specialty by using yellow pages.
- *Chamber of Commerce.* The Chamber of Commerce in your area can provide a list of local businesses and organizations.
- *Direct contact with companies.* Information about available positions can be obtained from personally visiting a business. Keep in mind, however, that this is a "fact-gathering" visit. From the visit, a position-related cover/application letter and résumé can be prepared. An applicant should take a generic application letter and résumé, in case there is an opportunity to speak with a manager. A clean, neat, professional appearance will make a favorable impression.

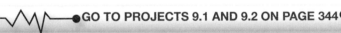

GO TO PROJECTS 9.1 AND 9.2 ON PAGE 344

9.2 COMPLETING AN ONLINE AND A TRADITIONAL APPLICATION

It is common for prospective employers to ask candidates to fill out an application prior to interviewing. Information requested on an application frequently is more complete than information provided on a résumé. A complete educational and work history, such as exact dates of employment, complete company addresses, supervisors' names and contact information, and salary or wage amounts, is commonly requested. This information is typically summarized on a résumé. Applications serve as a snapshot of the applicant, which helps employers choose interview candidates. Additionally, applicants must attest to the completeness and truthfulness of the presented application data by signing a statement of authenticity on the application. Individuals have been hired for a position and later fired because they provided false information on an application and/or a résumé.

Online applications are an effective and efficient method of submitting data. An advantage of submitting electronically is the opportunity to correct data. When preparing an application traditionally, applicants must either key the information in on a computer or fill it in by hand. If a computer is used to fill out an application and print it, errors can be easily corrected; however, applications prepared by hand require more effort to submit correctly. Correction fluid may be used to correct the occasional error on a handwritten application, but unless the applicant is skilled with using correction fluid, the correction will be obvious. It is best to redo the application. For this reason, when an applicant knows the application will be prepared by hand, additional copies of the application should be available. Blue or black ink should be used to complete an application. Be sure to look for specific instructions on the application concerning ink color. Data on a handwritten application should be printed and neat.

Whether the application is filed electronically or traditionally, several tips apply:

- Determine the information you will be need and have it accessible. Samples of information include the following:
  — *Personal information*: In addition to complete name and address, an applicant's Social Security number may be requested, but date of birth is not. Daytime and evening telephone numbers and cell phone number are requested.
  — *Name of position desired*: State the name of the position or positions to which the application applies; whether full-time, part-time, seasonal, or shift work is desired; the date you are available to begin work; and the desired salary. So that you do not eliminate yourself from possible employment because of a stated salary requirement, it is best to answer "Open" or "Negotiable" to the desired salary. While it is easiest to state "Open" or "Negotiable," you should research similar positions in the geographic region and have an idea of the salary requirements, to help you avoid under- or overpricing yourself for the available position. However, if you require a certain amount and will consider nothing less, then state your desired amount.
  — *Work history information*: Your work history is your employers' names and complete addresses, your supervisors' names and contact information, your dates of employment, beginning and ending salary or wage information, your responsibilities, your titles, and your reasons for leaving (if separated from employment). If you were fired or laid off, it is best not to place blame when stating the reason for leaving. Statements such as "My professional goal became different from the company's goal" or "The organization went through realignment" show a positive attitude.

    Address any gaps in your work history. Individuals have a variety of reasons for not being in the workforce. Reasons should be very brief statements, such as attending school, caring for aging parents, and the like. Be prepared to address reasons for frequent changes in jobs. Reasons such as seasonal work or temporary positions should be listed. If you have more work history than there is room for on the application, the short statement "Additional work experience is available upon request" may be used on the application. Most applications ask for work experience in reverse chronological order.
  — *Criminal history*: Honesty is the best policy. State the facts—what happened and how you have changed from the experience.
  — *Military history*: Be prepared to record dates and ranks.
  — *Education*: Have available postsecondary education information. Applications usually ask for the names and addresses of institutions, dates attended, degrees/credentials earned, hours completed, and grade point average (GPA) or ranking in class. Some employers also request high school information, including the name and

address of the high school, diploma or GED, and class ranking or GPA. Any specialized training, awards, or honors may also be requested.

— *References:* Stating "References are available upon request" is not a best practice for completing an application. A minimum of three references are typically requested. After asking permission, list three (or the requested number) individuals who know your work ethic, skills, and personal aptitudes. Relatives or clergy should not be listed as references. Fellow workers and committee members with whom you have served are good candidates for references. Sometimes an applicant has been out of the workforce, training for a new career. In this case, a fellow long-term classmate or an instructor may be used as a reference. Whomever you use, be sure of what they will say! Provide each person's name, title, address, and phone number. State how long you and the reference have known each other, as well as any company information for professional references.

- Spell every word correctly and use proper grammar.
- Fill in every question. If the question does not apply, then mark "Not Applicable" or "N/A" in the blank.
- Follow all directions on the application.
- Use only positive wording. Also, use wording on the application which reflects desired requirements of the position, such as Web design training and electronic health records experience. This is discussed in more detail later in the chapter.
- Describe your skills using action verbs and concrete nouns. Consider using "keys at 70 words per minute with no errors" instead of "good keyboarding skills" or "interpersonal verbal and communication skills" instead of "good with people."
- Refrain from using acronyms. Spell them out completely.
- Sign and date the application.

Continue the same style of wording when preparing all employment documents—applications, cover letters, résumés, and follow-up letters.

9.3 PREPARING A COVER/APPLICATION LETTER

The purpose of a **cover letter** is to personalize the application process by introducing the applicant to the employer and to gain an interview. It is also referred to as an application letter. The letter places a name and snapshot of relevant information in front of the reader and should entice the prospective employer to schedule an interview. An application may or may not accompany the cover letter.

Prior to writing a cover/application letter, do research to gather data about the company and the position(s). Learn specific job requirements and try to locate the name of the person to whom you will address your letter. The more your know about a company, the better prepared you will be to write a cover/application letter and to link your skills or traits to specific position requirements. Information can be obtained through the Internet, local business chambers of commerce, libraries, and newspapers, as well as the human resources departments of organizations. If it is a small company and the position has been advertised, information can be obtained through an office manager. However, if the position has not yet been advertised, obtain information and submit an application on the first day that applications are being accepted.

Although there are variations of cover/application letters, correct format, grammar, spelling, and punctuation are essential. The format style should be consistent in the cover/application letter, résumé, and follow-up letter. Left-justified letters and résumés are standard. However, modified-block letter style may also be used with a modified-block-style résumé and follow-up letter. When preparing the three employment documents, print them on the same color of high-quality paper. Bright colors (pink, purple, orange) should not be used. Neutral pastel colors, such as beige, wheat, or gray, are easier to read.

The parts of a cover/application letter are the letterhead or return address, inside address, salutation, typical three-paragraph body, and closing.

- *Letterhead or return address:* Many cover/application letters contain personally created letterheads with the applicant's name, address, phone number, and e-mail address. The format should be professional and not distract from the body of the letter. E-mail addresses should always be professional and not offensive. For example, the e-mail address hotmom@hotmail.com or ivoryqueen@gmail.com should not be used as contact information.

- *Date:* If the date that you composed the letter is different from the date that you are sending it, use the date you send the letter.

- *Inside address:* This is the name and address of the organization to which you are applying. Through prior research, you should know the name of the person to whom you will address the cover/application letter.

- *Salutation:* Correctly spell the name of the individual and use *Mr., Mrs., Ms., Dr.,* and so on with the name. Since this is a professional business letter, a colon (:) should follow the salutation. It is not professionally appropriate to use "To Whom It May Concern:" or "Dear Human Resources:". This sets a negative tone—one of not caring enough to find out the receiver's name. Sometimes, after extensively researching but not finding a name, the writer may use "Dear Members of the Search Committee:" or address the letter to the manager of a specific department, such as "Dear Coding Department Manager:".

- *Three-paragraph body:* Extensive work experience or education may necessitate a four-paragraph format, although it is usually possible to use concise wording and maintain a three-paragraph format. Prepare the body of the letter in the "you" approach and refrain from the "I" approach. In other words, state how the organization will benefit from your skills and traits.

  - Paragraph one is the most important position of the letter. The opening sentence should be professional yet grab the reader's attention. State the position for which you are applying and how, where, and when you learned of the position; also, refer to the position title and how your qualifications match those of the position. Also state if someone has referred you for the position.

    - Ineffective example:"I heard about your administrative medical assistant position and would like to apply for the job." This example is missing how, where, and when the applicant learned of the position and is written in the "I" approach.

    - Instead use "Your advertisement in the October 23, 2011, *Washington Central Post* seeks an administrative medical assistant, and the 11 years that I have worked in a progressive medical environment will be an asset to your established office. Please consider this letter as application for your administrative medical assistant position."

  - Use paragraph two to sell your skills and qualities to the employer. Three main topics are addressed: work experience/traits/skills, education, and résumé. Each of the topics should be related to the job requirements, placing first the category that most closely relates to the position. Use concrete nouns and action verbs to create a specific verbal portrait.

    - Ineffective example:"I am creative and able to multi-task." The example uses the "I" approach and soft-skills wording.

    - Instead use "During a rapid patient-growth period, I redesigned limited office space to maximize office work flow. This was accomplished while also implementing a new electronic health records system."

    - Avoid repeating information that will be contained in the résumé.

Compare the following two second-paragraph examples for their overall effectiveness.

EXAMPLE ONE (INEFFECTIVE)

"I have had 11 years of medical office experience, where I was able to work with people, function as a team member, and learn new duties. I received an associate degree in office systems with an emphasis in medical coding and billing. My résumé is enclosed."

EXAMPLE TWO (EFFECTIVE)

"Serving as a liaison between patients and insurance carriers enabled me to enhance my analytical and problem-solving skills. The result was an overall yearly increase in collectible accounts of 43%. During a five-year period, my democratic leadership style led the office team in developing requirements for and implementing an electronic health records system. Computer technology, medical office, and coding skills acquired through my associate degree training have and will continue to be an asset in technological environments, such as Anywhere Medical Center. You may further review relevant work experience and education on the enclosed résumé."

— Paragraph three is the "action" paragraph. The primary focus of paragraph three is a polite request for an interview. Provide contact times and phone numbers through which the employer may contact you. If the greeting on your contact phone is not professional, change it to a more appropriate greeting. A statement of appreciative anticipation of the next step or of further discussion about the position can be added to the third paragraph. Following is an example of a correctly worded third paragraph.

- "Putting my skills to work in a highly reputable medical office such as yours is an opportunity that I have been seeking. May I discuss my qualifications with you further during an interview? Please use the phone number in the letterhead to contact me Monday through Saturday prior to 10 P.M. to schedule a time for us to meet."

Closing: Many acceptable closings may be used in a cover/application letter, including "Yours sincerely," "Sincerely," and "Respectfully." Follow the closing with a comma and leave room for the signature. How much room is left depends on the software being used. No less than three spaces should be left. If the letter is being submitted electronically, attach the electronic signature to the letter. Be sure to include the "Enclosure" notation under the name for the enclosed résumé. The following is an example of a proper closing.

Sincerely,

Nenna Bayes

Enclosure

Figure 9.2 provides an example of a cover/application letter of an applicant who is applying for the position of medical insurance specialist in an orthopedic surgeon's office.

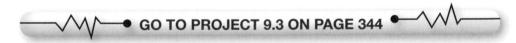

GO TO PROJECT 9.3 ON PAGE 344

9.4   PREPARING RÉSUMÉS

Investing time and energy into preparing a professional résumé pertinent to your career goal(s) is time and energy well spent. The primary goal of a résumé is not to obtain a position but to gain an interview with the employer and to convey what you can do for

Figure 9.2

Cover/Application Letter

```
1234 Any Street
Somewhere, US 12345-5555
October 23, 2012

Dr. Mike Doe
5555 St. Christopher's Street
Somewhere, US 12345-5555

Dear Dr. Doe:

During our October monthly medical coders' meeting, Nancy Smith re-
ferred me to your office vacancy for a medical insurance specialist.
After discussing the position requirements with Nancy, I am confident
that the skills and experience I possess would match those required in
the position, and I am, therefore, applying for the position of medical
insurance specialist.

Your position requires a certified coder. Since graduating from
Anywhere Community and Technical College with an associate degree in
health information technology, I have attained two national credentials
(Certified Professional Coder [CPC] and Chart Auditing) and have worked
with local physicians to implement policies and procedures that pro-
actively detect auditing errors. This has resulted in fewer rejected
claims and increased revenue. During the same 10-year period, I worked
with the medical office team to develop patient satisfaction surveys,
analyze results, and incorporate changes into the office environment.
The enclosed résumé lists further work and educational achievement.

During an interview we can further discuss how to put these and other
qualifications to work for your orthopedic practice. Please contact me
at (555) 555-5555 or at nennabayes@anyspace.com Monday through Saturday
prior to 9 P.M. to arrange a time for an interview.

Sincerely,


Nenna Bayes

Enclosure
```

the employer. Employers may have numerous résumés to review and only a few seconds to spend on each one. Résumés should be brief, easy to read and/or scan for relevant information, and well written. Just one typographical or grammatical error could land the résumé in "File 13"—the trash can. Investing time to learn about the company and available position and developing a résumé are the first steps to passing through the initial sorting process.

Various formats, which will be discussed later in this section, are used to present résumé data. Whichever format is chosen, there are basic do's and don'ts for résumé preparation.

Do

- Use **power words**/action verbs to showcase skills—"increased accounts receivable revenue by 23 percent in a six-month period." Power words are verbs that emphasize actions within a job position and should follow bullets (use professional bullets, not cute bullets) within the résumé—for example,
  - Billed and collected $15,000 from previously uncollectible accounts receivable"
  - Developed history and physical and other patient documentation forms for newly implemented electronic health records system
- Use correct tense. For activities that are still being performed, use present tense. For completed activities, use past tense.

- List military service, collegiate sports, leadership roles, and volunteer work. Military candidates are often viewed as responsible and reliable, with very good work ethics. Involvement in collegiate sports demonstrates teamwork and willingness to follow instructions. The ability to assume responsibility is evident through leadership positions and volunteer projects.
- Supply complete employment information, including company names, company locations (addresses, including phone numbers), and dates.
- Maintain a consistent, uncluttered format.
- Use left-justification, not right-justification.
- Use high-quality paper. If you prepare a cover/application letter, use the same high-quality paper for both the letter and the résumé.
- Prepare different résumés tailored to various career opportunities; rearrange bulleted items to fit the available position's requirements and skills. Have a traditional résumé even if you also have a scannable/electronic résumé.
- Include professional recognitions and awards; educational honors and a grade point average of 3.0 or higher may be listed.
- Limit the use of bold and other functional fonts to highlight data and a font size no larger than 13.
- Confine résumé data, if possible, to one page—use no more than two pages. Administrative positions, such as office manager, may require more pages.
- Ask a qualified individual to proofread the résumé for format, grammar, and content.
- Review social network sites for any comments, postings, photographs, statuses, and so on that may reflect badly on your image. What may have seemed funny at the time may suggest a lack of good judgment or immaturity to a prospective employer.

Don't

- Don't handwrite a résumé!
- Don't use complete sentences or add unnecessary wording. This is referred to as "fluff."
- Don't go back too far for work experience. The rule of thumb is approximately 10 years unless the last position is the only position listed.
- Don't lie about or overstate résumé data. This can lead to dismissal.
- Don't provide personal information such as age (including birth year), marital status, race, religion, marital status, physical data (weight/height, etc.), family, sexual orientation, or Social Security number.
- Don't break up words with hyphens. Hard return and move the complete word to the next line.
- Don't use first-person pronouns.
- Don't use a work e-mail or professionally distasteful e-mail address, such as singlegal@yahoo.com or loserboy@hotmail.com.
- Don't list numerous classes on the résumé—have a transcript available, if applicable.
- Don't list references but prepare a list in case an employer requests one.
- Don't list salary data on the résumé.
- Don't supply reasons for leaving previous positions but be prepared to discuss these issues. Also, be prepared to discuss gaps in employment history.

Résumé Formats

After investing time in researching the company and available career opportunities, the next step is to match your employment, education, and other relevant history to the position requirements. Compile the information and decide which résumé format is best suited to display the information. Basically, there are two categories—chronological and functional. A third format option is a scannable/electronic résumé, which is prepared in either chronological or functional format (or a combination of both) and formatted for optical character reading (OCR). The most widely used file format for submitting resumes over the Internet is the plain-text format.

Chronological Format. The traditional and most common résumé style is the **chronological résumé**. One advantage of this style is that employers can quickly view educational and employment-related information. However, gaps in these areas are also evident. Another advantage of this format is that it is relatively easy to compose. The following sections are included in a chronological format: a heading, a career objective, a summary of qualifications (a recent addition to résumé formats), education, work history, and optional components.

- *Heading:* This section contains identifying and contact information. State your name, address, phone numbers, and e-mail address. List your complete name, including your middle initial. Use a slightly larger font for the name. An address should include the street address, P.O. Box number, city, state, and zip code. List the phone number(s) to be used when more information is needed or to arrange for an interview. Include area codes with the phone number. As stated previously, e-mail addresses should be professional and not distasteful. Do not include a work e-mail on the résumé.

- *Career objective:* Opinions are divided as to whether a career objective should be included. If you choose to include a career objective, it should be specific to the position and written from the employer's perspective. A concisely written objective should be limited to no more than three lines. Consider the following examples.
  - Instead of "To obtain an administrative medical assistant position in a progressive medical office where I can use my training and skills"
  - Consider "Seeking an administrative medical assistant position where my training in medical front office and clinical skills can contribute to the efficient team dynamics of patient care"

- Summary of qualifications: As with the career objective, this is also an optional section. However, the inclusion of a well-written summary of qualifications can entice the employer to read further. Evaluate your experience (work, education, awards, accomplishments, technical and soft skills, etc.) and write a summary that targets the position's qualifications. A rule of thumb is to limit the number of bulleted items to five or six. **Keywords**, words used throughout the résumé that directly relate to the position's requirements, should be used in this section. If a position requirement is "use of Medisoft® software," consider using "Trained using Medisoft® software" instead of "medical office software training." Keywords are especially important when résumés will be scanned.

- *Education:* List your education in reverse chronological order (the most current first)—for many, this is collegiate information. List the school name and complete address as well as your major and minor. Grade point averages (GPAs) may be listed if they are at least 3.0 or higher. Academic awards and recognitions may be listed in this section or in a separate, later section. Only list classes that directly relate to the position, and the list should be concise. A transcript of classes should be made available for review. If college information is listed, it is not necessary to include high school information. If no college information is listed, supply the same data for high school education. If you obtained a GED, list the date on the GED.

- *Work history:* List employment in reverse chronological order. If work experience is most relevant to the available position, place it before the education section. List work experience and/or transfer skills, such as electronic health records experience, that demonstrate qualification for the position. For each position, list (1) employer's name and complete address; (2) dates of employment; (3) your most significant job title; and

(4) significant duties, accomplishments, and promotions. An employment application may require complete work history, but a résumé can be selective. If selective employment is listed, be prepared to explain the gaps in employment. A statement such as "Other employment experience is available upon request" may be added to the bottom portion of this section. If this statement is added, have the additional listing prepared using the same format and style as the résumé. Use power words and action verbs to describe job responsibilities. Do not list every responsibility, only those that relate to the position you are seeking. Avoid using personal pronouns and complete sentences.

- *Optional components:* Special skills and capabilities, community service, professional affiliations and/or activities, military service, awards/honors/achievements, and references are examples of optional sections within a chronological résumé. Employers seek individuals who not only are qualified for the position but also demonstrate a sense of community interest and self-enhancement. Opinions are divided on whether or not to include the notation "References available upon request." Whether you place such a notation on the résumé or not, a reference page should be prepared and available for the employer. Prior to placing anyone on a reference list, always ask that person's permission, and be sure the individual will give a positive recommendation. List three to five references on a separate sheet prepared in the same format and on the same high-quality paper as the résumé. Most, if not all, of the references should be **professional references**, individuals who know your work skills. If necessary, a **personal reference**, someone who knows your ethics, honesty, and trustworthiness may be used. For each reference, include

  — The reference's name, with a courtesy title, such as Mr., Mrs., or Ms. (many names can be either male or female).
  — The reference's position title, if applicable.
  — The name and complete address of the company.
  — The reference's phone number(s) with area code(s).
  — The reference's e-mail address, if given to you by the reference.

Figure 9.3 provides a sample of a chronological résumé, and Figure 9.4 shows a reference list.

Functional Format. **Functional résumés** organize skills and accomplishments into data groups that directly support the position goal, such as management, patient care, or software implementation. Being able to group skills together is one advantage of a functional résumé; however, it takes a little more thought and time to compose this style of résumé. It can best serve individuals who are changing fields and/or have gaps in their employment history. The typical organization of a functional résumé includes the following sections:

- Heading
- Summary of qualifications/skills (optional)
- Skills heading (use bulleted skills)
- Work experience with contact information; since skills will be listed in the previous section, only list the company name, dates of employment, and title
- Education—if education is most relevant to the position, list it prior to the work experience or skills section
- Optional sections

Figure 9.5 shows an example of a functional résumé. The same information was used to prepare both the chronological résumé (Figure 9.3) and the functional résumé samples. Notice the different placement of the information, such as the education section, in each résumé.

Figure 9.3

Chronological Résumé

NENNA L. BAYES

1234 Any Street
Somewhere, US 12345-5555

Cell Phone: 555-555-5555
E-mail: nennabayes@anyspace.com

OBJECTIVE

A position in a medical facility in which medical billing and coding experience can be used to sustain and increase revenue from accounts receivable and increase positive patient satisfaction

SUMMARY OF QUALIFICATIONS

- Nationally certified professional coder (CPC)
- Nationally certified chart auditor
- Developed, implemented, and analyzed patient satisfaction policies and procedures
- Implemented revenue-collection strategies that increased revenue by 23 percent in a six-month period

EDUCATION

2008–Present, Pursuing Bachelor of Science in Health Information Technology, Anywhere University, Somewhere, US 12345-5555

- Anticipated graduation date of 2012
- Presidential Scholarship for Academic Achievement
- 112 of 128 hours completed

1998–2000, Associate of Applied Science degree awarded May 2000, Anywhere Community and Technology College, Somewhere, US 12345-5555

- National Collegiate Honor Society
- GPA 3.98 on a 4.0 scale

Technical skills include

- Microsoft Office Suite 2003 and 2007 Certification (Word, Excel, Access, Outlook, and PowerPoint)
- Proficient in medical office software (Medisoft®)
- Input technology—Keyboarding skills of 85 corrected words per minute, voice-recognition software, and various scanning devices
- Records and database management

EXPERIENCE

May 2000–Present

- MEDICAL INSURANCE SPECIALIST AND ADMINISTRATIVE COORDINATOR FOR PHYSICIANS' CENTER OF SOMEWHERE, 8888 CENTER STREET, SOMEWHERE, US 12345-5555
  - Created and implemented revenue-intensive procedures that reduced uncollectible debt by 23 percent
  - Conducted certified continuing education workshops for physicians and staff
  - Streamlined staff workload to increase staff and patient satisfaction
  - Annually and quarterly updated all coding reference and source materials

COMMUNITY SERVICE

- Chairperson for SkillsUSA
- Organized Zumba Community Fitness Fair
- Conducted update training for Somewhere area medical coders
- Volunteer for Humane Society

PROFESSIONAL AFFILIATION

- American Academy of Professional Coders
- American Federation of Office Administrators

Figure 9.4

Reference Page

NENNA L. BAYES

1234 Any Street
Somewhere, US 12345-5555

Cell Phone: 555-555-5555
E-mail: nennabayes@anyspace.com

PROFESSIONAL REFERENCES

- Mr. Mark Someone, Office Manager
  Physician's Center of Somewhere
  8888 Center Street
  Somewhere, US 12345-5555
  555-555-5555
  e-mail—marksomeone@pcos.com

- Ms. Susie Sunshine, Medical Assistant
  Physician's Center of Somewhere
  8888 Center Street
  Somewhere, US 12345-5555
  555-555-5555
  e-mail—susiesunshine@pcos.com

- Mr. Allan Anyone, Regional President
  AAPC Organization
  9999 Local Avenue
  My Town, US 55555-4444
  444-444-4444
  e-mail—anyone@aapcky.org

- Mrs. Annie Okley, Vice Chair
  Medical Assistants Foundation
  7777 National Boulevard
  Professionals, US 44444-3333
  333-333-3333
  e-mail—aokley@maf.edu

Figure 9.5

Functional Résumé

NENNA L. BAYES

1234 Any Street
Somewhere, US 12345-5555

Cell Phone: 555-555-5555
E-mail: nennabayes@anyspace.com

OBJECTIVE

A position in a medical facility in which medical billing and coding experience can be used to sustain and increase revenue from accounts receivable and increase positive patient satisfaction

SUMMARY OF QUALIFICATIONS

- Nationally certified professional coder (CPC)
- Nationally certified chart auditor
- Developed, implemented, and analyzed patient satisfaction policies and procedures
- Implemented revenue-collection strategies that increased revenue by 23 percent in a six-month period

Figure 9.5

continued

NENNA L. BAYES   **Page 2**

ACHIEVEMENTS
- Billing and Coding Skills
  - Created and implemented revenue-intensive procedures that reduced uncollectible debt by 23 percent
  - Conducted certified continuing education workshops for physicians and staff
  - Streamlined staff workload to increase staff and patient satisfaction
  - Annually and quarterly updated all coding reference and source materials

- Administrative Skills
  - Supervised nine employees within the medical billing and coding department
  - Resolved patient complaints by taking direct, proactive action and conducted follow-up to resolution
  - Established work team and developed patient satisfaction survey—used results to implement patient satisfaction policies and procedures
  - Reorganized workflow within department, resulting in 45 percent, measurable increased productivity

- Technical Skills
  - Microsoft Office Suite 2003 and 2007 Certification (Word, Excel, Access, Outlook, and PowerPoint)
  - Proficient in medical office software (Medisoft®)
  - Input technology—Keyboarding skills of 85 corrected words per minute, voice-recognition software, and various scanning devices
  - Records and database management

EXPERIENCE

May 2000–Present
- MEDICAL INSURANCE SPECIALIST AND ADMINISTRATIVE COORDINATOR FOR PHYSICIANS CENTER OF SOMEWHERE, 8888 CENTER STREET, SOMEWHERE, US 12345-5555

EDUCATION

2008–Present, Pursuing Bachelor of Science in Health Information Technology, Anywhere University, Somewhere, US 12345-5555
- Anticipated graduation date of 2012
- Presidential Scholarship for Academic Achievement
- 112 of 128 hours completed

1998–2000, Associate of Applied Science degree awarded May 2000, Anywhere Community and Technology College, Somewhere, US 12345-5555
- National Collegiate Honor Society
- GPA 3.98 on a 4.0 scale

COMMUNITY SERVICE
- Chairperson for Skills USA
- Organized Zumba Community Fitness Fair
- Conducted update training for Somewhere area medical coders
- Volunteer for Humane Society

PROFESSIONAL AFFILIATION
- American Academy of Professional Coders
- American Federation of Office Administrators

There may be a situation in which the best style to use is a combination of chronological and functional formats. If you choose to combine formats, be sure to use the proper format for each section but format the entire résumé in a consistent style, such as underlining all side headings.

Scannable and Plain-Text Résumés. In today's technological workplace, résumés frequently are scanned into a database and referenced for interviews. An applicant should be prepared to submit two, differently formatted résumés: (1) a traditionally formatted chronological, functional, or combined chronological/functional résumé and (2) a scannable résumé. When preparing a **scannable résumé** for electronic (OCR) scanning, all of the formatting elements should be removed. Use only white paper and do not fold or attach anything to it. A folded résumé can lead to misreads by the OCR. Use black ink and a high-quality laser or jet-ink printer. The following are more tips for preparing a scannable résumé:

- Use one of the sans serif fonts or Times New Roman.
- Use 10- to 14-point type font.
- Avoid using italics, underlining, shading, and other unusual elements. Most OCRs can read solid bullets, asterisks, and bold, but use them sparingly.
- Place phone numbers on separate lines—the OCR may read numbers on the same line as one number.
- Use plenty of white space.
- Refrain from using columns.
- Limit the résumé to one page, if possible.

A **plain-text résumé**, a résumé with simplified formatting and electronically saved as a .txt file, can be e-mailed or cut and pasted into an online résumé drop box. A resume prepared using guidelines for scannable formatting but not saved as a plain-text file may transmit misinformation. When preparing a résumé to be sent as a plain-text file, use the same simplified formatting features used to prepare a scannable résumé and save the file as a plain-text file (save the resume using a .txt file). Plain-text is the most widely used file format for submitting résumés via the Internet. When submitting through an e-mail, be sure the subject specifically states the purpose of the message. Use all the previously mentioned tips for a scannable résumé but also

- Use shorter lines.
- Format all text to the left.
- Remove all tabs. If indentations are desired, use the space bar.
- Save the résumé as "Plain Text" or "Text Only."
- After saving the résumé, correct any errors.

Figure 9.6 shows an example of the previous résumé saved in plain-text format.

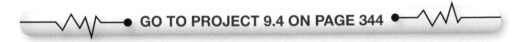

GO TO PROJECT 9.4 ON PAGE 344

HIPAA TIPS

As part of the externship process, medical offices may require students to sign a HIPAA agreement stating that no personal patient information will be shared with anyone outside the office. Every staff member or volunteer is responsible for adhering to HIPAA privacy and security regulations to ensure that protected health information (PHI) is secure and confidential. Violation of HIPAA law can result in both civil and criminal penalties.

What is the difference between a civil and a criminal penalty?

Figure 9.6

Plain-Text Résumé

NENNA L. BAYES

1234 Any Street
Somewhere, US 12345-5555
Cell Phone: 555-555-5555
E-mail: nennabayes@anyspace.com

OBJECTIVE

A position in a medical facility in which medical billing and coding experience can be used to sustain and increase revenue from accounts receivable and increase positive patient satisfaction

SUMMARY OF QUALIFICATIONS

· Nationally certified professional coder (CPC)
· Nationally certified chart auditor
· Developed, implemented, and analyzed patient satisfaction policies and procedures
· Implemented revenue-collection strategies that increased revenue by 23 percent in a six-month period

EDUCATION

2008-Present, Pursuing Bachelor of Science in Health Information Technology, Anywhere University, Somewhere, US 12345-5555

· Anticipated graduation date of 2012
· Presidential Scholarship for Academic Achievement
· 112 of 128 hours completed

1998-2000, Associate of Applied Science degree awarded May 2000, Anywhere Community and Technology College, Somewhere, US 12345-5555

· National Collegiate Honor Society
· GPA 3.98 on a 4.0 scale

Technical skills include
· Microsoft Office Suite 2003 and 2007 Certification (Word, Excel, Access, Outlook, and PowerPoint)
· Proficient in medical office software (Medisoft®)
· Input technology—Keyboarding skills of 85 corrected words per minute, voice-recognition software, and various scanning devices
· Records and database management

EXPERIENCE

May 2000-Present

· MEDICAL INSURANCE SPECIALIST AND ADMINISTRATIVE COORDINATOR FOR PHYSICIANS' CENTER OF SOMEWHERE, 8888 CENTER STREET, SOMEWHERE, US 12345-5555
  · Created and implemented revenue-intensive procedures that reduced uncollectible debt by 23 percent
  · Conducted certified continuing education workshops for physicians and staff
  · Streamlined staff workload to increase staff and patient satisfaction
  · Annually and quarterly updated all coding reference and source materials

COMMUNITY SERVICE

· Chairperson for SkillsUSA
· Organized Zumba Community Fitness Fair
· Conducted update training for Somewhere area medical coders
· Volunteer for Humane Society

PROFESSIONAL AFFILIATION

· American Academy of Professional Coders
· American Federation of Office Administrators

An interview may be one of the most stressful steps of the employment process if the applicant has not prepared. Even with preparation, will the applicant be nervous? Yes! Will the interviewer know the applicant is nervous? Yes! However, there is a way to make the interview less stressful and as successful as possible, and that is to do the "3 Ps"—prepare, prepare, and prepare.

Do the Research

It is more efficient to match skills to job requirements if the job seeker knows something about the company or office. Doing research will enable the applicant to learn more about the company's philosophy, profitability, stability, community service, and reputation. Also, knowing information about the organization will enable the applicant to formulate answers to anticipated interview questions and to ask questions during the interview. Several sources of company information are available.

Network Individuals. Person-to-person information is a valuable resource. Former and current employees of a company are important sources of first-hand information. However, listen carefully to distinguish between facts about the company and individuals' feelings. College placement offices and former students who are employed in your field of interest can also supply up-to-date information. As mentioned earlier, local chapters of professional organizations can provide information about local employers.

The Internet. Searching the Internet can yield a wealth of information. If the company has blogs and/or messages boards, read through the postings, and remember to look for facts. If negative statements are posted, gather information from other sources, such as newspaper articles, to determine if the postings are valid. If you decide to post, only post professional questions about company facts—steer clear of any negative postings.

Company Printed Resources. Most larger companies make available published literature, such as mission statements/philosophies and community involvement activities. These

Figure 9.7

The Interview

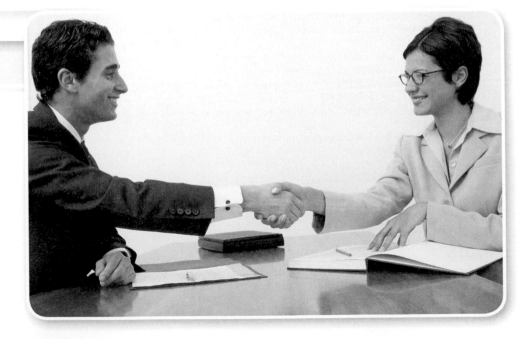

may also be published on their Web sites. Financial statements, organizational structures, and position descriptions also provide company details.

Preparing for the Interview

Remember the "3Ps"—prepare, prepare, and prepare. After researching the company, it is time to start preparing physically and mentally for the interview. Before the day of the interview, call the company for directions and make a trial run. As you travel to the interview site, note how long it takes to arrive. On the way, observe any detour or construction signs, school buses, or other factors that require more travel time. Look for parking areas, observing the availability of spaces and cost. Plan to arrive at least 10 minutes prior to the scheduled interview time and add those 10 minutes into the travel time. Also, if taking a bus or subway, add wait time. When traveling the route, look for alternate ways to the company—plan for the unexpected!

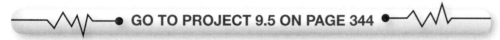

GO TO PROJECT 9.5 ON PAGE 344

Gather Materials. If necessary, purchase a two-pocket folder to use for interview materials. In it, place *copies* (not originals) of your résumé, your reference listing, recommendation letters, a list of additional work experience, your transcript, and examples of your work. De-identify any medical examples. These items may also be placed into a portfolio binder. If everything is equal between two competing applicants, the applicant who has expended the time and effort to assemble information into a portfolio may have the advantage. Take a pen or pencil and a notepad to the interview. The interviewer may ask for additional documents or information, which you should make note of. In today's technological age, it is also acceptable to take notes on a small, handheld device, such as a PDA. An applicant who is prepared to take notes appears organized. If using a cell phone to take notes, be sure to turn the ringer off.

Dress Appropriately. Clean and pressed—this should be the interviewee's overall physical presentation. The person's attire should reflect what he or she would wear if employed in the position. However, there are some exceptions. When interviewing for a position that requires a uniform (such as scrubs), professional office dress, not the uniform (scrubs), is

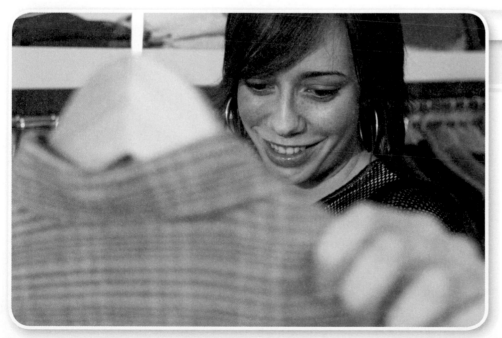

Figure 9.8

Dressing for the Interview

appropriate. If you are unsure about how to dress, it is best to be conservative. In other words, when in doubt, don't! Here are some basic rules or thumb guidelines for female and male interview attire.

Female Attire

- Business dress should have a modest length and neckline. Select a color that is not too flashy. Red and pink are examples of less favorable colors for an interview. Business pants or a skirt and blouse are also appropriate.
- Stockings (hose) should be worn with a dress or skirt. Wear closed-toed shoes with a modest heel—no sandals. Be sure shoes are clean and free of scuff marks.
- Nails should be clean, trimmed, and a modest length. If wearing nail polish, use clear or neutral colors.
- Rings and other jewelry should be limited. Many companies have a policy concerning the type and amount of jewelry to be worn. Check prior to the interview and follow any company policy. If one does not exist, follow these suggestions: no more than one ring per hand—engagement and wedding band are considered one ring; one bracelet (which does not make noise); a watch, if desired; no more than two modest earrings in each ear-lobe; and a conservative necklace. Tattoos should be covered for the interview—the applicant should investigate the company's policy on body art. Also, nose rings, tongue rings, or other body piercings (excluding earrings) should be removed for the interview, and again, the company policy on body piercings should be known prior to the inter-view. What is trendy in one social circle may not be considered professional dress.
- Perfume and/or scented lotions should be a very light scent or not worn at all to the in-terview. The interviewer may be allergic to the scent.
- Undergarments should be worn but should never be visible through clothing.
- Hair should be clean and conservatively styled. Keep hair away from the face and out of the eyes.

Male Attire

- Pants (cotton, wool, etc.) should be clean and free of wrinkles and a business-conserva-tive color, such as black or blue. Wear a collared, tucked-in shirt that matches the pants. If wearing a suit, select a professional, button-up shirt and matching tie. Be sure socks are the same color as the pants.
- Shoes should be casual if wearing business casual pants and shirt; however, a more pro-fessional shoe, such as a Wingtip shoe, should be worn with a business suit. Make sure shoes are clean and free of any scuff marks—no sandals.
- Fingernails, piercings, and tattoos should follow the same guidelines as those previously listed for females.
- Hair should be clean and well styled. Keep hair out of the face and eyes. Trim facial hair according to company policy.

Purchasing appropriate clothing for the interview does not have to be expensive. Many thrift and secondhand consignment shops offer a wide variety of business clothes at a frac-tion of new-store prices. Determine a budget and stick to it. Be a better consumer by using store advertisements and coupons.

Be aware of your personal hygiene. Take a shower or bath the day of the interview, use deodorant, clean your nails, and wash and style your hair. Oral hygiene is also important—brush your teeth and tongue and use mouthwash. Take breath mints and use them just before the interview. When nervous, some individuals have sweaty palms—take tissues to absorb the moisture. To help you feel alert, get at least eight hours of productive sleep the night before. It is best not to smoke prior to the interview; smoke smell tends to attach to clothing and hair. Check documents, such as the résumé, to be sure they are free of smoke smell.

Prepare for Interview Questions. Another way to prepare for an interview is by anticipating the questions the interviewer may ask and developing appropriate responses ahead of time. Employers want to know about the applicant's skills, training, experience, availability, and future plans. Although not every question can be anticipated, the following are some common, general interview questions and statements:

- Tell me about yourself.
- Why should we hire you?
- What is your strongest asset?
- Tell me what experience you have that relates to this position.
- Why do you want to work for our company?
- Can you travel?
- Are you willing to relocate?
- What do you see as your greatest weakness, and what have you done or are planning to do to overcome this?
- Do you work better individually or as part of a team?
- Why are you looking for a position?
- What have you learned from past mistakes?
- Professionally, where do you see yourself in five years?
- Do you plan to continue your education?
- Do you view yourself as a leader or as a follower?
- Have you ever been fired from a position? (Be honest and tactful when you answer this question. Placing blame on another individual may give the impression that you cannot take responsibility. State the reason for the separation and what you have learned from the experience.)
- What are the two most important accomplishments in your life so far?
- How would another person describe you?

Practice answering these and other interview questions several times before the actual interview. Even though the wording may be different, the intended content will probably be the same. For many interview questions, there is no right or wrong answer. Most questions are subjective, allowing interviewees to display their work ethics and character through their answers.

In an interview, it is illegal to ask questions about certain areas of an applicant's life. If such a question is asked, the interviewee has three options: (1) let the situation go and answer the question, (2) mention that the question is illegal and choose either to answer or not to answer the question, or (3) file a complaint. The choice is up to the interviewee.

Sometimes the wording of the question itself, not the intention, makes it illegal. Such questions are legal only if their content directly relates to a position's requirements. Illegal questions can be grouped into 11 categories:

- Affiliations
  - *Not Allowed:* "To which organizations do you belong?"
  - *Allowed:* "Do you belong to any professional organizations that you feel are relevant to this position?"
- Age
  - *Not Allowed:* "How old are you?" "Are you a Baby Boomer?" "When did you graduate from high school?"
  - *Allowed:* "Are you over the age of 18?"
- Arrest Record
  - *Not Allowed:* "Have you ever been arrested?"
  - *Allowed:* "Have you ever been convicted of one of the following crimes?" (The crime must be related to the position, such as a drug conviction relating to a position in a medical office.)

- Citizenship
  - *Not Allowed:* "Are you a U.S. citizen?"
  - *Allowed:* "Do you have the proper paperwork to work in the United States?"

- Health and/or Disabilities
  - *Not Allowed:* "Do you have any disabilities?" "Have you been hospitalized for any major illness in the last three years?" "Are you under the care of a mental health professional or have you ever been treated for any type of mental illness?"
  - *Allowed:* Upon completion of the interview and after receiving a thorough description of the job's duties, the applicant may be asked if he or she can perform the essential functions of the position. Many employers require a medical examination after the applicant has been hired. There are also stipulations regarding the release of the information obtained from these exams.

- Gender
  - *Not Allowed:* "Do you have any problem with having a male/female supervisor?" "What is your opinion of office romances?"
  - *Allowed:* "Please tell me about any previous supervising experience."

- Height/Weight
  - *Not Allowed:* "How tall are you?" "How much do you weigh?"
  - *Allowed:* "Are you able to lift a 100-pound patient from the examination table back into a wheelchair?" (Questions concerning height and weight are allowed only if they relate to minimum position requirements.)

- Marital and/or Family Status
  - *Not Allowed:* "Are you married?" "Are you single?" "How many children do you have?" "Do you plan to have children or more children?"
  - *Allowed:* "Are you willing to work overtime as needed?" "Can you travel?" (If asked of one candidate, these questions must be asked of each candidate applying for the position.)

- Military
  - *Not Allowed:* "Did you receive an honorable or a dishonorable discharge from your military service?"
  - *Allowed:* "What type of training did you receive while in the service?"

- National Origin or Race
  - *Not Allowed:* "Where are you from?" "Were you born in the United States?" "Your name is unusual—what is the origin of your name?"
  - *Allowed:* "Have you ever worked under a different name?"

- Religion
  - *Not Allowed:* "Where do you go to church?" "Which religious holidays do you celebrate?"
  - *Allowed:* "Are you a member of any organizations that you feel are relevant to and would enhance your performance in this position?"

Keep in mind, this list is not inclusive of all illegal questions and legal wordings, but it is meant to be a guide. Positions, such as those in security or medical facilities, do require the interviewer(s) to extract the candidate's position-related knowledge and qualifications in some of these areas but the questions must be directly related to the position requirements. Credit history and background checks are commonly performed on applicants in certain areas. Also, social networks are considered a source of public information and are being referenced by employers to access public information posted by applicants.

Conducting the Interview

During the interview is when the applicant presents his or her skills, training, and experience to the employer. The employer will determine the applicant's suitability for the position through a series of questions and observations. It is basically a question and answer session. Most of the work has already been completed—the applicant has gathered information, compiled the necessary documents, practiced questions and answers, and made physical preparations (e.g., dress, rest). The old saying "you never get a second chance to make a first impression" is extremely important during the interview process. The interviewer will be assessing not only the applicant's verbal communication skills but also his or her nonverbal communication. The interviewer will evaluate the applicant's confidence, respect, and attentiveness through various ordinary actions, such as a handshake. When you are asked to enter the interview area, wait until a hand is offered before shaking hands. It is a sign of respect to wait for the interviewer to first extend a handshake. Use a firm, but not crushingly firm, handshake. Shake using the whole hand and avoid the "finger" shake (only touching the tips of another individual's fingers).

Be aware of nervous habits or the perception of nervous habits. Consider the following real-life example. During an interview, an applicant was asked if she was a nervous individual. She responded that normally she was not but that today she was. The applicant inquired of the interviewer why the question was asked. The interviewer answered that he had noticed the applicant's very short fingernails and had thought them to be a sign of chronic nervousness. The applicant then explained that she played the piano and needed her nails to be short, a sign of practicality that had been misinterpreted as a sign of nervousness.

Address the interviewer using a courtesy title, such as Mr., Ms., or Dr., and allow the interviewer to be seated and to extend an invitation to be seated before sitting down. This is another sign of respect and courtesy. The following are some more guidelines for being successful in an interview:

- Be on time. Arrive approximately 10 minutes early—and alone. Don't take a friend into the interview venue.
- Refrain from chewing gum, eating candy, or drinking a beverage. However, it is acceptable to take a bottle of water into the interview. Remember to take it with you when the interview is over.
- Maintain consistent eye contact with the interviewer.
- Maintain good posture, both when standing and when sitting. Sit up straight and do not lean. Place your feet flat on the floor or crossed at the ankle. Crossing the legs may be interpreted as too relaxed and, for females wearing a skirt or dress, modesty may be jeopardized. Keep your hands still and comfortably folded in your lap or placed at your side.
- Smile! Smile sincerely and frequently during the interview. Fake smiles are noticeable.
- Listen attentively to the interviewer. Active listening will help you formulate questions for the interviewer.
- Use concrete nouns and action verbs when discussing your experience, your training, and other related position information.
- Avoid saying "um" and "like" when answering questions.
- Turn off your cell phone. Even when a cell phone is placed on vibrate or silent mode, the incoming call or message may still be a distraction. As mentioned earlier, if you use the phone to take notes, turn off the ringer and let the interviewer know you are taking notes on the phone.
- Ask questions of the interviewer at the point, usually near the end of the interview, when you are asked if you have any questions. Never say no. This conveys disinterest in the position. Instead, ask questions that will help you gain more knowledge of the position and its requirements. Questions concerning job duties, workload, schedule, evaluation strategies,

company structure, and immediate supervisor are all applicable. Salary and benefits questions are best left for the next level—the job offer. Sample questions include the following:

— Will my duties also include taking patient histories?
— Are periodic meetings conducted for clinical and administrative medical staff?
— Should I supply my own blood pressure cuff and stethoscope?
— Does the practice have a mentor assigned to new employees?

An applicant may be presented with different types of interviews. Panel interviews (a group of interviewers) will ask the applicant interview questions. Some panels are set up to ask questions in a predetermined sequence, while other panels are designed for members to randomly ask questions. You should greet each panel member with a smile and direct eye contact. Shake hands with each panel member. Prepare for a panel interview in the same manner as you would prepare for a one-on-one interview: use good posture, take notes, answer questions fully, be prepared to ask questions of the panel, and so on. Look at each panel member; do not focus on just one or a few members.

Phone interviews are becoming more common in today's global and fast-paced society. Mentally and physically prepare for a phone interview just as you would for a face-to-face meeting. Prior to the phone interview, confirm the interview time—be sure to consider differences in time zones. Locate a quiet place where you can fully concentrate on the interview without interruptions. Assemble all your employment credentials (e.g., résumé, transcript, and samples of work). Be sure to have pen and paper to take notes and a glass of water to clear your throat. Dress professionally for the phone interview—no jeans or sweatpants.

During a phone interview, follow these tips:

- Disable the call-waiting feature.
- Do not use speaker phone.
- Listen for and eliminate any background noises, such as a fan, prior to the phone interview.
- Smile and use good posture. This will give you a feeling of physically presenting yourself to the interviewer in a positive nonverbal manner. If you prefer, stand.
- Concentrate totally on the phone interview—do not try to multi-task.
- Listen attentively to questions and ask for clarification if you did not understand.
- Speak at a slightly slower pace than normal.
- Refrain from chewing or eating during the phone interview.
- Keep your answers to less than two minutes in length. It is easier to continue talking on the phone than in person.
- Apologize if you accidentally interrupt and allow the interviewer to finish.

Ending the Interview

After all questions have been asked and answered, it is time to conclude the interview. The interviewer normally will nonverbally signal the end by standing or by verbally thanking the applicant. This is a good time, if not answered earlier, to ask what action is next and the anticipated time frame. It is also an opportune time for the applicant to reiterate his or her desire and qualifications for the position. When offered, shake the interviewer's hand and thank the interviewer by name. Also, thank others who were involved, such as an administrative assistant or a receptionist, when leaving the interview.

 THE FOLLOW-UP CONTACT LETTER

After leaving an interview, you should immediately make notes of what happened during the interview, the information you gave and received, the names of people you met, and other details. Write a thank-you letter to the interviewer within a time frame of no more

Figure 9.9

Follow-up Contact Letter

1234 Any Street
Somewhere, US 12345-5555
October 26, 2012

Dr. Mike Doe
5555 St. Christopher's Street
Somewhere, US 12345-5555

Dear Dr. Doe:

Talking with you on Wednesday, October 26, about the medical insurance
specialist position was informative and interesting. Your medical
facility is progressive, and interviewing with you confirmed my belief
that our professional goals are the same. Thank you for describing
details of the position.

Your recent implementation of electronic health records at Advanced
Treatment Center utilizies a software program with which I have previously worked and updated. Designing the history and physical interface
was both challenging and rewarding and was an experience that your
facility can utilize to increase physician/patient productivity and
satisfaction. Our discussion on accounts receivable reinforced my
interest in becoming an integral part of your medical office team.
Since the interview, I have considered different options for conducting
internal documentation auditing on a consistent basis and am anxious
to discuss the two different plans with you.

It is exciting to be considered for the medical insurance specialist
position with Advanced Treatment Center, and I look forward to joining
your staff. If you have additional questions or would like to discuss
the position further with me, please contact me at 555-555-5555 or at
nennabayes@anyspace.com.

Sincerely,

Nenna Bayes

than two days. A thank-you letter serves two purposes. It (1) expresses gratitude to the interviewer and (2) places the applicant's name and qualifications in front of the interviewer one more time.

Prepare the follow-up contact letter using the same format and paper quality as you used for your cover/application letter and résumé. Use very few, if any, first-person pronouns at the beginnings of sentences. Like the cover/application letter, the thank-you follow-up letter should have three paragraphs:

- Paragraph one expresses gratitude for the interview opportunity.
- Paragraph two emphasizes the applicant's qualifications and any information you may have forgotten during the interview. Refer to specific topics discussed in the interview.
- Paragraph three is forward looking in content. Show enthusiasm and eagerness to join the office team.

Figure 9.9 shows a sample follow-up letter.

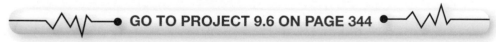

GO TO PROJECT 9.6 ON PAGE 344

It is easy to become discouraged during an employment search. Rejection is inherently part of the process; however, view rejection as an opportunity to learn, to improve, and to move forward. Rejection may have nothing to do with your level of skill or education but with timing, and a rejection becomes an opportunity to seek other career possibilities.

Chapter Projects

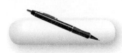

Project 9.1   Preparing Interview Questions

Imagine that you have the opportunity to interview a number of administrative medical assistants about their jobs. What information would you like to learn from them? With a partner, brainstorm a list of questions to ask the administrative medical assistants. Divide your list into questions about tasks, skills, and personal attributes. Be prepared to discuss your findings in class and submit your project findings to your instructor

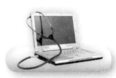

Project 9.2   Locating Positions

Using the Internet, research and describe three available positions for administrative medical assistants. If possible, locate the job opportunities in your geographical area by visiting the Web sites of your state's department of labor and those of local newspapers.

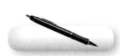

Project 9.3   Preparing a Cover/Application Letter

Using the data you collected in Project 9.1, compose a cover/application letter for the position of administrative medical assistant.

Use block-style formatting for the letter. Prepare it in the three-paragraph format discussed in this chapter.

Project 9.4   Preparing a Résumé

Prepare a résumé to accompany the cover/application letter you prepared in Project 9.3. Select the style (chronological or functional) that best suits your qualifications. After preparing the résumé, save it and reopen it. Save a copy of the résumé as plain text.

Project 9.5   Researching Potential Employers

Research various sources of available medical office positions and select a position. Research the company and collect data, which you will use to compose your employment credentials.

Project 9.6   Composing a Follow-up Letter

You have just completed an interview for the position in Project 9.3. Prepare a follow-up thank-you letter addressed to your interviewer, using that person's name. If you were not able to obtain an individual's name, address the letter to Dr. Karen Larsen.

9.1 List and explore visible and hidden career-employment resources. Pages 320–322	• Many rich sources of employment opportunities are available for job seekers. Examples of visible/traditional markets include classified advertisements, professional journals, career job fairs, job boards, the Internet, temporary employment agencies, and employment services. • Less common markets for career opportunities include telephone directories, chambers of commerce, company Web sites, and social/professional networks.
9.2 Assimilate information and prepare an employment application Pages 322–324	• Complete and accurate information is needed when completing an employment application: — Personal information — Employment—including dates of employment and addresses—information — Educational information — Reference information • Complete all blanks. • Print legibly using blue or black ink. • Be truthful. • Sign and date the application.
9.3 Compose a cover/ application letter. Pages 324–326	• The first impression of a potential employee is frequently made through an application letter. • Use a properly formatted letter containing correct grammar and punctuation. Block-style format is common. • Prepare the letter using a suggested three-paragraph format: — Paragraph one informs the reader from whom, where, and when the applicant heard of the position—the company may have more than one position to fill; actually state which position you are applying for. — Paragraph two presents your qualifications (experience/education), linked to the available position. Refer to the enclosed résumé. If electronic, refer to the résumé attachment. — In paragraph three—an action paragraph—request an interview and provide contact data for the reader. • Use high-quality paper. • Proofread, proofread, and proofread! • Sign the letter using blue or black ink. If electronic, use an electronic signature.

9.4 Assimilate data and compose résumés using different formats.
Pages 326–335
	- The main purpose of a résumé is to secure an interview.
	- Data compiled for an application, such as personal information, addresses and dates of employment, and education information, may be used to compose a résumé.
	- Résumés take the "snapshot picture" provided on the application or within the application letter to the next level by providing more detail.
	- Formats are chronological and functional. Sometimes a combination of chronological and functional formats is used.
	  — Chronological format supplies data within categories (i.e., education) in reverse chronological order (the most current is placed first).
	  — Functional format supplies data in related skills and experience categories, such as management or administration.
	- Plain-text format résumés should be prepared for electronic or electronically read submission.
	- Categories commonly included in résumés are header, objective, summary of qualifications, work experience, education, and optional categories (such as awards and community service).
	  — References should be listed on a separate reference page containing three to five professional references. The reference page should be available when requested.

9.5 Assemble personal information, professional information, and appropriate dress for the interview process and conduct a mock interview. Pages 336–342	- Gather all requested and/or anticipated interview materials and assemble them for review into a hardcopy portfolio or into an electronic portfolio. In addition to a cover/application letter and résumé, supply examples of professional work and educational documentation (transcript). Be prepared to leave information with the interviewer—take copies, not originals (unless an original transcript or other documentation is requested). - Dress should be professional and conservative. Check company policy on dress and accessories, such as rings, earrings and other piercings, and tattoos.

Copyright © 2012 McGraw-Hill Higher Education

	<ul><li>Use good personal hygiene—bathe/shower and use deodorant, brush teeth and use mouthwash, clean hair and nails, and refrain from using strong colognes and/or scented lotions.</li><li>Assemble a list of anticipated interview questions and questions to ask the interviewer.</li><li>Practice shaking hands, sitting, and standing.</li></ul>
9.6 Compose a follow-up thank-you letter. Pages 342–343	<ul><li>Within 24 hours—no more than 2 days—after the interview, compose and send a thank-you letter to the interviewer. The letter serves two purposes:<ul><li>— Expression of gratitude</li><li>— Reminder of your qualifications</li></ul></li><li>Use the same format for the follow-up letter as you used for the cover/application letter. If you used block style for the cover/application letter, use block style for the follow-up letter.</li><li>Prepare the follow-up letter using the same high-quality paper you used for the cover/application letter and résumé.</li><li>Construct the letter using a three-paragraph format:<ul><li>— In paragraph one, express gratitude for the interview.</li><li>— In paragraph two, remind the reader of your qualifications.</li><li>— In paragraph three, express your anticipation of employment with the company.</li></ul></li></ul>

Soft Skills Success

Interpersonal Skills

Interpersonal skills are all the behaviors and feelings that exist within all of us that influence our interactions with others. These skills are also referred to as communication skills, people skills, and/or soft skills. We learn them by watching our parents, the television, and our peers. Healthy interpersonal skills reduce stress, reduce conflict, improve communication, increase understanding, and promote joy. Improving these skills builds confidence and enhances our relationships with others. **How can interpersonal skills improve your chances when applying for a job? Can interpersonal skills make or break your interview?**

Positive Attitude

A positive attitude helps you cope more easily with daily life and helps you avoid worry. A positive attitude makes you happier and more successful. With a positive attitude, you see the bright side of life and expect the best. If your attitude is positive enough, it becomes contagious. Choose to be happy. Find reasons to smile more often, and associate with happy people. **Why is surrounding yourself with positive people so important?**

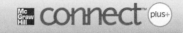
USING TERMINOLOGY

Match the term or phrase on the left with the correct answer on the right.

_____ 1. (LO 9.1) Hidden job market

_____ 2. (LO 9.3) Cover/application letter

_____ 3. (LO 9.4) Chronological résumé

_____ 4. (LO 9.4) Professional reference requirements

_____ 5. (LO 9.4) Functional résumé

_____ 6. (LO 9.4) Keywords

a. Document that concisely presents an applicant's specific traits that match a career opportunity

b. Career opportunity resources that are less visible

c. Words that are directly related to position

d. Data presented in categories, with the most recent listed first

e. Individual who can attest to an applicant's work ethic

f. Data organized by categories that directly support a position goal

CHECK YOUR UNDERSTANDING

Select the most correct answer.

1. (LO 9.1) Latisha recently graduated from a medical office program. While attending school, she worked part-time during evenings in the records department at a local hospital. She is now ready to seek full-time employment in her field of study. Where could she go to begin compiling employment possibilities?

   a. Friends and social networks
   b. Web site for the hospital where she works
   c. School career center
   d. All of the above are correct.

2. (LO 9.2) When filling out an employment application, periods of unemployment should be

   a. Left off the application.
   b. Placed on the application with a short explanation, such as "attending college."
   c. Placed on the application and left blank.
   d. Placed on the application and highlighted, so that it can be discussed during the interview.

3. (LO 9.2) Which of the following would not be considered an appropriate reference for an application or a résumé?

   a. Work colleague of the applicant
   b. Applicant's instructor during recent training
   c. Applicant's priest
   d. Fellow committee member

4. (LO 9.3) Which of the following is an example of a sentence composed using the "you" approach?

   a. "Training during the past two years in the medical office program at Anywhere Community and Technical College has provided me with skills that can be used to complement your HIT department."

   b. "I have attended school during the past two years at Anywhere Community and Technical College."

   c. "My skills and training in the medical office program during the past two years can be used by your HIT Department."

   d. "I recently became certified in medical records and would like to use my skills in your HIT department."

5. (LO 9.3) As Latisha composes a cover/application letter, she is unsure of where to mention her résumé. In which paragraph should she place a reference to her enclosed résumé?

   a. First
   b. Second
   c. Third
   d. Second and third

6. (LO 9.4) During her search for employment opportunities, Latisha found an open HIT position with a multi-physician clinic. The résumé is to be submitted online. Which format should she use to submit her online résumé?

   a. Functional, because she likes it better and already has a résumé prepared using this format
   b. Chronological with bold side headings
   c. Chronological, because her recent educational training and certification directly relate to the position requirements
   d. Chronological/plain-text format, because her recent educational training and certification directly relate to the position requirements

7. (LO 9.4) Which of the following statements is composed using power wording?

   a. "Implemented revenue collection strategies that increased the collection ratio from 22 percent to 62 percent during a nine-month period."
   b. "Assisted in increasing the collection ratio from 22 percent to 62 percent."
   c. "Increased the collection ratio from 22 percent to 62 percent."
   d. "Worked with the office team to increase the collection ratio rate."

8. (LO 9.5) During an interview for a medical coding position, which requires AHIMA or AAPC coding certification, which of the following questions may legally be asked of the interviewee?

   a. "To which organizations do you belong?"
   b. "Are you a certified coder through AHIMA or AAPC?"
   c. "Do you hold membership in coding organizations?"
   d. "May I see a list of all the organizations to which you belong?"

9. (LO 9.5) Which of the following questions should not be asked by the applicant during the first interview?

   a. "How many patients does the practice see during a normal working day?"
   b. "Will I be cross trained with other members of the medical office team?"
   c. "Do you prefer I wear scrubs or other office dress?"
   d. "Will I receive a yearly cost-of-living salary increase?"

10. (LO 9.6) Which of the following salutations should be used for a follow-up thank-you letter?

    a. Dear Human Resource Director:

    b. To Whom It May Concern:

    c. Dear Mr. Sanders:

    d. Dear Allen,

THINKING IT THROUGH

These questions cover the most important points in this chapter. Using your critical-thinking skills, play the role of an administrative medical assistant as you answer each question. Be prepared to present your response.

1. Donna Smith is an administrative medical assisting student who is currently finishing her education and preparing to seek employment in the healthcare field. Donna does not have transportation, so she has to rely on others for transportation, or she uses public transportation. As a result of this issue, she has arrived late to several interviews.

   Now, it is your turn to think it through!

       a. Should Donna discuss her lack of transportation during the interview? Why or why not?

       b. If Donna has a problem with transportation, should she be seeking employment?

       c. Due to Donna's transportation issue, she was repeatedly tardy for her last job. Should this information be shared during the interview process? Why or why not?

2. Nathan was granted an interview for an administrative medical assistant position. During the interview, the employer asked Nathan how the medical office's mission statement (displayed in the waiting area and on the facility's Web site) aligned with Nathan's professional goal(s). Also, Nathan's résumé, which was referred to during his interview, contained the old name of the medical practice. Nathan was not offered the position. Why do you think Nathan was not offered the position? Why is it important to learn about a potential employer before attending a job interview?

3. Addison was nervous during her interview and consistently looked from the floor to a picture located to the right of the interviewer, Ms. Jackson. Ms. Jackson asked Addison if something was bothering her, since she seemed to be distracted. Why is good eye contact important when meeting and speaking with potential employers?

4. "Getting a job is a full-time job in itself." Do you agree with this statement? Why or why not?

5. Why is being late for an interview one of the most serious mistakes a job applicant can make?

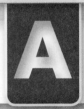

Introduction to **medisoft**®

Medisoft® is a widely used patient accounting program for medical offices. In this text you are studying the administrative tasks of the medical assistant. When you work as an administrative medical assistant, it is likely that you will encounter some sort of patient accounting software. The Medisoft® program includes the basic operations of all patient accounting software programs. Familiarizing yourself with Medisoft® will enable you to learn almost any similar software in a very brief period of time.

THE STUDENT DATA FILE

Before a medical office begins using Medisoft®, basic information about the practice and its patients must be entered in the computer. This preliminary work has been done for you. Dr. Karen Larsen's practice information is stored in the student data file located at the book's Online Learning Center (www.mhhe.com/bayes7e). The student data file contains all the data you will need to complete the Medisoft® projects and simulations in the text.

Check with your instructor to determine whether this file has already been loaded on your computer. If your instructor has not already loaded the file, go to the Online Learning Center at www.mhhe.com/bayes7e to download it. You will need to download the student data before you begin the Medisoft® projects and simulations in the text.

Backup Procedures

When entering data in Medisoft®, it is important to back up your work regularly for safekeeping. A backup copy of the database files prevents you from losing your work if the hard drive fails, or if you accidentally delete data while working. If you are in a school environment where you share computers, it is essential that you make a backup copy of your work after each Medisoft® session. This ensures that you can restore your work during the next session and you will be able to use your own data even if another student uses the computer after you or if, for any reason, the files on the school computer are changed or corrupted. This section provides instructions on backing up and restoring data in Medisoft®.

Backing Up Data

By default, whenever the Exit button on the toolbar or the Exit option on the File menu is selected, Medisoft® displays the Backup Reminder dialog box. This box reminds the user to back up the currently active data set before exiting the program. Other options in the Backup Reminder dialog box include exiting the Medisoft® program without backing up the data and canceling the Exit command and returning to the main Medisoft® window.

While working through the Medisoft® projects in *Medical Office Procedures, always* select the Back Up Data Now option to back up your work whenever you exit the program. The backup procedure is as follows.

1. To end the current session, click the Exit button on the toolbar (the last button on the right) or click Exit on the File menu.

2. The Backup Reminder dialog box appears.

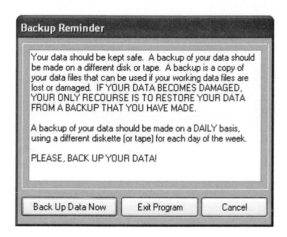

For the purposes of this text, it is recommended that you back up your work to the drive and folder where you are storing your work for this course. For example, in these instructions, a folder has been created under C:\ … \My Documents, called MOP, for backing up data. Click the Back Up Data Now button.

3. The Medisoft Backup dialog box is displayed. By default, the Destination File Path and Name box at the top of the dialog box shows the name of the drive and folder that was last used. If the correct location is not shown, click the Find button to select the drive and folder where you would like to store your work.

4. After the correct destination folder is displayed in the Medisoft Backup dialog box, you are ready to key in the name of the backup file at the end of the path name. We will name the backup file *KLarsen.mbk*, after the practice name in the text. Depending on the last time the program was used, the end of the path may or may not display a file with the .mbk extension (for Medisoft backup file). To check whether a backup file exists, press the right arrow key on your keyboard to move the cursor to the end of the path name. If no file with an .mbk extension appears, simply key in the new file name, *KLarsen.mbk*. If a backup file is already displayed, use the backspace key to delete the old file name and key in the new name. The end of the path should now read: \KLarsen.mbk, as shown here. (Note: If you are sharing a computer, you may also want to add your initials to the beginning of the file name.)

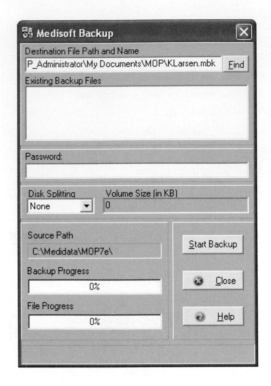

5. Medisoft® displays the location of the database files to be backed up in the Source Path box in the lower half of the dialog box automatically (C:\Medidata\MOP7e). Click the Start Backup button.

6. The program backs up the latest database files and displays an Information dialog box indicating the backup is complete. Click the OK button to close the Information dialog box, and then click the Close button to close the Medisoft Backup dialog box.

7. The Medisoft Backup dialog box disappears, and the Medisoft® program closes.

If you are not sharing a computer with other students, the backup file serves as an extra copy of your work for safekeeping. As in most offices, the extra time it takes to make a backup copy in a medical office can save countless hours later.

If you are sharing a computer with other students, the backup file serves an additional purpose. You will use the backup file to restore your work when you begin the next Medisoft® session. The steps required to perform a restore are as follows.

Restoring Data

If you are sharing a computer in an instructional environment, you must perform a restore before each new Medisoft® session to be certain you are working with your own data. The following steps are used to restore the latest backup file.

To restore the file *KLarsen.mbk* to C:\Medidata\MOP7e:

1. Copy your backup file from your external storage device to the assigned location on your hard drive.

2. Start Medisoft®.

3. Check the program's title bar at the top of the screen to make sure the MOP7e data set is the active data set. (If it is not, use the Open Practice option on the File menu to select it.)

4. Open the File menu and click Restore Data.

5. When the Warning box appears, click OK.

6. The Restore dialog box appears.

7. Use the Find button to locate your assigned storage folder (the folder used in step 1). Locate *KLarsen.mbk* in the list of existing backup files displayed for that folder, and click on it to attach it to the Backup File Path and Name at the top of the dialog box. The end of the path name should now read \ … \KLarsen.mbk, as shown here.

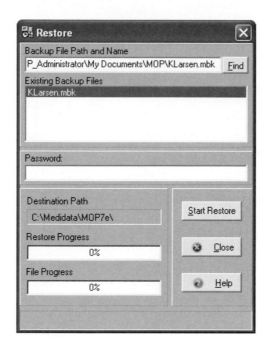

8. The Destination Path at the bottom of the box will automatically display C:\Medidata\MOP7e.

9. Click the Start Restore button.

10. When the Confirm box appears, click OK.

11. An Information dialog box appears, indicating the restore is complete. Click OK to continue, and then click the Close button to close the Restore dialog box.

12. The Restore dialog box closes. The latest data has been restored for the next session.

MEDISOFT® MENUS

Medisoft® offers choices of actions through a series of menus. Commands are issued by clicking an option on the menu bar or by clicking a shortcut button on the toolbar. All data, whether a patient's address or a charge for a procedure, is entered into Medisoft® through the menus on the menu bar or through the buttons on the toolbar. Selecting an option from the menus or toolbar brings up a dialog box. The Tab key is used to move between text boxes within a dialog box.

The menu bar lists the names of the menus in Medisoft®: File, Edit, Activities, Lists, Reports, Tools, Window, and Help. Beneath each menu name is a pull-down menu of one or more options.

File Menu. The File menu is used to enter information about the medical office practice when first setting up Medisoft® (see Figure A.1). It is also used to back up data, maintain files, and set program options.

Edit Menu. The Edit menu contains the basic commands needed to move, change, or delete information (see Figure A.2). These commands are Cut, Copy, Paste, and Delete.

Figure A.1

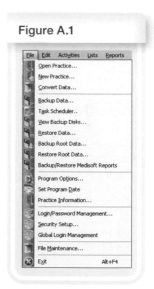

Figure A.2

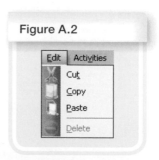

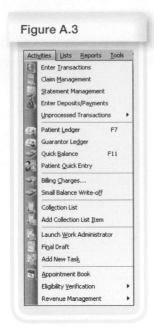

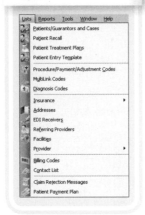

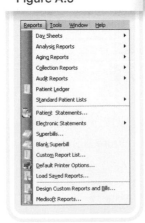

Activities Menu. Most medical office data collected on a day-to-day basis is entered through options on the Activities menu (see Figure A.3). This menu is used to enter financial transactions, including charges and payments; to create insurance claims; and to manage patient statements. Office Hours, Medisoft®'s built-in appointment book, is also accessed via the Activities menu.

Lists Menu. Information on new patients, such as name, address, and employer, is entered through the Lists menu (see Figure A.4). The Lists menu also provides access to lists of codes, insurance carriers, and providers.

Reports Menu. The Reports menu is used to print reports about patients' accounts and other reports about the practice (see Figure A.5).

Tools Menu. The calculator is accessed through the Tools menu (see Figure A.6). Other options on the Tools menu can also be used to view the contents of a file as well as a profile of the computer system.

Window Menu. Using the Window menu, it is possible to switch back and forth among several open windows (see Figure A.7).

Help Menu. The Help menu is used to access Medisoft®'s Help feature (see Figure A.8).

Dates in Medisoft®

Medisoft® is a date-sensitive program. The dates set in Medisoft® must be accurate, or the data entered will be of little value to the practice. Many times in medical offices date-sensitive information is not entered into Medisoft® on the same day that the event or transaction occurs. For example, Friday's office visits may not be entered into Medisoft® until Monday. If the program date is not changed to Friday's date before entering the data, all the information entered on Monday will be associated with Monday's date. For this reason, it is important to know how to change the Medisoft® Program Date.

For most of the exercises in this book, you will need to change the Medisoft® Program Date to the date specified in the project or simulation. The following steps are used to change the Medisoft® Program Date:

1. Click Set Program Date on the File menu, or click the date displayed on the status bar. A pop-up calendar is displayed.
2. Click the name of the month that is currently displayed. A pop-up menu appears. Click the desired month on the pop-up menu.
3. Select the desired year by clicking the year that is currently displayed. A pop-up menu appears. Click the desired year on the pop-up menu.
4. Select the desired date by clicking that date in the calendar.
5. The changes to the Medisoft® Program Date are automatically saved.

Answering Future Date Messages

For the Medisoft® projects and simulations in this textbook, which take place in the year 2014, you will need to change the Medisoft® Program Date to a specified date that is later than the current date on your computer (the Windows System Date). When a date is entered that is in the future, the program recognizes that a future date has been entered and displays one of several dialog boxes in response (see Figures A.9a, A.9b, A.9c, and A.9d).

Depending on where in the program the date is entered, the dialog box will vary. If a change is made to the pop-up calendar, for example, when entering a deposit, the Confirm dialog box in Figure A.9a appears as a notification that the date selected is in the future and asks whether the date should be changed. To keep the future date, the No button must be clicked.

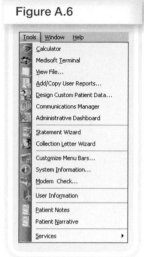

Figure A.6

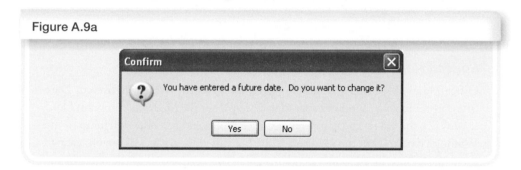

Figure A.9a

When entering patient office visit transactions, the Date of Service Validation dialog box appears and asks whether the transaction should be saved (see Figure A.9b). To keep the future date and save the transaction, it is necessary to click the Yes button.

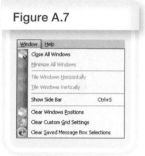

Figure A.7

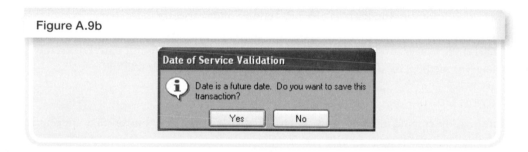

Figure A.9b

When entering a signature date for a patient, a Warning dialog box states that the date you entered is in the future (see Figure A.9c). To continue, the OK button is clicked.

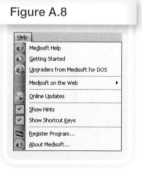

Figure A.8

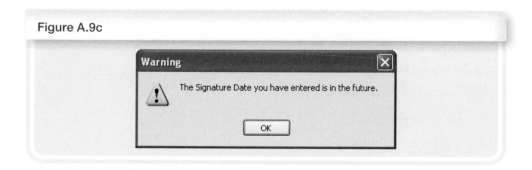

Figure A.9c

When simply changing the Medisoft® program date, an Information dialog box appears (see Figure A.9d) as a notification that the date selected is in the future. To keep the future date, click the OK button.

Figure A.9d

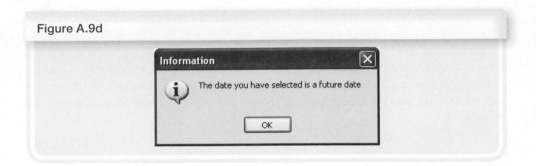

Special Note on Office Hours Dates

Office Hours, Medisoft®'s scheduling program, uses the Windows System Date (the date set in your Windows operating system), not the Medisoft® Program Date. If you click the Go to Today button in Office Hours, the calendar will jump to the Windows date and not the Medisoft® date. For this reason, you will need to change the date in the Office Hours calendar regularly to correspond to the dates in the projects and simulations in the text.

In most Medisoft® dialog boxes, if a pop-up calendar is not used, dates are entered in the MMDDCCYY format. The MMDDCCYY format is a specific way in which dates must be keyed. "MM" stands for the month, "DD" stands for the day, "CC" represents century, and "YY" stands for the year. Each day, month, century, and year entry must contain two digits, and no punctuation can be used. For example, the date of February 1, 2008, would be keyed "02012008." Alternatively, slashes can be used to separate the parts of the date. For example, using this method, the date of February 1, 2008, would be keyed "2/1/2008."

Saving Data

Information entered into Medisoft® is saved by clicking the Save button that appears in most dialog boxes (those in which data is input).

Deleting Data

In most Medisoft® dialog boxes, there are buttons for the purpose of deleting data. Data can also be deleted by highlighting an entry or a transaction and then clicking the right mouse button. A shortcut menu is displayed that contains an option to delete the entry. Medisoft® will ask for confirmation before deleting the data.

Exiting Medisoft®

Medisoft® is exited by clicking Exit on the File menu or by clicking the Exit button on the toolbar.

Using Medisoft® Help

Medisoft® offers users three different types of help.

Hints. As the cursor moves over certain fields, hints appear on the status bar at the bottom of the screen. The hints explain the purpose of the corresponding item.

Built-in Help. For more detailed help, Medisoft® has an extensive help feature built into the program itself, which is accessed through the Help menu.

Online Help. The Help menu also provides access to Medisoft® help available on the Medisoft® corporate website www.medisoft.com. The website contains a searchable knowledge base, which is a collection of up-to-date technical information about Medisoft® products.

ENTERING PATIENT INFORMATION

Patient information is entered in the Patient/Guarantor dialog box. To access this dialog box, first the Patients/Guarantors and Cases option is clicked on the Lists menu. Clicking this option displays the Patient List dialog box, which contains a list of established patients. Information on a new patient is added by clicking the New Patient button at the bottom of the dialog box. When the New Patient button is clicked, the Patient/Guarantor dialog box appears. It contains two tabs for entering information on a new patient: (1) the Name, Address tab and (2) the Other Information tab.

Name, Address Tab

The Name, Address tab (see Figure A.10) is completed with information from a new Patient Information Form. Most of the information is demographic: name, address, e-mail, phone numbers, birth date, sex, and Social Security number. Phone numbers must be entered without parentheses or hyphens. Similarly, the nine-digit Social Security number is entered without hyphens. Some of the boxes, such as the e-mail and cell phone number boxes, are optional.

Figure A.10

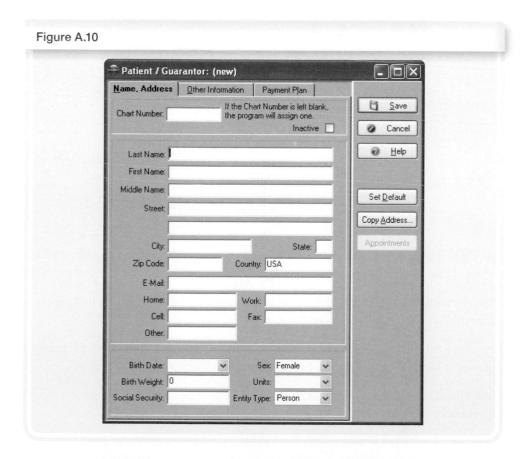

Chart Number. The chart number is a unique number that identifies each patient. The most common method of assigning a number is to use the first five letters of the last name, the first two letters of the first name, and the digit 0, which represents the head of house-hold, or guarantor, in the family. If additional family members are added to the database, the same chart number is used for each member, except that the final digit, 0, changes to 1, 2, 3, and so on. If the person's last name has fewer than five letters, use more letters of the first name and even letters of the middle name, if necessary.

Other Information Tab

The Other Information tab (see Figure A.11) contains facts about a patient's employment and other miscellaneous information. The following are the major fields in the Other Information tab.

Figure A.11

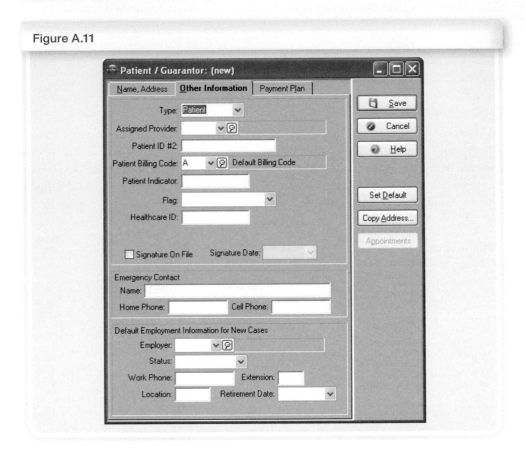

Type. The Type drop-down list designates whether, for billing purposes, an individual is a patient or guarantor. A guarantor is someone who is responsible for insurance and payment.

Assigned Provider. The code for the specific doctor who provides care to this patient is selected.

Signature on File. A check mark in a Signature on File check box means that the patient's signature is on file for the purpose of submitting insurance claims.

Signature Date. The date keyed in the Signature Date box is the date the patient signed the insurance release form.

Employer. The code for the patient's employer is selected from the drop-down list of employers that are in the database.

CASES

Information about a patient's insurance coverage, billing account, diagnosis, and condition is stored in cases. When a patient comes for treatment, a case is created. Cases are set up to contain the transactions that relate to a particular condition. For example, all treatments and procedures for bronchial asthma would be stored in a case called "Bronchial asthma." Services performed and charges for those services are entered in the system linked to the bronchial asthma case.

In Medisoft®, cases are created, edited, and deleted from within the Patient List dialog box. When the Case radio button in the Patient List dialog box is clicked, the following buttons appear at the bottom of the Patient List dialog box: Edit Case, New Case, Delete Case, Copy Case, Print Grid, Quick Entry, and Close. These buttons perform their respective functions on cases. For example, to create a new case, the New Case button is clicked.

Entering Case Information

Information on a patient is entered in 11 different tabs within the Case dialog box: Personal, Account, Diagnosis, Policy 1, Policy 2, Policy 3, Condition, Miscellaneous, Medicaid and Tricare, Comment, and EDI (see Figure A.12). After data is recorded in the appropriate tabs, it is stored by clicking the Save button on the right side of the dialog box.

Figure A.12

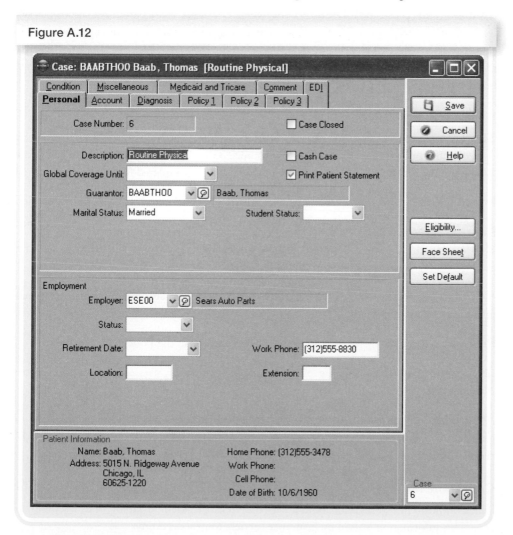

Personal Tab

The Personal tab contains basic information about a patient and his or her employment. The following are the most important boxes that must be completed in the Personal tab.

Description. Information entered in the Description box indicates a patient's complaint, or reason for seeing a physician.

Guarantor. The Guarantor box lists the name of the person responsible for paying the bill.

Account Tab

The Account tab includes information on a patient's assigned provider, referring provider, referral source, and other information that may be used in some medical practices but not others. The following is the most important box that must be completed in the Account tab.

Assigned Provider. The Assigned Provider box is automatically filled in with the code number and name of the assigned provider listed in the Patient/Guarantor dialog box.

Diagnosis Tab

The Diagnosis tab contains a patient's diagnosis, information about allergies, and electronic claim (EDI) notes. The following are the most important boxes that must be completed in the Diagnosis tab.

Principal Diagnosis and Default Diagnosis 2, 3, and 4. A patient's diagnosis is selected from the drop-down list of diagnoses. If a patient has more than one diagnosis for the same condition, the primary diagnosis is entered in the Principal Diagnosis field. Additional diagnoses are entered in the Default Diagnosis 2, 3, and 4 fields. The program options can be changed to display up to eight diagnoses if required.

Policy 1, 2, and 3 Tabs

The Policy tabs are where information about a patient's insurance carrier and coverage is recorded. If a patient has more than one insurance policy, the Policy 2 and 3 tabs are used. The following are the most important boxes that must be completed in the Policy tabs.

Insurance 1. The Insurance 1 box lists the code number and name of the insurance carrier.

Policy Holder 1. This box lists the person who is the policyholder for a particular policy. For example, if the patient is a child covered under his or her parent's insurance plan, the parent's chart number is entered in this box.

Relationship to Insured. This box describes a patient's relationship to the individual listed in the Insured 1 box.

Policy Number. The insurance policy number is entered in the Policy Number box.

Group Number. If there is a group number for the policy, it is entered in the Group Number box.

Assignment of Benefits/Accept Assignment. For physicians who are participating in an insurance plan, a check mark in this box indicates that the provider accepts payment directly from the insurance carrier.

Condition Tab

The Condition tab stores data about a patient's illness, accident, disability, and hospitalization. This information is used by insurance carriers to process claims.

Miscellaneous Tab

The Miscellaneous tab records a variety of miscellaneous information about the patient and his or her treatment, including outside lab work, prior authorization numbers, and other information.

Medicaid and Tricare Tab

For patients covered by Medicaid and Tricare, this tab is used to enter additional information about the government program.

Comment Tab

The Comment tab is used to enter case notes.

EDI Tab

The EDI tab is used to enter information for electronic claims specific to this case. Only fields that are relevant for the particular case need to be completed.

TRANSACTION ENTRY

Transactions are entered in the Transaction Entry dialog box, which is accessed by clicking Enter Transactions on the Activities menu (see Figure A.13). The Transaction Entry dialog box lists existing transactions—both charges and payments—and provides options for editing existing transactions as well as creating new transactions.

Figure A.13

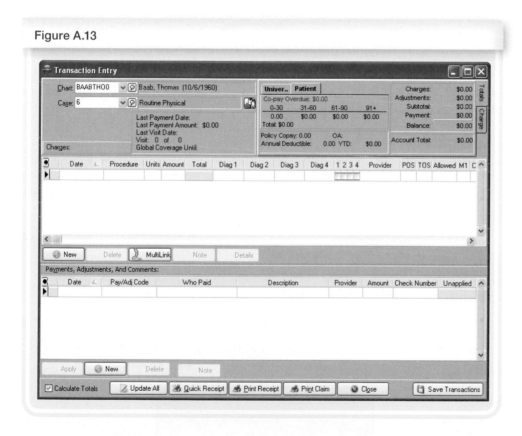

Entering Charges

To begin entering a new charge transaction, a patient's chart number is clicked on the drop-down list in the Chart box. After the chart number has been selected, the Case box displays a case number and description for a particular patient. If a patient has more than one open case, the drop-down list displays the full list of cases.

After the chart and case numbers have been entered, a new transaction is created by clicking the New button in the Charges section in the middle of the Transaction Entry dialog box.

Dates. When the New button is clicked, the program automatically enters the current date—that is, the Medisoft® Program Date—in the Date box. If this date is not the date the procedures were performed, the Medisoft® Program Date must be reset accordingly using the pop-up calendar inside the Date box. The date can also be changed by keying over the information that is already in the Date box. After the date is selected, the Tab key is pressed to move the cursor to the Procedure box.

Procedure. The procedure code for a service performed is selected from the drop-down list of CPT codes already entered in the system. Clicking inside the Procedure box displays a triangle button. When the triangle button is clicked, the drop-down list of procedure codes stored in the database is displayed. Only one procedure code can be selected for each transaction. If multiple procedures were performed for a patient, each one must be entered as a separate transaction.

After the CPT code is selected from the drop-down list and the Tab key is pressed, the charge for the procedure is displayed in the Amount box automatically.

Units. The Units box defaults to "1," but it can be changed if necessary.

Amount. The Amount box lists the charge amount for a procedure performed. The amount is entered automatically once a CPT code is entered.

Total. This field displays the total charges for the procedures performed. The system multiplies the number in the Units box by the number in the Amount box.

Diagnosis. The Diag 1, 2, 3, and 4 boxes correspond to the information in the Diagnosis tab of the Case folder. The patient's diagnoses are displayed automatically.

Provider. The Provider box lists the code number for a patient's assigned provider.

The remaining boxes in the Charges section display other information about the procedure selected. When all the charge information has been entered and checked for accuracy, it must be saved by clicking the Save Transactions button at the bottom of the Transaction Entry dialog box.

Special Note on Saving Transactions

As mentioned earlier, if the date of the transactions you are saving is later than the current date on your computer system (the Windows System Date), Medisoft® will display a Date of Service Validation box when you save the transactions you enter. This box asks you to confirm that you want to save the transactions, even though they have a future date. For the purposes of the projects and simulations in this text, which take place in 2014, click Yes each time this box appears.

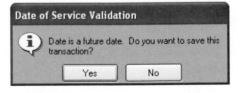

Entering Payments

Payments are entered in the Payments, Adjustments, And Comments section in the lower portion of the Transaction Entry dialog box. Just as when entering charges, a patient's chart number and case number must be selected before a transaction can be entered. A new payment transaction can be created or an existing transaction can be edited. To create a new payment transaction, the New button is clicked at the bottom of the Payments, Adjustments, And Comments section.

Date. When the New button is clicked, the program automatically enters the current date in the Date box. If this date is not the date the payment is being entered in the program, it must be edited. Once the correct date is displayed, the Tab key is pressed to move the cursor to the Pay/Adj Code box.

Pay/Adj Code. From the drop-down list in the Pay/Adj Code box, the type of payment is selected. For purposes of this text, the payment codes are

INSPAY	Insurance carrier payment
PACPAY	Patient payment, cash
PATPAY	Patient payment, check

Who Paid. After the code is selected and the Tab key is pressed, the program automatically completes the Who Paid box based on information stored in the database. The party that made the payment is selected from a drop-down list of guarantors and insurance carriers that are assigned in the patient case folder.

Description. The Description field can be used to enter a description of the payment received, if desired.

Amount. The amount of a payment is entered in the Amount box.

Check Number. If a payment is made by check, the check number is entered in this box.

After the boxes in the Payments, Adjustments, And Comments section of the Transaction Entry dialog box have been completed and checked for accuracy, the payment must be applied to charges. This is accomplished by clicking the Apply button at the bottom of the dialog box.

Clicking the Apply button displays the Apply Payment to Charges dialog box, which lists information about all unpaid charges for a patient, including the date of the procedure, the document number, the procedure code, the charge, the balance, and the total amount paid. In the top right corner of the dialog box, the amount of payment that has not yet been applied to charges is listed in the Unapplied box. Clicking the zeros in the This Payment box selects them, indicating that the box is active and ready for entry. The amount of the payment is entered and the Enter key is pressed.

Clicking the Close button exits the Apply Payment to Charges dialog box, and the Transaction Entry dialog box is again displayed. The payment is now listed in the list of transactions at the bottom of the dialog box with the Unapplied box at the end of the transaction line reduced to $0.00.

As with a charge transaction, when all the information on a payment transaction has been entered and checked for accuracy, it must be saved by clicking the Save Transactions button at the bottom of the Transaction Entry dialog box.

Printing Walkout Receipts

After transactions have been entered and saved in the Transaction Entry dialog box, a walkout receipt can be printed for a patient by clicking the Print Receipt button at the bottom of the Transaction Entry dialog box. (*Note:* Although the Quick Receipt button can also be used to print receipts, because of the likely difference in your computer's system date and the date used in the projects and simulations, the Print Receipt button should be used.)

The Open Report dialog box is displayed. Click Walkout Receipt (All Transactions) to select the report title, and then click the OK button.

Medisoft® then asks whether the report is to be previewed on the screen, sent directly to the printer, or exported to a file. If the report is to be previewed on screen, it can subsequently be printed directly from the Preview Report window. After the preview or print option is selected, the Data Selection Questions dialog box is displayed, confirming the date of the transaction. Clicking the OK button produces the report on screen or on paper.

Editing and Deleting Transactions

Transactions in the Transaction Entry dialog box are edited by clicking inside the appropriate box and then making the desired change. Transactions are deleted by clicking anywhere inside the transaction line and then clicking the Delete button at the bottom of the corresponding section—either the Charges section or the Payments, Adjustments, And Comments section. After changes or deletions are made, the data is saved by clicking the Save Transactions button.

OFFICE HOURS

The Office Hours scheduling program has its own menu bar and toolbar (see Figure A.14). The Office Hours menu bar lists the menus available: File, Edit, View, Lists, Reports, Tools, and Help. Under the menu bar is a toolbar with shortcut buttons. The functions of Office Hours are accessed by selecting a choice from one of the menus or by clicking a shortcut button.

Figure A.14

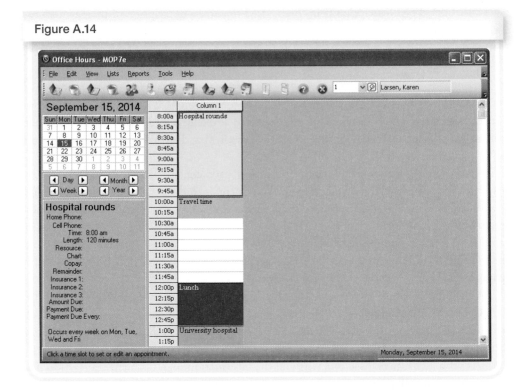

The Office Hours program uses the Windows System Date (rather than the Medisoft® Program Date) as the default date. Therefore, you will need to change the date in the Office Hours calendar regularly to correspond to the dates in the projects and simulations in this text.

The left half of the Office Hours screen displays the current date and a calendar of the current month. The current date is highlighted on the calendar. Clicking a different date on the calendar switches the schedule on the right side of the screen to the new day. Clicking the Go to Today shortcut button resets the screen to the current date (the Windows System Date).

The Office Hours schedule, shown in the right half of the screen, is a listing of time slots for a particular day for a specific provider.

Figure A.15

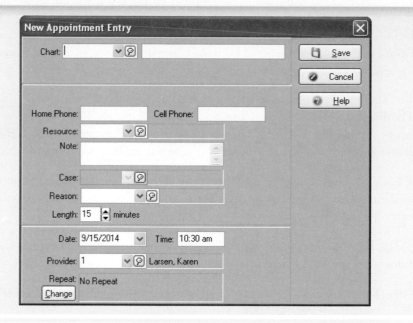

Starting and Exiting Office Hours

Office Hours can be started from within Medisoft® or directly from Windows. To access Office Hours from within Medisoft®, Appointment Book is clicked on the Activities menu. Office Hours can also be started by clicking the corresponding shortcut button on the Medisoft® toolbar.

To start Office Hours without entering Medisoft® first:

1. Click the Start button on the Windows task bar.
2. Click Medisoft® on the Program submenu.
3. Click Office Hours on the Medisoft® submenu.

The Office Hours program is closed by clicking Exit on the Office Hours File menu, or by clicking the Exit button on its toolbar. If Office Hours was started from within Medisoft®, exiting will return you to Medisoft®. If Office Hours was started directly from Windows, clicking Exit will return you to the Windows desktop.

Entering Appointments

Entering an appointment begins with selecting the provider for whom the appointment is being scheduled. The current provider is listed in the Provider box at the top right of the screen. Clicking the triangle button displays a drop-down list of providers in the system. To choose a different provider, click the name of the provider on the drop-down list.

After the provider is selected, the date of the desired appointment must be chosen. Dates are changed by clicking the Day, Week, Month, and Year right and left arrow buttons located under the calendar. After the provider and date have been selected, patient appointments can be entered.

Appointments are entered by clicking the Appointment Entry shortcut button or by double-clicking in a time slot on the schedule. When either action is taken, the New Appointment Entry dialog box is displayed (see Figure A.15). The program automatically enters information in the Length, Date, Time, and Provider fields.

The following are the main fields in the New Appointment Entry dialog box.

Chart. A patient's chart number is chosen from the Chart drop-down list. To select the desired patient, click the name and press the Enter or Tab key. If you are setting up an appointment for a new patient who has not been assigned a chart number, skip this box and key the patient's name in the Name box, the blank box to the right of the Chart box.

Once a patient's chart is selected from the Chart drop-down list and the Enter or Tab key is pressed, Medisoft® completes several other fields, including Name, Phone, and Case.

Length. The amount of time an appointment will take (in minutes) is entered in the Length box. The default entry is 15 minutes. To change the time, highlight 15 and key a new number (it must be a 15-minute increment, such as 30, 45, or 60). If an appointment is more than 15 minutes, the time slots below the first 15-minute slot on the schedule will be shaded.

Date. The Date box displays the date that is currently displayed on the calendar. If this is not the desired date, it may be changed by keying in a different date or by clicking the calendar button and selecting a date.

Time. The Time box displays the appointment time that is currently selected on the schedule. If this is not the desired time, it may be changed by keying in a different time.

Provider. The provider who will be treating the patient during this appointment is selected from the drop-down list of providers.

After the boxes in the New Appointment Entry dialog box have been completed, clicking the Save button enters the information on the schedule. The patient's name appears in the time slot corresponding to the appointment time. In addition, information about the appointment appears in the lower left corner of the Office Hours window.

Looking for a Future Date

Often a patient will need a follow-up appointment at a certain time in the future. For example, suppose a physician has seen a certain patient on a particular day and would like a checkup appointment in three weeks. The most efficient way to search for a future appointment in Office Hours is to use the Go to a Date shortcut button on the toolbar. (This feature can also be accessed on the Edit menu.)

Clicking the Go to a Date shortcut button displays the Go to Date dialog box. Within the dialog box, the Date From box indicates the current date in the appointment search. Four other boxes offer options for locating a date a specific number of days, weeks, months, or years in the future from the date indicated in the Date From box. After a number is entered in one of the four boxes, clicking the Go button closes the dialog box and begins the search. The system locates the future date and displays the calendar schedule for that date.

Searching for an Available Appointment Time

Often it is necessary to search for available appointment space on a particular day of the week and at a specific time. For example, a patient needs a 30-minute appointment and would like it to be during his lunch hour, which is from 12:00 P.M. to 1:00 P.M. He can get away from the office only on Mondays and Fridays. Office Hours makes it easy to locate an appointment slot that meets these requirements with the Search for Open Time Slot shortcut button.

Entering Appointments for New Patients

When a new patient phones the office for an appointment, the appointment can be scheduled in Office Hours before the patient information is entered in Medisoft®. Simply key the patient's information in the Name and Phone boxes in the New Appointment Entry dialog box. You do not need to assign a chart number at this time. The rest of the necessary information will be gathered when the patient comes in for the appointment and fills out a patient information form.

Creating Breaks

Office Hours provides features for inserting standard breaks in providers' schedules. The Office Hours break is a block of time when a physician is unavailable for appointments with patients. Examples of breaks include lunch breaks, meetings, surgery, and vacation. To set up a break, the desired provider is selected from the drop-down list in the Office Hours Provider box and then the Break Entry shortcut button is clicked (the second button from the left, which looks like a coffee cup in front of an appointment book). When the New Break Entry dialog box appears (see Figure A.16), the Name and Length fields are filled in to define the desired break.

Figure A.16

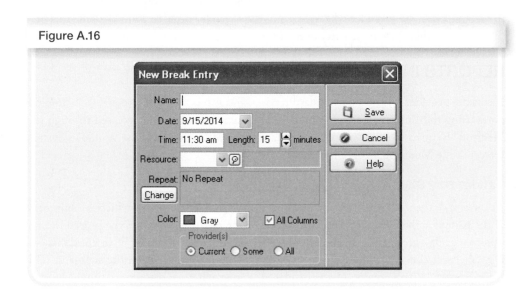

If the break is to be repeated (daily, weekly, monthly, or yearly), the Change button is used to define the frequency. When the Save button is clicked, the dialog box closes and the program enters the break in Office Hours automatically.

Changing or Deleting Appointments

It is often necessary to change a patient's appointment or cancel an appointment. Changing an appointment is accomplished with the Cut and Paste commands on the Office Hours Edit menu.

The following steps are used to reschedule an appointment:

1. Locate the appointment that needs to be changed. Make sure the appointment slot is visible on the schedule.

2. Click on the existing time-slot box. A black border surrounds the slot to indicate that it is selected.

3. Click Cut on the Edit menu. The appointment disappears from the schedule.

4. Click the date on the calendar when the appointment is to be rescheduled.

5. Click the desired time-slot box on the schedule. The slot becomes active.

6. Click Paste on the Edit menu. The patient's name appears in the new time-slot box.

The following steps are used to cancel an appointment without rescheduling:

1. Locate the appointment on the schedule.

2. Click the time-slot box to select the appointment.

3. Click Cut on the Edit menu. The appointment disappears from the schedule.

Previewing and Printing Schedules

In most medical offices, providers' schedules are printed on a daily basis. To view a list of all appointments for a provider for a given day, click Appointment List on the Office Hours Reports menu. The report can be previewed on screen, sent directly to the printer, or exported to a file. If the preview option is selected, the appointment list is displayed in a preview window. Various buttons are used to view the schedule at different sizes, to move from page to page, to print the schedule, and to save the schedule as a file. Clicking the Close button closes the preview window.

The schedule can also be printed by clicking the Print Appointment List shortcut button on the Office Hours toolbar, without using the Preview option. (Office Hours prints the schedule for the provider who is listed in the Provider box. To print the schedule of a different provider, change the entry in the Provider box before printing the schedule.)

REPORTS IN THE MEDICAL OFFICE

Medisoft® provides a variety of standard reports, and it has the ability to create custom reports using the Report Designer. Standard and custom reports are accessed through the Medisoft® Reports menu. Most of the standard Medisoft® reports use the Windows System Date, not the Medisoft® Program Date, as a default.

Patient Day Sheet

At the end of the day, many medical practices print a patient day sheet, which is a summary of the patient activity on that day. Medisoft®'s version of this report lists the procedures for a particular day, grouped by patient, in order by chart number. To print a patient day sheet, Day Sheets is clicked on the Reports menu and Patient Day Sheet on the submenu. The Print Report Where? dialog box is displayed, asking whether the report should be previewed on the screen, sent directly to the printer, or exported to a file.

When the Start button is clicked, the Search dialog box is displayed. This dialog box provides the opportunity to select the patients, dates, and providers for whom a report is being generated. If any box is left blank, all values are included in the report. When these selection boxes have been completed, the OK button is clicked and Medisoft® generates the report.

Procedure Day Sheet

A procedure day sheet lists all the procedures performed on a particular day and gives the dates, patients, document numbers, places of service, debits, and credits relating to these procedures. Procedures are listed in numeric order. Procedure day sheets are printed by clicking Day Sheets on the Reports menu and then Procedure Day Sheet on the submenu. The same Print Report Where? dialog box used for a patient day sheet is displayed. The report can be previewed on the screen, printed directly, or exported to a file.

Patient Statements

A patient statement lists the amount of money a patient owes, organized by the amount of time the money has been owed, the procedures performed, and the dates the procedures were performed. For the purposes of this text, the default statement format, known as Patient Statement (30, 60, 90), is used. The bottom of the report lists the total balance due, as well as the amount that is past due 30 days, 60 days, and 90 days.

Custom Reports

Clicking Custom Report List on the Reports menu displays a list of custom reports available in Medisoft®. The custom report list is used to view or print out a large variety of reports, including lists (such as patient lists and insurance carrier lists), insurance forms, and superbills.

AAMA (American Association of Medical Assistants) A national association providing continuing education, professional networking opportunities, and certification examinations to its members.

abandonment The physician's failure to furnish care for a particular illness for as long as it is required unless the patient has been discharged in an appropriate manner.

absolute accuracy Correctness that is 100 percent; correctness without error, required for handling financial transactions.

accepting assignment The agreement by a healthcare provider who participates in an insurance plan to accept the allowed charge as payment in full for services.

accession book A book containing a list of consecutive numbers used to assign each patient a number in practices where a numeric filing system is used; see also *numeric filing*.

accounting A system used to classify, record, and summarize financial transactions.

accounts payable (A/P) The unpaid amounts of money owed by the practice to creditors and/or suppliers.

accounts receivable (A/R) The unpaid amounts of money owed to the medical practice by patients and third-party payers.

accrual method The accounting method whereby income is recorded as soon as it is earned, whether or not payment is received; expenses are recorded when they are incurred.

accuracy Correctness, including attention to detail; the trait often ranked most important in assistants by physicians.

active files Those records belonging to patients currently seeing the physician.

administrative medical assistant The title given to medical office professionals who perform administrative tasks in a wide variety of settings.

agenda An outline of a meeting, specifying location, time, date, and major topics to be discussed.

aging reports Reports that show the passage of time between the issuing of a request for payment (invoice) and the receipt of payment; used to determine late payments and collect them.

AHDI (Association for Healthcare Documentation Integrity) A national organization that promotes professional standards and growth for the field of medical transcription.

AHIMA (American Health Information Management Association) A national organization that serves health information management professionals, keeps professionals current with legislation, and provides consumers of health services with topics of interest to them.

allowed charge The maximum amount that an insurer will pay for a service or procedure; also called "allowable," "maximum."

alphabetic filing A system of filing whereby documents are kept according to names, titles, or classifications in alphabetic order.

AMT (American Medical Technologists) A national organization that promotes professional standards and growth; certification available through the association's examination.

annotate The act of making notes that are either helpful or necessary in the margins of communications before forwarding them to the physician.

annual summary A report providing the monthly charges and payments for an entire year.

application software Computer programs that apply the computer's capabilities to specific uses, such as word processing, graphics, database management, and spreadsheets.

arbitration The process whereby a neutral third party judges the merits of a complaint by one party against another, with the consent of the parties; serves as an alternative to trial and the judgment is binding.

ARMA (Association of Records Managers and Administrators) An international association that includes among its members information managers, archivists, librarians, and educators; sets standards for filing, record retention, and other aspects of records management.

assault The clear threat of injury to another.

assertiveness The ability to step forward to make a point in a confident, positive manner.

assessment The physician's interpretation of subjective and objective findings as contained in the SOAP record; also called "diagnosis" or "impression."

assignment of benefits The permission given by a policyholder that allows a third-party payer to pay benefits directly to the healthcare provider.

audit A review of all financial data by an independent party outside the practice—the IRS or an accountant—to ensure the accuracy and completeness of all financial transactions.

authoritarian/autocratic A leadership style that provides clear and definitive expectations to team members.

authorization Expressed (stated) permission given by the physician and required to convey information about a patient to anyone (including the patient).

balance billing Collecting payment from the insured patient of the difference between a provider's usual fee and a payer's lower allowed charge.

balance sheet A report for a stated period indicating the practice's complete assets, liabilities, and capital.

bank reconciliation The process of comparing the balance on the monthly bank statement with the checkbook balance to determine whether there is agreement or a difference in the amounts.

basic insurance plan A policy that generally includes coverage of hospitalization, laboratory tests, surgery, and x-rays.

battery Any bodily contact without permission; in medicine, interpreted to include procedures performed without the patient's consent or those that go beyond the degree of consent given.

bibliography A list of all references used by an author in the preparation of a manuscript; listed in a separate section at the end of the text.

bioethics The branch of ethics that deals specifically with medical treatment, technology, and procedure; see also ethics.

birthday rule A guideline for determining which of two parents with medical coverage has the primary insurance for a child; states that the policy held by the insured with the earliest birthday in the calendar year is the primary policy.

blank endorsement The presence of only a signature to enable a check to be cashed or deposited; the most common form of endorsement.

block-style letter Arrangement of a letter so that all lines, including those beginning new paragraphs, begin at the left margin.

Blue Cross and Blue Shield Association (BCBS) One of the largest private-sector insurers in the United States; offers both indemnity and managed care plans with many variations.

bookkeeping The accurate recording of financial transactions.

Bound Printed Matter The classification of mail used for any material permanently bound by materials such as glue, staples, or spiral binding; at least 90 percent of the mailed materials must be imprinted materials composed by means other than handwriting; or typewriting; items may weigh up to 15 pounds and cost is determined by weight, distance, and shape.

capitation A form of payment made by the insurance company in advance of medical services received; the prepayment by the insurance carrier of a fixed amount to a physician to cover services for a member of a particular plan.

carrier An insurance company; also known as a third-party payer.

cash basis The system of accounting whereby charges for services are not recorded as income to the practice until payment is received and expenses are not recorded until they are paid.

CD-ROM drive An optical storage medium using a compact disk (CD); read only memory (ROM) means that the disk cannot record information but may be used to copy new programs onto the hard drive or to store information.

Centers for Medicare and Medicaid Services (CMS) The federal agency responsible for setting up the terms of Medicare and reviewing managed care plans that want to become Medicare-covered providers; part of the Department of Health and Human Services, CMS was called the Health Care Financing Administration (HCFA) before 2001.

Certificate of Mailing A receipt purchased at the time of mailing that documents the date the material was presented for mailing to the U.S. Postal Service.

certification An essential minimum standard of competence in a particular medical specialty, awarded by The American Board of Specialties; achieved through academic in-hospital training and successful completion of a comprehensive examination.

certified mail A service offered by the U.S. Postal Service whereby the Postal Service keeps a record of delivery and the sender receives a mailing receipt.

CHAMPVA Acronym for The Civilian Health and Medical Program of the Veteran's Administration; the government health insurance program that covers the medical expenses of families of veterans with total, permanent, service-connected disabilities; covers spouses and dependents of veterans who die as a result of injuries sustained in the line of duty.

channel The chosen method of transmitting the message.

charge/receipt slips Records of the doctor's services to each patient and the charges, combined with a tear-off receipt for the patient.

check A written order to a bank to pay a specific amount of money.

CHEDDAR A system of documenting medical data in a patient's chart using seven sequential categories: chief complaint, history, exam, details of problem/complaint, drug data, assessment, and return visit or referral.

chief complaint (CC) The reason for the patient's visit to seek the physician's advice.

chronological résumé The traditional and most common résumé style, which lists information in reverse chronological order.

clean claim A medical insurance claim that is free of errors and that can be adjudicated.

clearinghouse A service bureau that collects electronic claims from many different medical practices and forwards the claims to the appropriate insurance carriers.

closed files The records of those patients who have moved away from the area, died, or terminated their relationship with the physician.

cluster scheduling A method that brings several patients in at the same time, such as on the hour, to be seen by the provider; also known as wave scheduling.

CMS-1500 claim form A paper claim for physician services.

code linkage The connection between the diagnostic and procedural information, examined by insurance carriers to evaluate the medical necessity of the reported charges.

coding (1) The placing of a number, letter, color, or underscore beneath a word to indicate where a document should be filed; (2) the process of assigning codes to diagnoses and treatments based on standard code sets.

coinsurance The percentage of each claim that the insured person must pay; the percentage to be paid by the carrier is usually stated first as in "a rate of 80-20."

collection agency A business whose purpose is to collect unpaid debts for the creditor; usually used once other methods of securing payment have failed.

collection at the time of service The payment for services by patients at the time of the visit, by cash, check, or credit card where acceptable; the payment method required for insurance copayments.

collection ratio A percentage used to show the effectiveness of collection practices; the higher the collection ratio, the better the collection practices.

Collect on Delivery (COD) The U.S. Postal Service delivery service that collects postal and other fees from the recipient when the postal material is delivered.

color coding The organization of files according to a system of colored file folders.

compliance The act of adhering to legal rules and regulations as well as high ethical standards through practices and procedures within the medical practice, in all aspects of medical care.

confidentiality The legal requirement that a patient's medical information be kept secret except in certain clearly defined instances.

contributory negligence The failure of a patient to follow the advice and/or instructions of the physician, thus contributing to neglect or an outcome that may not be satisfactory.

coordination of benefits (COB) The clause in insurance policies which states that the insured who has two insurance policies may have only a maximum of 100 percent of the health costs.

copayment (copay) The set charge, required by HMOs and some other insurers, to be paid by patients every time they visit the physician's office.

cover/application letter A letter that introduces the applicant to the employer by supplying relevant information about the applicant as it relates to the available position.

CPT The initials used for *Current Procedural Terminology,* a book published by the American Medical Association and updated annually; contains the most commonly used system of procedure codes.

cross-reference sheet The indication, made on a sheet of paper or card, of other files where a copy of a particular document may be found.

customary fee A physician's charge for a procedure or service determined by what physicians with similar training and experience in a certain geographic area typically charge.

cuts Positions of tabs on folders.

cycle billing A method of billing patients designed to stabilize cash flow and workload; involves dividing patients into groups of a size roughly equal to the number of times that billing will take place during the month.

daily journal A record of services rendered by the physician, daily fees charged, and payments received; also called "general journal" or "daily earnings record."

database The complete history of a patient as contained in a problem-oriented medical record (POMR): includes the problem, medical, social, and family histories, a review of systems, and the physician's conclusions; also, any collection of related data, sets, or subsets of information.

database management application A software program that helps the user enter data and sort the data into useful subsets of information.

dead storage An area reserved for records that have been closed or that must be stored permanently; usually physically separate from where active files are kept.

decoding The application of meaning by the receiver of a transmitted message.

deductible A certain amount of medical expense the insured must incur before the insurance carrier will begin paying benefits.

deductions The amounts of money withheld from earnings to cover required taxes, insurance, and so on.

Defense Enrollment Eligibility Reporting System (DEERS) The system used to list individuals covered through TRICARE.

defensive medicine Those practices of the physician designed to help him or her avoid incurring lawsuits, such as ordering additional tests to confirm a diagnosis, as well as follow-up visits.

delegative/laissez faire A leadership style that uses a "hands-off" policy and tends to allow other office team members to make their own decisions.

Delivery Confirmation The U.S. Postal Service delivery service that provides the date and time of delivery or attempted delivery.

dependability The ability to complete work on schedule, do required tasks without complaint, and always communicate willingness to help; closely related to accuracy and thoroughness.

dependent A person related to a policyholder, such as a spouse or child.

deposition A sworn statement to the court before any trial begins and usually made outside of court.

deposits Checks or cash put into a bank account.

diagnosis (Dx) A term used interchangeably with "assessment" or "impression"; gives a name to the condition from which the patient is suffering.

diagnosis-related groups (DRGs) A system used by Medicare to establish payment for hospital stays; based on groupings of diagnostic codes that show the relative value of medical resources used throughout the nation for patients with similar conditions.

direct earnings Salaries paid to employees; see also *indirect earnings*.

disability insurance A plan that provides reimbursement for income lost when the insured person is unable to work because of illness or injury.

double-booking appointments The practice used, when the schedule is full, of entering overflow patient appointments in a second column beside regular appointments; in some cases, triple columns are used.

durable power of attorney A legal document giving a stated person the legal right to make decisions for another. This can be for medical decisions, financial decisions, or both.

editing The assessment of a document to determine its clarity, consistency, and overall effectiveness.

efficiency The ability to use time and other resources to avoid waste and unnecessary effort.

EFT The automatic withdrawal of employees' net pay from the practice account and the deposit to each employee's account; arranged for with the bank by the physician.

electronic claims Claims that are completed and transmitted to insurance companies by computer, with the assembling of data and completion of claims done using medical billing software.

electronic health records (EHRs) Healthcare databases compiled over the course of different patient encounters.

electronic mail service A service offered by the U.S. Postal Service allowing the secure transmission of documents over the Internet.

e-mail A telecommunications system for exchanging written messages through a computer network; also known as electronic mail.

emergency A medical status in which the delay of care of a serious injury or illness would threaten the patient's life or body part.

empathy Sensitivity to the feelings and situations of others that allows one to mentally put oneself in the other person's situation.

employer identification number (EIN) A tax identification number that employers are required to have by the Internal Revenue Service (IRS).

encoding Using words and gestures to convey a message.

endnotes References that the author may have used as background or relevant information, placed on a separate page following the text of the manuscript.

EOB The report sent to the patient and the healthcare provider by the insurance carrier informing them of the final reimbursement determination, explaining the decision, and appending reimbursement due the provider; used for paper claims.

ERA The report sent to the patient and healthcare provider by the insurance carrier informing them of the final reimbursement determination, and containing the same additional information as the EOB; used for electronic claims.

ergonomics The science of designing the work environment to meet the needs of the human body, while reducing the risks of injury or hazards without decreasing output.

established patient (EP) A patient who has seen the physician or a physician of the same specialty within the same practice group for three or more years.

e-signature A unique identifier created for each person through computer code; has the same legal standing as a printed signature.

ethics The standards of conduct that grow out of one's understanding of right and wrong.

ethnocentrism The tendency to believe that one's own race or ethnic group is the most important and that some or all aspects of its culture are superior to those of other groups.

etiquette Those behaviors and customs that are standards for what is considered good manners.

express consent The patient's approval, which may be given either orally or in writing; required for procedures that are not part of routine care.

Express Mail Service offered by the U.S. Postal Service that provides next day delivery of items.

family history (FH) Facts about the health of the patient's parents, siblings, and other blood relatives that might be significant to the patient's condition.

fee adjustment The reduction of a fee based on the physician's decision of the patient's need; see also *write off*.

feedback A receiver's response(s) to a message.

fee-for-service A payment method through an insurance carrier whereby the patient (policyholder) pays for medical services at the time of receiving them and is reimbursed by the insurance company once it has reviewed and approved a claim describing the services; alternately, the policyholder's directive that the carrier pay the service provider directly once services are received.

fee schedule A list maintained by each physician or medical practice of the usual procedures the office performs and the corresponding charges.

FICA The law that governs the Social Security system and requires that a certain amount of money be withheld for Social Security benefits; employer pays half the amount withdrawn and employee pays the other half.

file server A central computer within a computer network, used to store the computer programs and data that must be shared by all the computers in the network; also called, simply, a "server."

first-class mail The classification of mail weighing 13 ounces or less, which includes all correspondence, whether handwritten or typewritten, such as bills and statements of account, and is sealed against postal inspection.

first draft The first complete keying of a manuscript.

fixed office hours Designated hours during which the doctor is available for appointments; patients sign in with the receptionist and are seen in the order in which they arrive and sign in.

flexibility Adaptability to new or changing requirements.

folders Containers used to hold those items that are to be filed; frequently made of a sturdy material to withstand handling.

footnotes Notes, usually at the bottom of a page, used to cite sources of information or quotations used in the text.

fraud An intentionally dishonest practice that deprives others of their rights, such as falsifying credentials or submitting false or duplicate insurance claims.

full endorsement The signature on a check indicating the person, account number, or bank to which the check is being transferred, and the payee's name.

functional résumé The résumé format in which skills and accomplishments are organized into data groups that directly support the position goal.

FUTA The federal law that requires employers to pay a percentage of each employee's salary; the amount paid provides a fund for employees once they are unemployed and seeking new jobs.

good judgment The ability to use knowledge, experience, and logic to assess all aspects of a situation in order to reach a sound decision.

Good Samaritan Act A law designed to protect a physician who provides emergency care from liabilities for civil damages that may arise from the circumstances.

graphics application A software program that allows the user to manipulate images and to create original images electronically.

guarantor The insurance policyholder for a patient.

guide A rigid divider placed at the end of a section of files to indicate where a new section or category of files begins.

hard drive A nonremovable disk built into the computer that serves as the computer's central "filing cabinet."

HCFA-1500 See *CMS-1500 claim form.*

HCPCS Pronounced "hic-pics"; stands for Health Care Financing Administration's Common Procedure Coding System, for use in coding services for Medicare patients.

Health Insurance Portability and Accountability Act (HIPAA) The federal law that protects the security and privacy of health information by regulating how electronic patient information is stored and shared.

hidden job markets Employment markets that are less obvious and require more initiative by the job seekers to access.

history of present illness (HPI) Information taken from the patient about symptoms: when they began, what factors affect them, what the patient thinks is the cause, remedies tried, and any past treatment for the symptoms.

HMO (health maintenance organization) The oldest form of managed care; a medical center or designated group of physicians provides medical services to insured persons for a monthly or annual premium.

honesty Truth telling, expressed in words and actions; a quality that enables the person to be trusted at all times and in all situations.

hospital insurance Provides protection against the cost of hospital care and generally provides a room allowance for a maximum number of days per year; provisions exist for operating room charges, x-rays, lab work, drugs, and other necessary items during the patient's hospital stay.

IAAP A worldwide organization that sponsors continuing education and a certification examination with the successful completion earning the designation of Certified Professional Secretary (CPS); also works with employers to promote excellence; formerly known as Professional Secretaries International (PSI).

ICD-9-CM (International Classification of Diseases, 9th Revision, Clinical Modification) A list of codes for diseases and conditions required for use in government healthcare programs and generally adopted by the healthcare profession.

implied consent The patient's agreement that is not stated outright but is shown by the patient's having gone to the doctor's office for treatment.

impression A term used interchangeably with "assessment" or "diagnosis"; gives a name to the condition from which the patient is suffering.

inactive files The records of those patients who have not seen the doctor for six months or longer.

income statement A financial statement showing profit and loss for a stated period of time, such as a quarter or a year.

indemnity plan An insurance plan that provides a percentage of payment to the physician on a fee-for-service basis; the patient assumes responsibility for the remaining portion of the cost.

indexing The process of selecting the name, title, or classification under which a document or an item will be filed.

indirect earnings Amounts of money other than salary supplied to the employee, such as paid leave; also benefits such as employer-paid benefit programs that are worth amounts of money.

informed consent The ability of the patient to make a sound decision to agree because the problem has been explained in clear language and the physician has given both treatment options and a prognosis.

initiative The exercise of one's power to act independently.

input Data and instructions from a computer user, provided to the computer through input devices, the most common of which is the keyboard.

inspecting documents The act of checking each item received for filing to be sure that the information is complete and that the item is in good physical condition.

insured May be the person who takes out an insurance policy and is responsible for the payments; may also refer to anyone, such as a spouse or dependent, covered by an insurance policy.

insured mail Articles sent through the U.S. Postal Service or other carriers that are covered against loss or damage through the purchase or provision of insurance.

interest Money paid by the bank to depositors in return for the use of the depositor's money.

Internet A vast, worldwide computer network that links millions of computers; enables almost instantaneous sharing of information in various digital forms—text, graphics, sound, video, and so on.

itinerary A daily schedule of events for a traveler, containing such information as flight numbers and times and hotel and car arrangements.

keywords Words used throughout the résumé that directly relate to the position requirements.

label An oblong piece of paper, frequently adhesive, used to identify a file by title or subject.

laptop A portable computer, designed to fit into a briefcase; able to run on either plug-in current or batteries.

lateral files Drawers or shelves that open horizontally where files are arranged sideways from left to right instead of from front to back.

liability Legal responsibility.

licensure The act of the state whereby healthcare providers, and those in other professions, are granted licenses to practice

under certain conditions, including meeting the requirements of education and training.

litigation The bringing of lawsuits against an individual or other entity.

living will A written document providing directions for medical care to be given if a competent adult becomes incapacitated or otherwise unable to make decisions personally; also know as an advance directive.

mainframe A computer designed to store massive databases that many users may all access at the same time.

major medical insurance A policy that offers protection from large medical expenses.

malpractice An act that a reasonable and prudent physician would not do, or the failure to do some act that such a physician would do.

managed care A system that combines the financing and delivery of healthcare services to members.

management qualifications Usually regarded, for the administrative medical assistant, as the ability to be a team player; the ability to do strategic planning; and the ability to increase productivity.

maturity Emotional and psychological integrity composed of many qualities and skills.

Media Mail The rate used by the U.S. Postal Service for the mailing of books, videotapes, looseleaf pages, and binders; also called "Book Rate."

Medicaid A health benefit program, jointly funded by federal and state governments, designed for people with low incomes who cannot afford medical care.

medical insurance Insurance that covers benefits for outpatient medical care.

medical practice acts The laws of each state governing who must be licensed to give care, the rules for obtaining licensure, the grounds for revoking licenses, and the reports required by state law.

Medicare The federal health plan that provides insurance to citizens and permanent United States residents 65 years and older, people with disabilities (including kidney failure), and dependent widows; divided into Part A, hospitalization insurance, and Part B, medical insurance.

medicolegal A type of document that provides evidence of patient care and is considered a legal document in a court of law.

meeting minutes Official record of a meeting, including the major pieces of business conducted; the names and contributions of any attendees who spoke; the date, place, and time of the meeting; those present and absent; and the duration of the meeting.

Message ideas formulated by the sender to be received by the recipient.

micrographics The process of storing records in miniaturized images, usually in a microfiche sheet or ultrafiche format, viewed on readers that enlarge the image.

minicomputer A computer having less power than a mainframe; may operate for a single user or along with many terminals.

mobile-aisle files Open-shelf files that are moved manually or by motor.

modem A computer component that allows computers to communicate through telephone lines.

modified-block-style letter The arrangement of a letter whereby the date line, complimentary closing, and signature all begin at the center of the page and all other lines begin at the left margin.

monitor The display screen attached to the computer that shows to the user the results of commands, instructions to the computer, and data input.

monthly billing The system of sending each patient an updated statement of payments made and charges owed to the physician once per month; these are all sent from the office at the same time every month.

monthly summary The report that shows the daily charges and payments for the entire month.

networking A means of communicating, exchanging information, and pooling resources among a group of electronically linked computers.

new patient (NP) A patient who has not seen the physician or a physician of the same specialty within the same practice group for three or more years.

no shows A patient who, without notifying the physician's office, fails to show up for an appointment.

noise Internal and external interference with the communication process.

numeric filing A system of document storage in which each patient is assigned a number; see also *accession book*.

objective The physician's examination of the patient contained in the SOAP record; results of the examination may be shown under the heading "Physical Examination (PE)."

OCR Optical character reader equipment used to scan materials for data, such as a ZIP code.

online Connected to a computer network for purposes of communicating, gathering, or exchanging information.

open office hours A method of seeing patients during hours when the physician is available and no appointment is made, such as from 10 a.m. to noon; patients are seen on a first-come-first-seen basis.

open punctuation No punctuation used outside the body of a letter unless the line ends with an abbreviation.

open-shelf files Shelves that hold files, may be adjustable or fixed, and may extend from floor to ceiling; shelves accept files placed sideways with identifying tabs protruding.

operating system The internal programming that tells the computer how to use its own components by controlling the basic functions of the computer and directing the computer to interact with the user and with input and output devices.

out guide A card placed as a substitute for a file folder; indicates that a file has been removed.

output Processed data sent back to the user by the computer through output devices, such as a monitor.

output device A device used to display electronic data.

outside services file A list of professional and other resources kept in either a paper or electronic format.

palm computer A version of the personal computer small enough to be held in the palm of the hand; less powerful than other personal computers but usually has e-mail, fax, and other features; also called "palmtop" or, technically, "personal digital assistant (PDA)."

participating (PAR) provider A physician who joins an insurance plan and agrees to provide services according to the rules and payment schedules of the insurance plan.

parcel post The classification of mail for items 70 pounds or less and no more than 130 inches in length and girth; mailing fee is based on weight, distance to travel, and shape.

participative/democratic A leadership style in which the leader offers advice but also participates in the team dynamics and seeks input from other team members.

password A code assigned to a computer user as a security measure; limits access to computer files and safeguards information.

past medical history (PMH) A listing of any illnesses the patient has had in the past; includes treatments and procedures performed.

patient education materials Printed materials provided to patients to give information on caring for their health, lists of resources, descriptions of frequently requested tests and procedures, and the like.

patient encounter form The list made of procedures, diagnoses, and charges during any particular patient visit.

patient information brochure A booklet that provides vital information about the practice, such as services offered; qualifications of the physicians; instructions for making appointments; and ordering refills of prescriptions.

patient information form A form used to collect a patient's personal and insurance information; usually updated at least every 12 months.

patient statement   The copy provided to the patient of all charges incurred by the patient and all payments made by the patient or the patient's insurance company; also called the "patient bill."

payroll   The total earnings of all the employees in the practice.

perfectionism   setting unrealistic expectations and goals and being dissatisfied with anything less.

personal computer   A computer designed for one user; may reside on a desktop or may be portable, as laptop and notebook computers are; referred to as "PCs" or, less frequently, as "microcomputers."

personal reference   An individual who knows a job seeker's personal ethics, honesty, and trustworthiness.

petty cash fund   A fund containing small amounts of cash used for expenses so minor that checks would not be written to pay them: postage stamps, cab fares, and the like.

physical exam (PE)   A complete examination of the patient in which findings for each of the major areas of the body are stated or an examination that covers only the body systems pertinent to that particular visit.

plan   The treatment, as stated in the SOAP record, listing prescribed medication, instructions given to the patient, and recommendation for surgery or hospitalization.

plain text résumés   résumés with simplified formatting; used to submit an online résumé.

policies and procedures manual   An employee handbook that contains job descriptions, job responsibilities, instructions for completing routine tasks, personnel policies, and so on.

Postnet   A bar code interpretation of the ZIP code or the ZIP+4 consisting of a series of long and short vertical lines which is placed on the lower portion of the mailing address.

posting   The activity of transferring an amount from one record to another.

power words   Action verbs used to showcase your skills.

PPO (preferred provider organization)   A popular type of managed care plan that contracts to perform services for members at specified rates, usually lower than fees charged to regular patients; also provides members with a list of healthcare providers from which to receive services at lower PPO rates.

practice analysis report   The report used to analyze the revenue of the practice during any specified length of time; contains lab charges, patient payments, copayments, adjustments, and so on.

preauthorization   The requirement by HMOs and some other insurance plans that the physician obtain permission from the insurance plan before delivering certain types of services.

premium   The rate charged to a person who holds an insurance policy; usually paid on a regular basis, monthly or quarterly.

primary care provider (PCP)   The physician who coordinates the patient's overall care and ensures that various medical services are necessary; described as a "gatekeeper" and is often an internist or a general practitioner.

printer   A computer output device that produces a hardcopy of electronic information or images.

Priority Mail   A service offered by the U.S. Postal Service; two-day delivery service within most domestic destinations.

problem-oriented medical record (POMR)   A patient record organized around a list of the patient's complaints or problems; contains a database of the patient's history, initial plan, and problem list.

problem-solving   The ability to find solutions through flexibility, advice seeking, information gathering, and good judgment.

procedure day sheet   A numeric listing of all the procedures performed on a given day; includes patient names, document numbers, and places of service; may be a computerized journal form.

professional image   The appearance, manner, and bearing that reflect health, cleanliness, and wholesomeness; shown by evidence of healthful habits, good grooming, and appropriate dress.

professional reference   An individual who knows a job seeker's work ethics and skills.

proofreading   The careful reading and examination of a document for the sole purpose of finding and correcting errors.

provider   A physician or other healthcare professional.

punctuality   The ability to be on time.

reasonable fee   A charge for the physician's service that is a usual and stated charge and/or the charge by physicians in the geographic area with similar experience.

records management   The systematic control of the steps in the life of a record, from its creation through its maintenance to its disposition.

Red Flag Requirements   Mandated federal regulations that must be implemented by creditors to protect covered financial accounts from identity theft.

referral   The recommendation from the primary care provider (PCP) that the patient use a specialist for a specific service; in the referral document, the PCP names the provider and states the service.

registered mail   Items sent through the U.S. Postal Service for which a delivery record is maintained at the mailing post office; receipt is given to the sender at the time of mailing.

registration   A permit granted to a physician for prescribing and dispensing pharmaceutical medications.

relative value scale (RVS)   The assignment of values to medical services based on an analysis of the skill and time required to provide them; values are multiplied by a dollar conversion factor to calculate fees.

release of information Written permission signed by the patient, authorizing the proper transfer of information to those who have made a legitimate request or have a legitimate need; often called simply a "release."

releasing The indication, by initial or by some other agreed–upon mark, that a document has been inspected and acted upon and is ready for filing.

reprints Copies of an already published article; available from the publisher for a small fee or free when the physician is the author.

resource-based relative value scale The payment system used by Medicare; establishes relative value units for services based on what each service costs to provide.

Restricted Delivery Direct delivery through the U.S. Postal Service; item delivered only to the addressee or addressee's authorized agent.

restrictive endorsement Signing, or endorsing, of a check by writing, or stamping "For Deposit Only," the account number to which the check should be deposited, and the signature.

retention The length of time that records are kept; regulated in many cases by state law; also regulated by Medicare regulations.

return receipt A piece of paper provided by the U.S. Postal Service to give the sender proof of delivery.

review of systems (ROS) The physician's specific questions to the patient about each of the body's systems.

ROM (read-only memory) The permanent memory of the computer.

rotary circular file A small desktop file designed to rotate, thus permitting the use of both sides of an index card.

rule out (R/O) A possible diagnosis that must be proved or "ruled out" by further tests.

scannable résumé A format style used for résumés read by optical character readers.

scanner A computer input device that takes a picture of a printed page or graphic and copies it into the computer's memory.

screening calls The practice of evaluating calls to decide on appropriate appointment action.

scrubber program Software used to detect and correct medical insurance claims prior to being submitted to the insurance carrier.

self-motivation The quality expressed by willingness to contribute without being asked or required to undertake a task.

settlement An agreement by parties on opposing sides; may be the result of a court decision or an agreement arrived at without trial; may involve compensation to the complaining party.

simplified-style letter The arrangement of a letter in such a way that all lines begin at the left margin, a subject line substitutes for the salutation, and the complimentary closing is eliminated; open punctuation is used and the writer's name is in all capital letters on one line.

Signature Confirmation of Delivery U. S. Postal Service delivery service that provides the date, ZIP, time of delivery (or attempt), and signature of the person who accepted the delivery.

SOAP An acronym used to refer to the most common system for outlining and structuring notes on a patient's chart; the acronym stands for the headings used: Subjective, Objective, Assessment, and Plan.

social history (SH) Information that may be pertinent to treatment regarding the patient's marital history, occupation, interests, and eating, drinking, and smoking habits.

sorting The arrangement of documents in the order in which they will be filed.

sponsor The TRICARE and CHAMPVA term for enlisted military personnel through whom medical coverage is provided.

spreadsheet programs Software used for financial planning and budgeting.

standard punctuation The placing of a colon after the salutation of a letter and the placing of a comma after the complimentary closing.

statute of limitations A law made by each state government setting a time limit beyond which the collection of a debt, or the prosecution of many kinds of crimes, is not subject to legal action; varies from three to eight years.

statutory reports Information of a confidential nature that is required by law to be filed with state departments of health or social services.

storing The placement of an item in its correct place in a file; also called "filing."

stress Emotional and/or physiological reactions to external motivators.

subject filing A system of document storing whereby the placement of related material is alphabetic by subject categories.

subjective The patient's description of the problem or complaint, including symptoms, when symptoms began, associated factors, remedies tried, and past medical history.

subpoena A legal document ordering that all materials related to a lawsuit be delivered to court; also, a legal document requiring people to divulge information.

subpoena duces tecum A legal order for a person to appear, testify, and present specified documents.

summons A written notice to the person being sued (defendant), ordering the person to answer charges presented in the document.

supercomputer The most powerful computers available.

surgical insurance Provides protection for the cost of the surgeon's fee for performing surgery; generally includes coverage for the cost of anesthesia.

tab A projection that extends beyond the rest of the file folder so that the folder may be labeled and easily viewed.

tact The ability to speak and act considerately, especially in difficult situations.

team player One who is generous with his of her time, helping other staff members when necessary; who observes both the written and unwritten rules of the office; and who practices professional and personal courtesy.

telephone etiquette A set of skills and attitudes used when answering the phone that allows the assistant to sound alert, interested, and concerned.

template A standard electronic version of a frequently used document; may be altered slightly from one use to the next; saves user time in keying and formatting commonly used documents and forms.

terminated account The account of a patient from whom it has not been possible to extract payment; also the status of accounts at the end of the patient-physician relationship for other reasons.

third-party liability The assumption of responsibility for charges related to a patient by someone other than the patient—for example, children of aged parents.

third-party payer An insurance company that agrees to carry the risk of paying for medical services for the insured.

thoroughness The ability to perform tasks with attention to completeness, correctness, and detail.

title page The first manuscript page, which contains the title of the manuscript and the author's name, degree and/or title, and affiliation.

transcription A method of recording data whereby the medical provider dictates data into a recording device and an individual trained in medical keyboarding skills keys the information into documentation format.

travel agent A professional, often certified by the travel industry, who may work independently or within a travel company; handles all aspects of travel arrangements at no charge to the customer.

triage The determination of how soon a patient needs to be seen by the physician based on whether the patient's condition requires immediate attention.

TRICARE The Department of Defense health insurance plan for military personnel and their families; coverage extends to active or retired members of the U.S. Army, Navy, Marines, Air Force, Coast Guard, Public Health Service, and National Oceanic and Atmospheric Administration, and dependents of military personnel killed on active duty; formerly called CHAMPUS.

urgent A medical injury or illness, though not life threatening, that needs prompt medical attention within a 24-hour time period in order to prevent serious decline of the patient's condition

usual fee A healthcare provider's average charge for a certain procedure or service, usually shown on the physician's fee schedule.

vertical files Drawer files, contained in cabinets of various sizes; files are arranged from front to back.

visible job markets Employment markets composed of resources that are traditional and most obvious.

virus A malicious computer program written with the intent of harming other data, software, and/or computers.

voice recognition technology A program used along with a word processing application to transcribe spoken words into text without the use of a keyboard.

wave scheduling Fixed office hours combined with scheduled office appointments for a specific number of patients.

wireless communication The use of radio waves rather than wires or cables to transmit data through a computer network.

word processing program Software used to enter, edit, format, and print documents.

work ethic The collective habits and skills that help the worker deal effectively with work tasks and with people.

workers' compensation State law and insurance plan requiring employers to obtain insurance in case of employee accident or injury.

write-off The subtraction of an amount from a patient's bill; entered into the patient ledger as an adjustment.

ZIP abbreviation for Zone Improvement Plan which is a system of the U.S. Postal Service of designating delivery of mail based on numerical codes.

ZIP+4 an extension of the postal ZIP system that adds an additional four codes which represent a geographic segment such as a building number to the original ZIP code.

Zip drive A small disk drive that may be installed inside a PC or operated externally; stores large files or creates archives of files for long-term storage.

Blackett, Karine B. *Career Achievement: Growing Your Goals.* New York: McGraw-Hill, 2011.

Clinical and Admininistrative Skills of the AMA (AAMA). November 2009. American Association of Medical Assistants, The CMA (AAMA). 6 July 2010. http://aama-ntl.org/resources/library/OA.pdf.

Cultural Clues Communicating with Your Deaf Patient. April 2007. University of Washington Medical Center. 6 July 2010. http://depts.washington.edu/pfes/PDFs/DeafCultureClue.pdf.

Eischen, Clifford, and Lynn Eischen. *Resumes, Cover Letters, Networking, and Interviewing.* 3d ed. Mason: South-Western Cengage Learning, 2010.

Informed Consent. July 2009. American Cancer Society. 6 July 2010. www.cancer.org/Treatment/FindingandPayingforTreatment/UnderstandingFinancialandLegalMatters/InformedConsent/index.htm.

Interagency Security Committee. *Best Practices for Safe Mail Handling.* U.S. Department of Homeland Security. 6 July 2010. www.oca.gsa.gov or www.dhs.gov/xlibrary/assets/isc_safe_mail_handling-2007.pdf.

Official "Do Not Use" List. March 2009. The Joint Commission. 6 July 2010. www.jointcommission.org/NR/rdonlyres/2329F8F5-6EC5-4E21-B932-54B2B7D53F00/0/dnu_list.pdf.

Sabin, William A. *The Gregg Reference Manual Tribute Edition.* 11th ed. New York: McGraw-Hill, 2011.

Stein, Loren. *Glossary of Medical Specialties.* February 2009. Blue Cross Blue Shield of Massachusetts, Consumer Health Interactive. 6 July 2010. www.ahealthyme.com/topic/medglossary.

U.S. Department of Labor, Bureau of Labor Statistics. *Occupational Outlook Handbook, 2010–11 Edition.* 28 June 2010. www.bls.gov/oco/ocos164.htm.

Yena, Donna J. *Career Directions: The Path to Your Ideal Career.* 5th ed. New York: McGraw-Hill, 2011.

Photo Credits

Index

A

AAMA. *See* American Association of Medical Assistants
AAMT (American Association of Medical Transcription), 18
AAPC (American Academy of Professional Coders), 18–19, 37
Abandonment, 45
Abbreviations
    medical, 166–168
    of patient names, 159
    state, 114
    in transcription, B-4
ABN (advance beneficiary notice for uncovered services), 274
Absence of doctor, duties related to, 199–200
Absolute accuracy, 298
Acceptable use policy (AUP), 133
Accepting assignment, 231–233
Access to information, 44, 47–50
Accession book, 161
Account tab (Medisoft®), A-11
Accounting, 292
Accounting software, 293, 295
Accounts payable (A/P), 292
Accounts receivable (A/R), 292
"Accounts Receivable Control" section, 293
Accrual method, 292
Accuracy
    of banking tasks, 298
    of claim information, 265–266
    of documentation, 12, 58
    of financial records, 293
Acknowledgement letters, 79
Acknowledgment of Receipt of Notice of Privacy Practices, 54
Acquired immunodeficiency syndrome (AIDS), 56
Acronyms, medical, 166–168
Action verbs, 327
Active files, 149
Add-on codes, 239
Adjustment factor, 233
Administrative duties, 5, 187. *See also* Office management; *specific duty*
Administrative medical assistant, 3–28
    employment opportunities, 9–11
    ethical responsibility, 36–37
    interpersonal skills, 7, 19–24
    personal attributes, 7–9
    professional growth and certification, 17–19, 40
    professional image, 15–17
    role in compliance, 6, 22, 58
    skills, 5–7
    tasks, 4–5
    work ethic, 11–15
Administrative Simplification (HIPAA), 50

Admissions, hospital, 111–112
Advance beneficiary notice for uncovered services (ABN), 274
Advertisements, job, 320
Agenda, meeting, 201–202
Aging-family caregiver, 190
Aging reports, 260, 295–296
AHDI (Association for Healthcare Documentation Integrity), 18, 40, B-2
AHIMA. *See* American Health Information Management Association
AIDS (acquired immunodeficiency syndrome), 56
Allowed charge, 231
Alphabetic filing, 157–161
Alphabetic Index *(ICD-9-CM)*, 235–238
AMA. *See* American Medical Association
American Academy of Professional Coders (AAPC), 18–19, 37
American Association of Medical Assistants (AAMA), 18
    certification, 17
    Code of Ethics and Creed, 36–37
    Role Delineation Chart, 4
American Association of Medical Transcription (AAMT), 18
American Board of Specialties, 40
American Health Information Management Association (AHIMA), 18
    certification, 18–19
    code of ethics, 37
    record retention guidelines, 150, 151
American Medical Association (AMA)
    Council on Ethical and Judicial Affairs, 147
    Current Procedural Coding (See CPT-4)
    journals, 196–197
    Manual of Style, 86
    medical specialties, 9–10
    Principles of Medical Ethics, 36–37
American Medical Technologists (AMT), 18
Anger management, 193
Annotation, 113
Annual summary, 292
Answering services, 96
Appealing claims, 264–265
Appearance, 75
Application software, 135
Applications. *See* Job applications
Appointment(s)
    canceling, 110
    emergency, 108
    extended, 109
    irregular, 108–109
    length of time required for, 102–103
    next, 110–111
    no shows, 104, 110
    out-of-office, 111–112
    patient arrival registration, 21–22, 109–110, 189

    patients late for, 108–109
    rescheduling, 110, 128
    same-day, 104, 106, 107
    scheduled, 103, 105
    stat, 104, 106
    See also Scheduling
Appointment cards, 111
Arabic numerals, 160, B-5
Arbitration, 47
ARMA (Association of Records Managers and Administrators), 151, 158
Arrivals, registering, 21–22, 109–110, 189
Assault, 45–46
Assertiveness, 15
Assessment, 143
Assignment of benefits, 231–233
Association for Healthcare Documentation Integrity (AHDI), 18, 40, B-2
Association of Records Managers and Administrators (ARMA), 151, 158
Attire, 75, 211, 337–338
Audit, 58, 292
Audit trails, inspection of, 137–138
AUP (acceptable use policy), 133
Authoritarian/autocratic leader, 195
Authorization, 47–48, 55
Automated phone systems, 98

B

Backing up data, 138
Backup procedures (Medisoft®), A-1 to A-3
Balance billing, 231
Balance sheet, 293
Bank reconciliation, 301–303
Banking, 298–304
    accuracy in, 298
    checks and checking, 272, 298–300
    electronic, 303–304
    office policy, 301
Basic insurance plan, 223
Battery, 45–46
BCBS (Blue Cross and Blue Shield Association), 11, 227, 262
Benefit policies (employee), 211
Best Practices for Safe Mail Handling, 113
Bibliography, 86
Billing, 256–260
    AMA tasks, 5
    balance, 231
    compliance issues, 57, 231, 261, 269, 273
    computerized, 132, 259–260, 266
    confidentiality issues, 230, 269, 275, 292
    for copied medical records, 148
    delinquent accounts (*See* Collection(s))
    fee schedules, 231, 233, 258
    patient encounter form, 234–235, 256–258

patient statements, 258–259, 272, A-20
policy and procedures, 209
schedules, 272
See also Payment(s)
Bioethics, 37–38
Birthday rule, 223
Blank endorsement, 299
Block-style letter, 76–77
Blue Cross and Blue Shield Association (BCBS), 11, 227, 262
Board certification, 40
Body language, 5, 7, 74–75
The Book of Style for Medical Transcription (AHDI), B-2
Bookkeeping, 292, 294–295
Bound Printed Matter, 114
Bullet (•), 239
Bullet inside circle (⊙), 239
Bulletin boards (e-mail), 196
Business associates, HIPAA compliance, 51, 54
Business names, alphabetic filing rules, 159–160

C

CAAHEP (Commission on Accreditation for Allied Health Education Programs), 17
Calendars, 193
Cancellations
fees, 273
patient appointments, 110
travel arrangements, 199
CAP (Certified Administrative Professional), 18
Capitalization, B-3
Capitation payments, 224–225
Care facilities, employment opportunities, 11
Career fairs, 320–321
Career objective, 329
Caregivers, stress on, 190–191
Carrier (insurance), 222
Cash basis, 292
Cash payments, 272, 300, 304
CC (chief complaint), 103, 142
CCA (Certified Coding Association), 18
CCS (Certified Coding Specialist), 18
CCS-P (Certified Coding Specialist-Physician Based), 18
Centers for Medicare and Medicaid Services (CMS), 51, 231
CMS-1500 claim form, 261–262, 266–268
Centralized files, 152
Certificate of Mailing, 114, 115
Certification
of administrative medical assistants, 17–19, 40
of medical specialists, 40
retention of, 150
Certified Administrative Professional (CAP), 18
Certified Coding Association (CCA), 18
Certified Coding Specialist (CCS), 18

Certified Coding Specialist-Physician Based (CCS-P), 18
Certified Interventional Radiology Cardiovascular Coder (CIRCC), 18
Certified Mail, 114
Certified Medical Administrative Specialist (CMAS), 18
Certified Medical Assistant (CMA), 17
Certified Medical Transcriptionist (CMT), 18, 40
Certified Professional Coder (CPC), 18, 40
Certified Professional Coder-Outpatient Hospital (CPC-H), 18
Certified Professional Coder-Payer (CPC-P), 18
Certified Professional Secretary (CPS), 18
CEUs (continuing education units), 40
Chamber of Commerce, 322
CHAMPUS (TRICARE), 11, 228
CHAMPVA, 228
Channel, 72–73
Charge/receipt slips, 292
Charge slip (patient encounter form), 234–235, 256–258
Charges section (Medisoft®), A-12 to A-13
Chart notes, 139–140
appointment changes, 110
format, 141–147
telephone messages, 101, 140
See also Medical records
Chart number (Medisoft®), A-9
Checks and checking, 272, 298–300
CHEDDAR method, 145–146
Cheerfulness, 8
Chicago Manual of Style, 86
Chief complaint (CC), 103, 142
Chief compliance officer, 58
Chronological résumé, 329–331
CIGNA, 11
CIRCC (Certified Interventional Radiology Cardiovascular Coder), 18
Circular communication cycle, 72–73
Civil law, 46
Claims. *See* Medical insurance claims
Clean claim, 369
Clearinghouse, 51, 269
Clinical forms, 140
Clinical work, computers in, 133
Clinics, employment opportunities, 11
Closed files, 150
Clothing, 75, 211, 337–338
Cluster (wave) scheduling, 103–104, 105
CMA (Certified Medical Assistant), 17
CMAS (Certified Medical Administrative Specialist), 18
CMS (Centers for Medicare and Medicaid Services), 51, 231
CMS-1500 claim form, 261–262, 266–268
CMT (Certified Medical Transcriptionist), 18, 40
COB (coordination of benefits), 222–223
COD (Collect on Delivery), 115
Code linkage, 243
Code of Ethics and Creed (AAMA), 36–37

Code Set Standards (HIPAA), 52
Coding of files, 156
Coding systems, 234–245
compliance issues, 57, 238, 241, 243–244
crosswalk, 244–245
diagnostic (*See* Diagnostic coding)
procedural (*See* Procedural coding)
standard code sets, 52, 244
Coinsurance, 225
Collect on Delivery (COD), 115
Collection(s), 274–278
communicating with patients about, 274–275
computers in, 132
course of action, 275–276
credit arrangements, 278
laws governing, 275
by letter, 276–277
office policy on, 275
payment guidelines, 275
policy and procedures, 210
statute of limitations, 278
by telephone, 276
Collection agency, 276, 278
Collection at the time of service, 271
Collection ratio, 275
Colons (:), B-3
Color-coding, 162
Comma (,), B-2 to B-3
Comment tab (Medisoft®), A-12
Commission on Accreditation for Allied Health Education Programs (CAAHEP), 17
Communicable disease control, 56
Communication, 5, 70–125
barriers to, 73–74
in collections process, 274–275
compliance and, 58
confidentiality issues, 22
cycle of, 72–74
electronic (*See* Electronic communications)
interpersonal, 7, 19–24
language barriers and, 23–24
legal aspects, 47–50 (*See also* Confidentiality; HIPAA)
nonverbal, 5, 7, 74–75
phone (*See* Telephone skills)
written (*See* Written communications)
Compact disks, 196
Compassion, 38
Compliance, 57–59
AMA's role in, 6, 22, 58
audit trails, 137–138
billing, 57, 231, 261, 269, 273
coding, 57, 238, 241, 243–244
documentation of communication, 94
HIPAA, 50–51, 53–54
plans for, 57–58
records management, 58, 141, 149, 157
Red Flag requirements, 297–298
release of information, 49, 53–54, 80, 130, 138, 148
scheduling, 102, 107, 109

Compliance Program Guidance for Individual and Small Group Physician Practices (OIG), 57, 58
Computer(s), 128–139
    billing using, 132, 259–260, 266
    categories of, 133–134
    clinical usage, 133
    communication via (*See* Electronic communications)
    data input technologies, 166–170
    electronic medical records, 129
    ergonomics, 134–135
    financial usage, 131–133, 293, 295
    in office management, 212
    proofreading on, 86
    scheduling using, 104, 106, 128–129
    security, 22, 50, 54, 56, 128, 137–139
    software (*See* Software)
Computer networks, 130–131
Computer skills, 6–7
Condition tab (Medisoft®), A-11
Confidentiality, 21–23
    access to information, 47–50
    billing, 230, 269, 275, 292
    computer security, 22, 50, 54, 56, 137–139
    electronic communication, 49–50, 102
    exceptions to, 49, 55–56
    fax machines, 49, 98–100
    filing systems and, 157
    helping to ensure, 49, 59
    HIPAA provisions, 50, 52–56
    medical histories, 22
    outside office environment, 22, 53
    sign-in log, 21–22, 109–110, 189
    telephone use, 12, 22, 90, 95
    written communications, 76
Conflict management, 193
Consent, 41–44
    liability and, 45–46
Consultation codes, 241
Consultation letters, 79–80, 140
Consumer Credit Card Protection Act, 278
Contact letters, follow-up, 342–343
Continuation pages, 78
Continuing education units (CEUs), 40
Contracts
    medical insurance, 222–223
    in physician's practice, 40–41
    termination of, 45, 277
Contributory negligence, 46–47
Conversation, with patients, 20–21
Coordination of benefits (COB), 222–223
Copayment (copay), 225, 271, 273
Corrections, to medical records, 141, 149, 166
Corrective action, for compliance offenses, 58
Correspondence
    defined, 152
    filing systems (*See* Filing)
    in medical records, 140
    types of, 79–83
    See also specific type of correspondence

Council of Biology Editors, *Scientific Style and Format,* 86
Council on Ethical and Judicial Affairs (AMA), 147
Court order, release of information under, 55
Cover/application letters, 324–327
Covered entities (HIPAA), 50–51, 54
CPC (Certified Professional Coder), 18, 40
CPC-H (Certified Professional Coder-Outpatient Hospital), 18
CPC-P (Certified Professional Coder-Payer), 18
CPS (Certified Professional Secretary), 18
CPT-4, 238–243
    coding evaluation and management services, 240–241
    HCPCS codes, 52, 242
    immunizations, 242
    laboratory procedures, 241
    notes and modifiers, 239–240
    surgical procedures, 241
    symbols and format, 239
    using, 242–243
Credit arrangements, 278
Credit card payments, 272
Creditors, Red Flag requirements, 297–298
Criminal law, 46
Cross-reference sheets, 155–156
Cross-referencing, 160
Crosswalk (coding), 244–245
Cultural diversity, 23–24, 74–75
Current Procedural Terminology. See CPT-4
Custom reports (Medisoft®), A-20
Customary fees, 233
Cycle billing, 272

D

"Daily Cash" section, 293
Daily journal, 292–294
Daily report (day sheet), 260, A-19
Daily routine, 207–208
Data backup, 138, A-1 to A-3
Data code sets (HIPAA), 52. *See also* Coding
Data entry log, inspection of, 137–138
Data entry skills, 6, 58, 167–168, 293
Data input technologies, 166–170
Database(s), 132
    online, 196
    problem-oriented medical records, 147
Database management software, 137
Date(s)
    in Medisoft®, A-5 to A-7
    in transcription, B-2
Day sheet (daily report), 260, A-19
De-identified health information, 56
DEA (Drug Enforcement Administration), 40
Dead storage, 151
Deaf patients, 23–24
Debit card payments, 272
Decentralized files, 152
Decimal points, B-5
Decoding, 73
Deductibles, 225, 228, 273

Deductions, 304–306
Defendant, 46
Defense Enrollment Eligibility Reporting System (DEERS), 228
Defensive medicine, 44
Delayed schedule, open slots for, 111
Delegating tasks, 192, 195
Delegative/laissez-faire leader, 196
Delinquent accounts. *See* Collection(s)
Delivery Confirmation, 115
Democratic/participative leader, 195
Dental insurance, 224
Dental services, code sets for, 52
Dependability, 12
Dependent children, 274
Deposit(s), 300
    direct, 307
Deposition, 46
Designated record set, 55
Diagnosis (Dx), 143
    primary, 235
Diagnosis tab (Medisoft®), A-11
Diagnostic coding, 13, 234–238
    basic steps in, 238
    compliance issues, 57, 238, 243–244
    defined, 234
    ICD-9-CM, 52, 234–238
    ICD-10-CM, 13, 52, 244
Diagnostic procedures, scheduling, 112
Diagnostic-related groups (DRGs), 233
Dictation equipment, B-1
Difficult patients, 20–21
Direct deposit, 307
Direct earnings, 305
Directories
    office personnel, 206
    telephone, 97, 321
Disability insurance, 224
Disciplinary directives, 58
Disclosure of information, 54, 138
Discounted fee-for-service payment schedule, 224
Disposition of records, 151
DNR (Do Not Resuscitate), 44
"Do Not Use" list (abbreviations and symbols), 168
Doctors. *See* Physician(s)
Documentation
    accuracy of, 12, 58
    compliance plan for, 57
    inspecting, 156
    releasing, 156
    of telephone calls, 94, 100–101
    See also Written communications; *specific document type*
Double-booking appointments, 104
Double-column schedule, 105
Double-entry bookkeeping, 294–295
DPA (durable power of attorney), 41, 44
Drafts, first, 83
Dress, 75, 211, 337–338
DRGs (diagnostic-related groups), 233
Drug Enforcement Administration (DEA), 40
Durable power of attorney (DPA), 41, 44
Dx (diagnosis), 143
    primary, 235

E

E codes, 234–238
E/M (evaluation and management) services, 240–241
E-mail, 102, 130
  confidentiality and, 50, 102
  format, 82–83
E-mail bulletin boards, 196
E-signature, 303
EDI tab (Medisoft®), A-12
Edit menu (Medisoft®), A-4, A-5
Editing
  defined, 86
  techniques, 88–89
Editorial research projects, 196–197
Education
  employee, 58, 206
  patient, 205–206
Educational qualifications, 329
Efficiency, 12–13, 76
EFT (electronic funds transfer), 133, 263, 304, 307
EHRs (electronic health records), 129, 164–166, 258
EIN (Employer Identification Number), 56, 305
Electronic banking, 303–304
Electronic claims, 132–133, 262
  versus paper claims, 266–269
Electronic communications, 129–131
  appointment notifications, 111, 128
  confidentiality and, 49–50, 262
  skills required for, 5
  See also E-mail
Electronic funds transfer (EFT), 133, 263, 304, 307
Electronic health records (EHRs), 129, 164–166, 258
Electronic job applications, 322–324
Electronic payroll, 307
Electronic records, versus paper records, 150–151, 164–166
Electronic remittance advice (ERA), 262, 270
Electronic scheduling systems, 104, 106, 128–129
Electronic signature systems, 138, 303
Electronic voice mail, 102
Emergencies, out-of-office, 109
Emergency appointments, 108
Emergency calls, 94
Empathy, 8–9
Employee(s)
  benefit policies, 211
  earnings (See Payroll)
  education, 58, 206
  evaluation policies, 210
  hiring policies, 210
  safety of, 44
  stress management, 190–192
Employee handbook. See Policies and procedures manual
Employee Retirement Income Security Act of 1974 (ERISA), 50
Employee's Withholding Allowance Certification (Form W-4), 305

Employer Identification Number (EIN), 56, 305
Employer Identifier (HIPAA), 56
Employment Eligibility Verification Form (Form I-9), 305
Employment opportunities, 9–11
  applications (See Job applications)
  sources of, 320–322
Employment preparation, 319–351
Employment services, 321
Encoding, 72
Encounter form, 234–235, 256–258
Encryption, 138
Endorsement
  check, 299–300
  in licensing process, 39
EOB (explanation of benefits), 262–263, 270
EP (established patient), 107, 240–241
Equipment
  computerized, 133
  filing, 152–156
  inventory of, 210
  transcription, B-1
Equipment skills, 6–7
ERA (electronic remittance advice), 262, 270
Ergonomics, 134–135, 189
ERISA (Employee Retirement Income Security Act of 1974), 50
Errors
  coding, 243–244
  in financial records, 293
  on insurance claims, 269–270
  in medical records, 141, 149, 166
  proofreading, 88
Established patient (EP), 107, 240–241
Ethics. See Medical ethics
Ethnocentrism, 23
Etiquette, 38–39
  telephone, 89–91
Evaluation
  employee, 210
  of skills and goals, 320
Evaluation and management (E/M) services, 240–241
Exemptions (payroll), 306
Expenses, 293, 304
Explanation of benefits (EOB), 262–263, 270
Express consent, 41
Express Mail, 114
Extended appointments, 109
Externship, 334
Eye contact, 74–75

F

Facial expression, 74
Facing triangles (►◄), 239
Fair Debt Collection Practices Act, 275
Familiarity with patients, 19
Family caregivers, stress on, 190–191
Family history (FH), 143
Fax (facsimile) machines, 49, 98–100
Federal Employee Health Benefit Program (FEHBP), 227
Federal Employee Program (FEP), 227
Federal Equal Credit Opportunity Act, 278

Federal Insurance Contributions Act (FICA), 305–306
Federal Trade Commission, 297
Federal Unemployment Tax Act (FUTA), 306
Fee adjustment, 272–273
Fee-for-service payment, 224, 228
Fee schedules, 231, 233, 258
Feedback, 73
FEHBP (Federal Employee Health Benefit Program), 227
FEP (Federal Employee Program), 227
FH (family history), 143
FICA tax, 305–306
File(s)
  active, 149
  centralized, 152
  closed, 150
  decentralized, 152
  inactive, 149–150
  lateral, 153–154
  missing, 163
  mobile-aisle, 154–155
  open-shelf, 152–153
  outside services, 211
  tickler, 149, 157
  vertical, 153
  See also Medical records
File backup, 138, A-1 to A-3
File menu (Medisoft®), A-4
File server, 131
Filing, 151–163
  equipment and supplies, 152–156
  methods of, 157–163
  procedures manual, 208–209
  steps in, 156–157
Filing cabinets, 153
Final manuscripts, 83–84
Final privacy rule, 47
Financial pressures, stress caused by, 191
Financial records, 291–296
  computerized, 133
  retention of, 150
Firewalls, 138
First-class mail, 114
First draft, 83
Fixed/open office hours, 103, 105
Flexibility, 13
Folders, 154–155
Follow-up
  in filing, 156–157
  insurance claims, 270–271
  tickler file, 149, 157
Follow-up calls, 100–101, 111
Follow-up letters, 80, 342–343
Foot pedal, B-1
Footnotes, 85–86
"For Deposit Only" annotation, 272, 299–300
Form(s)
  advance beneficiary notice for uncovered services, 274
  bank reconciliation, 302
  claim
    CMS-1500, 261–262, 266–268
    completing and transmitting, 265–269

Form(s)—*Cont.*
  clinical, 140
  medical release, 44, 48, 80, 138, 148
  patient encounter, 234–235, 256–258
  precertification, 226
  samples and instructions for, 210
Format
  chart notes, 141–147
  e-mail, 82–83
  interoffice memorandums, 81–82
  letters, 76–78
    cover/application, 325–326
    fax cover, 99
    follow-up contact, 343
  policies and procedures manual, 206
  professional reports, 83–86
  résumés, 328–335
  transcription, B-2 to B-6
Fraud, 46, 58, 273, 297–298
Front desk tasks, 4
Full disclosure policy, 138
Full endorsement, 299
Functional résumé, 330, 332–333
FUTA (Federal Unemployment Tax Act), 306

G

General Equivalency Mapping (GEM), 244–245
Gestures, 74–75
Good judgment, 13
Good Samaritan Act, 47
Government names, alphabetic filing rules, 160–161
Grammar checkers, 87, 136
Graphics applications, 136
Greetings, telephone, 90–91
The Gregg Reference Manual, 79
Grooming, 16, 75
Gross earnings, 306
Guarantor, 274
Guides, 155

H

Hash symbol (#), 239
HCFA-1500 claim form (CMS-1500 claim form), 261–262, 266–268
HCPCS (Health Care Financing Administration Common Procedure Coding System), 52, 242
Headings
  reports, 85
  résumés, 329
Headphones, B-1
Health care clearinghouse, 51, 269
Health Care Financing Administration Common Procedure Coding System (HCPCS), 52, 242
Health care providers
  HIPAA compliance, 50, 53–54, 57
  See also Physician(s)
Health information (HI), 53
  de-identified, 56
  protected, 53–54, 56
Health insurance. *See* Medical insurance

Health Insurance Portability and Accountability Act. *See* HIPAA
Health maintenance organizations (HMOs), 225–226
Health management, 15–16, 192, 193–194
Health Plan Identifier (HIPAA), 57
Health plans, HIPAA compliance, 50
Hearing impaired patients, 23–24
Help menu (Medisoft®), A-5
HHS. *See* U.S. Department of Health and Human Services
HI. *See* Health information
Hidden job markets, 320, 321–322
HIPAA (Health Insurance Portability and Accountability Act), 50–57
  Administrative Simplification, 50
  billing, 230, 261, 270, 275, 292
  compliance, 50–51, 53–54
  computer security, 128
  electronic communication, 49–52, 262
  externship, 334
  flexibility and, 13
  National Identifiers, 56–57
  ownership of medical records, 148
  patient sign-in log, 21, 189
  Privacy Rule, 50, 52–56
    exceptions to, 55–56
  release of information, 44, 53–54, 148
  Security Rule, 56
  telephone usage, 12, 90
  Transaction and Code Set Standards, 51–52
Hippocratic oath, 36
Hiring policies, 210
Histories, confidentiality of, 22
History and physical (H&P), 140
History of present illness (HPI), 142
HIV (human immunodeficiency virus), 56
HMOs (health maintenance organizations), 225–226
Honesty, 13–14, 38
Honorable behavior, 38
Hospital(s)
  admissions, 111–112
  employment opportunities, 11
Hospital insurance, 224, 227
Hospital-related services, code sets for, 52
Hours, office, 102, 103, 105
H&P (history and physical), 140
HPI (history of present illness), 142
Human immunodeficiency virus (HIV), 56
Hyphenated names, 159
Hyphens (-), B-4

I

IAAP (International Association of Administrative Professionals), 18
ICD-9-CM, 52, 234–237
ICD-10-CM, 13, 52, 244
ICD-10-PSC, 52, 244
Identity theft, 297–298
Illustrations, 86
Immunizations, coding, 242
Implied consent, 41
Impression, 143

Inactive files, 149–150
Income statement, 293
Incoming mail, 112–113
Incoming telephone calls, 90–96
  answering services, 96
  emergency, 94
  etiquette, 90–91
  message-taking (*See* Message-taking)
  screening, 91–94
  transferring, 93
Indemnity plans, 225
Indexing of files, 156–163
Indirect earnings, 305
Inducements, improper, 57
Information
  access to, 44, 47–50
  disclosure of, 54, 138
  electronic transmission of, 49–52, 102, 132–133, 138 (*See also* Electronic communications)
  release of, 44, 47–48, 53–54, 80, 130, 138, 148
  use of, 54
Information letters, 79
Informed consent, 41–43
Initiative, 14
Inpatient hospital services, code sets for, 52
Input devices, 166–170
Inspecting documents, 156
Insurance
  AMA tasks, 5, 222
  health (*See* Medical insurance)
  liability, 46
  workers' compensation, 55, 229
Insurance policies, retention of, 150
Insured, 222
Insured Mail, 115
Interest, 298
Internal Revenue Service (IRS), 292, 304, 305
International Association of Administrative Professionals (IAAP), 18
International Classification of Diseases
  ICD-9-CM, 52, 234–237
  ICD-10-CM, 13, 52, 244
  ICD-10-PSC, 52, 244
Internet, 131
  job listings on, 321
  resources on, 212, 336
  security issues, 139
  service providers, 170
  See also Electronic communications
Interoffice memorandums, 81–82, 100
Interpersonal skills, 7, 19–24
Interviews, 336–342
  conducting, 341–342
  ending, 342
  follow-up letters, 342–343
  preparing for, 337–340
  types of, 342
Intimate zone, 75
Inventory, 210
Irregular appointments, 108–109
IRS (Internal Revenue Service), 292, 304, 305
Italics, 85
Itinerary (travel), 198–199

J

JAMA (Journal of the American Medical Association), 196–197
Job advertisements, 320
Job applications, 322–324
    cover letters, 324–327
    interview (*See* Interviews)
    résumés, 326–335
Job boards, 321
Job descriptions, 206
Job fairs, 320–321
Journal(s)
    employment advertisements in, 320
    medical, 196–197
Journal of the American Medical Association (JAMA), 196–197
Judgment, 13

K

Keyboards, 135
Keywords, 329
Kickbacks, 57

L

Lab reports, 133, 140
Label(s), 155
Label method, of patient sign-in, 21–22, 109
Laboratory procedures, coding, 241
Laissez-faire/delegative leader, 196
Language barriers, 23–24
Laptops, 134
Late patients, 108–109
Lateral files, 153–154
Leadership styles, 195–196
Ledgers, 292
Legal competency, 41
Legal issues. *See* Litigation; Medical law
Legal majority, 41
Letters
    of acknowledgment, 79
    collection by, 276–277
    consultation, 79–80, 140
    continuation pages, 78
    cover/application, 324–327
    fax cover, 99
    follow-up, 80, 342–343
    formatting, 76–78
    of information, 79
    punctuation, 78
    referral, 79–81, 140
    withdrawal, 45
    See also Mail
Liability, 44–47
    abandonment, 45
    assault and battery, 45–46
    defined, 44
    fraud, 46
    malpractice, 44–45
    termination, 45
    third-party, 274
Liability insurance, 46
Library, research at, 196
Licensure, 39–40, 150
Listening techniques, 74, B-1

Lists menu (Medisoft®), A-5
Litigation, 46–47
    alternatives to trial, 47
    Good Samaritan Act, 47
    malpractice, 44–45
    physician's response to, 46–47
    safeguards against, 59
    statute of limitations, 47
    steps in, 46

M

Mail, 112–115
    incoming, 112–113
    outgoing, 113–115
    safe handling of, 113
    See also Letters
Mainframe computers, 133–134
Maintenance, office, 211
Major medical insurance, 224
Majority, legal, 41
Malpractice, 44–45, 59
Malware, 138–139
Managed care, 11, 225–227
Management qualifications, 187. *See also* Office management
Manual of Style (AMA), 86
Manuscripts
    draft, 83
    final, 83–84
Master patient index (MPI), 161
Mathematics skills, 5
Maturity, 17
Media Mail, 114
Medicaid, 11, 228
Medicaid tab (Medisoft®), A-12
Medical abbreviations, 166–168
Medical centers, employment opportunities, 11
Medical compliance plans, 57–58
Medical ethics, 36–39
    AAMA code, 36–37
    bioethics, 37–38
    defined, 36
    patient records and, 147–148
    principles of, 36–37
Medical insurance, 221–233
    contract, 222–223
    coverage types, 223–224
    fee schedules, 231, 233, 258
    payers, 227–229
    payment methods, 231–233, 273–274
    payment types, 224–225
    plan participation, 229–230
    plan types, 225–227
Medical insurance claims, 260–271
    appealing, 264–265
    clean, 269
    coding (*See* Coding systems)
    completing and transmitting forms, 265–269
    electronic, 132–133, 262, 266–269
    following up on, 270–271
    procedures manual, 210
    process overview, 260–265

Medical insurance companies, 222, 227–229
    employment opportunities, 11
    See also specific company
Medical journals, 196–197
Medical labs, computer usage in, 133
Medical law, 39–50
    collections, 275, 278
    communications, 47–50
    on confidentiality (*See* Confidentiality; HIPAA)
    defined, 39
    liability (*See* Liability)
    litigation (*See* Litigation)
    patient records, 139, 150
    physician's practice and, 40–44
Medical practice acts, 39
Medical records, 139–141
    access to, 44, 47–50
    chart notations (*See* Chart notes)
    compliance issues, 58, 141, 149
    confidentiality of (*See* Confidentiality)
    contents of, 139–140, 149
    corrections to, 141, 149, 166
    data input, 166–170
    disclosure of, 44, 47–48, 53–55, 138
    documentation formats, 142–147
    electronic, 129
    filing systems (*See* Filing)
    as legal documents, 139
    ownership of, 147–148
    quality assurance, 149
    reasons for maintaining, 140–141
    retention of, 149–151
    telephone messages in, 94, 100–101, 140
    transcription (*See* Transcription)
    transferring, 209
Medical release form, 44, 48, 80, 138, 148
Medical reports, 140
Medical specialties, 9–10, 40
Medical terminology, 166
Medical transcription. *See* Transcription
Medicare, 11, 227–228
    advance beneficiary notice for uncovered services, 274
    coding (*See* Coding systems)
    fee schedules, 231, 233
    HIPAA compliance and, 51
    Part A, 227
    Part B, 227
    Part C (Advantage Plans), 227
    Part D, 228
Medication list, 140
Medisoft®, A-1 to A-20
    backup procedures, A-1 to A-3
    billing functions, 132, 259–260
    cases, A-10 to A-12
    dates in, A-5 to A-7
    deleting data, A-7
    entering patient information, A-8 to A-9
    exiting, A-7
    filing systems, 158, 161–162
    help functions, A-7 to A-8
    menus, A-4 to A-5

Medisoft®—*Cont.*
  Office Hours, 104, 106, 129, A-7, A-15 to A-19
  procedure day sheet, 293–294, A-19 to A-20
  reports, A-19 to A-20
  restoring data, A-3 to A-4
  saving data, A-7
  student data file, A-1 to A-4
  transaction entry, A-12 to A-15
MEDLINE, 196
Meeting arrangements, 200–202
Meeting minutes, 202–205
Meeting schedule, 211
Memorandums, interoffice, 81–82, 100
Message, 72–73
Message-taking (telephone), 94–96
  answering services, 96
  appropriate situations for, 92–93
  medical records and, 94, 100–101, 140
  message slips, 95, 96, 100–101
  verifying information, 95
Microcomputers (personal computers), 134
Micrographics, 150–151
Military treatment facilities (MTFs), 228
Minicomputers, 134
Minimum necessary standard, 54
Minors
  guarantors for, 274
  legal consent, 41–42
Minutes of meetings, 202–205
Miscellaneous tab (Medisoft®), A-12
Misconduct, 39
Missing files, 163
Mistakes. *See* Errors
Mobile-aisle files, 154–155
Modified-block letter, 77–78
Modifiers *(CPT)*, 239–230
Money orders, 272
Monitor (computer), 22, 54, 135, 137
Monitoring programs, for compliance, 58
Monthly billing, 272
Monthly reports, 260
Monthly summary, 292
Moral values, 38
MPI (master patient index), 161
MTFs (military treatment facilities), 228
Multi-career family units, 191

N

Name, Address tab (Medisoft®), A-8
Names, alphabetic filing rules, 158–161
Narcotics registration, 40
National Board of Medical Examiners, 39
National conversion factor, 233
National Identifiers (HIPAA), 56–57
National Provider Identifier (NPI), 57
Necessary data, for scheduling, 107–108
Necessary services, 57
Negligence, contributory, 46–47
Negotiable checks, 299
Net earnings, 306
Net pay statement, 306
Network (computer), 130–131
Networking, 321–322, 336

New patient (NP), 107, 109, 209
  CPT codes, 240–241
  Notice of Privacy Practices, 54
  orientation procedures, 209
Next appointment, 110–111
No shows, 104, 110
Nonparticipating provider (nonPAR), 232
Nonpatients
  communication with, 24
  disclosure of patient information to, 44
"Nonsufficient Funds" (NSF) notation, 300
Nonverbal communication, 5, 7, 74–75
Notes
  chart (*See* Chart notes)
  CPT, 239–240
  in reports, 85–86
Notice of Privacy Practices, 54
NP. *See* New patient
NPI (National Provider Identifier), 57
NSF ("Nonsufficient Funds") notation, 300
Number(s), in transcription, B-4 to B-5
Number method, for patient sign-in, 22
Numbering, of report pages, 84
Numeric filing, 161–162

O

Objective findings, 143
OCR (Office of Civil Rights), 55
OCR (optical character reader), 115, 267, 329, 334
Office communications. *See* Communication
Office dress code, 211
Office environment, 188–189
Office hours, 102, 103, 105
Office Hours (Medisoft®), 104, 106, 129, A-7, A-15 to A-19
Office management, 187–218
  editorial research projects, 196–197
  patient education materials, 205–206
  personal management skills, 190–194
  policies and procedures (*See* Policies and procedures manual)
  travel and meeting arrangements, 197–205
Office manager
  resources and responsibilities, 212
  role of, 194–196
Office of Civil Rights (OCR), 55
Office of the Inspector General (OIG), 57, 58
Office personnel directory, 206
Office policy
  banking, 301
  collections, 275
  information disclosure, 138
  manual of (*See* Policies and procedures manual)
  for scheduling appointments, 102–103
  transcription, B-1
Office safety, 44, 211
OIG (Office of the Inspector General), 57, 58
Online, 130. *See also* Internet; *under electronic*
Online databases, 196
Online job applications, 322–324
Open/fixed office hours, 103, 105

Open punctuation, 78
Open-shelf files, 152–153
Open slots, in scheduling, 111
Operating system, 135–136
Optical character reader (OCR), 115, 267, 329, 334
Oral communication
  versus written communication, 76
  See also Telephone skills
Oral consent, 41
Ordering procedures, 210
Organizational names, alphabetic filing rules, 159–160
Organizational skills, 5–6
Other Information tab (Medisoft®), A-9
Out guides, 155
Out-of-office appointments, 111–112
Out-of-office emergencies, 109
Outgoing mail, 113–115
Outgoing telephone calls, 96–100
  fax machines, 49, 98–100
  following through on, 100–101
  placing, 98
  planning, 96–97
  resources for, 97
Outpatient, 223
Outside services file, 211
Outstanding checks, 303

P

"Paid in Full" annotation, 299
Panel interviews, 342
Paper records, versus electronic records, 150–151, 164–166
PAR (participating provider), 230, 232
Parcel Post, 114
Parent code, 239
Participating provider (PAR), 230, 232
Participative/democratic leader, 195
Passwords, 22, 100, 128, 138
Past medical history (PMH), 143
Patient(s)
  abandonment of, 45
  appointments (*See* Appointment(s); Scheduling)
  billing, 263–264
  communication with, 7–9, 19–24
  conversation with, 20–21
  cultural diversity, 23–24, 74–75
  difficult, 20–21
  established, 107, 240–241
  familiarity with, 19
  medical records (*See* Medical records)
  new (*See* New patient)
  payments from, 271–274
    delinquent (*See* Collection(s))
  physician relationship with (*See* Physician-patient relationship)
  privacy issues (*See* Confidentiality)
  social relationships with, 20
  terminally ill, 21
Patient care, policy and procedures, 209
Patient day sheet (Medisoft®), A-19
Patient education materials, 205–206
Patient encounter form, 234–235, 256–258

Patient/Guarantor dialog box (Medisoft®), A-8
Patient identifier standard, 57
Patient information brochure, 205–206
Patient information form, 261
Patient ledger cards, 292
Patient names, alphabetic filing rules, 158–159
Patient rights, 55
Patient sign-in log, 21–22, 109–110, 189
Patient statements, 258–259, 272, A-20
Patient waiting area, 188–189
Payment(s)
    delinquent (See Collection(s))
    medical insurance, 224–225, 231–233, 273–274
    from patients, 271–274
    third-party liability, 274
    See also Billing
Payment plans, 272
Payments section (Medisoft®), A-13
Payroll, 304–307
    calculating, 306
    deductions, 304–306
    electronic, 307
    employer's tax responsibilities, 306
    identification numbers, 305
    records management, 305, 307
PCPs (primary care providers), 226
PCs (personal computers), 134
PDA (personal digital assistant), 134, 170
PE (physical exam), 143
Pegboard accounting system, 294
Perfectionism, 192
Period (.), B-2
Personal calls, 94
Personal computers (PCs), 134
Personal digital assistant (PDA), 134, 170
Personal references, 330, 332
Personal tab (Medisoft®), A-11
Personal titles, 19, 159
Personal zone, 75
Petty cash fund, 304
Pharmaceutical sales representatives, 24
PHI (protected health information), 53–54, 56, 109
Phone skills. See Telephone skills
Physical attributes, 15–16, 75
Physical environment, 188–189
Physical exam (PE), 143
Physician(s)
    absence of, 199–200
    liability (See Liability)
    medical specialties, 9–10
    travel and meeting arrangements, 197–205
Physician-patient relationship
    abandonment and, 45
    legal aspects of, 40–41
    termination of, 45, 277
Physician practice
    employment opportunities, 9
    financial management (See Billing; Financial records; Payment(s))
    HIPAA compliance, 51
    legal issues, 40–44

management records, 152
office management (See Office management)
policies (See Office policy)
Physicians' services, code sets for, 52
Plain-text résumé, 334–335
Plaintiff, 46
Plan (treatment), 144, 147
Planning
    payment, 272
    strategic, 195
    telephone calls, 96–97
    travel and meeting arrangements, 197–205
Plus sign (+), 239
PMH (past medical history), 143
Policies and procedures manual, 206–211
    collections, 275–276
    as compliance plan, 58
    contents, 206–211
    format, 206
    rules of etiquette, 39
Policy. See Office policy
Policy tabs (Medisoft®), A-11
Policyholder, 222
POMR (problem-oriented medical record), 147–148
Postal service, 114
Postdated checks, 299
Posting, 292, 293
POSTNET, 115
Posture, 75
Power words, 327
PPOs (preferred provider organizations), 226–227, 258
Practice analysis report, 295–296
Practice management records, 152
Preauthorization (precertification), 225–226
Predated checks, 299
Preferred provider organizations (PPOs), 226–227, 258
Prefixes, in surnames, 158–159
Premium, 222
Prescriptions
    Medicare coverage, 228
    narcotics, 40
Presentation software, 136
Primary care providers (PCPs), 226
Primary diagnosis, 235
Priorities, setting, 192
Priority Mail, 114
Privacy, 47. See also Confidentiality
Privacy Rule (HIPAA), 50, 52–56
    exceptions to, 55–56
Private-sector payers, 227
Problem-oriented medical record (POMR), 147–148
Problem-solving skills, 14, 195
Procedural coding, 238–243
    basic steps in, 242–243
    compliance issues, 57, 241, 243–244
    defined, 234
    standard code sets, 52 (See also CPT-4)
Procedure day sheet, 293–294
Procedures manual. See Policies and procedures manual

Procrastination, avoiding, 192–193
Productivity, 194–195
Professional courtesy, prohibition of, 273
Professional growth, 17–19
Professional image, 15–17
Professional licenses, 39–40, 150
Professional references, 330, 332
Professional reports, 83–86
Professional Secretaries International (PSI), 18
Professional titles, 19, 159
Promptness, in answering telephone calls, 90
"Proof of Posting" section, 293
Proofreading, 86–89
    common errors, 88
    defined, 86
    methods, 86–87
    symbols, 87
    techniques, 88
Protected health information (PHI), 53–54, 56, 109
Provider, 222
    participating, 230, 232
PSI (Professional Secretaries International), 18
Public zone, 75
Publication Manual of the American Psychological Association, 86
PubMed, 196
Punctuality, 14
Punctuation, 78

Q

Quality assurance, in records management, 149
Questions, interview, 339–340
Quotations, 85, B-2

R

R/O (rule out), 143
RBRVS (resource-based relative value scale), 233
Reasonable and necessary services, 57
Reasonable fees, 233
Receipt(s)
    for patient payments, 271–272
    retention of, 150
    walkout (Medisoft®), A-14 to A-15
Receipt/charge slips, 292
Receiver, 73
Reception area, 189
Reconciliation (bank), 301–303
Recorder, of meeting minutes, 204
Records management, 128–181
    AHIMA guidelines, 150–151
    AMA tasks, 4–5
    compliance issues, 58, 141, 149, 157
    defined, 151
    destruction of records, 151
    filing systems (See Filing)
    paper versus electronic, 150–151, 164–166
    payroll, 305, 307

Records management—*Cont.*
    responsibility for, 212
    security issues, 22, 56
    See also Financial records; Medical
        records
Red Flag requirements, 297–298
References, 330, 332
Referral(s)
    CPT coding, 241
    in managed care, 226
    outside services file for, 211
    self-, 57
Referral letters, 79–81, 140
Registered Health Information
    Administrator (RHIA), 18
Registered Health Information Technician
    (RHIT), 18
Registered Mail, 115
Registered Medical Assistant (RMA), 18
Registered Medical Transcriptionist (RMT), 18
Registration
    of narcotics, 40
    of patient arrivals, 21–22, 109–110, 189
Reimbursement details, checking, 262–263
Relative value scale (RVS), 233
Relative value unit (RVU), 233
Release of information, 44, 47–48, 53–54,
    80, 130, 138, 148
Releasing documents, 156
Relicensure, 39–40
Reports
    financial, 260, 293–296
    lab, 133, 140
    medical, 140
    Medisoft®, A-19 to A-20
    professional, 83–86
    statutory, 49, 55–56
Reports menu (Medisoft®), A-5
Reprints, 197
Rescheduling appointments, 110, 128
Research
    computer usage for, 133
    for job interview, 336–337
Research data, 56
Research projects, 196–197
Reservations, travel, 198–199
Residents, 40
Resource-based relative value scale
    (RBRVS), 233
Resources
    employment opportunities, 320–321, 336
    office management, 195, 212
Responsibilities
    ethical, 36–38
    of office manager, 212
    payroll tax, 306
    for records, 212
Restoring data (Medisoft®), A-3 to A-4
Restricted Delivery, 115
Restrictive endorsement, 300
Résumés, 326–335
    formats, 328–335
Retention
    financial records, 150
    medical records, 149–151
    payroll records, 307

Return Receipt, 115
Returned checks, 300
Review of systems (ROS), 143
RHIA (Registered Health Information
    Administrator), 18
RHIT (Registered Health Information
    Technician), 18
Right to practice, 39
Rights of patient, 55
RMA (Registered Medical Assistant), 18
RMT (Registered Medical
    Transcriptionist), 18
Role Delineation Chart (AAMA), 4
Roman numerals, 160, B-5
ROS (review of systems), 143
Routing slip (patient encounter form),
    234–235, 256–258
Rule out (R/O), 143
RVS (relative value scale), 233
RVU (relative value unit), 233

S

Safety
    mail handling, 113
    office, 44, 211
    See also Security
Sales representatives, 24
Same-day appointments (SDA), 104,
    106, 107
Scannable résumé, 334
Scheduling, 4, 102–112
    adjustments to, 108–111
    computer, 104, 106, 128–129
    guidelines for, 106
    necessary data, 107–108
    out-of-office appointments, 111–112
    patients' preferences for, 107
    physician preferences for, 103
    physician's policy on, 102–103
    procedures manual, 209
    screening (triage), 104–107
    types of, 103–104
    See also Appointment(s)
SCHIP (State Children's Health Insurance
    Program), 228
Scientific Style and Format (Council of
    Biology Editors), 86
Screen savers, 22, 137
Screening
    mail, 112–113
    for scheduling (triage), 104–107
    telephone calls, 91–94
Scrubber programs, 269
SDA (same-day appointments), 107
Security
    computer, 22, 50, 54, 56, 128, 137–139
    HIPAA provisions, 50
    payments, 272
    record, 22, 56
    Red Flag requirements, 297–298
    travel, 197–198
Security Rule (HIPAA), 56
Self-motivation, 14
Self-pay, 222
Self-referrals, 57

Semicolon (;), B-2 to B-3
Sender, 72
Server (file), 131
Service form (patient encounter form),
    234–235, 256–258
Settlement, 47
SH (social history), 143
Sign-in log, 21–22, 109–110, 189
Signature(s)
    on checks, 301
    electronic, 138, 303
    on interoffice memorandums, 82
    patient sign-in log, 21–22, 109–110, 189
    on release of information, 80, 138, 148
Signature Confirmation of Delivery, 114, 115
Signature on file (SOF), 231
Simulations, 182–185, 288–289, 315–316
Single-entry bookkeeping, 294–295
Single-parent providers, 190
Skill evaluation, 320
SOAP method, 142–147
Social history (SH), 143
Social relationships, with patients, 20
Social Security, 305
Social zone, 75
SOF (signature on file), 231
Software, 135–137
    accounting, 293, 295
    banking, 303–304
    billing, 132, 259–260
    database management, 137
    electronic health records, 164–166
    filing systems, 158, 161–162
    graphics, 136
    operating system, 135–136
    payroll, 306
    scheduling, 104, 106
    spell and grammar checkers, 87, 136
    spreadsheet, 137, 295, 306
    virus checkers, 138–139
    voice-recognition, 169–170
    word processing, 130, 136
    See also Medisoft®
Sorting of files, 156
Space, personal, 75
Speaker (meeting), 201
Speakerphones, 12, 95–96
Special Handling, 115
Specialties, medical, 9–10, 40
Speed-dial feature, 98
Spell checkers, 87, 136
Sponsors, 228
Spreadsheet programs, 137, 295, 306
Standard punctuation, 78
Stat appointments, 104, 106
State abbreviations, 114
State Children's Health Insurance Program
    (SCHIP), 228
Statements
    bank, 301–303
    financial, 293
    patient billing, 258–259, 272, A-20
    payroll, 306
Statute of limitations, 47, 278
Statutory reports, 49, 55–56
Storing of files, 156

Straight-numeric filing, 161
Strategic planning, 195
Stress management, 190–192, 194
Student data file (Medisoft®), A-1 to A-4
Style manuals, 86
Subject filing, 162–163
Subjective findings, 142
Subpoena, 46, 55
Subterms (ICD-9-CM), 236
Summaries, 292, 293, 295
Summons, 46
Superbill (patient encounter form), 234–235, 256–258
Supercomputers, 133
Supplementary insurance, 227
Supplementary terms (ICD-9-CM), 236
Supplies
    for filing system, 152–156
    ordering procedures, 210
Surgical insurance, 224
Surgical procedures
    coding, 241
    scheduling, 112
Suspicious mailings, 113
Symbols
    CPT-4, 239
    medical, 168
    proofreading, 87
    transcription, B-5 to B-6

T

Tab(s), 154
Tab cuts, 154–155
Tabular List (ICD-9-CM), 235–238
Tact, 15
Taxes
    payroll, 305–306
    records management, 150, 293
Team player, 15, 194
Telephone Consumer Protection Act, 275
Telephone directories, 97, 321
Telephone interviews, 342
Telephone skills, 89–102
    collections, 276
    confidentiality issues, 12, 22, 90, 95
    documentation, 94, 100–101
    etiquette, 89–91
    incoming calls (See Incoming telephone calls)
    oral consent, 41
    outgoing calls (See Outgoing telephone calls)
    policy and procedures, 209
    speakerphones, 12, 95–96
Telephone systems, 98
Template, 136
Temporary employment agencies, 321
Terminal-digit filing, 161
Terminally ill patients, 21
Terminated account, 277
Termination, of physician-patient relationship, 45, 277
Terminology, medical, 166
Third-party checks, 299
Third-party liability, 274

Third-party payer, 222, 233, 262
Thoroughness, 12
Thunderbolt symbol, 239
Tickler file, 149, 157
Time management, 192–193
Title(s)
    of doctors, 19, 159, B-2
    of patients, 19, 159
Title page, 83, 85
To-do list
    follow-through notation on, 101
    for stress management, 191
Today appointments, 104, 106, 107
Tone of voice, 74, 90
Tools menu (Medisoft®), A-5
TPO (treatment, payment, and operations), 53–54
Transaction Entry dialog box (Medisoft®), A-12 to A-15
Transaction Standards (HIPAA), 51
Transactions, recording, 256–260
Transcription, 167–168
    guidelines, B-2 to B-6
    listening techniques, B-1
    office policy, B-1
Transferring
    patient records, 209
    telephone calls, 93
Transmission of message, 73
    electronic (See Electronic communications)
Transportation Security Administration (TSA), 197
Travel agents, 198
Travel arrangements, 197–200
    changes in, 198–199
    duties related to physician's absence, 199–200
    reservations, 198–199
Treatment, payment, and operations (TPO), 53–54
Triage, 104–107
Triangle (▲), 239
TRICARE, 11, 228
TRICARE tab (Medisoft®), A-12
Trojans, 139
Truth in Lending Act, 278

U

UCR (usual, customary, and reasonable) fees, 233
Uncollectible accounts, 278
Underscoring, 85
Unemployment taxes, 306
U.S. Department of Health and Human Services (HHS)
    Centers for Medicare and Medicaid Services, 51, 231, 261
    code set rules, 52
    Office of Civil Rights (OCR), 55
    Office of the Inspector General (OIG), 57, 58
    privacy complaints, 55
U.S. Department of Homeland Security, 113

United States Postal Service (USPS), 114–115
Units of measure, B-5 to B-6
University of Chicago, Chicago Manual of Style, 86
Urgent cases, 108
Use of information, 54
Usual fees, 233

V

V codes, 234–237
Vertical files, 153
Veterans Administration, Civilian Health and Medical Program, 228
Videotaping, consent for, 43
Virus checkers, 138–139
Visible job markets, 320–321
Vitae (biographical and credentialing information), 201
Voice, tone of, 74, 90
Voice mail, electronic, 102
Voice-recognition technology, 169–170
Voluntary deductions, 306

W

W-2 forms, 306
W-4 forms, 305
Waiting area, 188–189
Walk-in patient, 108
Walkout receipts (Medisoft®), A-14 to A-15
Wave (cluster) scheduling, 103–104, 105
"Whatever" category, 192
Window menu (Medisoft®), A-5
Wireless communication, 131, 170
Withdrawal letter, 45
Withholding, 306
Word processing programs, 130, 136
Work area, 189
Work ethic, 11–15
Work history, 329–330
Work-life balance, 192
Workers' compensation, 55, 229
Workplace expectations, 190
World Health Organization (WHO), 244
Worm virus, 139
Write-off, 272–273, 278
Written communications, 75–89
    confidentiality of, 76
    in litigation, 46–47
    versus oral communication, 76
    proofreading and editing, 86–89
    security issues, 22, 50, 54, 56
    skills needed for, 6
    See also Letters; specific document type

X

X12 (HIPAA electronic transactions), 51–52
X-ray reports, 140

Z

ZIP codes, 114, 115

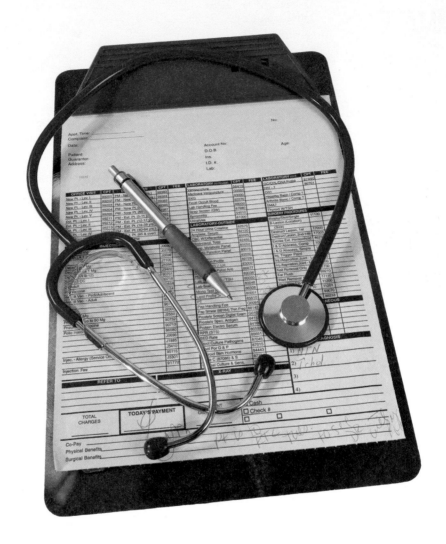

WORKING PAPERS

WP Number	Title
1	Work Ethic and Interpersonal Relationships
2	Physician's Obligations and Medical Law
3	Medical Liability and Communications
4	Legal Terms
5–6	Composing a Referral Letter
7–8	Proofing and Editing Reports
9–16	Taking Messages
17	Scheduling Decision Making
18–34	Setting Up Dr. Larsen's Practice
35	Rescheduling Appointments
36	Out-of-Office Scheduling
37	Communications Terms
38	Computer Terms
39	Computer Technology
40	A Lesson in EHR
41	Insurance Terminology
42	Insurance Plan, Payers, and Payment Methods
43	*ICD-9-CM* Diagnostic Codes
44–45	Updating Patient Statements
46–49	Updating Daily Journals
50	Deposits
51–52	Patient Information Forms
53	Records Release Form
54	Telephone Log
55	To-Do List
56	Telephone Log
57	To-Do List
58	Letter from Dr. Tai
59	Receipts
60	Florence Sherman's Patient Encounter Form
61	Stephen Villano's Patient Encounter Form
62	Gary Robertson's Patient Encounter Form
63	Monica Armstrong's Patient Encounter Form

WP Number	Title
64	Doris Casagranda's Patient Encounter Form
65	Cheng Sun's Patient Encounter Form
66	Charles Jonanthan III's Patient Encounter Form
67	Sara Babcock's Patient Encounter Form
68	Gene Sinclair's Patient Encounter Form
69	Laura Lund's Patient Encounter Form
70	Ana Mendez's Patient Encounter Form
71	Donald Mitchell's Patient Encounter Form
72	Theresa Dayton's Patient Encounter Form
73	Raymond Murrary's Patient Encounter Form
74	Telephone Log
75	To-Do List
76	Marc Phan's Patient Encounter Form
77	Sarah Morton's Patient Encounter Form
78	Doris Casagranda's Patient Encounter Form
79	Randy Burton's Patient Encounter Form
80	Gary Robertson's Patient Encounter Form
81	Checks received
82	Daily journal #106
83	Monica Armstrong's Patient Encounter Form
84	Jeffrey Kramer's Patient Encounter Form
85	Cheng Sun's Patient Encounter Form
86	Checks received
87	Daily journal #107
88	Thomas Baab's Patient Encounter Form
89	Theresa Dayton's Patient Encounter Form
90	Ardis Matthews' Patient Encounter Form
91	Ana Mendez's Patient Encounter Form
92	Gary Robertson's Patient Encounter Form
93	Florence Sherman's Patient Encounter Form
94	Checks received
95	Daily journal #108

WORK ETHIC AND INTERPERSONAL RELATIONSHIPS

Directions: Match the term in Column 2 with its definition in Column 1.

Column 1

_____ **1.** On time and ready to work.

_____ **2.** Inspired to increase knowledge and to advance.

_____ **3.** Able to produce work with few or no errors.

_____ **4.** Able to understand how a patient feels.

_____ **5.** Careful to pay attention to detail.

_____ **6.** Truthful; trustworthy.

_____ **7.** Privacy for all patient information.

_____ **8.** Ability to take independent action.

_____ **9.** The correct appearance for the job.

_____ **10.** Able to present ideas and information without offending.

_____ **11.** A person who works well with associates and pitches in when needed.

_____ **12.** Able to make good use of time and materials and to be organized.

_____ **13.** Able to present ideas to others with confidence.

_____ **14.** Pleasant and friendly.

_____ **15.** Able to adapt to new conditions; willing to try new ideas.

Column 2

a. accurate

b. assertive

c. cheerful

d. confidentiality

e. efficient

f. empathetic

g. flexible

h. honest

i. initiative

j. professional image

k. punctual

l. self-motivated

m. tactful

n. team player

o. thorough

PHYSICIAN'S OBLIGATIONS AND MEDICAL LAW

Directions: The following items refer to the obligations of the physician and/or medical law. Mark each statement with either "T" for *true* or "F" for *false*. Be prepared to discuss your answers in class.

_____ 1. The Principles of Medical Ethics states that the physician may refuse to accept a new patient.

_____ 2. A license to practice is good for the life of the physician.

_____ 3. A physician must obtain an annual permit for narcotic registration.

_____ 4. The physician is legally obligated to inform a patient of all possible reactions to a medication.

_____ 5. A physician must obtain a written consent before seeing a new patient.

_____ 6. A physician is legally obligated to seek a referral if the conditions are beyond the physician's scope of knowledge.

_____ 7. A physician's license to practice medicine is valid in all 50 states.

_____ 8. Medical practice acts, established by law, govern the practice of medicine.

_____ 9. The physician cannot refuse to perform a procedure on a patient because of that physician's moral beliefs.

_____ 10. The Drug Education Administration issues narcotic registration and annual renewals.

_____ 11. When a patient visits a physician for an appointment, he or she is establishing implied consent.

_____ 12. A physician must obtain the maximum amount of education in a particular medical specialty before becoming certified in that specialty.

_____ 13. The adult age as defined by law is known as *majority*.

_____ 14. Express consent is not required in an emergency situation.

_____ 15. A physician must sign a consent form before performing any procedure.

MEDICAL LIABILITY AND COMMUNICATIONS

Directions: The following items refer to medical liability and communications. Mark each statement with either "T" for *true* or "F" for *false.* Be prepared to discuss your answers in class.

_____ 1.   The charge of battery exists when there is a clear threat of injury to another.

_____ 2.   A subpoena orders the defendant to answer the stated charges.

_____ 3.   Contributory negligence may exist if the patient has failed to follow the physician's advice and treatment.

_____ 4.   Access to health records is the form that contains written permission to release patient information.

_____ 5.   Defensive medicine means the physician is dissolving legal responsibility.

_____ 6.   An authorization for release of information does not have the physician's signature.

_____ 7.   A statute of limitations controls the time limit for starting a lawsuit.

_____ 8.   Using e-mail to transmit medical documents is preferred over faxing documents.

_____ 9.   In a lawsuit, the burden of proof that malpractice exists rests on the patient.

_____ 10.   The physician may be charged with abandonment if the physician discontinues care without sending proper notification to the patient.

_____ 11.   Statutory reports require that the patient's condition be reported to the patient's insurance.

_____ 12.   Operating beyond the patient's expressed consent may establish a charge of battery.

_____ 13.   A deposition is sent to the defendant requiring the defendant's appearance in court.

_____ 14.   A Good Samaritan act states that a patient may start a lawsuit upon reaching majority.

_____ 15.   HIPAA is a federal law that protects the security and privacy of a patient's electronic health information.

Working Papers

LEGAL TERMS

Directions: Match the term in Column 2 with its definition in Column 1.

Column 1

_____ **1.** Standards of right and wrong conduct.

_____ **2.** Adherence to rules and regulations.

_____ **3.** Patient's permission for treatment when he or she enters a doctor's office.

_____ **4.** Legal responsibility.

_____ **5.** Testimony under oath, usually outside of court.

_____ **6.** Behavior and customs that are considered good manners.

_____ **7.** Time limit for a lawsuit to start.

_____ **8.** Physician's leaving a case before the patient is recovered.

_____ **9.** State law that governs the state's practice of medicine.

_____ **10.** Patient's written agreement to have a procedure performed.

_____ **11.** Clear threat of injury.

_____ **12.** Depriving others of their rights by dishonest means.

_____ **13.** A lawsuit.

_____ **14.** Legal document ordering all relevant documents to be submitted to the court.

_____ **15.** Authorization to send the patient's information to another physician.

_____ **16.** Operating beyond the patient's given consent.

_____ **17.** Written notice sent to the defendant asking for an answer to the charges.

_____ **18.** Resolution of a case brought about by an unbiased third party.

_____ **19.** Protection for the physician from liability of civil damages in emergency care.

_____ **20.** Confidential information that must be submitted to the state department.

Column 2

a. abandonment

b. arbitration

c. assault

d. battery

e. compliance

f. deposition

g. ethics

h. etiquette

i. express consent

j. fraud

k. Good Samaritan act

l. implied consent

m. liability

n. litigation

o. medical practice act

p. release of information

q. statute of limitations

r. statutory report

s. subpoena

t. summons

OUTSIDE SERVICES

Hugh Arnold, MD 2785 South Ridgeway Avenue, Suite 440 Chicago, IL 60647-2700 312-555-6800 **Internist**	Martinez Transcription Service 2200 South Ridgeway Avenue Chicago, IL 60623-2000 312-555-2424 **Betze Martinez**
Jason Berger, MD 5000 North Oak Park Drive Chicago, IL 60634-0005 312-555-7050 **Personal Friend**	Elizabeth Miller-Young, MD 2901 West Fifth Avenue, Suite 205 Chicago, IL 60612-9002 312-555-3500 **OB/GYN**
Consumer Pharmacy Pharmacists: Dale Geddal, MD 312-555-1252 Joy Rishard, MD **Pharmacy in medical center**	Mark Newman, MD 2785 South Ridgeway Avenue Chicago, IL 60647-2700 312-555-2700 **On-call doctor**
Lynn Corbett, MD Professional Buildng 8672 South Ridgeway Avenue, Suite 300 Chicago, IL 60623-2240 312-555-2300 **Cardiologist**	Margery Pierce, MD 6452 North Ridgeway Avenue, Suite 209 Chicago, IL 60626-5462 312-555-4880 **Pediatrician**
Richard Diangelis, MD 2785 South Ridgeway Avenue, Suite 280 Chicago, IL 60647-2700 312-555-1575 **Ophthalmologist**	Laura Sinn, MD 2901 West Fifth Avenue, Suite 100 Chicago, IL 60612-9002 312-555-7850 **Urologist**
Greg Koski, MD Professional Building 8672 South Ridgeway Avenue, Suite 350 Chicago, IL 60623-2240 312-555-4500 **Orthopedic Surgeon**	Theresa Townsend, MD 500 South Dearborn Street Chicago, IL 60605-0005 **Chairperson** 312-555-2200 **Chicago Medical Society**
University Hospital 5500 North Ridgeway Avenue Chicago, IL 60625-1200 312-555-2500	**Education services:** Juanita Yates 312-555-2950 **Human Resources:** 312-555-1200 **Resident services:** Lee Eaton 312-555-3043

CHART NOTE

Sherman, Florence   312-555-1217
DOB: 05/22/19--   Age: 65

10/08/20--
CHIEF COMPLAINT: Trouble with vision.

SUBJECTIVE: Patient is a 65-year-old female who had two episodes during
the last week of jagged lights occurring in central visual field. These
lasted 15—20 minutes; no other symptoms. Patient has long history of
migraines.

OBJECTIVE: Within normal limits; specifically, no evidence of tear or hole
in the retina.

ASSESSMENT: Migraine equivalent vs. posterior vitreous detachment.

PLAN: 1. Discussed with ophthalmologist, Richard Diangelis, MD. Patient
             advised about signs and symptoms of detachment of the retina
             and told to seek immediate medical attention should any of
             these signs appear.
          2. Trial of Midrin for migraines.
          3. Recheck in one to two months.
          4. Patient requests referral to Dr. Diangelis.

Karen Larsen, MD/ls

Doublespace body.
Page numbers on upper
right starting on page 2.

↓ 2

RUBELLA (GERMAN MEASLES)

DEFINITION

Rubella (german measles) is a *highly* communicable viral disease characterized by diffuse, punctate, macular rash. Rubella is a relatively benign viral illness un_less there is transplacental transmission. (Define the following terms: *communicable, diffuse, punctate, transplacental,* and *macular*.)

ETIOLOGY

Rubella is caused by rubella virus (*Rubivirus*) ~~that is~~ spread by air_borne direct contact with nasopharyngeal secretion*s*. This disease is communicable from one week before *the* rash appears to five days after the rash disappears. Rubella is most common in children but may also affect adults ~~who were~~ not infected during childhood. (Define the following terms: airborne, direct contact, and nasopharyngeal.)

INCIDENCE

Rubella occurs most often in the spring, but there are major epidemics occurring in 6 to 9 year cycles. (Investigate recent epidemics vs. the use of the vaccine.)

PATHOPHYSIOLOGY

The virus invades the nasopharynx and travels to the lymph #glands, causing lymphadenopathy. Then in 5 to seven days it enters the blood_stream stimulating an immune response causing the *skin* rash. This rash lasts about three days.

(Define lymphadenopathy.)

CLINICAL SYSTEMS

The first ^ Clinical symptoms of rubella include swollen *l* gands, fever, sore throat, cough, and fatigue. The *often* pruritic rash generally starts in 1 to 5 days after the prodrome. The rash begins on the face and *the* trunk and spreads to the upper and lower extremities. Symptom*s* of headache and conjunctivitis may occur after the rash. (Define conjunctivitis, pruritic, and swollen glands.)

ADDITIONAL ASSIGNMENT:

Investigate what complication*s* may occur to a fetus and a child with rubella, describing each complication plus its incidence.

¶ Investigate what complication*s* may occur in adult*s* with rubella, describing each complication plus its incidence.

Investigate what diagnostic testing can be done for the occurrence *of* rubella.

Investigate treatment options.

MUMPS (INFECTIOUS PAROTITIS)

DEFINITION

Mumps is an _acute_ viral disease that may include myalgia, anorexia, malaise, headache, low-grade fever, _and_ parotid gland tenderness and unilateral or bilateral swelling, although many other organs can be involved. (Define the following terms: _myalgia, anorexia,_ and _malaise._)

ETIOLOGY

Mumps is caused _by_ paramyxovirus transmitted in saliva droplets or direct contact. The virus lives in the saliva six to 9 days before the parotid gland swelling. The highest communicable period is 48 hours before the on set of swelling but continues until swelling is decreased. Incubation period range_s_ from 14 to 25 days.

INCIDENCE

(Investigate the incidence in the past 10 years.)

PATHOPHYSIOLOGY

During the incubation period, the virus invades _the_ salivary glands which causes tissue edema and infiltration of lymphocytes. Degeneration of cells in the glandular tissue produce_s_ necrotic debris that plugs the ducts.

CLINICAL SYMPTOMS

The prodrome _of mumps_ generally begins with ~~generally begins~~ myalgia, anorexia, malaise, headache, and low-grade fever. Next the patient may have an ear ache aggravated by chewing, temperature of 101° to 104° F, and pain from chewing food or drinking acidic liquid. Both the parotid gland and other salivary glands _may_ become swollen. (Define _prodrome._)

ADDITIONAL ASSIGNMENT:

Investigate what complications may occur with mumps in _both_ children and adults.

Summarize how mumps would be diagnosed.

Summarize outpatient and inpatient complications of treatment.

MESSAGE

TO _____
DATE _____ TIME _____
FROM _____
PHONE _____
☐ PLEASE CALL ☐ RETURNED YOUR CALL ☐ WILL CALL AGAIN
REGARDING _____
_____
_____
_____
TAKEN BY _____

MESSAGE

TO _____
DATE _____ TIME _____
FROM _____
PHONE _____
☐ PLEASE CALL ☐ RETURNED YOUR CALL ☐ WILL CALL AGAIN
REGARDING _____
_____
_____
_____
TAKEN BY _____

MESSAGE

TO _____
DATE _____ TIME _____
FROM _____
PHONE _____
☐ PLEASE CALL ☐ RETURNED YOUR CALL ☐ WILL CALL AGAIN
REGARDING _____
_____
_____
_____
TAKEN BY _____

MESSAGE

TO _____
DATE _____ TIME _____
FROM _____
PHONE _____
☐ PLEASE CALL ☐ RETURNED YOUR CALL ☐ WILL CALL AGAIN
REGARDING _____
_____
_____
_____
TAKEN BY _____

MESSAGE

TO _____

DATE _____ TIME _____

FROM _____

PHONE _____

☐ PLEASE CALL ☐ RETURNED YOUR CALL ☐ WILL CALL AGAIN

REGARDING _____

_____

_____

_____

TAKEN BY _____

MESSAGE

TO _____

DATE _____ TIME _____

FROM _____

PHONE _____

☐ PLEASE CALL ☐ RETURNED YOUR CALL ☐ WILL CALL AGAIN

REGARDING _____

_____

_____

_____

TAKEN BY _____

MESSAGE

TO _____

DATE _____ TIME _____

FROM _____

PHONE _____

☐ PLEASE CALL ☐ RETURNED YOUR CALL ☐ WILL CALL AGAIN

REGARDING _____

_____

_____

_____

TAKEN BY _____

MESSAGE

TO _____

DATE _____ TIME _____

FROM _____

PHONE _____

☐ PLEASE CALL ☐ RETURNED YOUR CALL ☐ WILL CALL AGAIN

REGARDING _____

_____

_____

_____

TAKEN BY _____

MESSAGE

TO _____

FROM _____

PHONE _____

DATE _____ TIME _____

☐ PLEASE CALL   ☐ RETURNED YOUR CALL   ☐ WILL CALL AGAIN

REGARDING _____

_____

_____

_____

TAKEN BY _____

MESSAGE

TO _____

FROM _____

PHONE _____

DATE _____ TIME _____

☐ PLEASE CALL   ☐ RETURNED YOUR CALL   ☐ WILL CALL AGAIN

REGARDING _____

_____

_____

_____

TAKEN BY _____

MESSAGE

TO _____

FROM _____

PHONE _____

DATE _____ TIME _____

☐ PLEASE CALL   ☐ RETURNED YOUR CALL   ☐ WILL CALL AGAIN

REGARDING _____

_____

_____

_____

TAKEN BY _____

MESSAGE

TO _____

FROM _____

PHONE _____

DATE _____ TIME _____

☐ PLEASE CALL   ☐ RETURNED YOUR CALL   ☐ WILL CALL AGAIN

REGARDING _____

_____

_____

_____

TAKEN BY _____

MESSAGE

TO _____
FROM _____
PHONE _____
DATE _____ TIME _____
☐ PLEASE CALL   ☐ RETURNED YOUR CALL   ☐ WILL CALL AGAIN
REGARDING _____
_____
_____
_____
_____
_____
TAKEN BY _____

MESSAGE

TO _____
FROM _____
PHONE _____
DATE _____ TIME _____
☐ PLEASE CALL   ☐ RETURNED YOUR CALL   ☐ WILL CALL AGAIN
REGARDING _____
_____
_____
_____
_____
_____
TAKEN BY _____

MESSAGE

TO _____
FROM _____
PHONE _____
DATE _____ TIME _____
☐ PLEASE CALL   ☐ RETURNED YOUR CALL   ☐ WILL CALL AGAIN
REGARDING _____
_____
_____
_____
_____
_____
TAKEN BY _____

MESSAGE

TO _____
FROM _____
PHONE _____
DATE _____ TIME _____
☐ PLEASE CALL   ☐ RETURNED YOUR CALL   ☐ WILL CALL AGAIN
REGARDING _____
_____
_____
_____
_____
_____
TAKEN BY _____

MESSAGE

TO _____
FROM _____
PHONE _____
☐ PLEASE CALL   ☐ RETURNED YOUR CALL   ☐ WILL CALL AGAIN
REGARDING _____
_____
_____
_____
DATE _____   TIME _____
TAKEN BY _____

MESSAGE

TO _____
FROM _____
PHONE _____
☐ PLEASE CALL   ☐ RETURNED YOUR CALL   ☐ WILL CALL AGAIN
REGARDING _____
_____
_____
_____
DATE _____   TIME _____
TAKEN BY _____

MESSAGE

TO _____
FROM _____
PHONE _____
☐ PLEASE CALL   ☐ RETURNED YOUR CALL   ☐ WILL CALL AGAIN
REGARDING _____
_____
_____
_____
DATE _____   TIME _____
TAKEN BY _____

MESSAGE

TO _____
FROM _____
PHONE _____
☐ PLEASE CALL   ☐ RETURNED YOUR CALL   ☐ WILL CALL AGAIN
REGARDING _____
_____
_____
_____
DATE _____   TIME _____
TAKEN BY _____

MESSAGE

TO _____ DATE _____ TIME _____

FROM _____

PHONE _____

☐ PLEASE CALL   ☐ RETURNED YOUR CALL   ☐ WILL CALL AGAIN

REGARDING _____

_____

_____

_____

TAKEN BY _____

MESSAGE

TO _____ DATE _____ TIME _____

FROM _____

PHONE _____

☐ PLEASE CALL   ☐ RETURNED YOUR CALL   ☐ WILL CALL AGAIN

REGARDING _____

_____

_____

_____

TAKEN BY _____

MESSAGE

TO _____ DATE _____ TIME _____

FROM _____

PHONE _____

☐ PLEASE CALL   ☐ RETURNED YOUR CALL   ☐ WILL CALL AGAIN

REGARDING _____

_____

_____

_____

TAKEN BY _____

MESSAGE

TO _____ DATE _____ TIME _____

FROM _____

PHONE _____

☐ PLEASE CALL   ☐ RETURNED YOUR CALL   ☐ WILL CALL AGAIN

REGARDING _____

_____

_____

_____

TAKEN BY _____

MESSAGE

TO _____

FROM _____

PHONE _____

DATE _____ TIME _____

☐ PLEASE CALL ☐ RETURNED YOUR CALL ☐ WILL CALL AGAIN

REGARDING _____

_____

_____

TAKEN BY _____

MESSAGE

TO _____

FROM _____

PHONE _____

DATE _____ TIME _____

☐ PLEASE CALL ☐ RETURNED YOUR CALL ☐ WILL CALL AGAIN

REGARDING _____

_____

_____

TAKEN BY _____

MESSAGE

TO _____

FROM _____

PHONE _____

DATE _____ TIME _____

☐ PLEASE CALL ☐ RETURNED YOUR CALL ☐ WILL CALL AGAIN

REGARDING _____

_____

_____

TAKEN BY _____

MESSAGE

TO _____

FROM _____

PHONE _____

DATE _____ TIME _____

☐ PLEASE CALL ☐ RETURNED YOUR CALL ☐ WILL CALL AGAIN

REGARDING _____

_____

_____

TAKEN BY _____

MESSAGE

TO _____

DATE _____ TIME _____

FROM _____

PHONE _____

☐ PLEASE CALL ☐ RETURNED YOUR CALL ☐ WILL CALL AGAIN

REGARDING _____

_____

_____

TAKEN BY _____

MESSAGE

TO _____

DATE _____ TIME _____

FROM _____

PHONE _____

☐ PLEASE CALL ☐ RETURNED YOUR CALL ☐ WILL CALL AGAIN

REGARDING _____

_____

_____

TAKEN BY _____

MESSAGE

TO _____

DATE _____ TIME _____

FROM _____

PHONE _____

☐ PLEASE CALL ☐ RETURNED YOUR CALL ☐ WILL CALL AGAIN

REGARDING _____

_____

_____

TAKEN BY _____

MESSAGE

TO _____

DATE _____ TIME _____

FROM _____

PHONE _____

☐ PLEASE CALL ☐ RETURNED YOUR CALL ☐ WILL CALL AGAIN

REGARDING _____

_____

_____

TAKEN BY _____

SCHEDULING DECISION MAKING

Directions: The following calls in Column 1 are for a family practice physician. The physician does see emergencies in the office. Choose the appropriate response from Column 2 to indicate when an appointment should be made for **STAT, Today, Tomorrow, Later,** or a message taken—**Take message.**

Column 1

_____ **1.** Loni Kayen desires weight control, 312-555-9834.

_____ **2.** North Lab's report on prothrombin time for Walter Boone; control was 11.6; patient, 18, 312-555-6757.

_____ **3.** Hank Holm at 312-555-4432 wants to talk to the doctor about his left leg cast; it seems too tight, feels numbness in his toes.

_____ **4.** Brian Verk at 312-555-2389 needs diabetes recheck.

_____ **5.** Kay Frank, bee sting, left face check, swelling and a hard spot in the middle; she has no allergies; 312-555-6734.

_____ **6.** Beth Cater has a urinary problem, hurts to urinate, no blood in urine, 312-555-9823.

_____ **7.** True Value Drug, 312-555-9877, prescription refill Diane Yvon, Coumadin 5 mg q.d., #60, last filled two months ago.

_____ **8.** Hu Grangdon, rash over abdomen times 2 days, itching, no new foods or meds, 312-555-3341.

_____ **9.** Ben Jones, BP recheck, 312-555-3478.

_____ **10.** Dana Lund, annual Pap smear, 312-555-0043.

_____ **11.** Donna Kelly, son Alex got hit in head with a bat, bleeding, swelling, 312-555-9823.

_____ **12.** North X-ray, 312-555-6757, chest x-ray on Ann Tyn is negative.

_____ **13.** Pamela Bond, 6-week checkup for baby Keith, 312-555-5636.

_____ **14.** Rein Los Ames, age 2 months, cranky, pulling right ear, slight temperature, 312-555-3223.

_____ **15.** Tom Urness, 312-555-5574, age 47, noticed blood in stools, very concerned, read about colon cancer in recent magazine.

_____ **16.** Karin Olsson, age 72, infected hangnail with green pus, hurts, swollen, 312-555-9966.

_____ **17.** Wendy Rinke, age 8, something in her eye, red, watering. Father was sanding where she was playing, 312-555-7845.

Column 2

a. STAT

b. Today

c. Tomorrow

d. Later

e. Take message

KAREN LARSEN, MD, OFFICE SCHEDULE

2235 South Ridgeway Avenue
Chicago, IL 60623-2240
312-555-6022
Fax: 312-555-0025

Monday, Tuesday, and Wednesday

Hospital rounds	8:00 A.M. – 10:00 A.M.
Travel time	10:00 A.M. – 10:30 A.M.
Patient appointments	10:30 A.M. – 12 noon
Lunch	12 noon – 1:00 P.M.
Teach and work at University Hospital	1:00 P.M. – 5:00 P.M.

Thursday

Teach and work at University Hospital	8:00 A.M. – 5:00 P.M.

Friday

Hospital rounds	8:00 A.M. – 10:00 A.M.
Travel time	10:00 A.M. – 10:30 A.M.
Office for dictation, messages, writing, and course preparation	10:30 A.M. – 12 noon
Office closed	12 noon – 5:00 P.M.

Length of Appointments

Complete physical examination	1 hour
All other appointments, unless designated	15 minutes

Appointment Abbreviations

abd	abdominal
BP	blood pressure
✓	checkup
Dx	diagnosis
ECG	electrocardiogram
F/U	follow-up visit
FX	fracture
GI	gastrointestinal
N & V	nausea and vomiting
NP	new patient
CPE, PE	physical examination
preop	preoperative
postop	postoperative

Monday, October 13

8:00	
8:15	
8:30	
8:45	
9:00	
9:15	
9:30	
9:45	
10:00	
10:15	
10:30	
10:45	
11:00	Seminar
11:15	
11:30	University
11:45	
12:00	
12:15	
12:30	
12:45	
1:00	
1:15	
1:30	
1:45	
2:00	
2:15	
2:30	
2:45	
3:00	
3:15	
3:30	
3:45	
4:00	
4:15	
4:30	
4:45	
5:00	

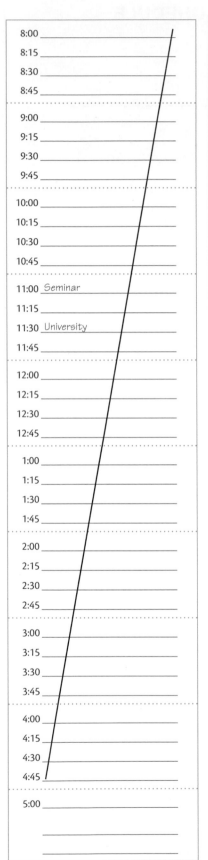

Tuesday, October 14

8:00	
8:15	
8:30	
8:45	Hospital
9:00	Rounds
9:15	
9:30	
9:45	
10:00	Travel
10:15	
10:30	
10:45	
11:00	
11:15	
11:30	
11:45	
12:00	
12:15	Lunch
12:30	
12:45	
1:00	
1:15	
1:30	
1:45	University
2:00	Hospital
2:15	
2:30	
2:45	
3:00	
3:15	
3:30	
3:45	
4:00	
4:15	
4:30	
4:45	
5:00	

8 p.m. Chicago Medical Society

Wednesday, October 15

8:00	
8:15	
8:30	
8:45	Hospital
9:00	Rounds
9:15	
9:30	
9:45	
10:00	Travel
10:15	
10:30	
10:45	
11:00	
11:15	
11:30	
11:45	
12:00	
12:15	Lunch
12:30	
12:45	
1:00	
1:15	
1:30	
1:45	University
2:00	Hospital
2:15	
2:30	
2:45	
3:00	
3:15	
3:30	
3:45	
4:00	
4:15	
4:30	
4:45	
5:00	

Thursday, October 16

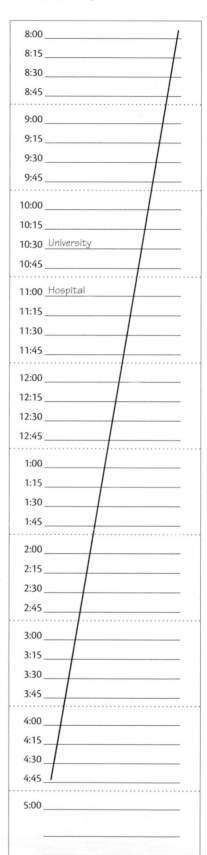

8:00	
8:15	
8:30	
8:45	
9:00	
9:15	
9:30	
9:45	
10:00	
10:15	
10:30	University
10:45	
11:00	Hospital
11:15	
11:30	
11:45	
12:00	
12:15	
12:30	
12:45	
1:00	
1:15	
1:30	
1:45	
2:00	
2:15	
2:30	
2:45	
3:00	
3:15	
3:30	
3:45	
4:00	
4:15	
4:30	
4:45	
5:00	

Friday, October 17

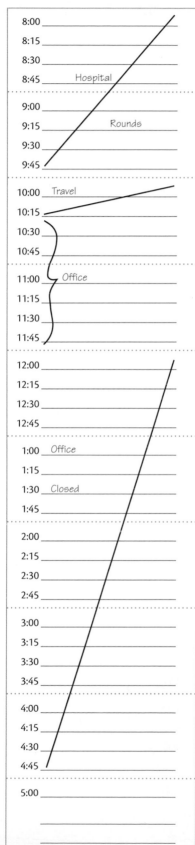

8:00	
8:15	
8:30	
8:45	Hospital
9:00	
9:15	Rounds
9:30	
9:45	
10:00	Travel
10:15	
10:30	
10:45	
11:00	Office
11:15	
11:30	
11:45	
12:00	
12:15	
12:30	
12:45	
1:00	Office
1:15	
1:30	Closed
1:45	
2:00	
2:15	
2:30	
2:45	
3:00	
3:15	
3:30	
3:45	
4:00	
4:15	
4:30	
4:45	
5:00	

October

S	M	T	W	T	F	S
			1	2	3	4
5	6	7	8	9	10	11
12	13	14	15	16	17	18
19	20	21	22	23	24	25
26	27	28	29	30	31	

November

S	M	T	W	T	F	S
						1
2	3	4	5	6	7	8
9	10	11	12	13	14	15
16	17	18	19	20	21	22
23	24	25	26	27	28	29
30						

December

S	M	T	W	T	F	S
	1	2	3	4	5	6
7	8	9	10	11	12	13
14	15	16	17	18	19	20
21	22	23	24	25	26	27
28	29	30	31			

Monday, October 20	Tuesday, October 21	Wednesday, October 22
8:00	8:00	8:00
8:15	8:15	8:15
8:30	8:30	8:30
8:45 Hospital	8:45 Hospital	8:45 Hospital
9:00	9:00	9:00
9:15 Rounds	9:15 Rounds	9:15 Rounds
9:30	9:30	9:30
9:45	9:45	9:45
10:00 Travel	10:00 Travel	10:00 Travel
10:15	10:15	10:15
10:30	10:30	10:30
10:45	10:45	10:45
11:00	11:00	11:00
11:15	11:15	11:15
11:30	11:30	11:30
11:45	11:45	11:45
12:00	12:00	12:00
12:15 Lunch	12:15 Lunch	12:15 Lunch
12:30	12:30	12:30
12:45	12:45	12:45
1:00	1:00	1:00
1:15	1:15	1:15
1:30	1:30	1:30
1:45 University	1:45 University	1:45 University
2:00 Hospital	2:00 Hospital	2:00 Hospital
2:15	2:15	2:15
2:30	2:30	2:30
2:45	2:45	2:45
3:00	3:00	3:00
3:15	3:15	3:15
3:30	3:30	3:30
3:45	3:45	3:45
4:00	4:00	4:00
4:15	4:15	4:15
4:30	4:30	4:30
4:45	4:45	4:45
5:00	5:00	5:00

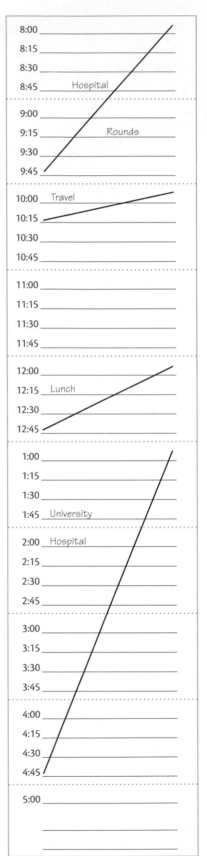

Working Papers

Thursday, October 23

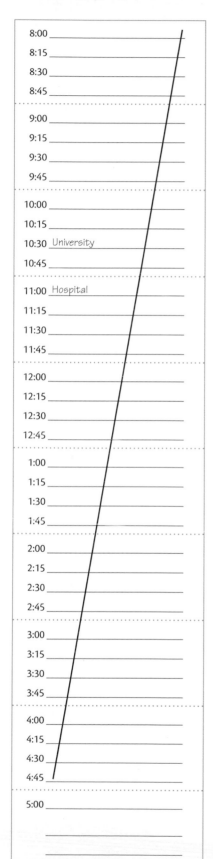

8:00 _____
8:15 _____
8:30 _____
8:45 _____

9:00 _____
9:15 _____
9:30 _____
9:45 _____

10:00 _____
10:15 _____
10:30 University _____
10:45 _____

11:00 Hospital _____
11:15 _____
11:30 _____
11:45 _____

12:00 _____
12:15 _____
12:30 _____
12:45 _____

1:00 _____
1:15 _____
1:30 _____
1:45 _____

2:00 _____
2:15 _____
2:30 _____
2:45 _____

3:00 _____
3:15 _____
3:30 _____
3:45 _____

4:00 _____
4:15 _____
4:30 _____
4:45 _____

5:00 _____

_____
_____

Friday, October 24

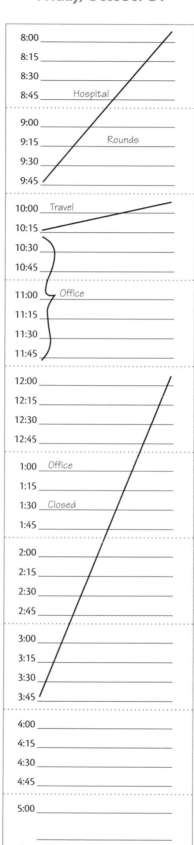

8:00 _____
8:15 _____
8:30 _____
8:45 Hospital _____

9:00 _____
9:15 Rounds _____
9:30 _____
9:45 _____

10:00 Travel _____
10:15 _____
10:30 _____
10:45 _____

11:00 Office _____
11:15 _____
11:30 _____
11:45 _____

12:00 _____
12:15 _____
12:30 _____
12:45 _____

1:00 Office _____
1:15 _____
1:30 Closed _____
1:45 _____

2:00 _____
2:15 _____
2:30 _____
2:45 _____

3:00 _____
3:15 _____
3:30 _____
3:45 _____

4:00 _____
4:15 _____
4:30 _____
4:45 _____

5:00 _____

_____
_____

October

S	M	T	W	T	F	S
			1	2	3	4
5	6	7	8	9	10	11
12	13	14	15	16	17	18
19	20	21	22	23	24	25
26	27	28	29	30	31	

November

S	M	T	W	T	F	S
						1
2	3	4	5	6	7	8
9	10	11	12	13	14	15
16	17	18	19	20	21	22
23	24	25	26	27	28	29
30						

December

S	M	T	W	T	F	S
	1	2	3	4	5	6
7	8	9	10	11	12	13
14	15	16	17	18	19	20
21	22	23	24	25	26	27
28	29	30	31			

Monday, October 27

8:00 _____
8:15 _____
8:30 _____
8:45 _____ Hospital _____

9:00 _____
9:15 _____ Rounds _____
9:30 _____
9:45 _____

10:00 Travel _____
10:15 _____
10:30 _____
10:45 _____

11:00 _____
11:15 _____
11:30 _____
11:45 _____

12:00 _____
12:15 Lunch _____
12:30 _____
12:45 _____

1:00 _____
1:15 _____
1:30 _____
1:45 _____ University _____

2:00 Hospital _____
2:15 _____
2:30 _____
2:45 _____

3:00 _____
3:15 _____
3:30 _____
3:45 _____

4:00 _____
4:15 _____
4:30 _____
4:45 _____

5:00 _____

_____
_____

Tuesday, October 28

8:00 _____
8:15 _____
8:30 _____
8:45 _____ Hospital _____

9:00 _____
9:15 _____ Rounds _____
9:30 _____
9:45 _____

10:00 Travel _____
10:15 _____
10:30 _____
10:45 _____

11:00 _____
11:15 _____
11:30 _____
11:45 _____

12:00 _____
12:15 Lunch _____
12:30 _____
12:45 _____

1:00 _____
1:15 _____
1:30 _____
1:45 _____ University _____

2:00 Hospital _____
2:15 _____
2:30 _____
2:45 _____

3:00 _____
3:15 _____
3:30 _____
3:45 _____

4:00 _____
4:15 _____
4:30 _____
4:45 _____

5:00 _____

_____
_____

Wednesday, October 29

8:00 _____
8:15 _____
8:30 _____
8:45 _____ Hospital _____

9:00 _____
9:15 _____ Rounds _____
9:30 _____
9:45 _____

10:00 Travel _____
10:15 _____
10:30 _____
10:45 _____

11:00 _____
11:15 _____
11:30 _____
11:45 _____

12:00 _____
12:15 Lunch _____
12:30 _____
12:45 _____

1:00 _____
1:15 _____
1:30 _____
1:45 _____ University _____

2:00 Hospital _____
2:15 _____
2:30 _____
2:45 _____

3:00 _____
3:15 _____
3:30 _____
3:45 _____

4:00 _____
4:15 _____
4:30 _____
4:45 _____

5:00 _____

_____
_____

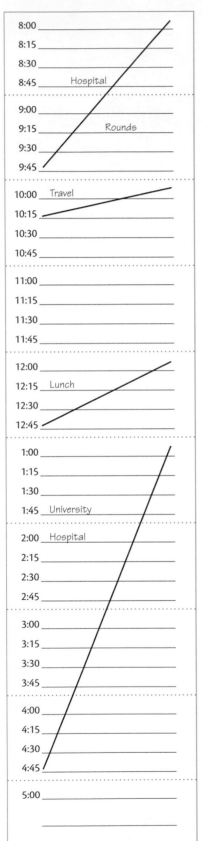
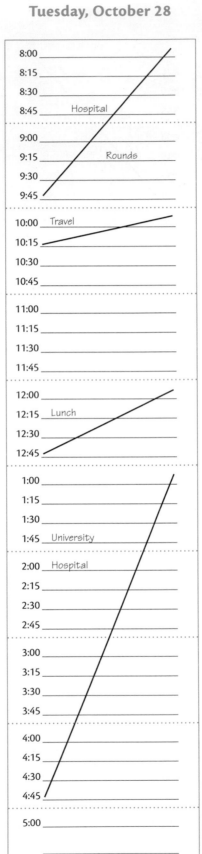

Thursday, October 30   **Friday, October 31**

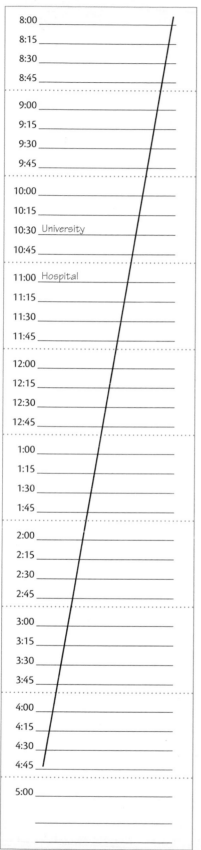
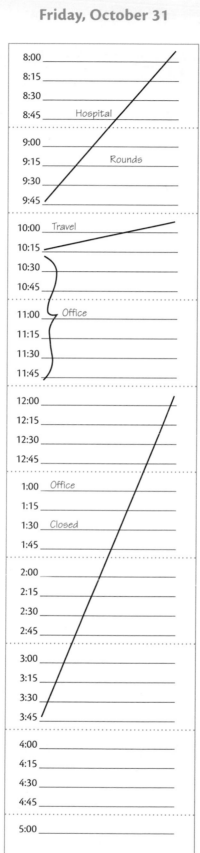

	Thursday, October 30
8:00	
8:15	
8:30	
8:45	
9:00	
9:15	
9:30	
9:45	
10:00	
10:15	
10:30	University
10:45	
11:00	Hospital
11:15	
11:30	
11:45	
12:00	
12:15	
12:30	
12:45	
1:00	
1:15	
1:30	
1:45	
2:00	
2:15	
2:30	
2:45	
3:00	
3:15	
3:30	
3:45	
4:00	
4:15	
4:30	
4:45	
5:00	

	Friday, October 31
8:00	
8:15	
8:30	
8:45	Hospital
9:00	
9:15	Rounds
9:30	
9:45	
10:00	Travel
10:15	
10:30	
10:45	
11:00	Office
11:15	
11:30	
11:45	
12:00	
12:15	
12:30	
12:45	
1:00	Office
1:15	
1:30	Closed
1:45	
2:00	
2:15	
2:30	
2:45	
3:00	
3:15	
3:30	
3:45	
4:00	
4:15	
4:30	
4:45	
5:00	

October

S	M	T	W	T	F	S
		1	2	3	4	
5	6	7	8	9	10	11
12	13	14	15	16	17	18
19	20	21	22	23	24	25
26	27	28	29	30	31	

November

S	M	T	W	T	F	S
						1
2	3	4	5	6	7	8
9	10	11	12	13	14	15
16	17	18	19	20	21	22
23	24	25	26	27	28	29
30						

December

S	M	T	W	T	F	S
	1	2	3	4	5	6
7	8	9	10	11	12	13
14	15	16	17	18	19	20
21	22	23	24	25	26	27
28	29	30	31			

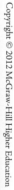

Monday, November 3

8:00	
8:15	
8:30	
8:45	Hospital
9:00	
9:15	Rounds
9:30	
9:45	
10:00	Travel
10:15	
10:30	
10:45	
11:00	Joseph Castro, CPE
11:15	555-1020
11:30	
11:45	
12:00	
12:15	Lunch
12:30	
12:45	
1:00	
1:15	
1:30	
1:45	University
2:00	Hospital
2:15	
2:30	
2:45	
3:00	
3:15	
3:30	
3:45	
4:00	
4:15	
4:30	
4:45	
5:00	

Tuesday, November 4

8:00	
8:15	
8:30	
8:45	Hospital
9:00	
9:15	Rounds
9:30	
9:45	
10:00	Travel
10:15	
10:30	
10:45	
11:00	
11:15	
11:30	
11:45	
12:00	
12:15	Lunch
12:30	
12:45	
1:00	
1:15	
1:30	
1:45	University
2:00	Hospital
2:15	
2:30	
2:45	
3:00	
3:15	
3:30	
3:45	
4:00	
4:15	
4:30	
4:45	
5:00	

Wednesday, November 5

8:00	
8:15	
8:30	
8:45	Hospital
9:00	
9:15	Rounds
9:30	
9:45	
10:00	Travel
10:15	
10:30	Clarence Rogers, CPE
10:45	555-5297
11:00	
11:15	
11:30	
11:45	
12:00	
12:15	Lunch
12:30	
12:45	
1:00	
1:15	
1:30	
1:45	University
2:00	Hospital
2:15	
2:30	
2:45	
3:00	
3:15	
3:30	
3:45	
4:00	
4:15	
4:30	
4:45	
5:00	

Working Papers

Thursday, November 6

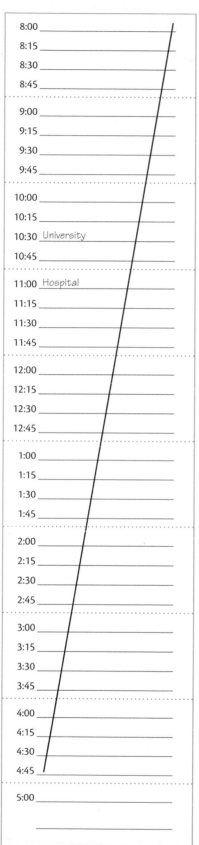

8:00	
8:15	
8:30	
8:45	
9:00	
9:15	
9:30	
9:45	
10:00	
10:15	
10:30	University
10:45	
11:00	Hospital
11:15	
11:30	
11:45	
12:00	
12:15	
12:30	
12:45	
1:00	
1:15	
1:30	
1:45	
2:00	
2:15	
2:30	
2:45	
3:00	
3:15	
3:30	
3:45	
4:00	
4:15	
4:30	
4:45	
5:00	

Friday, November 7

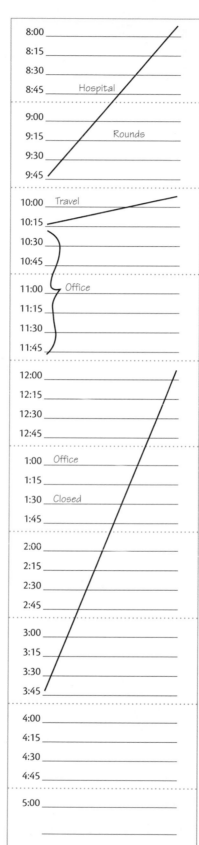

8:00	
8:15	
8:30	
8:45	Hospital
9:00	
9:15	Rounds
9:30	
9:45	
10:00	Travel
10:15	
10:30	
10:45	
11:00	Office
11:15	
11:30	
11:45	
12:00	
12:15	
12:30	
12:45	
1:00	Office
1:15	
1:30	Closed
1:45	
2:00	
2:15	
2:30	
2:45	
3:00	
3:15	
3:30	
3:45	
4:00	
4:15	
4:30	
4:45	
5:00	

October

S	M	T	W	T	F	S
			1	2	3	4
5	6	7	8	9	10	11
12	13	14	15	16	17	18
19	20	21	22	23	24	25
26	27	28	29	30	31	

November

S	M	T	W	T	F	S
						1
2	3	4	5	6	7	8
9	10	11	12	13	14	15
16	17	18	19	20	21	22
23	24	25	26	27	28	29
30						

December

S	M	T	W	T	F	S
	1	2	3	4	5	6
7	8	9	10	11	12	13
14	15	16	17	18	19	20
21	22	23	24	25	26	27
28	29	30	31			

Monday, November 10

8:00	
8:15	
8:30	
8:45	Hospital
9:00	
9:15	Rounds
9:30	
9:45	
10:00	Travel
10:15	
10:30	
10:45	
11:00	
11:15	
11:30	
11:45	
12:00	
12:15	Lunch
12:30	
12:45	
1:00	
1:15	
1:30	
1:45	University
2:00	Hospital
2:15	
2:30	
2:45	
3:00	
3:15	
3:30	
3:45	
4:00	
4:15	
4:30	
4:45	
5:00	

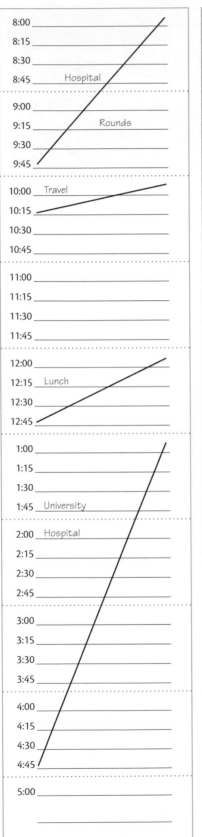

Tuesday, November 11

8:00	
8:15	
8:30	
8:45	Hospital
9:00	
9:15	Rounds
9:30	
9:45	
10:00	Travel
10:15	
10:30	
10:45	Raymond Murrary, CPE
11:00	555-6343
11:15	
11:30	
11:45	
12:00	
12:15	Lunch
12:30	
12:45	
1:00	
1:15	
1:30	
1:45	University
2:00	Hospital
2:15	
2:30	
2:45	
3:00	
3:15	
3:30	
3:45	
4:00	
4:15	
4:30	
4:45	
5:00	

8 p.m. Chicago Medical Society

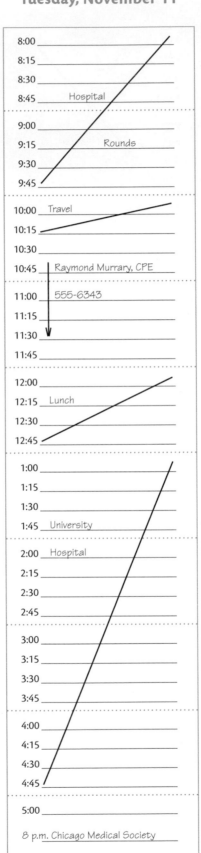

Wednesday, November 12

8:00	
8:15	
8:30	
8:45	Hospital
9:00	
9:15	Rounds
9:30	
9:45	
10:00	Travel
10:15	
10:30	
10:45	
11:00	
11:15	
11:30	
11:45	
12:00	
12:15	Lunch
12:30	
12:45	
1:00	
1:15	
1:30	
1:45	University
2:00	Hospital
2:15	
2:30	
2:45	
3:00	
3:15	
3:30	
3:45	
4:00	
4:15	
4:30	
4:45	
5:00	

Thursday, November 13 **Friday, November 14**

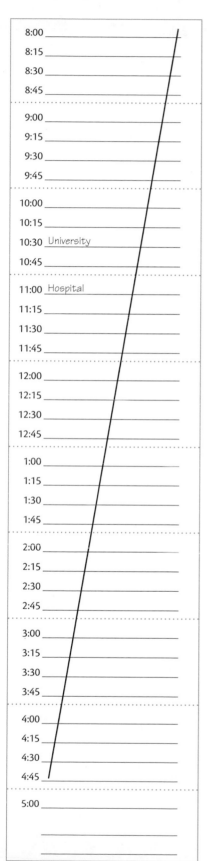

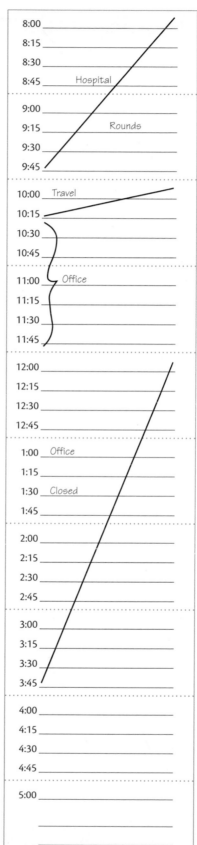

8:00	_____
8:15	_____
8:30	_____
8:45	_____
9:00	_____
9:15	_____
9:30	_____
9:45	_____
10:00	_____
10:15	_____
10:30 University	_____
10:45	_____
11:00 Hospital	_____
11:15	_____
11:30	_____
11:45	_____
12:00	_____
12:15	_____
12:30	_____
12:45	_____
1:00	_____
1:15	_____
1:30	_____
1:45	_____
2:00	_____
2:15	_____
2:30	_____
2:45	_____
3:00	_____
3:15	_____
3:30	_____
3:45	_____
4:00	_____
4:15	_____
4:30	_____
4:45	_____
5:00	_____

8:00	_____
8:15	_____
8:30	_____
8:45 Hospital	_____
9:00	_____
9:15 Rounds	_____
9:30	_____
9:45	_____
10:00 Travel	_____
10:15	_____
10:30	_____
10:45	_____
11:00 Office	_____
11:15	_____
11:30	_____
11:45	_____
12:00	_____
12:15	_____
12:30	_____
12:45	_____
1:00 Office	_____
1:15	_____
1:30 Closed	_____
1:45	_____
2:00	_____
2:15	_____
2:30	_____
2:45	_____
3:00	_____
3:15	_____
3:30	_____
3:45	_____
4:00	_____
4:15	_____
4:30	_____
4:45	_____
5:00	_____

October

S	M	T	W	T	F	S
			1	2	3	4
5	6	7	8	9	10	11
12	13	14	15	16	17	18
19	20	21	22	23	24	25
26	27	28	29	30	31	

November

S	M	T	W	T	F	S
						1
2	3	4	5	6	7	8
9	10	11	12	13	14	15
16	17	18	19	20	21	22
23	24	25	26	27	28	29
30						

December

S	M	T	W	T	F	S
	1	2	3	4	5	6
7	8	9	10	11	12	13
14	15	16	17	18	19	20
21	22	23	24	25	26	27
28	29	30	31			

Monday, November 17	Tuesday, November 18	Wednesday, November 19
8:00	8:00	8:00
8:15	8:15	8:15
8:30	8:30	8:30
8:45 Hospital	8:45 Hospital	8:45 Hospital
9:00	9:00	9:00
9:15 Rounds	9:15 Rounds	9:15 Rounds
9:30	9:30	9:30
9:45	9:45	9:45
10:00 Travel	10:00 Travel	10:00 Travel
10:15	10:15	10:15
10:30	10:30	10:30
10:45	10:45	10:45
11:00	11:00	11:00
11:15	11:15	11:15
11:30	11:30	11:30
11:45	11:45	11:45
12:00	12:00	12:00
12:15 Lunch	12:15 Lunch	12:15 Lunch
12:30	12:30	12:30
12:45	12:45	12:45
1:00	1:00	1:00
1:15	1:15	1:15
1:30	1:30	1:30
1:45 University	1:45 University	1:45 University
2:00 Hospital	2:00 Hospital	2:00 Hospital
2:15	2:15	2:15
2:30	2:30	2:30
2:45	2:45	2:45
3:00	3:00	3:00
3:15	3:15	3:15
3:30	3:30	3:30
3:45	3:45	3:45
4:00	4:00	4:00
4:15	4:15	4:15
4:30	4:30	4:30
4:45	4:45	4:45
5:00	5:00	5:00

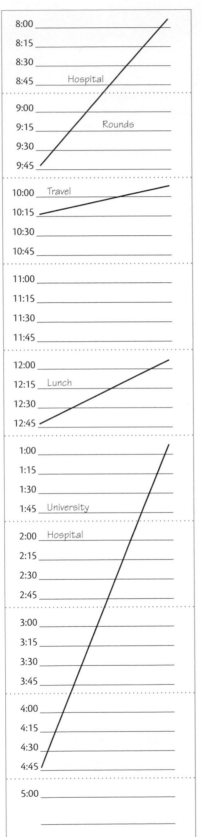

Working Papers

Thursday, November 20 **Friday, November 21**

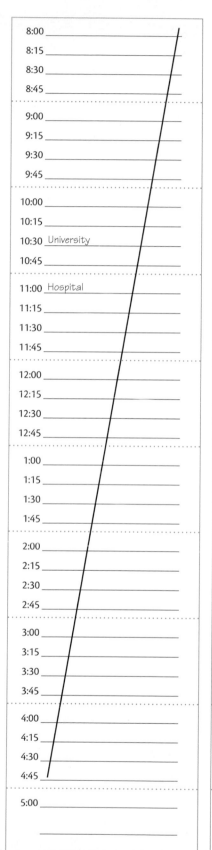

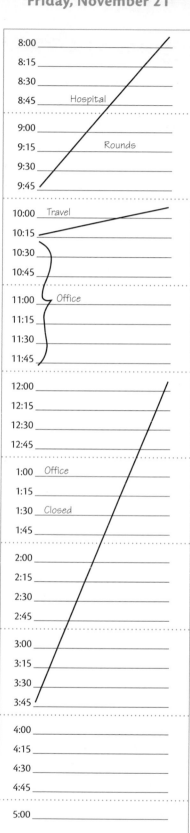

8:00 _____	8:00 _____
8:15 _____	8:15 _____
8:30 _____	8:30 _____
8:45 _____	8:45 Hospital _____
9:00 _____	9:00 _____
9:15 _____	9:15 Rounds _____
9:30 _____	9:30 _____
9:45 _____	9:45 _____
10:00 _____	10:00 Travel _____
10:15 _____	10:15 _____
10:30 University _____	10:30 _____
10:45 _____	10:45 _____
11:00 Hospital _____	11:00 Office _____
11:15 _____	11:15 _____
11:30 _____	11:30 _____
11:45 _____	11:45 _____
12:00 _____	12:00 _____
12:15 _____	12:15 _____
12:30 _____	12:30 _____
12:45 _____	12:45 _____
1:00 _____	1:00 Office _____
1:15 _____	1:15 _____
1:30 _____	1:30 Closed _____
1:45 _____	1:45 _____
2:00 _____	2:00 _____
2:15 _____	2:15 _____
2:30 _____	2:30 _____
2:45 _____	2:45 _____
3:00 _____	3:00 _____
3:15 _____	3:15 _____
3:30 _____	3:30 _____
3:45 _____	3:45 _____
4:00 _____	4:00 _____
4:15 _____	4:15 _____
4:30 _____	4:30 _____
4:45 _____	4:45 _____
5:00 _____	5:00 _____

October

S	M	T	W	T	F	S
			1	2	3	4
5	6	7	8	9	10	11
12	13	14	15	16	17	18
19	20	21	22	23	24	25
26	27	28	29	30	31	

November

S	M	T	W	T	F	S
						1
2	3	4	5	6	7	8
9	10	11	12	13	14	15
16	17	18	19	20	21	22
23	24	25	26	27	28	29
30						

December

S	M	T	W	T	F	S
	1	2	3	4	5	6
7	8	9	10	11	12	13
14	15	16	17	18	19	20
21	22	23	24	25	26	27
28	29	30	31			

Monday, November 24

8:00	
8:15	
8:30	
8:45	Hospital
9:00	
9:15	Rounds
9:30	
9:45	
10:00	Travel
10:15	
10:30	
10:45	
11:00	
11:15	
11:30	
11:45	
12:00	
12:15	Lunch
12:30	
12:45	
1:00	
1:15	
1:30	
1:45	University
2:00	Hospital
2:15	
2:30	
2:45	
3:00	
3:15	
3:30	
3:45	
4:00	
4:15	
4:30	
4:45	
5:00	

Tuesday, November 25

8:00	
8:15	
8:30	
8:45	Hospital
9:00	
9:15	Rounds
9:30	
9:45	
10:00	Travel
10:15	
10:30	
10:45	
11:00	
11:15	
11:30	
11:45	
12:00	
12:15	Lunch
12:30	
12:45	
1:00	
1:15	
1:30	
1:45	University
2:00	Hospital
2:15	
2:30	
2:45	
3:00	
3:15	
3:30	
3:45	
4:00	
4:15	
4:30	
4:45	
5:00	

Wednesday, November 26

8:00	
8:15	
8:30	
8:45	Hospital
9:00	
9:15	Rounds
9:30	
9:45	
10:00	Travel
10:15	
10:30	
10:45	
11:00	
11:15	
11:30	
11:45	
12:00	
12:15	Lunch
12:30	
12:45	
1:00	
1:15	
1:30	
1:45	University
2:00	Hospital
2:15	
2:30	
2:45	
3:00	
3:15	
3:30	
3:45	
4:00	
4:15	
4:30	
4:45	
5:00	

Working Papers

Thursday, November 27

8:00	
8:15	
8:30	
8:45	
9:00	
9:15	
9:30	
9:45	
10:00	
10:15	
10:30	
10:45	Office
11:00	Closed
11:15	Thanksgiving
11:30	
11:45	
12:00	
12:15	
12:30	
12:45	
1:00	
1:15	
1:30	
1:45	
2:00	
2:15	
2:30	
2:45	
3:00	
3:15	
3:30	
3:45	
4:00	
4:15	
4:30	
4:45	
5:00	

Friday, November 28

8:00	
8:15	
8:30	
8:45	
9:00	
9:15	
9:30	
9:45	
10:00	
10:15	
10:30	
10:45	Office
11:00	Closed
11:15	Thanksgiving
11:30	
11:45	
12:00	
12:15	
12:30	
12:45	
1:00	
1:15	
1:30	
1:45	
2:00	
2:15	
2:30	
2:45	
3:00	
3:15	
3:30	
3:45	
4:00	
4:15	
4:30	
4:45	
5:00	

October

S	M	T	W	T	F	S
			1	2	3	4
5	6	7	8	9	10	11
12	13	14	15	16	17	18
19	20	21	22	23	24	25
26	27	28	29	30	31	

November

S	M	T	W	T	F	S
						1
2	3	4	5	6	7	8
9	10	11	12	13	14	15
16	17	18	19	20	21	22
23	24	25	26	27	28	29
30						

December

S	M	T	W	T	F	S
	1	2	3	4	5	6
7	8	9	10	11	12	13
14	15	16	17	18	19	20
21	22	23	24	25	26	27
28	29	30	31			

Monday, December 1

8:00 _____
8:15 _____
8:30 _____
8:45 ____Hospital_____

9:00 _____
9:15 _____Rounds_____
9:30 _____
9:45 _____

10:00 __Travel_____
10:15 _____
10:30 _____
10:45 _____

11:00 _____
11:15 _____
11:30 _____
11:45 _____

12:00 _____
12:15 __Lunch_____
12:30 _____
12:45 _____

1:00 _____
1:15 _____
1:30 _____
1:45 __University_____

2:00 __Hospital_____
2:15 _____
2:30 _____
2:45 _____

3:00 _____
3:15 _____
3:30 _____
3:45 _____

4:00 _____
4:15 _____
4:30 _____
4:45 _____

5:00 _____

_____
_____

Tuesday, December 2

8:00 _____
8:15 _____
8:30 _____
8:45 ____Hospital_____

9:00 _____
9:15 _____Rounds_____
9:30 _____
9:45 _____

10:00 __Travel_____
10:15 _____
10:30 _____
10:45 _____

11:00 _____
11:15 _____
11:30 _____
11:45 _____

12:00 _____
12:15 __Lunch_____
12:30 _____
12:45 _____

1:00 _____
1:15 _____
1:30 _____
1:45 __University_____

2:00 __Hospital_____
2:15 _____
2:30 _____
2:45 _____

3:00 _____
3:15 _____
3:30 _____
3:45 _____

4:00 _____
4:15 _____
4:30 _____
4:45 _____

5:00 _____

_____
_____

Wednesday, December 3

8:00 _____
8:15 _____
8:30 _____
8:45 ____Hospital_____

9:00 _____
9:15 _____Rounds_____
9:30 _____
9:45 _____

10:00 __Travel_____
10:15 _____
10:30 _____
10:45 _____

11:00 _____
11:15 _____
11:30 _____
11:45 _____

12:00 _____
12:15 __Lunch_____
12:30 _____
12:45 _____

1:00 _____
1:15 _____
1:30 _____
1:45 __University_____

2:00 __Hospital_____
2:15 _____
2:30 _____
2:45 _____

3:00 _____
3:15 _____
3:30 _____
3:45 _____

4:00 _____
4:15 _____
4:30 _____
4:45 _____

5:00 _____

_____
_____

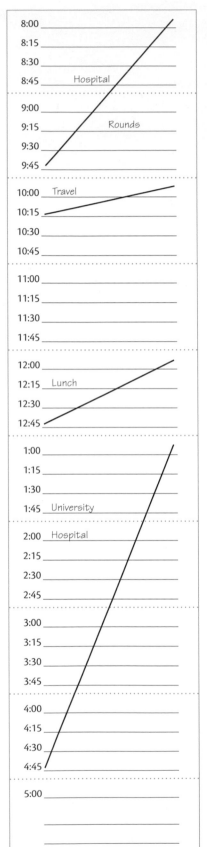

Thursday, December 4

8:00	
8:15	
8:30	
8:45	
9:00	
9:15	
9:30	
9:45	
10:00	
10:15	
10:30	University
10:45	
11:00	Hospital
11:15	
11:30	
11:45	
12:00	
12:15	
12:30	
12:45	
1:00	
1:15	
1:30	
1:45	
2:00	
2:15	
2:30	
2:45	
3:00	
3:15	
3:30	
3:45	
4:00	
4:15	
4:30	
4:45	
5:00	

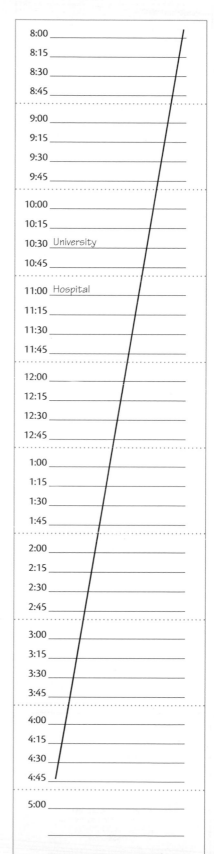

Friday, December 5

8:00	
8:15	
8:30	
8:45	Hospital
9:00	
9:15	Rounds
9:30	
9:45	
10:00	Travel
10:15	
10:30	
10:45	
11:00	Office
11:15	
11:30	
11:45	
12:00	
12:15	
12:30	
12:45	
1:00	Office
1:15	
1:30	Closed
1:45	
2:00	
2:15	
2:30	
2:45	
3:00	
3:15	
3:30	
3:45	
4:00	
4:15	
4:30	
4:45	
5:00	

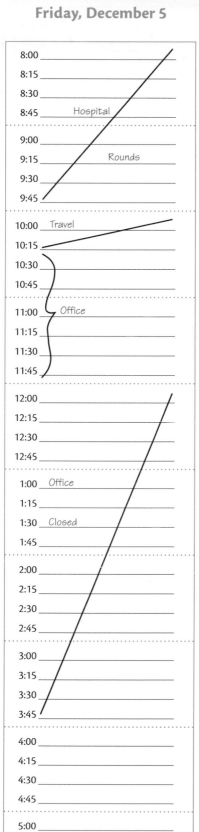

October

S	M	T	W	T	F	S
			1	2	3	4
5	6	7	8	9	10	11
12	13	14	15	16	17	18
19	20	21	22	23	24	25
26	27	28	29	30	31	

November

S	M	T	W	T	F	S
						1
2	3	4	5	6	7	8
9	10	11	12	13	14	15
16	17	18	19	20	21	22
23	24	25	26	27	28	29
30						

December

S	M	T	W	T	F	S
	1	2	3	4	5	6
7	8	9	10	11	12	13
14	15	16	17	18	19	20
21	22	23	24	25	26	27
28	29	30	31			

YOUR APPOINTMENT IS:

_____ AT _____

SPECIAL INSTRUCTIONS:

KAREN LARSEN, MD
2235 South Ridgeway Avenue
Chicago, IL 60623-2240
312-555-6022

PLEASE CALL IF YOU CANNOT KEEP THIS APPOINTMENT.

YOUR APPOINTMENT IS:

_____ AT _____

SPECIAL INSTRUCTIONS:

KAREN LARSEN, MD
2235 South Ridgeway Avenue
Chicago, IL 60623-2240
312-555-6022

PLEASE CALL IF YOU CANNOT KEEP THIS APPOINTMENT.

YOUR APPOINTMENT IS:

_____ AT _____

SPECIAL INSTRUCTIONS:

KAREN LARSEN, MD
2235 South Ridgeway Avenue
Chicago, IL 60623-2240
312-555-6022

PLEASE CALL IF YOU CANNOT KEEP THIS APPOINTMENT.

YOUR APPOINTMENT IS:

_____ AT _____

SPECIAL INSTRUCTIONS:

KAREN LARSEN, MD
2235 South Ridgeway Avenue
Chicago, IL 60623-2240
312-555-6022

PLEASE CALL IF YOU CANNOT KEEP THIS APPOINTMENT.

YOUR APPOINTMENT IS:

_____ AT _____

SPECIAL INSTRUCTIONS:

KAREN LARSEN, MD
2235 South Ridgeway Avenue
Chicago, IL 60623-2240
312-555-6022

PLEASE CALL IF YOU CANNOT KEEP THIS APPOINTMENT.

YOUR APPOINTMENT IS:

_____ AT _____

SPECIAL INSTRUCTIONS:

KAREN LARSEN, MD
2235 South Ridgeway Avenue
Chicago, IL 60623-2240
312-555-6022

PLEASE CALL IF YOU CANNOT KEEP THIS APPOINTMENT.

YOUR APPOINTMENT IS:

_____ AT _____

SPECIAL INSTRUCTIONS:

KAREN LARSEN, MD
2235 South Ridgeway Avenue
Chicago, IL 60623-2240
312-555-6022

PLEASE CALL IF YOU CANNOT KEEP THIS APPOINTMENT.

YOUR APPOINTMENT IS:

_____ AT _____

SPECIAL INSTRUCTIONS:

KAREN LARSEN, MD
2235 South Ridgeway Avenue
Chicago, IL 60623-2240
312-555-6022

PLEASE CALL IF YOU CANNOT KEEP THIS APPOINTMENT.

YOUR APPOINTMENT IS:

_____ AT _____

SPECIAL INSTRUCTIONS:

KAREN LARSEN, MD
2235 South Ridgeway Avenue
Chicago, IL 60623-2240
312-555-6022

PLEASE CALL IF YOU CANNOT KEEP THIS APPOINTMENT.

YOUR APPOINTMENT IS:

_____ AT _____

SPECIAL INSTRUCTIONS:

KAREN LARSEN, MD
2235 South Ridgeway Avenue
Chicago, IL 60623-2240
312-555-6022

PLEASE CALL IF YOU CANNOT KEEP THIS APPOINTMENT.

YOUR APPOINTMENT IS:

_____ AT _____

SPECIAL INSTRUCTIONS:

KAREN LARSEN, MD
2235 South Ridgeway Avenue
Chicago, IL 60623-2240
312-555-6022

PLEASE CALL IF YOU CANNOT KEEP THIS APPOINTMENT.

YOUR APPOINTMENT IS:

_____ AT _____

SPECIAL INSTRUCTIONS:

KAREN LARSEN, MD
2235 South Ridgeway Avenue
Chicago, IL 60623-2240
312-555-6022

PLEASE CALL IF YOU CANNOT KEEP THIS APPOINTMENT.

YOUR APPOINTMENT IS:

_____ AT _____

SPECIAL INSTRUCTIONS:

KAREN LARSEN, MD
2235 South Ridgeway Avenue
Chicago, IL 60623-2240
312-555-6022

PLEASE CALL IF YOU CANNOT KEEP THIS APPOINTMENT.

YOUR APPOINTMENT IS:

_____ AT _____

SPECIAL INSTRUCTIONS:

KAREN LARSEN, MD
2235 South Ridgeway Avenue
Chicago, IL 60623-2240
312-555-6022

PLEASE CALL IF YOU CANNOT KEEP THIS APPOINTMENT.

YOUR APPOINTMENT IS:

_____ AT _____

SPECIAL INSTRUCTIONS:

KAREN LARSEN, MD
2235 South Ridgeway Avenue
Chicago, IL 60623-2240
312-555-6022

PLEASE CALL IF YOU CANNOT KEEP THIS APPOINTMENT.

OUT-OF-OFFICE SCHEDULING

Directions: You are working for several physicians: Dr. R. Gain, a cardiologist; Dr. J. Brent, a family practice physician; and Dr. E. Oren, a general surgeon. Determine what element is missing in the situations in Column 1. Choose the appropriate response from Column 2.

Column 1

_____ **1.** Dr. Gain asks you to admit the patient, age 72, with a recent myocardial infarction to University Hospital today for controlled cardiovascular monitoring.

_____ **2.** Dr. Oren asks you to schedule a gastrectomy for Les Weiner, age 65, at University Hospital next Monday or Tuesday morning.

_____ **3.** Dr. Brent asks you to schedule Mary Maye for a bone marrow aspiration at University Hospital Lab because of her iron deficiency anemia.

_____ **4.** Peter Nu fractured his right wrist playing racquetball. Dr. Brent wants you to schedule an appointment with an orthopedic surgeon as soon as possible for possible surgery.

_____ **5.** Dr. Brent asks you to refer a 4-year-old patient, Jan Davis, with acute lymphocytic leukemia to an oncologist next week to start a program of chemotherapy.

_____ **6.** Dr. Oren wants you to schedule a short-stay surgery room at University Hospital for Tina Messer next Tuesday morning. Tina has a nodule in her right breast.

_____ **7.** Dr. Gain wants you to admit Ian Wenth to University Hospital. Ian has pulmonary insufficiency caused by pneumonia and will need intensive oxygen therapy.

_____ **8.** Patient Larry Phen has been diagnosed with emphysema. Dr. Gain now wants to refer Larry to a pulmonary specialist as soon as possible for therapeutic management.

_____ **9.** Dr. Brent wants to refer this patient as soon as possible to Dr. Henri Wilson, a neurologist. The patient's migraines have increased in frequency and in severity; her therapeutic program needs to be reevaluated.

_____ **10.** Dr. Oren wants you to admit Jane Hanson with appendicitis to University Hospital this morning.

Column 2

a. Specialist's name

b. Patient's name

c. Diagnosis or problem

d. When to be seen

e. Procedure to be performed

COMMUNICATIONS TERMS

Directions: Match the term in Column 2 with its definition in Column 1.

Column 1

_____ 1. The type of letter formatting that begins all parts of the letter at the left margin.

_____ 2. Manuscript sources at the bottom of the page on which the source is cited.

_____ 3. Careful reading and examination of a document to find and correct errors.

_____ 4. Style that has a colon after the salutation and a comma after the complimentary closing.

_____ 5. To skim a document and write notes in the margin.

_____ 6. Letter that begins the date line, complimentary closing, and signature line at the center point.

_____ 7. Fastest way to send heavier mail items that weigh less than 70 pounds.

_____ 8. Mail service providing the greatest security for valuables.

_____ 9. Style without punctuation after the salutation and complimentary closing.

_____ 10. Assessing a document to determine its clarity, consistency, and overall effectiveness.

_____ 11. Mail service that provides the sender with a mailing receipt.

_____ 12. Letter without a salutation or complimentary closing.

_____ 13. Rate used for books or film.

_____ 14. Fastest mail service, available 365 days a year.

_____ 15. Manuscript sources placed on a separate page following the last page of text.

Column 2

a. annotate

b. block-style letter

c. certified mail

d. editing

e. endnotes

f. Express Mail

g. footnotes

h. Media Mail

i. modified-block-style letter

j. open punctuation

k. Priority Mail

l. proofreading

m. registered mail

n. simplified-style letter

o. standard punctuation

COMPUTER TERMS

Directions: Match the term in Column 2 with its definition in Column 1.

Column 1

_____ **1.** Software that relates to specific tasks, such as word processing.

_____ **2.** Communications system for exchanging messages written on a computer over telephone lines.

_____ **3.** Portable, notebook-sized computers.

_____ **4.** The brain of a computer.

_____ **5.** Software that allows a person to edit a printed document.

_____ **6.** A display screen.

_____ **7.** Software that transcribes spoken words into text without using a keyboard.

_____ **8.** A system that allows a group of computers to communicate, exchange information, or pool resources.

_____ **9.** A personal computer small enough to fit in a person's hand.

_____ **10.** Software that allows the creation of images on the computer.

_____ **11.** A collection of related data.

_____ **12.** A removable storage medium.

_____ **13.** Temporary computer memory.

_____ **14.** Software that allows numerical data to be tabulated according to mathematical formulas.

_____ **15.** A device to input data.

Column 2

a. application software

b. CPU

c. database

d. flash drive

e. e-mail

f. graphics application

g. keyboard

h. monitor

i. networking

j. palm computer

k. laptops

l. RAM

m. spreadsheet program

n. voice-recognition software

o. word processing program

COMPUTER TECHNOLOGY

Directions: The following items refer to computer technology. Mark each statement with either "T" for *true* or "F" for *false*. Be prepared to discuss your answers in class.

_____ **1.** It is easier to locate open time slots for appointments on an electronic scheduler than on a paper schedule.

_____ **2.** Only one user at a time can access a file on a network.

_____ **3.** A mainframe computer is necessary to operate any doctor's office.

_____ **4.** A firewall prevents outsider parties from access to the office's particular files.

_____ **5.** ROM is temporary; everything in ROM disappears when the computer is shut down.

_____ **6.** When you are online, you are connected to a network.

_____ **7.** An electronic medical record must be backed up with a paper medical record.

_____ **8.** E-mail systems do not allow you to print messages.

_____ **9.** A transaction database contains data on a specific patient's visit, including such items as services rendered during that visit, necessary diagnosis and procedure codes, and so forth.

_____ **10.** The cost of filing an electronic insurance claim is higher than that of filing a paper copy.

_____ **11.** A scanner allows you to enter information into the computer's memory without keying it.

_____ **12.** Designing the work environment to conform to the physical needs of a user is ergonomics.

_____ **13.** A firewall turns data into unrecognizable information during transmission.

_____ **14.** Wireless communication transmits data through telephone wires.

_____ **15.** The most powerful computer available is the supercomputer.

_____ **16.** Virus checkers do not need to be updated.

_____ **17.** A screen saver protects data from being seen by others.

_____ **18.** Everyone in the medical office will be performing audit trails on computer usage.

_____ **19.** Passwords are designed to limit access to computer files.

_____ **20.** An office does not need a signed release-of-information form for use with electronic health records.

Working Papers

Knowledge of the EHR

Directions: The following items refer to insurance plans and processing claims. Mark each statement with either "T" for *true* or "F" for *false*. Be prepared to share your answers with the class.

_____ 1. The use of EHR has been an unnatural outgrowth of the widespread clinical use of computers in the healthcare industry.

_____ 2. For many facilities and private practices the cost of EHR is prohibitive.

_____ 3. Frequent and ongoing training for medical team members is imperative to ensure the integrity of the input data and the security of the system.

_____ 4. Policies and procedures for updating personnel and evidence of the training should be placed in the Personnel Manual.

_____ 5. Converting paper-based records to electronic health records requires the scanning of paper records into the electronic database.

_____ 6. Until electronic health records are fully implemented into the healthcare system, scanners will be provided.

_____ 7. After all office medical documents have been scanned into the system, hard copy lab reports, consultation letters, etc. will automatically be entered into the patient's electronic records.

_____ 8. Converting paper-based records to electronic health records requires the scanning of paper records into the electronic database.

_____ 9. Errors will not occur in EMR, only in the paper-based record.

_____ 10. There is no need for proofreading electronic medical data.

_____ 11. To correct an electronic medical record error, use the same method used to correct a paper-based medical record error.

_____ 12. An electronic signature or initials are not needed when correcting erroneous information in the EHR.

_____ 13. Completely removing electronic data is an acceptable practice when utilizing EHR.

_____ 14. There are many advantages to converting from paper-based medical records to electronic EHR.

_____ 15. Initial cost and contract fees are relatively inexpensive for healthcare providers.

INSURANCE TERMINOLOGY

Directions: Match the term in Column 2 with its definition in Column 1.

Column 1

_____ 1. Insurance through employment, with all employees having one master policy.

_____ 2. Person who is covered by an insurance policy.

_____ 3. Insurance company that provides insurance benefits.

_____ 4. Provides reimbursement for income lost because of insured's illness.

_____ 5. Rate charged for policy.

_____ 6. Healthcare professional who supplies the healthcare.

_____ 7. Ensures that payment for medical expenses will not exceed 100 percent of the medical expenses.

_____ 8. Generally covers hospitalization, lab tests, surgery, and x-rays.

_____ 9. A term used to describe an insurance company in the context of the doctor's and patient's relationship.

_____ 10. Covers medically necessary services while insured is an inpatient.

_____ 11. Covers physician's services for office visits.

_____ 12. Covers medical expenses in a catastrophic situation.

_____ 13. In a family with two family insurance contracts, determines which policy will be the primary carrier for the children.

_____ 14. Covers physician's fee for surgery.

_____ 15. Person in whose name the policy is written.

Column 2

a. basic insurance plan

b. birthday rule

c. carrier

d. COB

e. disability insurance

f. group insurance

g. hospital insurance

h. insured

i. major medical insurance

j. medical insurance

k. policyholder

l. premium

m. provider

n. surgical insurance

o. third-party payer

INSURANCE PLANS, PAYERS, AND PAYMENT METHODS

Directions: The following items refer to insurance plans and processing claims. Mark each statement with either "T" for *true* or "F" for *false*. Be prepared to discuss your answers in class.

_____ 1. Coinsurance is the amount of medical expense that the insured must pay before the insurance carrier begins paying benefits.

_____ 2. A government agency called the Centers for Medicare and Medicaid Services (CMS) administers the Medicare and Medicaid programs.

_____ 3. In an indemnity plan, patients receive medical services from a primary care physician who coordinates the patient's overall care.

_____ 4. Coinsurance is the percentage of each claim that the insured must pay, according to the terms of the insurance policy.

_____ 5. Everyone eligible for Medicare Part A (hospitalization insurance) automatically receives Medicare Part B (medical insurance).

_____ 6. *Balance billing* refers to billing the patient for any amount due on a provider's bill after the insurance company has taken care of its responsibility.

_____ 7. The customary fee, in insurance terms, is the most the insurance company will pay any provider for a given procedure.

_____ 8. Every time HMO and PPO members visit their physician, they pay a set charge called a copayment.

_____ 9. A PAR provider who agrees to accept the allowed charge set forth by the insurance company as payment in full is accepting assignment.

_____10. In a capitated plan, a physician may receive $35 per month for each patient assigned to him or her, even if the patient receives no care during that month.

_____11. A Medicare participating provider decides whether to accept assignment on a claim-by-claim basis.

_____12. RBRVS is the payment system used by Medicare for determining how much it will pay for inpatient care.

_____13. When the amount the physician charges is more than the insurance company's allowed charge, the difference must be absorbed by the insurance company or the provider.

ICD-9-CM DIAGNOSTIC CODES

Codes	Description	Codes	Description
626.0	Amenorrhea	785.6	Lymphadenopathy
285.9	Anemia	627.9	Menopausal symptom
413.9	Angina	626.9	Menstrual disorder
427.9	Arrhythmia	787.02	Nausea
716.90	Arthritis, NOS	278.00	Obesity
714.0	Arthritis, rheumatoid	733.0	Osteoporosis
715.90	Arthritis/DJD/Osteo	380.10	Otitis externa
493.90	Asthma	382.9	Otitis media
791.9	Bacteruria	789.00	Pain, abdominal
373.00	Blepharitis	724.9	Pain, back, NOS
490	Bronchitis	729.1	Pain, muscular
682.9	Cellulitis/Abscess	785.1	Palpitations
437.9	Cerebrovascular disease	625.9	Pelvic pain, female
786.50	Chest pain	462	Pharyngitis/Sore throat
428.0	CHF	486	Pneumonia
575.1	Cholecystitis	783.5	Polydipsia
372.30	Conjunctivitis	788.42	Polyuria
786.2	Cough	V72.4	Pregnancy test
692.9	Dermatitis	V72.83	Pre-op
V18.0	Diabetes family history	V70.0	Preventive, adult
250.01	Diabetes I—IDDM	V72.3	Preventive including GYN exam
250.00	Diabetes II—NIDDM	V20.2	Preventive, pediatric
787.91	Diarrhea	V70.3	Preventive, school admission
562.1	Diverticulitis	600	Prostatic hypertrophy, benign
780.4	Dizziness/Lightheadedness	601.9	Prostatitis
536.8	Dyspepsia	791.0	Proteinuria
788.1	Dysuria	790.93	PSA, elevated
782.3	Edema	782.1	Rash/Skin eruption
V70.5	Employment exam	786.09	Shortness of breath
784.7	Epistaxis	461.9	Sinusitis, acute
780.79	Fatigue	785.0	Tachycardia
780.6	Fever	795.3	Throat culture, positive
535.50	Gastritis	388.30	Tinnitus
558.9	Gastroenteritis	463	Tonsillitis, acute
008.8	Gastroenteritis, viral	556.2	Ulcerative colitis/Proctitis
530.1	Gastroesophageal reflux	465.9	URI
784.0	Headache	788.41	Urinary frequency
346.90	Headache, migraine	788.30	Urinary incontinence
V17.4	Heart disease family history	599.0	UTI
272.0	Hypercholesterolemia	616.10	Vaginitis
272.4	Hyperlipidemia	079.99	Viral infection
401.9	Hypertension	V73.99	Viral screening, unspecified
487.1	Influenza	787.03	Vomiting
780.52	Insomnia	288.8	wbc high
564.1	Irritable bowel	288.0	wbc low
719.40	Joint pain	783.2	Weight loss

Working Papers

No.	Date	Description	Charge	Credit		Current Balance
				Payment	Adjustment	
	03/11/20--	Annual exam/CBC/UA	185.00	25.00	-------	160.00

Patient Information

7921 W. 42d Street
Address

Chicago, IL 60632-1426
City, State, ZIP

312-555-4279   312-555-6264
Home phone   **Work phone**

same   self
Responsible person   **Relationship**

Blue Cross/Blue Shield   407-55-1275
Insurance   **Contract numbers**

Patient _____ Provost, Janet _____

Date: 03/11/20--   **Chart #**

Karen Larsen, MD
2235 S. Ridgeway Avenue
Chicago, IL 60623-2240

312-555-6022

Fax: 312-555-0025

Diagnoses:

1. ___ V70.0 ___

2. _____

3. _____

4. _____

OFFICE VISITS

New Patient	Established Patient

Preventive Medicine

	New Patient		Preventive Medicine		Established Patient		
		_____ 99381	under 1 year	_____ 99391			
_____ 99201		_____ 99382	1–4	_____ 99392		_____ 99211	
_____ 99202		_____ 99383	5–11	_____ 99393		_____ 99212	
_____ 99203		_____ 99384	12–17	_____ 99394		_____ 99213	
_____ 99204		_____ 99385	18–39	_136_ 99395		_____ 99214	
_____ 99205		_____ 99386	40–64	_____ 99396		_____ 99215	
		_____ 99387	65+	_____ 99397			

Hospital Visits
Initial:
_____ 99221
_____ 99222
_____ 99223
Subsequent:
_____ 99231
_____ 99232
_____ 99233
Nursing Facility
Initial:
_____ 99304
_____ 99305
_____ 99306

Other

_____
_____

Lab:
_____ 80048 Basic
metabolic panel
(SMA-8)
_____ 87110 Chlamydia
culture
_____ 85651 ESR;
nonautomated
_____ 83001 FSH
_____ 82947 Glucose,
blood
_25_ 85025 Hemogram
(CBC) with
differential
_____ 80076 Hepatic
function panel
_____ 85018 HGB
_____ 86701 HIV-1
_____ 83002 LH
_____ 80061 Lipid panel
_____ 86617 Lyme
antibody

_____ 86308 Monospot
test
_____ 88150 Pap
_____ 85610 Prothrombin
time
_____ 84152 PSA
_____ 86430 Rheumatoid
factor
_____ 82270 Stool
hemoccult x 3
_____ 87430 Strep screen
_____ 84478 Triglycerides
_____ 84443 TSH
_24_ 81001 UA with
microscopy
_____ 87088 UC
_____ 84550 Uric acid,
blood
_____ 81025 Urine
pregnancy test

_____
_____

Injections:
_____ 90471 admin 1 vac
_____ 90472 each add'l
vac
_____ 90716 Chickenpox
_____ 90702 DT
_____ 90701 DTP
_____ 90657 Influenza
6-35 months
_____ 90658 Influenza
3 years +
_____ 90665 Lyme
disease
_____ 90707 MMR
_____ 90704 Mumps
_____ 90713 Polio vac
inactivated (IPV)
_____ 90703 Tetanus Tox
ECG: _____ 93000 ECG

Other

_____
_____

Fee Schedule—Karen Larsen, MD

| New Patient | | Established Patient | |

Preventive Medicine

New Patient	Preventive Medicine		Established Patient	
	_139_ 99381	under 1 year	_110_ 99391	
_54_ 99201	_145_ 99382	1–4	_123_ 99392	_29_ 99211
_73_ 99202	_142_ 99383	5–11	_128_ 99393	_44_ 99212
_100_ 99203	_177_ 99384	12–17	_148_ 99394	_60_ 99213
_147_ 99204	_165_ 99385	18–39	_136_ 99395	_87_ 99214
_190_ 99205	_178_ 99386	40–64	_148_ 99396	_134_ 99215
	_199_ 99387	65+	_119_ 99397	

Hospital Visits

Initial:

_121_ 99221

_172_ 99222

_217_ 99223

Subsequent:

_65_ 99231

_90_ 99232

_132_ 99233

Nursing Facility

Initial:

_53_ 99304

_77_ 99305

_109_ 99306

Other

_____

_____

Lab:

_51_ 80048 Basic metabolic panel (SMA-8)

_74_ 87110 Chlamydia culture

_21_ 85651 ESR; nonautomated

_97_ 83001 FSH

_21_ 82947 Glucose, blood

_25_ 85025 Hemogram (CBC) with differential

_55_ 80076 Hepatic function panel

_13_ 85018 HGB

_77_ 86701 HIV-1

_97_ 83002 LH

_72_ 80061 Lipid panel

_86_ 86617 Lyme antibody

_33_ 86308 Monospot test

_33_ 88150 Pap

_23_ 85610 Prothrombin time

_91_ 84152 PSA

_30_ 86430 Rheumatoid factor

_15_ 82270 Stool hemoccult x 3

_39_ 87430 Strep screen

_21_ 84478 Triglycerides

_69_ 84443 TSH

_24_ 81001 UA with microscopy

_35_ 87088 UC

_20_ 84550 Uric acid, blood

_23_ 81025 Urine pregnancy test

_____

_____

_____

Injections:

_10_ 90471 admin 1 vac

_8_ 90472 each add'l vac

_133_ 90716 Chickenpox

_31_ 90702 DT

_78_ 90701 DTP

_30_ 90657 Influenza 6-35 months

_35_ 90658 Influenza 3 years +

_40_ 90665 Lyme disease

_104_ 90707 MMR

_51_ 90704 Mumps

_52_ 90713 Polio vac inactivated (IPV)

_26_ 90703 Tetanus Tox

ECG: _70_ 93000 ECG

Other

_____

_____

_____

DAILY JOURNAL

	RECEIPT NUMBER	DATE	DESCRIPTION CODE	CHARGE	PAYMENT	ADJUSTMENTS	BALANCE	PREVIOUS BALANCE	NAME
1	1090	10/20	OV	44 00	—	—	44 00	—	Sherman
2	1091	10/20	OV/Strep screen	83 00	16 60	—	66 40	—	Villano
3	1092	10/20	OV	44 00	—	—	147 00	103 00	Robertson
4	1093	10/20	OV/LAB	241 00	48 20	—	192 80	—	Armstrong
5	1094	10/20	OV	44 00	—	—	44 00	—	Casagranda
6									
7									
32									
33									
34									
			TOTALS	Column A	Column B	Column C	Column D	Column E	TOTALS

◄ ALL RECEIPTS MUST BE
IN NUMERICAL ORDER

Proof of Posting

Column E Total $ _____
Plus Column A Total $ _____
Subtotal $ _____
Minus Column B Total $ _____
Equals Column D Total $ _____

Accounts Receivable Control

Previous Balance $ ___6260.40___
Plus Column A $ _____
Subtotal $ _____
Minus Column B Total $ _____
Present Acc'ts Rec. Balance $ _____

Daily Cash

Opening Cash on Hand
at Beginning of Day $ ___–0–___
Cash Received During Day $ _____
Total $ _____

DAILY JOURNAL

DATE ___10/21/20--___   SHEET NO. ___103___

	RECEIPT NUMBER	DATE	DESCRIPTION CODE	CHARGE	PAYMENT	ADJUSTMENTS	BALANCE	PREVIOUS BALANCE	NAME
1	1095	10/21	OV (WC)	44 00	—	—	44 00	—	Sun, Cheng
2	1096	10/21	OV	44 00	—	—	44 00	—	Jonathan
3	1097	10/21	CPE/LAB	278 00	—	—	278 00	—	Babcock
4									
5									
6									
7									
32									
33									
34									
				Column A	Column B	Column C	Column D	Column E	TOTALS

◄ ALL RECEIPTS MUST BE IN NUMERICAL ORDER

Proof of Posting

Column E Total $	_____
Plus Column A Total $	_____
Subtotal $	_____
Minus Column B Total $	_____
Equals Column D Total $	_____

Accounts Receivable Control

Previous Balance $	_____
Plus Column A $	_____
Subtotal $	_____
Minus Column B Total $	_____
Present Acc'ts Rec. Balance $	_____

Daily Cash

Opening Cash on Hand at Beginning of Day $	_____
Cash Received During Day $	_____
Total $	_____

DAILY JOURNAL

DATE ___10/22/20--___   SHEET NO. ___104___

	RECEIPT NUMBER	DATE	DESCRIPTION CODE	CHARGE	PAYMENT	ADJUSTMENTS	BALANCE	PREVIOUS BALANCE	NAME
1	1098	10/22	OV	44 00	—	—			Sinclair
2	1099	10/22	OV	44 00	—	—			Lund
3	1100	10/22	OV	44 00	8 80	—			Mendez
4	1101	10/22	CPE/UA	163 00	—	—			Mitchell, D.
5	1102	10/22	OV	44 00	—	—			Dayton
6	1103	10/22	Nursing home visit	53 00	—	—			Murrary
7									
32									
33									
34									
TOTALS			Column A	Column B	Column C	Column D	Column E	

◄ ALL RECEIPTS MUST BE IN NUMERICAL ORDER

Proof of Posting

Column E Total $	_____
Plus Column A Total $	_____
Subtotal $	_____
Minus Column B Total $	_____
Equals Column D Total $	_____

Accounts Receivable Control

Previous Balance $	_____
Plus Column A $	_____
Subtotal $	_____
Minus Column B Total $	_____
Present Acc't's Rec. Balance $	_____

Daily Cash

Opening Cash on Hand at Beginning of Day $	_____
Cash Received During Day $	_____
Total $	_____

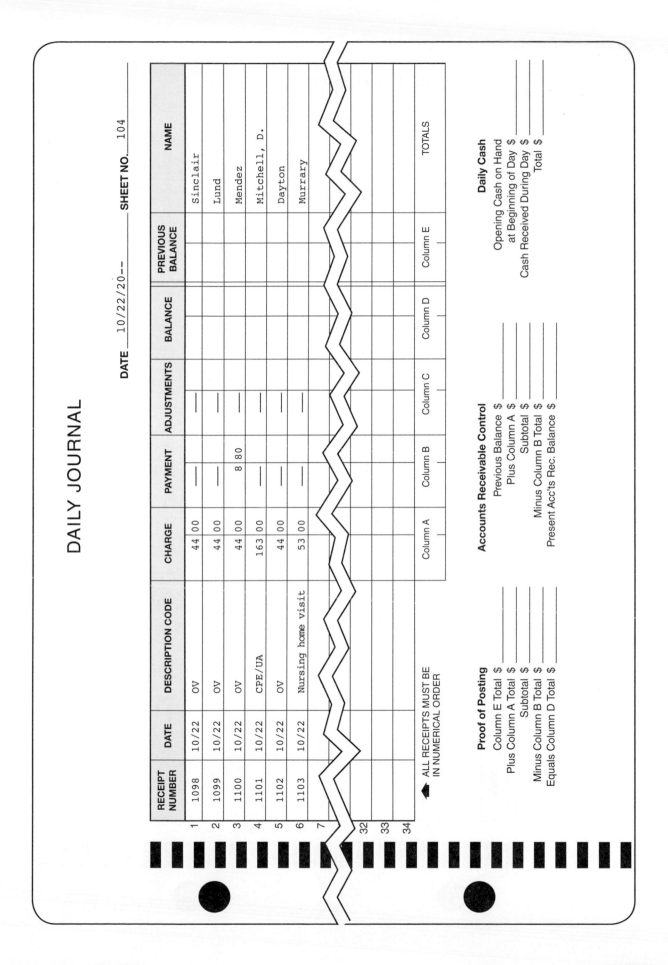

DAILY JOURNAL

DATE _____   SHEET NO. _____

RECEIPT NUMBER	DATE	DESCRIPTION CODE	CHARGE	PAYMENT	ADJUSTMENTS	BALANCE	PREVIOUS BALANCE	NAME
1								
2								
3								
4								
5								
6								
7								
32								
33								
34								
TOTALS			Column A	Column B	Column C	Column D	Column E	

➤ ALL RECEIPTS MUST BE IN NUMERICAL ORDER

Proof of Posting

Column E Total $	_____
Plus Column A Total $	_____
Subtotal $	_____
Minus Column B Total $	_____
Equals Column D Total $	_____

Accounts Receivable Control

Previous Balance $	_____
Plus Column A $	_____
Subtotal $	_____
Minus Column B Total $	_____
Present Acc'ts Rec. Balance $	_____

Daily Cash

Opening Cash on Hand at Beginning of Day $	_____
Cash Received During Day $	_____
Total $	_____

DEPOSITED IN

First National Bank
Chicago, IL 60623-2791

THIS DEPOSIT ACCEPTED UNDER AND SUBJECT TO THE PROVISIONS
OF THE UNIFORM COMMERCIAL CODE.

DATE _____

Karen Larsen, MD
2235 South Ridgeway Avenue
Chicago, IL 60623-2240

⑈0710 ⑊0062 242 ⑊027720 ⑈

	DOLLARS	CENTS
Cash..............		
Checks..........1 list separately		
2		
3		
4		
5		
6		
7		
8		

DEPOSITED IN

First National Bank
Chicago, IL 60623-2791

THIS DEPOSIT ACCEPTED UNDER AND SUBJECT TO THE PROVISIONS
OF THE UNIFORM COMMERCIAL CODE.

DATE _____

Karen Larsen, MD
2235 South Ridgeway Avenue
Chicago, IL 60623-2240

⑈0710 ⑊0062 242 ⑊027720 ⑈

	DOLLARS	CENTS
Cash..............		
Checks..........1 list separately		
2		
3		
4		
5		
6		
7		
8		

DEPOSITED IN

First National Bank
Chicago, IL 60623-2791

THIS DEPOSIT ACCEPTED UNDER AND SUBJECT TO THE PROVISIONS
OF THE UNIFORM COMMERCIAL CODE.

DATE _____

Karen Larsen, MD
2235 South Ridgeway Avenue
Chicago, IL 60623-2240

⑈0710 ⑊0062 242 ⑊027720 ⑈

	DOLLARS	CENTS
Cash..............		
Checks..........1 list separately		
2		
3		
4		
5		
6		
7		
8		

DEPOSITED IN

First National Bank
Chicago, IL 60623-2791

THIS DEPOSIT ACCEPTED UNDER AND SUBJECT TO THE PROVISIONS
OF THE UNIFORM COMMERCIAL CODE.

DATE _____

Karen Larsen, MD
2235 South Ridgeway Avenue
Chicago, IL 60623-2240

⑈0710 ⑊0062 242 ⑊027720 ⑈

	DOLLARS	CENTS
Cash..............		
Checks..........1 list separately		
2		
3		
4		
5		
6		
7		
8		

Welcome *Please complete this form using only ink. This information will remain confidential.*

PATIENT INFORMATION

Last name:	First name:	Initial:	Date of birth:	Home phone:

Address:	Marital status: (check appropriate box) S ☐ M ☐ D ☐ W ☐	Sex M F

City:	State:	ZIP:	Social Security number:

Patient's employer: (If student, name of school.)	Employment address: Business phone:

Bill to:	Relationship:

Address:	City:	State:	ZIP:

NOTIFY IN CASE OF EMERGENCY

Name:	Relationship:

Address:	Phone:

City:	State:	ZIP:	

INSURANCE INFORMATION

Primary insurance company:		Secondary insurance company:	
Subscriber's name:	DOB:	Subscriber's name:	DOB:
Policy #:	Group #:	Policy #:	Group #:

OTHER INFORMATION

Reason for visit:	Name of referring physician:

_____ Patient's signature/Parent or guardian's signature	Today's date

Welcome

Please complete this form using only ink. This information will remain confidential.

PATIENT INFORMATION

Last name:	First name:	Initial:	Date of birth:	Home phone:

Address:	Marital status: (check appropriate box) S ☐　M ☐　D ☐　W ☐	Sex M　　F

City:	State:	ZIP:	Social Security number:

Patient's employer: (If student, name of school.)	Employment address: Business phone:

Bill to:	Relationship:

Address:	City:	State:	ZIP:

NOTIFY IN CASE OF EMERGENCY

Name:	Relationship:

Address:	Phone:

City:	State:	ZIP:	

INSURANCE INFORMATION

Primary insurance company:	Secondary insurance company:

Subscriber's name:	DOB:	Subscriber's name:	DOB:

Policy #:	Group #:	Policy #:	Group #:

OTHER INFORMATION

Reason for visit:	Name of referring physician:

Patient's signature/Parent or guardian's signature	Today's date

RECORDS RELEASE

TO: _____ Healthcare provider

_____ Address

_____ City, State, ZIP

I authorize the above-named healthcare provider to release the specified information listed below to the following physician:

Karen Larsen, MD   312-555-6022
2235 South Ridgeway Avenue   Fax: 312-555-0025
Chicago, IL 60623-2240

PATIENT: _____   DOB: _____

_____   Address

_____   City, State, ZIP

Please include _____   specific records.

Signed _____   Date _____

RECORDS RELEASE

TO: _____ Healthcare provider

_____ Address

_____ City, State, ZIP

I authorize the above-named Healthcare provider to release the specified information listed below to the following physician:

Karen Larsen, MD   312-555-6022
2235 South Ridgeway Avenue   Fax: 312-555-0025
Chicago, IL 60623-2240

PATIENT: _____   DOB: _____

_____   Address

_____   City, State, ZIP

Please include _____   specific records.

Signed _____   Date _____

TELEPHONE LOG

Date _____

TIME	CALLER	TELEPHONE NUMBER	REASON	DONE

TO-DO LIST

Date _____

RUSH	ITEMS TO DO	DONE

TELEPHONE LOG

Date _____

TIME	CALLER	TELEPHONE NUMBER	REASON	DONE

TO-DO LIST

Date _____

RUSH	ITEMS TO DO	DONE

TAI CLINIC, INC.
Grace Tai, MD
100 Sun Valley Road, Lisle, IL 60532
312-555-9300

October 20, 20--

Karen Larsen, MD
2235 South Ridgeway Avenue
Chicago, IL 60623-2240

Dear Dr. Larsen:

RE: David Kramer   DOB: 4/28/20--

David is up to date on his immunizations. His immunization
record is as follows:

  DTP: 3 months (7/26/20--)   Oral polio: 3 months (7/26/20--)
       6 months (10/22/20--)   6 months (10/22/20--)
       9 months (1/29/20--)   9 months (1/29/20--)

  MMR: 2 years (5/2/20--)

David is due for a booster DTP before starting kindergarten.

If you have any questions, please contact our office.

Sincerely,

Grace Tai, MD

Grace Tai, MD

jz

KL
Please file.

No. 1214

To _____

Date _____

For _____

Amount _____

_____

No. 1214 _____ 20 _____

Received from _____

_____ Dollars

For _____

_____

$ _____

No. _____

To _____

Date _____

For _____

Amount _____

_____

No. _____ 20 _____

Received from _____

_____ Dollars

For _____

_____

$ _____

No. _____

To _____

Date _____

For _____

Amount _____

_____

No. _____ 20 _____

Received from _____

_____ Dollars

For _____

_____

$ _____

No. _____

To _____

Date _____

For _____

Amount _____

_____

No. _____ 20 _____

Received from _____

_____ Dollars

For _____

_____

$ _____

Working Papers

No.	Date	Description	Charge	Credit		Current Balance
				Payment	Adjustment	

Patient Information

6111 N. Lincoln Avenue

Address

Chicago, IL 60608-3173

City, State, ZIP

312-555-1217

Home phone   **Work phone**

self

Responsible person   **Relationship**

Medicare   669-35-2244

Insurance   **Contract numbers**

Patient _____ Florence Sherman _____

Date: 10/20/20--   **Chart #**

Karen Larsen, MD
2235 S. Ridgeway Avenue
Chicago, IL 60623-2240

312-555-6022

Fax: 312-555-0025

Diagnoses:

1. ___ V70.0 ___

2. ___

3. ___

4. ___

OFFICE VISITS

New Patient	Established Patient

Preventive Medicine

	_____ 99381	under 1 year	_____ 99391		
_____ 99201	_____ 99382	1–4	_____ 99392	_____ 99211	
_____ 99202	_____ 99383	5–11	_____ 99393	(99212)	
_____ 99203	_____ 99384	12–17	_____ 99394	_____ 99213	
_____ 99204	_____ 99385	18–39	_____ 99395	_____ 99214	
_____ 99205	_____ 99386	40–64	_____ 99396	_____ 99215	
	_____ 99387	65+	_____ 99397		

Hospital Visits

Initial:
_____ 99221
_____ 99222
_____ 99223

Subsequent:
_____ 99231
_____ 99232
_____ 99233

Nursing Facility

Initial:
_____ 99304
_____ 99305
_____ 99306

Other

_____
_____

Lab:
_____ 80048 Basic metabolic panel (SMA-8)
_____ 87110 Chlamydia culture
_____ 85651 ESR; nonautomated
_____ 83001 FSH
_____ 82947 Glucose, blood
_____ 85025 Hemogram (CBC) with differential
_____ 80076 Hepatic function panel
_____ 85018 HGB
_____ 86701 HIV-1
_____ 83002 LH
_____ 80061 Lipid panel
_____ 86617 Lyme antibody

_____ 86308 Monospot test
_____ 88150 Pap
_____ 85610 Prothrombin time
_____ 84152 PSA
_____ 86430 Rheumatoid factor
_____ 82270 Stool hemoccult x 3
_____ 87430 Strep screen
_____ 84478 Triglycerides
_____ 84443 TSH
_____ 81001 UA with microscopy
_____ 87088 UC
_____ 84550 Uric acid, blood
_____ 81025 Urine pregnancy test
_____
_____

Injections:
_____ 90471 admin 1 vac
_____ 90472 each add'l vac
_____ 90716 Chickenpox
_____ 90702 DT
_____ 90701 DTP
_____ 90657 Influenza 6-35 months
_____ 90658 Influenza 3 years +
_____ 90665 Lyme disease
_____ 90707 MMR
_____ 90704 Mumps
_____ 90713 Polio vac inactivated (IPV)
_____ 90703 Tetanus Tox
ECG: _____ 93000 ECG

Other
_____
_____

No.	Date	Description	Charge	Credit		Current Balance
				Payment	Adjustment	

Patient Information

3518 South 23d Street
Address

Chicago, IL 60623-7355
City, State, ZIP

	father
312-555-3493	312-555-8842
Home phone	**Work phone**

Juan Villano	father
Responsible person	**Relationship**

Employee Benefit Plan, 200-97-4811-02, 35A Grp
Insurance   **Contract numbers**

Patient _____ Stephen Villano _____

Date: 10/20/20--   **Chart #**

Karen Larsen, MD   **Diagnoses:**
2235 S. Ridgeway Avenue
Chicago, IL 60623-2240   1. __034.0__

312-555-6022   2. _____

Fax: 312-555-0025   3. _____

                                4. _____

OFFICE VISITS

New Patient	Established Patient

Preventive Medicine

New Patient		Age	Established Patient	
	____ 99381	under 1 year	____ 99391	
____ 99201	____ 99382	1–4	____ 99392	____ 99211
____ 99202	____ 99383	5–11	____ 99393	(99212)
____ 99203	____ 99384	12–17	____ 99394	____ 99213
____ 99204	____ 99385	18–39	____ 99395	____ 99214
____ 99205	____ 99386	40–64	____ 99396	____ 99215
	____ 99387	65+	____ 99397	

Hospital Visits
Initial:
____ 99221
____ 99222
____ 99223
Subsequent:
____ 99231
____ 99232
____ 99233

Nursing Facility
Initial:
____ 99304
____ 99305
____ 99306

Other
_____
_____

Lab:
____ 80048 Basic metabolic panel (SMA-8)
____ 87110 Chlamydia culture
____ 85651 ESR; nonautomated
____ 83001 FSH
____ 82947 Glucose, blood
____ 85025 Hemogram (CBC) with differential
____ 80076 Hepatic function panel
____ 85018 HGB
____ 86701 HIV-1
____ 83002 LH
____ 80061 Lipid panel
____ 86617 Lyme antibody

____ 86308 Monospot test
____ 88150 Pap
____ 85610 Prothrombin time
____ 84152 PSA
____ 86430 Rheumatoid factor
____ 82270 Stool hemoccult x 3
(87430) Strep screen
____ 84478 Triglycerides
____ 84443 TSH
____ 81001 UA with microscopy
____ 87088 UC
____ 84550 Uric acid, blood
____ 81025 Urine pregnancy test
_____
_____

Injections:
____ 90471 admin 1 vac
____ 90472 each add'l vac
____ 90716 Chickenpox
____ 90702 DT
____ 90701 DTP
____ 90657 Influenza 6-35 months
____ 90658 Influenza 3 years +
____ 90665 Lyme disease
____ 90707 MMR
____ 90704 Mumps
____ 90713 Polio vac inactivated (IPV)
____ 90703 Tetanus Tox
ECG: ____ 93000 ECG

Other
_____
_____

No.	Date	Description	Charge	Credit		Current Balance
				Payment	Adjustment	

Patient Information	Patient	Gary Robertson

3449 W. Foster Avenue

Address

Chicago, IL 60625-2377

City, State, ZIP

312-555-9565   312-555-8857

Home phone   **Work phone**

self

Responsible person   **Relationship**

Prudential Group Health   255-74-1021

Insurance   **Contract numbers**

Date: 10/20/20--   **Chart #**

Karen Larsen, MD
2235 S. Ridgeway Avenue
Chicago, IL 60623-2240

312-555-6022

Fax: 312-555-0025

Diagnoses:

1. _590.10_

2. _____

3. _____

4. _____

OFFICE VISITS

New Patient	Established Patient

Preventive Medicine

	_____ 99381	under 1 year	_____ 99391	
_____ 99201	_____ 99382	1–4	_____ 99392	_____ 99211
_____ 99202	_____ 99383	5–11	_____ 99393	(99212)
_____ 99203	_____ 99384	12–17	_____ 99394	_____ 99213
_____ 99204	_____ 99385	18–39	_____ 99395	_____ 99214
_____ 99205	_____ 99386	40–64	_____ 99396	_____ 99215
	_____ 99387	65+	_____ 99397	

Hospital Visits

Initial:

_____ 99221
_____ 99222
_____ 99223

Subsequent:

_____ 99231
_____ 99232
_____ 99233

Nursing Facility

Initial:

_____ 99304
_____ 99305
_____ 99306

Other

_____

_____

Lab:

_____ 80048 Basic metabolic panel (SMA-8)
_____ 87110 Chlamydia culture
_____ 85651 ESR; nonautomated
_____ 83001 FSH
_____ 82947 Glucose, blood
_____ 85025 Hemogram (CBC) with differential
_____ 80076 Hepatic function panel
_____ 85018 HGB
_____ 86701 HIV-1
_____ 83002 LH
_____ 80061 Lipid panel
_____ 86617 Lyme antibody

_____ 86308 Monospot test
_____ 88150 Pap
_____ 85610 Prothrombin time
_____ 84152 PSA
_____ 86430 Rheumatoid factor
_____ 82270 Stool hemoccult x 3
_____ 87430 Strep screen
_____ 84478 Triglycerides
_____ 84443 TSH
_____ 81001 UA with microscopy
_____ 87088 UC
_____ 84550 Uric acid, blood
_____ 81025 Urine pregnancy test

_____

_____

Injections:

_____ 90471 admin 1 vac
_____ 90472 each add'l vac
_____ 90716 Chickenpox
_____ 90702 DT
_____ 90701 DTP
_____ 90657 Influenza 6-35 months
_____ 90658 Influenza 3 years +
_____ 90665 Lyme disease
_____ 90707 MMR
_____ 90704 Mumps
_____ 90713 Polio vac inactivated (IPV)
_____ 90703 Tetanus Tox

ECG: _____ 93000 ECG

Other

_____

_____

No.	Date	Description	Charge	Credit		Current Balance
				Payment	**Adjustment**	

Patient Information

5518 Monroe Street
Address

Chicago, IL 60644-5519
City, State, ZIP

312-555-4413   312-555-8825
Home phone   **Work phone**

self
Responsible person   **Relationship**

Blue Cross/Blue Shield, 486-29-3789-1, 2458 Grp
Insurance   **Contract numbers**

Patient _____ Monica Armstrong _____

Date: 10/20/20-- | **Chart #**

Karen Larsen, MD
2235 S. Ridgeway Avenue
Chicago, IL 60623-2240

312-555-6022

Fax: 312-555-0025

Diagnoses:

1. _____

2. _____

3. _____

4. _____

OFFICE VISITS

New Patient	Established Patient

Preventive Medicine

	_____ 99381	under 1 year	_____ 99391	
_____ 99201	_____ 99382	1–4	_____ 99392	_____ 99211
_____ 99202	_____ 99383	5–11	_____ 99393	(99212)
_____ 99203	_____ 99384	12–17	_____ 99394	_____ 99213
_____ 99204	_____ 99385	18–39	_____ 99395	_____ 99214
_____ 99205	_____ 99386	40–64	_____ 99396	_____ 99215
	_____ 99387	65+	_____ 99397	

Hospital Visits
Initial:
_____ 99221
_____ 99222
_____ 99223
Subsequent:
_____ 99231
_____ 99232
_____ 99233
Nursing Facility
Initial:
_____ 99304
_____ 99305
_____ 99306

Other
_____
_____

Lab:
(80048) Basic metabolic panel (SMA-8)
_____ 87110 Chlamydia culture
_____ 85651 ESR; nonautomated
(83001) FSH
_____ 82947 Glucose, blood
(85025) Hemogram (CBC) with differential
_____ 80076 Hepatic function panel
_____ 85018 HGB
_____ 86701 HIV-1
_____ 83002 LH
_____ 80061 Lipid panel
_____ 86617 Lyme antibody

_____ 86308 Monospot test
_____ 88150 Pap
_____ 85610 Prothrombin time
_____ 84152 PSA
_____ 86430 Rheumatoid factor
_____ 82270 Stool hemoccult x 3
_____ 87430 Strep screen
_____ 84478 Triglycerides
_____ 84443 TSH
(81001) UA with microscopy
_____ 87088 UC
_____ 84550 Uric acid, blood
_____ 81025 Urine pregnancy test
_____
_____

Injections:
_____ 90471 admin 1 vac
_____ 90472 each add'l vac
_____ 90716 Chickenpox
_____ 90702 DT
_____ 90701 DTP
_____ 90657 Influenza 6-35 months
_____ 90658 Influenza 3 years +
_____ 90665 Lyme disease
_____ 90707 MMR
_____ 90704 Mumps
_____ 90713 Polio vac inactivated (IPV)
_____ 90703 Tetanus Tox
ECG: _____ 93000 ECG

Other
_____
_____

No.	Date	Description	Charge	Credit		Current Balance
				Payment	Adjustment	

Patient Information

3132 W. 42d Street
Address

Chicago, IL 60632-1406
City, State, ZIP

	father
312-555-1200	312-555-1245
Home phone	**Work phone**

George Casagranda | father
Responsible person | **Relationship**

National Insurance | 497-27-3367-05
Insurance | **Contract numbers**

Patient _____ Doris Casagranda _____

Date: 10/20/20-- | **Chart #**

Karen Larsen, MD
2235 S. Ridgeway Avenue
Chicago, IL 60623-2240

312-555-6022

Fax: 312-555-0025

Diagnoses:

1. _705.83_

2._____

3._____

4._____

OFFICE VISITS

New Patient	Established Patient

Preventive Medicine

New Patient				Established Patient	
	____ 99381	under 1 year		____ 99391	
____ 99201	____ 99382	1–4		____ 99392	____ 99211
____ 99202	____ 99383	5–11		____ 99393	(99212)
____ 99203	____ 99384	12–17		____ 99394	____ 99213
____ 99204	____ 99385	18–39		____ 99395	____ 99214
____ 99205	____ 99386	40–64		____ 99396	____ 99215
	____ 99387	65+		____ 99397	

Hospital Visits
Initial:
____ 99221
____ 99222
____ 99223
Subsequent:
____ 99231
____ 99232
____ 99233
Nursing Facility
Initial:
____ 99304
____ 99305
____ 99306

Other

_____
_____

Lab:
____ 80048 Basic metabolic panel (SMA-8)
____ 87110 Chlamydia culture
____ 85651 ESR; nonautomated
____ 83001 FSH
____ 82947 Glucose, blood
____ 85025 Hemogram (CBC) with differential
____ 80076 Hepatic function panel
____ 85018 HGB
____ 86701 HIV-1
____ 83002 LH
____ 80061 Lipid panel
____ 86617 Lyme antibody

____ 86308 Monospot test
____ 88150 Pap
____ 85610 Prothrombin time
____ 84152 PSA
____ 86430 Rheumatoid factor
____ 82270 Stool hemoccult x 3
____ 87430 Strep screen
____ 84478 Triglycerides
____ 84443 TSH
____ 81001 UA with microscopy
____ 87088 UC
____ 84550 Uric acid, blood
____ 81025 Urine pregnancy test

_____
_____

Injections:
____ 90471 admin 1 vac
____ 90472 each add'l vac
____ 90716 Chickenpox
____ 90702 DT
____ 90701 DTP
____ 90657 Influenza 6-35 months
____ 90658 Influenza 3 years +
____ 90665 Lyme disease
____ 90707 MMR
____ 90704 Mumps
____ 90713 Polio vac inactivated (IPV)
____ 90703 Tetanus Tox
ECG: ____ 93000 ECG

Other

_____
_____

No.	Date	Description	Charge	Credit		Current Balance
				Payment	Adjustment	

Patient Information

2235 W. School Street
Address

Chicago, IL 60618-5785
City, State, ZIP

312-555-3750   312-555-8149
Home phone   **Work phone**

Billings, Inc. Worker's Comp, employer
Responsible person   **Relationship**

Insurance   **Contract numbers**

Patient _____ Cheng Sun _____

Date: 10/21/20--   **Chart #**

Karen Larsen, MD
2235 S. Ridgeway Avenue
Chicago, IL 60623-2240

312-555-6022

Fax: 312-555-0025

Diagnoses:

1. ___915___

2. _____

3. _____

4. _____

OFFICE VISITS

New Patient	Established Patient

Preventive Medicine

	_____ 99381	under 1 year	_____ 99391	
_____ 99201	_____ 99382	1–4	_____ 99392	_____ 99211
_____ 99202	_____ 99383	5–11	_____ 99393	(99212)
_____ 99203	_____ 99384	12–17	_____ 99394	_____ 99213
_____ 99204	_____ 99385	18–39	_____ 99395	_____ 99214
_____ 99205	_____ 99386	40–64	_____ 99396	_____ 99215
	_____ 99387	65+	_____ 99397	

Hospital Visits
Initial:
_____ 99221
_____ 99222
_____ 99223
Subsequent:
_____ 99231
_____ 99232
_____ 99233

Nursing Facility
Initial:
_____ 99304
_____ 99305
_____ 99306

Other
_____
_____

Lab:
_____ 80048 Basic metabolic panel (SMA-8)
_____ 87110 Chlamydia culture
_____ 85651 ESR; nonautomated
_____ 83001 FSH
_____ 82947 Glucose, blood
_____ 85025 Hemogram (CBC) with differential
_____ 80076 Hepatic function panel
_____ 85018 HGB
_____ 86701 HIV-1
_____ 83002 LH
_____ 80061 Lipid panel
_____ 86617 Lyme antibody

_____ 86308 Monospot test
_____ 88150 Pap
_____ 85610 Prothrombin time
_____ 84152 PSA
_____ 86430 Rheumatoid factor
_____ 82270 Stool hemoccult x 3
_____ 87430 Strep screen
_____ 84478 Triglycerides
_____ 84443 TSH
_____ 81001 UA with microscopy
_____ 87088 UC
_____ 84550 Uric acid, blood
_____ 81025 Urine pregnancy test
_____
_____

Injections:
_____ 90471 admin 1 vac
_____ 90472 each add'l vac
_____ 90716 Chickenpox
_____ 90702 DT
_____ 90701 DTP
_____ 90657 Influenza 6-35 months
_____ 90658 Influenza 3 years +
_____ 90665 Lyme disease
_____ 90707 MMR
_____ 90704 Mumps
_____ 90713 Polio vac inactivated (IPV)
_____ 90703 Tetanus Tox
ECG: _____ 93000 ECG

Other
_____
_____

No.	Date	Description	Charge	Credit Payment	Credit Adjustment	Current Balance

Patient Information

5708 W. 63d Place
Address

Chicago, IL 60638-3391
City, State, ZIP

312-555-3097   312-555-8850
Home phone   **Work phone**

self
Responsible person   **Relationship**

Kaiser Insurance   444-02-4422, 991A Grp
Insurance   **Contract numbers**

Patient _____ Charles Jonathan III _____

Date: 10/21/20--   **Chart #**

Karen Larsen, MD
2235 S. Ridgeway Avenue
Chicago, IL 60623-2240

312-555-6022

Fax: 312-555-0025

Diagnoses:

1. ___ 719.46 ___

2. _____

3. _____

4. _____

OFFICE VISITS

New Patient	Established Patient

Preventive Medicine

	_____ 99381	under 1 year	_____ 99391	
_____ 99201	_____ 99382	1–4	_____ 99392	_____ 99211
_____ 99202	_____ 99383	5–11	_____ 99393	(99212)
_____ 99203	_____ 99384	12–17	_____ 99394	_____ 99213
_____ 99204	_____ 99385	18–39	_____ 99395	_____ 99214
_____ 99205	_____ 99386	40–64	_____ 99396	_____ 99215
	_____ 99387	65+	_____ 99397	

Hospital Visits
Initial:
_____ 99221
_____ 99222
_____ 99223
Subsequent:
_____ 99231
_____ 99232
_____ 99233
Nursing Facility
Initial:
_____ 99304
_____ 99305
_____ 99306

Other

_____
_____

Lab:
_____ 80048 Basic metabolic panel (SMA-8)
_____ 87110 Chlamydia culture
_____ 85651 ESR; nonautomated
_____ 83001 FSH
_____ 82947 Glucose, blood
_____ 85025 Hemogram (CBC) with differential
_____ 80076 Hepatic function panel
_____ 85018 HGB
_____ 86701 HIV-1
_____ 83002 LH
_____ 80061 Lipid panel
_____ 86617 Lyme antibody

_____ 86308 Monospot test
_____ 88150 Pap
_____ 85610 Prothrombin time
_____ 84152 PSA
_____ 86430 Rheumatoid factor
_____ 82270 Stool hemoccult x 3
_____ 87430 Strep screen
_____ 84478 Triglycerides
_____ 84443 TSH
_____ 81001 UA with microscopy
_____ 87088 UC
_____ 84550 Uric acid, blood
_____ 81025 Urine pregnancy test

_____
_____

Injections:
_____ 90471 admin 1 vac
_____ 90472 each add'l vac
_____ 90716 Chickenpox
_____ 90702 DT
_____ 90701 DTP
_____ 90657 Influenza 6-35 months
_____ 90658 Influenza 3 years +
_____ 90665 Lyme disease
_____ 90707 MMR
_____ 90704 Mumps
_____ 90713 Polio vac inactivated (IPV)
_____ 90703 Tetanus Tox
ECG: _____ 93000 ECG

Other

_____
_____

No.	Date	Description	Charge	Credit		Current Balance
				Payment	Adjustment	

Patient Information

131 N. Mason Avenue
Address

Chicago, IL 60644-4455
City, State, ZIP

312-555-5441   312-555-9966
Home phone   **Work phone**

self
Responsible person   **Relationship**

Kaiser Insurance   987-87-3759
Insurance   **Contract numbers**

Patient _____ Sara Babcock _____

Date: 10/21/20--   **Chart #**

Karen Larsen, MD   **Diagnoses:**
2235 S. Ridgeway Avenue
Chicago, IL 60623-2240   1. _V72.3_

312-555-6022   2. _112.1_

Fax: 312-555-0025   3. _V25.41_

                             4. _625.6_

OFFICE VISITS

New Patient	Established Patient

Preventive Medicine

New Patient			Established Patient	
	_____ 99381	under 1 year		
_____ 99201	_____ 99382	1–4	_____ 99391	
_____ 99202	_____ 99383	5–11	_____ 99392	_____ 99211
_____ 99203	_____ 99384	12–17	_____ 99393	_____ 99212
_____ 99204	_____ 99385	18–39	_____ 99394	_____ 99213
_____ 99205	_____ 99386	40–64	_____ (99395)	_____ 99214
	_____ 99387	65+	_____ 99396	_____ 99215
			_____ 99397	

Hospital Visits
Initial:
_____ 99221
_____ 99222
_____ 99223
Subsequent:
_____ 99231
_____ 99232
_____ 99233
Nursing Facility
Initial:
_____ 99304
_____ 99305
_____ 99306

Other
_____
_____

Lab:
_____ 80048 Basic metabolic panel (SMA-8)
_____ 87110 Chlamydia culture
_____ 85651 ESR; nonautomated
_____ 83001 FSH
_____ 82947 Glucose, blood
_____ 85025 Hemogram (CBC) with differential
_____ 80076 Hepatic function panel
_____ (85018) HGB
_____ 86701 HIV-1
_____ 83002 LH
_____ (80061) Lipid panel
_____ 86617 Lyme antibody

_____ 86308 Monospot test
_____ (88150) Pap
_____ 85610 Prothrombin time
_____ 84152 PSA
_____ 86430 Rheumatoid factor
_____ 82270 Stool hemoccult x 3
_____ 87430 Strep screen
_____ 84478 Triglycerides
_____ 84443 TSH
_____ (81001) UA with microscopy
_____ 87088 UC
_____ 84550 Uric acid, blood
_____ 81025 Urine pregnancy test
_____
_____

Injections:
_____ 90471 admin 1 vac
_____ 90472 each add'l vac
_____ 90716 Chickenpox
_____ 90702 DT
_____ 90701 DTP
_____ 90657 Influenza 6-35 months
_____ 90658 Influenza 3 years +
_____ 90665 Lyme disease
_____ 90707 MMR
_____ 90704 Mumps
_____ 90713 Polio vac inactivated (IPV)
_____ 90703 Tetanus Tox
ECG: _____ 93000 ECG

Other
_____
_____

No.	Date	Description	Charge	Credit		Current Balance
				Payment	**Adjustment**	

Patient Information

2721 W. 18th Street
Address

Chicago, IL 60608-6260
City, State, ZIP

312-555-4381
Home phone   **Work phone**

self
Responsible person   **Relationship**

Medicare   322-91-7722A
Insurance   **Contract numbers**

Patient _____ Gene Sinclair _____

Date: 10/22/20--   **Chart #**

Karen Larsen, MD
2235 S. Ridgeway Avenue
Chicago, IL 60623-2240

312-555-6022

Fax: 312-555-0025

Diagnoses:

1. _709.9_____

2. _____

3. _____

4. _____

OFFICE VISITS

New Patient	Established Patient

Preventive Medicine

	_____ 99381	under 1 year	_____ 99391	
_____ 99201	_____ 99382	1–4	_____ 99392	_____ 99211
_____ 99202	_____ 99383	5–11	_____ 99393	(99212)
_____ 99203	_____ 99384	12–17	_____ 99394	_____ 99213
_____ 99204	_____ 99385	18–39	_____ 99395	_____ 99214
_____ 99205	_____ 99386	40–64	_____ 99396	_____ 99215
	_____ 99387	65+	_____ 99397	

Hospital Visits
Initial:
_____ 99221
_____ 99222
_____ 99223
Subsequent:
_____ 99231
_____ 99232
_____ 99233
Nursing Facility
Initial:
_____ 99304
_____ 99305
_____ 99306

Other
_____
_____

Lab:
_____ 80048 Basic
    metabolic panel
    (SMA-8)
_____ 87110 Chlamydia
    culture
_____ 85651 ESR;
    nonautomated
_____ 83001 FSH
_____ 82947 Glucose,
    blood
_____ 85025 Hemogram
    (CBC) with
    differential
_____ 80076 Hepatic
    function panel
_____ 85018 HGB
_____ 86701 HIV-1
_____ 83002 LH
_____ 80061 Lipid panel
_____ 86617 Lyme
    antibody

_____ 86308 Monospot
    test
_____ 88150 Pap
_____ 85610 Prothrombin
    time
_____ 84152 PSA
_____ 86430 Rheumatoid
    factor
_____ 82270 Stool
    hemoccult x 3
_____ 87430 Strep screen
_____ 84478 Triglycerides
_____ 84443 TSH
_____ 81001 UA with
    microscopy
_____ 87088 UC
_____ 84550 Uric acid,
    blood
_____ 81025 Urine
    pregnancy test
_____
_____

Injections:
_____ 90471 admin 1 vac
_____ 90472 each add'l
    vac
_____ 90716 Chickenpox
_____ 90702 DT
_____ 90701 DTP
_____ 90657 Influenza
    6-35 months
_____ 90658 Influenza
    3 years +
_____ 90665 Lyme
    disease
_____ 90707 MMR
_____ 90704 Mumps
_____ 90713 Polio vac
    inactivated (IPV)
_____ 90703 Tetanus Tox
ECG: _____ 93000 ECG

Other
_____

No.	Date	Description	Charge	Credit		Current Balance
				Payment	Adjustment	

Patient Information

13419 S. Buffalo Avenue
Address

Chicago, IL 60633-2010
City, State, ZIP

	father
312-555-4106	312-555-8840
Home phone	**Work phone**

Lawrence Lund | father
Responsible person | **Relationship**

Employee Benefit Plan | 200-66-3980-01
Insurance | **Contract numbers**

Patient _____ Laura Lund _____

Date: 10/22/20-- | **Chart #**

Karen Larsen, MD
2235 S. Ridgeway Avenue
Chicago, IL 60623-2240

312-555-6022

Fax: 312-555-0025

Diagnoses:

1. _____ 847.0 _____

2. _____

3. _____

4. _____

OFFICE VISITS

New Patient	**Established Patient**

Preventive Medicine

New Patient	Preventive Medicine		Established Patient	
	_____ 99381	under 1 year	_____ 99391	
_____ 99201	_____ 99382	1–4	_____ 99392	_____ 99211
_____ 99202	_____ 99383	5–11	_____ 99393	(99212)
_____ 99203	_____ 99384	12–17	_____ 99394	_____ 99213
_____ 99204	_____ 99385	18–39	_____ 99395	_____ 99214
_____ 99205	_____ 99386	40–64	_____ 99396	_____ 99215
	_____ 99387	65+	_____ 99397	

Hospital Visits
Initial:
_____ 99221
_____ 99222
_____ 99223
Subsequent:
_____ 99231
_____ 99232
_____ 99233
Nursing Facility
Initial:
_____ 99304
_____ 99305
_____ 99306

Other

_____

_____

Lab:
_____ 80048 Basic metabolic panel (SMA-8)
_____ 87110 Chlamydia culture
_____ 85651 ESR; nonautomated
_____ 83001 FSH
_____ 82947 Glucose, blood
_____ 85025 Hemogram (CBC) with differential
_____ 80076 Hepatic function panel
_____ 85018 HGB
_____ 86701 HIV-1
_____ 83002 LH
_____ 80061 Lipid panel
_____ 86617 Lyme antibody

_____ 86308 Monospot test
_____ 88150 Pap
_____ 85610 Prothrombin time
_____ 84152 PSA
_____ 86430 Rheumatoid factor
_____ 82270 Stool hemoccult x 3
_____ 87430 Strep screen
_____ 84478 Triglycerides
_____ 84443 TSH
_____ 81001 UA with microscopy
_____ 87088 UC
_____ 84550 Uric acid, blood
_____ 81025 Urine pregnancy test

_____

_____

Injections:
_____ 90471 admin 1 vac
_____ 90472 each add'l vac
_____ 90716 Chickenpox
_____ 90702 DT
_____ 90701 DTP
_____ 90657 Influenza 6-35 months
_____ 90658 Influenza 3 years +
_____ 90665 Lyme disease
_____ 90707 MMR
_____ 90704 Mumps
_____ 90713 Polio vac inactivated (IPV)
_____ 90703 Tetanus Tox
ECG: _____ 93000 ECG

Other

_____

_____

No.	Date	Description	Charge	Credit		Current Balance
				Payment	Adjustment	

Patient Information

3457 W. 63d Place
Address

Chicago, IL 60629-4270
City, State, ZIP

312-555-3606
Home phone   **Work phone**

self
Responsible person   **Relationship**

Blue Cross & Blue Shield 295-99-3325, 354 Grp
Insurance   **Contract numbers**

Patient _____ Ana Mendez _____

Date: 10/22/20--   **Chart #**

Karen Larsen, MD
2235 S. Ridgeway Avenue
Chicago, IL 60623-2240

312-555-6022

Fax: 312-555-0025

Diagnoses:

1. __463__

2. __289.3__

3. _____

4. _____

OFFICE VISITS

New Patient		Established Patient

Preventive Medicine

	_____ 99381	under 1 year	_____ 99391	
_____ 99201	_____ 99382	1–4	_____ 99392	_____ 99211
_____ 99202	_____ 99383	5–11	_____ 99393	(99212)
_____ 99203	_____ 99384	12–17	_____ 99394	_____ 99213
_____ 99204	_____ 99385	18–39	_____ 99395	_____ 99214
_____ 99205	_____ 99386	40–64	_____ 99396	_____ 99215
	_____ 99387	65+	_____ 99397	

Hospital Visits
Initial:
_____ 99221
_____ 99222
_____ 99223
Subsequent:
_____ 99231
_____ 99232
_____ 99233
Nursing Facility
Initial:
_____ 99304
_____ 99305
_____ 99306

Other

_____

Lab:
_____ 80048 Basic
    metabolic panel
    (SMA-8)
_____ 87110 Chlamydia
    culture
_____ 85651 ESR;
    nonautomated
_____ 83001 FSH
_____ 82947 Glucose,
    blood
_____ 85025 Hemogram
    (CBC) with
    differential
_____ 80076 Hepatic
    function panel
_____ 85018 HGB
_____ 86701 HIV-1
_____ 83002 LH
_____ 80061 Lipid panel
_____ 86617 Lyme
    antibody

_____ 86308 Monospot
    test
_____ 88150 Pap
_____ 85610 Prothrombin
    time
_____ 84152 PSA
_____ 86430 Rheumatoid
    factor
_____ 82270 Stool
    hemoccult x 3
_____ 87430 Strep screen
_____ 84478 Triglycerides
_____ 84443 TSH
_____ 81001 UA with
    microscopy
_____ 87088 UC
_____ 84550 Uric acid,
    blood
_____ 81025 Urine
    pregnancy test

_____

Injections:
_____ 90471 admin 1 vac
_____ 90472 each add'l
    vac
_____ 90716 Chickenpox
_____ 90702 DT
_____ 90701 DTP
_____ 90657 Influenza
    6-35 months
_____ 90658 Influenza
    3 years +
_____ 90665 Lyme
    disease
_____ 90707 MMR
_____ 90704 Mumps
_____ 90713 Polio vac
    inactivated (IPV)
_____ 90703 Tetanus Tox
ECG: _____ 93000 ECG

Other

_____

_____

No.	Date	Description	Charge	Credit		Current Balance
				Payment	Adjustment	

Patient Information

5231 W. School Street
Address

Chicago, IL 60651-2248
City, State, ZIP

312-555-8153
Home phone

father
312-555-6141
Work phone

Alan Mitchell
Responsible person

father
Relationship

New York Mutual
Insurance

304253, 5245 Grp
Contract numbers

Patient Donald Mitchell

Date: 10/22/20--   **Chart #**

Karen Larsen, MD
2235 S. Ridgeway Avenue
Chicago, IL 60623-2240

312-555-6022

Fax: 312-555-0025

Diagnoses:

1. _____

2. _____

3. _____

4. _____

OFFICE VISITS

| **New Patient** | **Established Patient** |

Preventive Medicine

	_____ (99381) under 1 year	_____ 99391	
_____ 99201	_____ 99382 1–4	_____ 99392	_____ 99211
_____ 99202	_____ 99383 5–11	_____ 99393	_____ 99212
_____ 99203	_____ 99384 12–17	_____ 99394	_____ 99213
_____ 99204	_____ 99385 18–39	_____ 99395	_____ 99214
_____ 99205	_____ 99386 40–64	_____ 99396	_____ 99215
	_____ 99387 65+	_____ 99397	

Hospital Visits
Initial:
_____ 99221
_____ 99222
_____ 99223
Subsequent:
_____ 99231
_____ 99232
_____ 99233
Nursing Facility
Initial:
_____ 99304
_____ 99305
_____ 99306

Other
_____
_____

Lab:
_____ 80048 Basic metabolic panel (SMA-8)
_____ 87110 Chlamydia culture
_____ 85651 ESR; nonautomated
_____ 83001 FSH
_____ 82947 Glucose, blood
_____ 85025 Hemogram (CBC) with differential
_____ 80076 Hepatic function panel
_____ 85018 HGB
_____ 86701 HIV-1
_____ 83002 LH
_____ 80061 Lipid panel
_____ 86617 Lyme antibody

_____ 86308 Monospot test
_____ 88150 Pap
_____ 85610 Prothrombin time
_____ 84152 PSA
_____ 86430 Rheumatoid factor
_____ 82270 Stool hemoccult x 3
_____ 87430 Strep screen
_____ 84478 Triglycerides
_____ 84443 TSH
_____ (81001) UA with microscopy
_____ 87088 UC
_____ 84550 Uric acid, blood
_____ 81025 Urine pregnancy test
_____
_____

Injections:
_____ 90471 admin 1 vac
_____ 90472 each add'l vac
_____ 90716 Chickenpox
_____ 90702 DT
_____ 90701 DTP
_____ 90657 Influenza 6-35 months
_____ 90658 Influenza 3 years +
_____ 90665 Lyme disease
_____ 90707 MMR
_____ 90704 Mumps
_____ 90713 Polio vac inactivated (IPV)
_____ 90703 Tetanus Tox
ECG: _____ 93000 ECG

Other
_____
_____

No.	Date	Description	Charge	Credit		Current Balance
				Payment	Adjustment	

Patient Information

Address
105 W. Chestnut Street

City, State, ZIP
Chicago, IL 60610-2816

Home phone
312-555-2231

Work phone
312-555-2583

Responsible person
self

Relationship

Insurance
University Health Plan, 797-90-1128, S357C Grp.

Contract numbers

Patient _____ Theresa Dayton _____

Date: 10/22/20--   **Chart #**

Karen Larsen, MD
2235 S. Ridgeway Avenue
Chicago, IL 60623-2240

312-555-6022

Fax: 312-555-0025

Diagnoses:

1. _610.0_

2. _V25.9_

3. _____

4. _____

OFFICE VISITS

New Patient	Established Patient

Preventive Medicine

	_____ 99381 under 1 year	_____ 99391	
_____ 99201	_____ 99382 1–4	_____ 99392	_____ 99211
_____ 99202	_____ 99383 5–11	_____ 99393	(99212)
_____ 99203	_____ 99384 12–17	_____ 99394	_____ 99213
_____ 99204	_____ 99385 18–39	_____ 99395	_____ 99214
_____ 99205	_____ 99386 40–64	_____ 99396	_____ 99215
	_____ 99387 65+	_____ 99397	

Hospital Visits
Initial:
_____ 99221
_____ 99222
_____ 99223
Subsequent:
_____ 99231
_____ 99232
_____ 99233
Nursing Facility
Initial:
_____ 99304
_____ 99305
_____ 99306

Other
_____
_____

Lab:
_____ 80048 Basic metabolic panel (SMA-8)
_____ 87110 Chlamydia culture
_____ 85651 ESR; nonautomated
_____ 83001 FSH
_____ 82947 Glucose, blood
_____ 85025 Hemogram (CBC) with differential
_____ 80076 Hepatic function panel
_____ 85018 HGB
_____ 86701 HIV-1
_____ 83002 LH
_____ 80061 Lipid panel
_____ 86617 Lyme antibody

_____ 86308 Monospot test
_____ 88150 Pap
_____ 85610 Prothrombin time
_____ 84152 PSA
_____ 86430 Rheumatoid factor
_____ 82270 Stool hemoccult x 3
_____ 87430 Strep screen
_____ 84478 Triglycerides
_____ 84443 TSH
_____ 81001 UA with microscopy
_____ 87088 UC
_____ 84550 Uric acid, blood
_____ 81025 Urine pregnancy test
_____
_____

Injections:
_____ 90471 admin 1 vac
_____ 90472 each add'l vac
_____ 90716 Chickenpox
_____ 90702 DT
_____ 90701 DTP
_____ 90657 Influenza 6-35 months
_____ 90658 Influenza 3 years +
_____ 90665 Lyme disease
_____ 90707 MMR
_____ 90704 Mumps
_____ 90713 Polio vac inactivated (IPV)
_____ 90703 Tetanus Tox
ECG: _____ 93000 ECG

Other
_____
_____

No.	Date	Description	Charge	Credit		Current Balance
				Payment	Adjustment	

Patient Information

3908 N. Central Avenue
Address

Chicago, IL 60634-3276
City, State, ZIP

312-555-6343
Home phone   **Work phone**

self
Responsible person   **Relationship**

Medicare   555-88-3822B
Insurance   **Contract numbers**

Patient _____ Raymond Murrary _____

Date: 10/22/20--   **Chart #**

Karen Larsen, MD   **Diagnoses:**
2235 S. Ridgeway Avenue
Chicago, IL 60623-2240   1. _491.21_

312-555-6022   2. _490_

Fax: 312-555-0025   3. _____

          4. _____

OFFICE VISITS

New Patient		Established Patient	

Preventive Medicine

New Patient			Established Patient	
	_____ 99381	under 1 year	_____ 99391	
_____ 99201	_____ 99382	1–4	_____ 99392	_____ 99211
_____ 99202	_____ 99383	5–11	_____ 99393	_____ 99212
_____ 99203	_____ 99384	12–17	_____ 99394	_____ 99213
_____ 99204	_____ 99385	18–39	_____ 99395	_____ 99214
_____ 99205	_____ 99386	40–64	_____ 99396	_____ 99215
	_____ 99387	65+	_____ 99397	

Hospital Visits
Initial:
_____ 99221
_____ 99222
_____ 99223
Subsequent:
_____ 99231
_____ 99232
_____ 99233
Nursing Facility
Initial:
(99304)
_____ 99305
_____ 99306

Other
_____
_____

Lab:
_____ 80048 Basic metabolic panel (SMA-8)
_____ 87110 Chlamydia culture
_____ 85651 ESR; nonautomated
_____ 83001 FSH
_____ 82947 Glucose, blood
_____ 85025 Hemogram (CBC) with differential
_____ 80076 Hepatic function panel
_____ 85018 HGB
_____ 86701 HIV-1
_____ 83002 LH
_____ 80061 Lipid panel
_____ 86617 Lyme antibody

_____ 86308 Monospot test
_____ 88150 Pap
_____ 85610 Prothrombin time
_____ 84152 PSA
_____ 86430 Rheumatoid factor
_____ 82270 Stool hemoccult x 3
_____ 87430 Strep screen
_____ 84478 Triglycerides
_____ 84443 TSH
_____ 81001 UA with microscopy
_____ 87088 UC
_____ 84550 Uric acid, blood
_____ 81025 Urine pregnancy test
_____
_____

Injections:
_____ 90471 admin 1 vac
_____ 90472 each add'l vac
_____ 90716 Chickenpox
_____ 90702 DT
_____ 90701 DTP
_____ 90657 Influenza 6-35 months
_____ 90658 Influenza 3 years +
_____ 90665 Lyme disease
_____ 90707 MMR
_____ 90704 Mumps
_____ 90713 Polio vac inactivated (IPV)
_____ 90703 Tetanus Tox
ECG: _____ 93000 ECG

Other
_____
_____

TELEPHONE LOG

Date _____

TIME	CALLER	TELEPHONE NUMBER	REASON	DONE

TO-DO LIST

Date _____

RUSH	ITEMS TO DO	DONE

| No. | Date | Description | Charge | Credit | | Current Balance |
				Payment	Adjustment	

Patient Information

9340 S. Green Street
Address

Chicago, IL 60620-8129
City, State, ZIP

	father
312-555-3344	312-555-2577
Home phone	**Work phone**

Tam Phan	father
Responsible person	**Relationship**

University Health Plan, 888-90-8229 A287-05
Insurance   **Contract numbers**

Patient _____ Marc Phan _____

Date: 10/27/20--   **Chart #**

Karen Larsen, MD
2235 S. Ridgeway Avenue
Chicago, IL 60623-2240

312-555-6022

Fax: 312-555-0025

Diagnoses:

1. __490__

2. __691.0__

3. _____

4. _____

OFFICE VISITS

New Patient	Established Patient

Preventive Medicine

New Patient			Established Patient	
	_____ 99381	under 1 year	_____ 99391	
_____ 99201	_____ 99382	1–4	_____ 99392	_____ 99211
_____ 99202	_____ 99383	5–11	_____ 99393	(99212)
_____ 99203	_____ 99384	12–17	_____ 99394	_____ 99213
_____ 99204	_____ 99385	18–39	_____ 99395	_____ 99214
_____ 99205	_____ 99386	40–64	_____ 99396	_____ 99215
	_____ 99387	65+	_____ 99397	

Hospital Visits
Initial:
_____ 99221
_____ 99222
_____ 99223
Subsequent:
_____ 99231
_____ 99232
_____ 99233
Nursing Facility
Initial:
_____ 99304
_____ 99305
_____ 99306

Other
_____
_____

Lab:
_____ 80048 Basic
metabolic panel
(SMA-8)
_____ 87110 Chlamydia
culture
_____ 85651 ESR;
nonautomated
_____ 83001 FSH
_____ 82947 Glucose,
blood
_____ 85025 Hemogram
(CBC) with
differential
_____ 80076 Hepatic
function panel
_____ 85018 HGB
_____ 86701 HIV-1
_____ 83002 LH
_____ 80061 Lipid panel
_____ 86617 Lyme
antibody

_____ 86308 Monospot
test
_____ 88150 Pap
_____ 85610 Prothrombin
time
_____ 84152 PSA
_____ 86430 Rheumatoid
factor
_____ 82270 Stool
hemoccult x 3
_____ 87430 Strep screen
_____ 84478 Triglycerides
_____ 84443 TSH
_____ 81001 UA with
microscopy
_____ 87088 UC
_____ 84550 Uric acid,
blood
_____ 81025 Urine
pregnancy test

Injections:
_____ 90471 admin 1 vac
_____ 90472 each add'l
vac
_____ 90716 Chickenpox
_____ 90702 DT
_____ 90701 DTP
_____ 90657 Influenza
6-35 months
_____ 90658 Influenza
3 years +
_____ 90665 Lyme
disease
_____ 90707 MMR
_____ 90704 Mumps
_____ 90713 Polio vac
inactivated (IPV)
_____ 90703 Tetanus Tox
ECG: _____ 93000 ECG

Other
_____
_____

No.	Date	Description	Charge	Credit		Current Balance
				Payment	Adjustment	

Patient Information

723 W. Sixth Place

Address

Chicago, IL 60621-2314

City, State, ZIP

312-555-2324

Home phone

Responsible person Esther Morton

Insurance Northstar Insurance,

mother

312-555-8876

Work phone

mother

Relationship

300-29-1874 255-03

Contract numbers

Patient _____ Sarah Morton _____

Date: 10/27/20--

Chart #

Karen Larsen, MD
2235 S. Ridgeway Avenue
Chicago, IL 60623-2240

312-555-6022

Fax: 312-555-0025

Diagnoses:

1. _737.30_

2. _736.81_

3. _____

4. _____

OFFICE VISITS

New Patient		Established Patient	

Preventive Medicine

	_____ 99381	under 1 year	_____ 99391	
_____ 99201	_____ 99382	1–4	_____ 99392	_____ 99211
_____ 99202	_____ 99383	5–11	_____ 99393	(99212)
_____ 99203	_____ 99384	12–17	_____ 99394	_____ 99213
_____ 99204	_____ 99385	18–39	_____ 99395	_____ 99214
_____ 99205	_____ 99386	40–64	_____ 99396	_____ 99215
	_____ 99387	65+	_____ 99397	

Hospital Visits

Initial:
_____ 99221
_____ 99222
_____ 99223
Subsequent:
_____ 99231
_____ 99232
_____ 99233

Nursing Facility

Initial:
_____ 99304
_____ 99305
_____ 99306

Other

_____
_____

Lab:
_____ 80048 Basic metabolic panel (SMA-8)
_____ 87110 Chlamydia culture
_____ 85651 ESR; nonautomated
_____ 83001 FSH
_____ 82947 Glucose, blood
_____ 85025 Hemogram (CBC) with differential
_____ 80076 Hepatic function panel
_____ 85018 HGB
_____ 86701 HIV-1
_____ 83002 LH
_____ 80061 Lipid panel
_____ 86617 Lyme antibody

_____ 86308 Monospot test
_____ 88150 Pap
_____ 85610 Prothrombin time
_____ 84152 PSA
_____ 86430 Rheumatoid factor
_____ 82270 Stool hemoccult x 3
_____ 87430 Strep screen
_____ 84478 Triglycerides
_____ 84443 TSH
_____ 81001 UA with microscopy
_____ 87088 UC
_____ 84550 Uric acid, blood
_____ 81025 Urine pregnancy test
_____
_____

Injections:
_____ 90471 admin 1 vac
_____ 90472 each add'l vac
_____ 90716 Chickenpox
_____ 90702 DT
_____ 90701 DTP
_____ 90657 Influenza 6-35 months
_____ 90658 Influenza 3 years +
_____ 90665 Lyme disease
_____ 90707 MMR
_____ 90704 Mumps
_____ 90713 Polio vac inactivated (IPV)
_____ 90703 Tetanus Tox
ECG: _____ 93000 ECG

Other
_____
_____

No.	Date	Description	Charge	Credit		Current Balance
				Payment	Adjustment	

Patient Information

3132 W. 42d Street

Address

Chicago, IL 60632-1406

City, State, ZIP

	father
312-555-1200	312-555-1245
Home phone	**Work phone**

George Casagranda	father
Responsible person	**Relationship**

National Insurance	497-27-3367-05
Insurance	**Contract numbers**

Patient _____ Doris Casagranda _____

Date: 10/27/20--   **Chart #**

Karen Larsen, MD
2235 S. Ridgeway Avenue
Chicago, IL 60623-2240

312-555-6022

Fax: 312-555-0025

Diagnoses:

1. _705.83_

2. _____

3. _____

4. _____

OFFICE VISITS

New Patient	**Established Patient**

Preventive Medicine

	_____ 99381	under 1 year	_____ 99391		
_____ 99201	_____ 99382	1–4	_____ 99392	_____ 99211	
_____ 99202	_____ 99383	5–11	_____ 99393	(99212)	
_____ 99203	_____ 99384	12–17	_____ 99394	_____ 99213	
_____ 99204	_____ 99385	18–39	_____ 99395	_____ 99214	
_____ 99205	_____ 99386	40–64	_____ 99396	_____ 99215	
	_____ 99387	65+	_____ 99397		

Hospital Visits

Initial:

_____ 99221

_____ 99222

_____ 99223

Subsequent:

_____ 99231

_____ 99232

_____ 99233

Nursing Facility

Initial:

_____ 99304

_____ 99305

_____ 99306

Other

_____

_____

Lab:

_____ 80048 Basic metabolic panel (SMA-8)

_____ 87110 Chlamydia culture

_____ 85651 ESR; nonautomated

_____ 83001 FSH

_____ 82947 Glucose, blood

_____ 85025 Hemogram (CBC) with differential

_____ 80076 Hepatic function panel

_____ 85018 HGB

_____ 86701 HIV-1

_____ 83002 LH

_____ 80061 Lipid panel

_____ 86617 Lyme antibody

_____ 86308 Monospot test

_____ 88150 Pap

_____ 85610 Prothrombin time

_____ 84152 PSA

_____ 86430 Rheumatoid factor

_____ 82270 Stool hemoccult x 3

_____ 87430 Strep screen

_____ 84478 Triglycerides

_____ 84443 TSH

_____ 81001 UA with microscopy

_____ 87088 UC

_____ 84550 Uric acid, blood

_____ 81025 Urine pregnancy test

_____

_____

Injections:

_____ 90471 admin 1 vac

_____ 90472 each add'l vac

_____ 90716 Chickenpox

_____ 90702 DT

_____ 90701 DTP

_____ 90657 Influenza 6-35 months

_____ 90658 Influenza 3 years +

_____ 90665 Lyme disease

_____ 90707 MMR

_____ 90704 Mumps

_____ 90713 Polio vac inactivated (IPV)

_____ 90703 Tetanus Tox

ECG: _____ 93000 ECG

Other

_____

_____

No.	Date	Description	Charge	Credit		Current Balance
				Payment	Adjustment	

Patient Information

4345 W. Grace Street
Address

Chicago, IL 60641-6730
City, State, ZIP

312-555-7292
Home phone   **Work phone**

Paul Burton   father
Responsible person   **Relationship**

No insurance
Insurance   **Contract numbers**

Patient _____ Randy Burton _____

Date: 10/27/20--   **Chart #**

Karen Larsen, MD   **Diagnoses:**
2235 S. Ridgeway Avenue
Chicago, IL 60623-2240   1. __V20.2__

312-555-6022   2. _____

Fax: 312-555-0025   3. _____

                             4. _____

OFFICE VISITS

New Patient		**Established Patient**	

Preventive Medicine

	_____ 99381	under 1 year	_____ 99391	
_____ 99201	_____ 99382	1–4	_____ (99392)	_____ 99211
_____ 99202	_____ 99383	5–11	_____ 99393	_____ 99212
_____ 99203	_____ 99384	12–17	_____ 99394	_____ 99213
_____ 99204	_____ 99385	18–39	_____ 99395	_____ 99214
_____ 99205	_____ 99386	40–64	_____ 99396	_____ 99215
	_____ 99387	65+	_____ 99397	

Hospital Visits
Initial:
_____ 99221
_____ 99222
_____ 99223
Subsequent:
_____ 99231
_____ 99232
_____ 99233
Nursing Facility
Initial:
_____ 99304
_____ 99305
_____ 99306

Other
_____
_____

Lab:
_____ 80048 Basic
metabolic panel
(SMA-8)
_____ 87110 Chlamydia
culture
_____ 85651 ESR;
nonautomated
_____ 83001 FSH
_____ 82947 Glucose,
blood
_____ 85025 Hemogram
(CBC) with
differential
_____ 80076 Hepatic
function panel
_____ 85018 HGB
_____ 86701 HIV-1
_____ 83002 LH
_____ 80061 Lipid panel
_____ 86617 Lyme
antibody

_____ 86308 Monospot
test
_____ 88150 Pap
_____ 85610 Prothrombin
time
_____ 84152 PSA
_____ 86430 Rheumatoid
factor
_____ 82270 Stool
hemoccult x 3
_____ 87430 Strep screen
_____ 84478 Triglycerides
_____ 84443 TSH
_____ 81001 UA with
microscopy
_____ 87088 UC
_____ 84550 Uric acid,
blood
_____ 81025 Urine
pregnancy test
_____
_____

Injections:
_____ (90471) admin 1 vac
_____ (90472) each add'l
vac
_____ 90716 Chickenpox
_____ 90702 DT
_____ (90701) DTP
_____ 90657 Influenza
6-35 months
_____ 90658 Influenza
3 years +
_____ 90665 Lyme
disease
_____ 90707 MMR
_____ 90704 Mumps
_____ (90713) Polio vac
inactivated (IPV)
_____ 90703 Tetanus Tox
ECG: _____ 93000 ECG

Other
_____
_____

| No. | Date | Description | Charge | Credit | | Current Balance |
				Payment	Adjustment	

Patient Information

3449 W. Foster Avenue
Address

Chicago, IL 60625-2377
City, State, ZIP

312-555-9565   312-555-8857
Home phone   **Work phone**

self
Responsible person   **Relationship**

Prudential Group Health   255-74-1021
Insurance   **Contract numbers**

Patient _____ Gary Robertson _____

Date: 10/27/20--   **Chart #**

Karen Larsen, MD   **Diagnoses:**
2235 S. Ridgeway Avenue
Chicago, IL 60623-2240   1. __590.10__

312-555-6022   2. _____

Fax: 312-555-0025   3. _____

4. _____

OFFICE VISITS

New Patient	**Established Patient**

Preventive Medicine

		_____ 99381	under 1 year	_____ 99391		
_____ 99201		_____ 99382	1–4	_____ 99392	_____ 99211	
_____ 99202		_____ 99383	5–11	_____ 99393	_____ 99212	
_____ 99203		_____ 99384	12–17	_____ 99394	_____ 99213	
_____ 99204		_____ 99385	18–39	_____ 99395	_____ 99214	
_____ 99205		_____ 99386	40–64	_____ 99396	_____ 99215	
		_____ 99387	65+	_____ 99397		

Hospital Visits
Initial:
_____ 99221
_____ 99222
_____ 99223
Subsequent:
x 3 (99231)
_____ 99232
_____ 99233
Nursing Facility
Initial:
_____ 99304
_____ 99305
_____ 99306

Other
_____
_____

Visits:
    10/21
    10/23
    10/25

Lab:
_____ 80048 Basic
    metabolic panel
    (SMA-8)
_____ 87110 Chlamydia
    culture
_____ 85651 ESR;
    nonautomated
_____ 83001 FSH
_____ 82947 Glucose,
    blood
_____ 85025 Hemogram
    (CBC) with
    differential
_____ 80076 Hepatic
    function panel
_____ 85018 HGB
_____ 86701 HIV-1
_____ 83002 LH
_____ 80061 Lipid panel
_____ 86617 Lyme
    antibody

_____ 86308 Monospot
    test
_____ 88150 Pap
_____ 85610 Prothrombin
    time
_____ 84152 PSA
_____ 86430 Rheumatoid
    factor
_____ 82270 Stool
    hemoccult x 3
_____ 87430 Strep screen
_____ 84478 Triglycerides
_____ 84443 TSH
_____ 81001 UA with
    microscopy
_____ 87088 UC
_____ 84550 Uric acid,
    blood
_____ 81025 Urine
    pregnancy test

_____
_____

Injections:
_____ 90471 admin 1 vac
_____ 90472 each add'l
    vac
_____ 90716 Chickenpox
_____ 90702 DT
_____ 90701 DTP
_____ 90657 Influenza
    6-35 months
_____ 90658 Influenza
    3 years +
_____ 90665 Lyme
    disease
_____ 90707 MMR
_____ 90704 Mumps
_____ 90713 Polio vac
    inactivated (IPV)
_____ 90703 Tetanus Tox
ECG: _____ 93000 ECG

Other
_____
_____

Checks Received: Daily Journal #106

NO. 5321
20 – 62
710

October 24 20 --

PAY TO THE ORDER OF Karen Larsen, MD $ 44 00/100

Forty-four and no/100 _____ DOLLARS

First National Bank
Chicago, IL 60623-2791

FOR _____ *Charles Jonathan*

⑈0710⑈0062 242⑈046580⑈

NO. 10082
20 – 62
710

October 24 20 --

PAY TO THE ORDER OF Karen Larsen, MD $ 44 and no/100

Forty-four and no/100 _____ DOLLARS

First National Bank
Chicago, IL 60623-2791

FOR *Cheng Sun Worker's Comp* *Billings, Inc.*

⑈0710⑈0062 202⑈056232⑈

NO. 152462
20 – 62
710

October 24 20 --

PAY TO THE ORDER OF Karen Larsen, MD $ 143 and 20/100

One hundred forty-three and 20/100 _____ DOLLARS

Chicago Bank
Chicago, IL 60621

FOR *David Kramer* *New York Mutual*

⑈0710⑈0155 262⑈025592⑈

NO. 152463
20 – 62
710

October 24 20 --

PAY TO THE ORDER OF Karen Larsen, MD $ 90 and 40/100

Ninety and 40/100 _____ DOLLARS

Chicago Bank
Chicago, IL 60621

FOR *Erin Mitchell* *New York Mutual*

⑈0710⑈0155 262⑈025592⑈

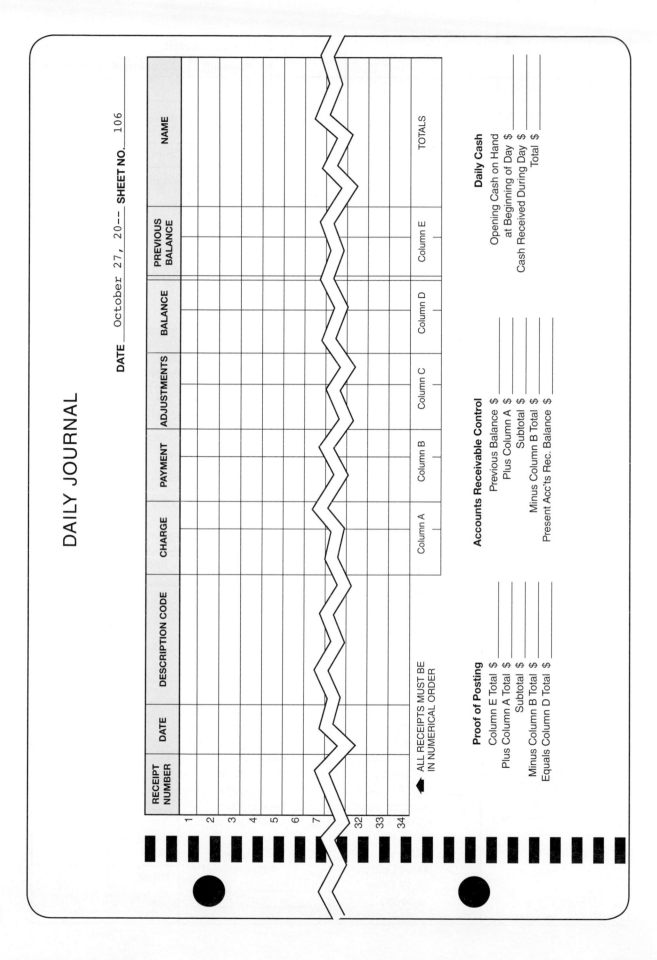

DAILY JOURNAL

DATE ___October 27, 20-- ___ **SHEET NO.** ___106___

RECEIPT NUMBER	DATE	DESCRIPTION CODE	CHARGE	PAYMENT	ADJUSTMENTS	BALANCE	PREVIOUS BALANCE	NAME
1								
2								
3								
4								
5								
6								
7								
32								
33								
34								
			Column A	Column B	Column C	Column D	Column E	TOTALS

◀ ALL RECEIPTS MUST BE IN NUMERICAL ORDER

Proof of Posting

Column E Total $ ____
Plus Column A Total $ ____
Subtotal $ ____
Minus Column B Total $ ____
Equals Column D Total $ ____

Accounts Receivable Control

Previous Balance $ ____
Plus Column A $ ____
Subtotal $ ____
Minus Column B Total $ ____
Present Acc'ts Rec. Balance $ ____

Daily Cash

Opening Cash on Hand
at Beginning of Day $ ____
Cash Received During Day $ ____
Total $ ____

No.	Date	Description	Charge	Credit		Current Balance
				Payment	Adjustment	

Patient Information

5518 Monroe Street
Address

Chicago, IL 60644-5519
City, State, ZIP

312-555-4413   312-555-8825
Home phone   **Work phone**

self
Responsible person   **Relationship**

Blue Cross/Blue Shield, 486-29-3789-1, 2458 Grp
Insurance   **Contract numbers**

Patient _____ Monica Armstrong _____

Date: 10/28/20--   **Chart #**

Karen Larsen, MD
2235 S. Ridgeway Avenue
Chicago, IL 60623-2240

312-555-6022

Fax: 312-555-0025

Diagnoses:

1. 626.2
2. 622.7
3. 785.2
4. _____

OFFICE VISITS

New Patient	Established Patient	

Preventive Medicine

	_____ 99381	under 1 year	_____ 99391	
_____ 99201	_____ 99382	1–4	_____ 99392	_____ 99211
_____ 99202	_____ 99383	5–11	_____ 99393	_____ 99212
_____ 99203	_____ 99384	12–17	_____ 99394	_____ 99213
_____ 99204	_____ 99385	18–39	_____ 99395	_____ 99214
_____ 99205	_____ 99386	40–64	(99396)	_____ 99215
	_____ 99387	65+	_____ 99397	

Hospital Visits
Initial:
_____ 99221
_____ 99222
_____ 99223
Subsequent:
_____ 99231
_____ 99232
_____ 99233
Nursing Facility
Initial:
_____ 99304
_____ 99305
_____ 99306

Other
_____
_____

Lab:
_____ 80048 Basic
 metabolic panel
 (SMA-8)
_____ 87110 Chlamydia
 culture
_____ 85651 ESR;
 nonautomated
_____ 83001 FSH
_____ 82947 Glucose,
 blood
_____ 85025 Hemogram
 (CBC) with
 differential
_____ 80076 Hepatic
 function panel
_____ 85018 HGB
_____ 86701 HIV-1
_____ 83002 LH
_____ 80061 Lipid panel
_____ 86617 Lyme
 antibody

_____ 86308 Monospot
 test
(88150 Pap)
_____ 85610 Prothrombin
 time
_____ 84152 PSA
_____ 86430 Rheumatoid
 factor
_____ 82270 Stool
 hemoccult x 3
_____ 87430 Strep screen
_____ 84478 Triglycerides
_____ 84443 TSH
_____ 81001 UA with
 microscopy
_____ 87088 UC
_____ 84550 Uric acid,
 blood
_____ 81025 Urine
 pregnancy test
_____
_____

Injections:
_____ 90471 admin 1 vac
_____ 90472 each add'l
 vac
_____ 90716 Chickenpox
_____ 90702 DT
_____ 90701 DTP
_____ 90657 Influenza
 6-35 months
_____ 90658 Influenza
 3 years +
_____ 90665 Lyme
 disease
_____ 90707 MMR
_____ 90704 Mumps
_____ 90713 Polio vac
 inactivated (IPV)
_____ 90703 Tetanus Tox
ECG: _____ 93000 ECG

Other
_____
_____

Working Papers

No.	Date	Description	Charge	Credit		Current Balance
				Payment	**Adjustment**	

Patient Information

510 N. Marine Drive
Address

Chicago, IL 60640-5607
City, State, ZIP

	father
312-555-1913	312-555-8820
Home phone	**Work phone**

Andrew Kramer   father
Responsible person   **Relationship**

Northstar Premium Insurance,
747-22-3401-02, Grp 411
Insurance   **Contract numbers**

Patient _____ Jeffrey Kramer _____

Date: 10/28/20-- | **Chart #**

Karen Larsen, MD
2235 S. Ridgeway Avenue
Chicago, IL 60623-2240

312-555-6022

Fax: 312-555-0025

Diagnoses:

1. 382.00

2. 380.10

3. _____

4. _____

OFFICE VISITS

New Patient	**Established Patient**

Preventive Medicine

New Patient		Preventive		Established	Established
	_____ 99381	under 1 year	_____ 99391		
_____ 99201	_____ 99382	1–4	_____ 99392		_____ 99211
_____ 99202	_____ 99383	5–11	_____ 99393		(99212)
_____ 99203	_____ 99384	12–17	_____ 99394		_____ 99213
_____ 99204	_____ 99385	18–39	_____ 99395		_____ 99214
_____ 99205	_____ 99386	40–64	_____ 99396		_____ 99215
	_____ 99387	65+	_____ 99397		

Hospital Visits
Initial:
_____ 99221
_____ 99222
_____ 99223
Subsequent:
_____ 99231
_____ 99232
_____ 99233
Nursing Facility
Initial:
_____ 99304
_____ 99305
_____ 99306

Other

_____

_____

Lab:
_____ 80048 Basic
  metabolic panel
  (SMA-8)
_____ 87110 Chlamydia
  culture
_____ 85651 ESR;
  nonautomated
_____ 83001 FSH
_____ 82947 Glucose,
  blood
_____ 85025 Hemogram
  (CBC) with
  differential
_____ 80076 Hepatic
  function panel
_____ 85018 HGB
_____ 86701 HIV-1
_____ 83002 LH
_____ 80061 Lipid panel
_____ 86617 Lyme
  antibody

_____ 86308 Monospot
  test
_____ 88150 Pap
_____ 85610 Prothrombin
  time
_____ 84152 PSA
_____ 86430 Rheumatoid
  factor
_____ 82270 Stool
  hemoccult x 3
_____ 87430 Strep screen
_____ 84478 Triglycerides
_____ 84443 TSH
_____ 81001 UA with
  microscopy
_____ 87088 UC
_____ 84550 Uric acid,
  blood
_____ 81025 Urine
  pregnancy test

_____

_____

Injections:
_____ 90471 admin 1 vac
_____ 90472 each add'l
  vac
_____ 90716 Chickenpox
_____ 90702 DT
_____ 90701 DTP
_____ 90657 Influenza
  6-35 months
_____ 90658 Influenza
  3 years +
_____ 90665 Lyme
  disease
_____ 90707 MMR
_____ 90704 Mumps
_____ 90713 Polio vac
  inactivated (IPV)
_____ 90703 Tetanus Tox
ECG: _____ 93000 ECG

Other

_____

_____

No.	Date	Description	Charge	Credit		Current Balance
				Payment	Adjustment	

Patient Information		Patient	Cheng Sun

2235 W. School Street
Address

Chicago, IL 60618-5785
City, State, ZIP

312-555-3750   312-555-8149
Home phone   **Work phone**

self

Responsible person   **Relationship**

Metro State Plan,   285-90-9125,35A Grp.
Insurance   **Contract numbers**

Date: 10/28/20--   **Chart #**

Karen Larsen, MD
2235 S. Ridgeway Avenue
Chicago, IL 60623-2240

312-555-6022

Fax: 312-555-0025

Diagnoses:

1. _V70.0_

2. _____

3. _____

4. _____

OFFICE VISITS

New Patient	Established Patient

Preventive Medicine

	_____ 99381	under 1 year	_____ 99391	
_____ 99201	_____ 99382	1–4	_____ 99392	_____ 99211
_____ 99202	_____ 99383	5–11	_____ 99393	_____ 99212
_____ 99203	_____ 99384	12–17	_____ 99394	_____ 99213
_____ 99204	_____ 99385	18–39	_____ 99395	_____ 99214
_____ 99205	_____ 99386	40–64	_____ (99396)	_____ 99215
	_____ 99387	65+	_____ 99397	

Hospital Visits
Initial:
_____ 99221
_____ 99222
_____ 99223
Subsequent:
_____ 99231
_____ 99232
_____ 99233
Nursing Facility
Initial:
_____ 99304
_____ 99305
_____ 99306

Other
_____
_____

Lab:
_____ (80048) Basic metabolic panel (SMA-8)
_____ 87110 Chlamydia culture
_____ 85651 ESR; nonautomated
_____ 83001 FSH
_____ 82947 Glucose, blood
_____ 85025 Hemogram (CBC) with differential
_____ 80076 Hepatic function panel
_____ 85018 HGB
_____ 86701 HIV-1
_____ 83002 LH
_____ (80061) Lipid panel
_____ 86617 Lyme antibody

_____ 86308 Monospot test
_____ 88150 Pap
_____ 85610 Prothrombin time
_____ (84152) PSA
_____ 86430 Rheumatoid factor
_____ (82270) Stool hemoccult x 3
_____ 87430 Strep screen
_____ 84478 Triglycerides
_____ 84443 TSH
_____ (81001) UA with microscopy
_____ 87088 UC
_____ 84550 Uric acid, blood
_____ 81025 Urine pregnancy test
_____
_____

Injections:
_____ 90471 admin 1 vac
_____ 90472 each add'l vac
_____ 90716 Chickenpox
_____ 90702 DT
_____ 90701 DTP
_____ 90657 Influenza 6-35 months
_____ 90658 Influenza 3 years +
_____ 90665 Lyme disease
_____ 90707 MMR
_____ 90704 Mumps
_____ 90713 Polio vac inactivated (IPV)
_____ 90703 Tetanus Tox
ECG: _____ 93000 ECG

Other
_____
_____

Working Papers

Checks Received: Daily Journal #107

NO. 1532106   20 – 62
710

October 24   20 --

PAY
TO THE
ORDER OF   Karen Larsen, MD $ 192 and 80/100

One hundred ninety-two and 80/100 _____ DOLLARS

First National Bank
Chicago, IL 60623-2791

FOR   Monica Armstrong   BC/BS

⑈0710⑈0062 242⑈046580 ⑈'

NO. 1909242   20 – 62
710

October 24   20 --

PAY
TO THE
ORDER OF   Karen Larsen, MD $ 93 and no/100

Ninety-three and no/100 _____ DOLLARS

First National Bank
Chicago, IL 60623-2791

FOR   Laura Lund   Employee Benefit

⑈0710⑈0062 202⑈056232 ⑈'

NO. 19646482   20 – 62
710

October 24   20 --

PAY
TO THE
ORDER OF   Karen Larsen, MD $ 222 and 40/100

Two hundred twenty-two and 40/100 _____ DOLLARS

Chicago Bank
Chicago, IL 60621

FOR   Sara Babcock   Kaiser Insurance

⑈0710⑈0155 262⑈025592 ⑈'

NO. 1227847   20 – 62
710

October 23   20 --

PAY
TO THE
ORDER OF   Karen Larsen, MD $ 147 and 00/100

One hundred forty-seven and 00/100 _____ DOLLARS

First National Bank
Chicago, IL 60623-2791

FOR   Gary Robertson   Prudential Group Health

⑈0710⑈0062 081⑈502249 ⑈'

DAILY JOURNAL

DATE October 28, 20-- **SHEET NO.** 107

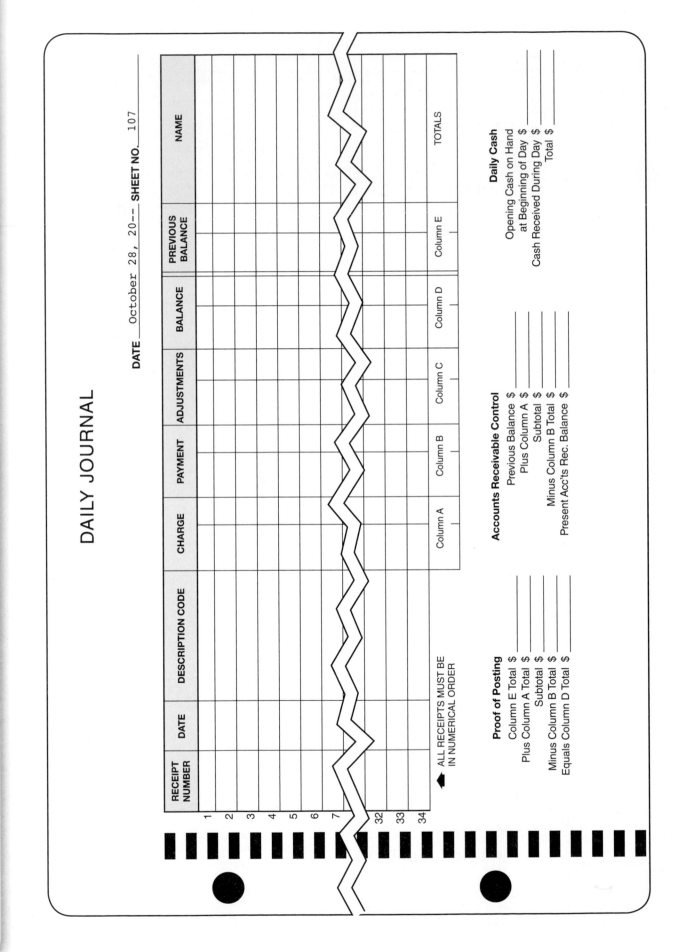

RECEIPT NUMBER	DATE	DESCRIPTION CODE	CHARGE	PAYMENT	ADJUSTMENTS	BALANCE	PREVIOUS BALANCE	NAME
1								
2								
3								
4								
5								
6								
7								
32								
33								
34								
			Column A	Column B	Column C	Column D	Column E	TOTALS

◄ ALL RECEIPTS MUST BE IN NUMERICAL ORDER

Proof of Posting

Column E Total $ ____
Plus Column A Total $ ____
Subtotal $ ____
Minus Column B Total $ ____
Equals Column D Total $ ____

Accounts Receivable Control

Previous Balance $ ____
Plus Column A $ ____
Subtotal $ ____
Minus Column B Total $ ____
Present Acc'ts Rec. Balance $ ____

Daily Cash

Opening Cash on Hand
at Beginning of Day $ ____
Cash Received During Day $ ____
Total $ ____

No.	Date	Description	Charge	Credit Payment	Adjustment	Current Balance

Patient Information

5015 N. Ridgeway Avenue
Address

Chicago, IL 60625-1220
City, State, ZIP

312-555-3478   312-555-8830
Home phone   **Work phone**

self

Responsible person   **Relationship**
University Health Plan,
                    581-57-0376-59, A87 Grp
Insurance   **Contract numbers**

Patient _____ Thomas Baab _____

Date: 10/29/20-- | **Chart #**

Karen Larsen, MD
2235 S. Ridgeway Avenue
Chicago, IL 60623-2240

312-555-6022

Fax: 312-555-0025

Diagnoses:

1. ___ V70.0 ___

2. _____

3. _____

4. _____

OFFICE VISITS

New Patient	Established Patient

Preventive Medicine

	_____ 99381	under 1 year	_____ 99391	
_____ 99201	_____ 99382	1–4	_____ 99392	_____ 99211
_____ 99202	_____ 99383	5–11	_____ 99393	(99212)
_____ 99203	_____ 99384	12–17	_____ 99394	_____ 99213
_____ 99204	_____ 99385	18–39	_____ 99395	_____ 99214
_____ 99205	_____ 99386	40–64	_____ 99396	_____ 99215
	_____ 99387	65+	_____ 99397	

Hospital Visits
Initial:
_____ 99221
_____ 99222
_____ 99223
Subsequent:
_____ 99231
_____ 99232
_____ 99233
Nursing Facility
Initial:
_____ 99304
_____ 99305
_____ 99306

Other
_____
_____

Lab:
_____ 80048 Basic
metabolic panel
(SMA-8)
_____ 87110 Chlamydia
culture
_____ 85651 ESR;
nonautomated
_____ 83001 FSH
_____ 82947 Glucose,
blood
_____ 85025 Hemogram
(CBC) with
differential
_____ 80076 Hepatic
function panel
_____ 85018 HGB
_____ 86701 HIV-1
_____ 83002 LH
_____ 80061 Lipid panel
_____ 86617 Lyme
antibody

_____ 86308 Monospot
test
_____ 88150 Pap
_____ 85610 Prothrombin
time
_____ 84152 PSA
_____ 86430 Rheumatoid
factor
_____ 82270 Stool
hemoccult x 3
_____ 87430 Strep screen
_____ 84478 Triglycerides
_____ 84443 TSH
_____ 81001 UA with
microscopy
_____ 87088 UC
_____ 84550 Uric acid,
blood
_____ 81025 Urine
pregnancy test

_____
_____

Injections:
_____ 90471 admin 1 vac
_____ 90472 each add'l
vac
_____ 90716 Chickenpox
_____ 90702 DT
_____ 90701 DTP
_____ 90657 Influenza
6-35 months
_____ 90658 Influenza
3 years +
_____ 90665 Lyme
disease
_____ 90707 MMR
_____ 90704 Mumps
_____ 90713 Polio vac
inactivated (IPV)
_____ 90703 Tetanus Tox
ECG: _____ 93000 ECG

Other
_____
_____

No.	Date	Description	Charge	Credit		Current Balance
				Payment	Adjustment	

Patient Information

105 W. Chestnut Street
Address

Chicago, IL 60610-2816
City, State, ZIP

312-555-2231   312-555-2583
Home phone   **Work phone**

self
Responsible person   **Relationship**

University Health Plan,
                     797-90-1128, S357C Grp.
Insurance   **Contract numbers**

Patient _____ Theresa Dayton _____

Date: 10/29/20--   **Chart #**

Karen Larsen, MD   **Diagnoses:**
2235 S. Ridgeway Avenue
Chicago, IL 60623-2240 1. _307.81_

312-555-6022   2. _____

Fax: 312-555-0025   3. _____

                            4. _____

OFFICE VISITS

New Patient	**Established Patient**

Preventive Medicine

	_____ 99381	under 1 year	_____ 99391	
_____ 99201	_____ 99382	1–4	_____ 99392	_____ 99211
_____ 99202	_____ 99383	5–11	_____ 99393	(99212)
_____ 99203	_____ 99384	12–17	_____ 99394	_____ 99213
_____ 99204	_____ 99385	18–39	_____ 99395	_____ 99214
_____ 99205	_____ 99386	40–64	_____ 99396	_____ 99215
	_____ 99387	65+	_____ 99397	

Hospital Visits
Initial:
_____ 99221
_____ 99222
_____ 99223
Subsequent:
_____ 99231
_____ 99232
_____ 99233
Nursing Facility
Initial:
_____ 99304
_____ 99305
_____ 99306

Other
_____
_____

Lab:
_____ 80048 Basic
metabolic panel
(SMA-8)
_____ 87110 Chlamydia
culture
_____ 85651 ESR;
nonautomated
_____ 83001 FSH
_____ 82947 Glucose,
blood
_____ 85025 Hemogram
(CBC) with
differential
_____ 80076 Hepatic
function panel
_____ 85018 HGB
_____ 86701 HIV-1
_____ 83002 LH
_____ 80061 Lipid panel
_____ 86617 Lyme
antibody

_____ 86308 Monospot
test
_____ 88150 Pap
_____ 85610 Prothrombin
time
_____ 84152 PSA
_____ 86430 Rheumatoid
factor
_____ 82270 Stool
hemoccult x 3
_____ 87430 Strep screen
_____ 84478 Triglycerides
_____ 84443 TSH
_____ 81001 UA with
microscopy
_____ 87088 UC
_____ 84550 Uric acid,
blood
_____ 81025 Urine
pregnancy test
_____
_____

Injections:
_____ 90471 admin 1 vac
_____ 90472 each add'l
vac
_____ 90716 Chickenpox
_____ 90702 DT
_____ 90701 DTP
_____ 90657 Influenza
6-35 months
_____ 90658 Influenza
3 years +
_____ 90665 Lyme
disease
_____ 90707 MMR
_____ 90704 Mumps
_____ 90713 Polio vac
inactivated (IPV)
_____ 90703 Tetanus Tox
ECG: _____ 93000 ECG

Other
_____
_____

Working Papers

No.	Date	Description	Charge	Credit		Current Balance
				Payment	Adjustment	

Patient Information

4443 W. Monroe Street

Address

Chicago, IL 60624-8966

City, State, ZIP

312-555-3178   312-555-8848

Home phone   **Work phone**

Earl Matthews   husband

Responsible person   **Relationship**

Arling Employee Plan,

294-82-8099-02, 33A Grp

Insurance   **Contract numbers**

Patient _____ Ardis Matthews _____

Date: 10/29/20--   **Chart #**

Karen Larsen, MD
2235 S. Ridgeway Avenue
Chicago, IL 60623-2240

312-555-6022

Fax: 312-555-0025

Diagnoses:

1. _008.8_____

2. _____

3. _____

4. _____

OFFICE VISITS

New Patient	**Established Patient**

Preventive Medicine

	_____ 99381	under 1 year	_____ 99391	
_____ 99201	_____ 99382	1–4	_____ 99392	_____ 99211
_____ 99202	_____ 99383	5–11	_____ 99393	(99212)
_____ 99203	_____ 99384	12–17	_____ 99394	_____ 99213
_____ 99204	_____ 99385	18–39	_____ 99395	_____ 99214
_____ 99205	_____ 99386	40–64	_____ 99396	_____ 99215
	_____ 99387	65+	_____ 99397	

Hospital Visits

Initial:
_____ 99221
_____ 99222
_____ 99223

Subsequent:
_____ 99231
_____ 99232
_____ 99233

Nursing Facility

Initial:
_____ 99304
_____ 99305
_____ 99306

Other

_____
_____

Lab:
_____ 80048 Basic metabolic panel (SMA-8)
_____ 87110 Chlamydia culture
_____ 85651 ESR; nonautomated
_____ 83001 FSH
_____ 82947 Glucose, blood
_____ 85025 Hemogram (CBC) with differential
_____ 80076 Hepatic function panel
_____ 85018 HGB
_____ 86701 HIV-1
_____ 83002 LH
_____ 80061 Lipid panel
_____ 86617 Lyme antibody

_____ 86308 Monospot test
_____ 88150 Pap
_____ 85610 Prothrombin time
_____ 84152 PSA
_____ 86430 Rheumatoid factor
_____ 82270 Stool hemoccult x 3
_____ 87430 Strep screen
_____ 84478 Triglycerides
_____ 84443 TSH
_____ 81001 UA with microscopy
_____ 87088 UC
_____ 84550 Uric acid, blood
_____ 81025 Urine pregnancy test
_____
_____

Injections:
_____ 90471 admin 1 vac
_____ 90472 each add'l vac
_____ 90716 Chickenpox
_____ 90702 DT
_____ 90701 DTP
_____ 90657 Influenza 6-35 months
_____ 90658 Influenza 3 years +
_____ 90665 Lyme disease
_____ 90707 MMR
_____ 90704 Mumps
_____ 90713 Polio vac inactivated (IPV)
_____ 90703 Tetanus Tox
ECG: _____ 93000 ECG

Other
_____
_____

No.	Date	Description	Charge	Credit		Current Balance
				Payment	Adjustment	

Patient Information

3457 W. 63d Place
Address

Chicago, IL 60629-4270
City, State, ZIP

312-555-3606
Home phone   **Work phone**

self
Responsible person   **Relationship**

Blue Cross & Blue Shield,
                      295-99-3325, 354 Grp.
Insurance   **Contract numbers**

Patient _____ Ana Mendez _____

Date: 10/29/20--   **Chart #**

Karen Larsen, MD   **Diagnoses:**
2235 S. Ridgeway Avenue
Chicago, IL 60623-2240   1. _____

312-555-6022   2. _____

Fax: 312-555-0025   3. _____

                                4. _____

OFFICE VISITS

New Patient	**Established Patient**

Preventive Medicine

New Patient	Preventive Medicine		Established Patient	
	_____ 99381	under 1 year	_____ 99391	
_____ 99201	_____ 99382	1–4	_____ 99392	_____ 99211
_____ 99202	_____ 99383	5–11	_____ 99393	(99212)
_____ 99203	_____ 99384	12–17	_____ 99394	_____ 99213
_____ 99204	_____ 99385	18–39	_____ 99395	_____ 99214
_____ 99205	_____ 99386	40–64	_____ 99396	_____ 99215
	_____ 99387	65+	_____ 99397	

Hospital Visits
Initial:
_____ 99221
_____ 99222
_____ 99223
Subsequent:
_____ 99231
_____ 99232
_____ 99233
Nursing Facility
Initial:
_____ 99304
_____ 99305
_____ 99306

Other
_____
_____

Lab:
_____ 80048 Basic
          metabolic panel
          (SMA-8)
_____ 87110 Chlamydia
          culture
_____ 85651 ESR;
          nonautomated
_____ 83001 FSH
_____ 82947 Glucose,
          blood
_____ 85025 Hemogram
          (CBC) with
          differential
_____ 80076 Hepatic
          function panel
_____ 85018 HGB
_____ 86701 HIV-1
_____ 83002 LH
_____ 80061 Lipid panel
_____ 86617 Lyme
          antibody

_____ 86308 Monospot
          test
_____ 88150 Pap
_____ 85610 Prothrombin
          time
_____ 84152 PSA
_____ 86430 Rheumatoid
          factor
_____ 82270 Stool
          hemoccult x 3
_____ 87430 Strep screen
_____ 84478 Triglycerides
_____ 84443 TSH
_____ 81001 UA with
          microscopy
_____ 87088 UC
_____ 84550 Uric acid,
          blood
_____ 81025 Urine
          pregnancy test

_____
_____

Injections:
_____ 90471 admin 1 vac
_____ 90472 each add'l
          vac
_____ 90716 Chickenpox
_____ 90702 DT
_____ 90701 DTP
_____ 90657 Influenza
          6-35 months
_____ 90658 Influenza
          3 years +
_____ 90665 Lyme
          disease
_____ 90707 MMR
_____ 90704 Mumps
_____ 90713 Polio vac
          inactivated (IPV)
_____ 90703 Tetanus Tox
ECG: _____ 93000 ECG

Other
_____
_____

No.	Date	Description	Charge	Credit		Current Balance
				Payment	Adjustment	

Patient Information

3449 W. Foster Avenue
Address

Chicago, IL 60625-2377
City, State, ZIP

312-555-9565   312-555-8857
Home phone   **Work phone**

self
Responsible person   **Relationship**

Prudential Group Health,   255-74-1021
Insurance   **Contract numbers**

Patient _____ Gary Robertson _____

Date: 10/29/20--   **Chart #**

Karen Larsen, MD   **Diagnoses:**
2235 S. Ridgeway Avenue
Chicago, IL 60623-2240   1. __590.80__

312-555-6022   2. _____

Fax: 312-555-0025   3. _____

4. _____

OFFICE VISITS

New Patient	**Established Patient**

Preventive Medicine

	_____ 99381	under 1 year	_____ 99391	
_____ 99201	_____ 99382	1–4	_____ 99392	_____ 99211
_____ 99202	_____ 99383	5–11	_____ 99393	(99212)
_____ 99203	_____ 99384	12–17	_____ 99394	_____ 99213
_____ 99204	_____ 99385	18–39	_____ 99395	_____ 99214
_____ 99205	_____ 99386	40–64	_____ 99396	_____ 99215
	_____ 99387	65+	_____ 99397	

Hospital Visits
Initial:
_____ 99221
_____ 99222
_____ 99223
Subsequent:
_____ 99231
_____ 99232
_____ 99233
Nursing Facility
Initial:
_____ 99304
_____ 99305
_____ 99306

Other

_____
_____

Lab:
_____ 80048 Basic metabolic panel (SMA-8)
_____ 87110 Chlamydia culture
_____ 85651 ESR; nonautomated
_____ 83001 FSH
_____ 82947 Glucose, blood
_____ 85025 Hemogram (CBC) with differential
_____ 80076 Hepatic function panel
_____ 85018 HGB
_____ 86701 HIV-1
_____ 83002 LH
_____ 80061 Lipid panel
_____ 86617 Lyme antibody

_____ 86308 Monospot test
_____ 88150 Pap
_____ 85610 Prothrombin time
_____ 84152 PSA
_____ 86430 Rheumatoid factor
_____ 82270 Stool hemoccult x 3
_____ 87430 Strep screen
_____ 84478 Triglycerides
_____ 84443 TSH
_____ 81001 UA with microscopy
_____ 87088 UC
_____ 84550 Uric acid, blood
_____ 81025 Urine pregnancy test

_____
_____

Injections:
_____ 90471 admin 1 vac
_____ 90472 each add'l vac
_____ 90716 Chickenpox
_____ 90702 DT
_____ 90701 DTP
_____ 90657 Influenza 6-35 months
_____ 90658 Influenza 3 years +
_____ 90665 Lyme disease
_____ 90707 MMR
_____ 90704 Mumps
_____ 90713 Polio vac inactivated (IPV)
_____ 90703 Tetanus Tox
ECG: _____ 93000 ECG

Other

_____
_____

No.	Date	Description	Charge	Credit		Current Balance
				Payment	**Adjustment**	

Patient Information	**Patient**	Florence Sherman

6111 N. Lincoln Avenue
Address

Chicago, IL 60608-3173
City, State, ZIP

312-555-1217
Home phone   **Work phone**

self
Responsible person   **Relationship**

Medicare   669-35-2244B
Insurance   **Contract numbers**

Date: 10/29/20--   **Chart #**

Karen Larsen, MD   **Diagnoses:**
2235 S. Ridgeway Avenue
Chicago, IL 60623-2240   1. _920_

312-555-6022   2. _923.03_

Fax: 312-555-0025   3. _____

                             4. _____

OFFICE VISITS

New Patient	**Established Patient**

Preventive Medicine

	_____ 99381	under 1 year	_____ 99391	
_____ 99201	_____ 99382	1–4	_____ 99392	_____ 99211
_____ 99202	_____ 99383	5–11	_____ 99393	(99212)
_____ 99203	_____ 99384	12–17	_____ 99394	_____ 99213
_____ 99204	_____ 99385	18–39	_____ 99395	_____ 99214
_____ 99205	_____ 99386	40–64	_____ 99396	_____ 99215
	_____ 99387	65+	_____ 99397	

Hospital Visits
Initial:
_____ 99221
_____ 99222
_____ 99223
Subsequent:
_____ 99231
_____ 99232
_____ 99233
Nursing Facility
Initial:
_____ 99304
_____ 99305
_____ 99306

Other
_____
_____

Lab:
_____ 80048 Basic
       metabolic panel
       (SMA-8)
_____ 87110 Chlamydia
       culture
_____ 85651 ESR;
       nonautomated
_____ 83001 FSH
_____ 82947 Glucose,
       blood
_____ 85025 Hemogram
       (CBC) with
       differential
_____ 80076 Hepatic
       function panel
_____ 85018 HGB
_____ 86701 HIV-1
_____ 83002 LH
_____ 80061 Lipid panel
_____ 86617 Lyme
       antibody

_____ 86308 Monospot
       test
_____ 88150 Pap
_____ 85610 Prothrombin
       time
_____ 84152 PSA
_____ 86430 Rheumatoid
       factor
_____ 82270 Stool
       hemoccult x 3
_____ 87430 Strep screen
_____ 84478 Triglycerides
_____ 84443 TSH
_____ 81001 UA with
       microscopy
_____ 87088 UC
_____ 84550 Uric acid,
       blood
_____ 81025 Urine
       pregnancy test
_____
_____

Injections:
_____ 90471 admin 1 vac
_____ 90472 each add'l
       vac
_____ 90716 Chickenpox
_____ 90702 DT
_____ 90701 DTP
_____ 90657 Influenza
       6-35 months
_____ 90658 Influenza
       3 years +
_____ 90665 Lyme
       disease
_____ 90707 MMR
_____ 90704 Mumps
_____ 90713 Polio vac
       inactivated (IPV)
_____ 90703 Tetanus Tox
ECG: _____ 93000 ECG

Other
_____
_____

Checks Received: Daily Journal #108

NO. 439205   20 – 62 / 710

October 22   20 --

PAY TO THE ORDER OF   Karen Larsen, MD $ 114 and no/100

One hundred fourteen and 00/100 _____ DOLLARS

First National Bank
Chicago, IL 60623-2791

FOR Todd Grant   Prudential Plan

⑆0710⑈0062 081⑈502249⑈

NO. 1983425   20 – 62 / 710

October 20   20 --

PAY TO THE ORDER OF   Karen Larsen, MD $ 42 and 40/100

Forty-two and 40/100 _____ DOLLARS

First National Bank
Chicago, IL 60623-2791

FOR Raymond Murrary   Medicare

⑆0710⑈0062 242⑈046580⑈

NO. 475   20 – 62 / 710

October 23   20 --

PAY TO THE ORDER OF   Karen Larsen, MD $ 86 and 20/100

Eighty-six and 20/100 _____ DOLLARS

First National Bank
Chicago, IL 60623-2791

FOR _____   Clarence Rogers

⑆0710⑈0062 202⑈056232⑈

NO. 704382   20 – 62 / 710

October 22   20 --

PAY TO THE ORDER OF   Karen Larsen, MD $ 66 and 40/100

Sixty-six and 40/100 _____ DOLLARS

Chicago Bank
Chicago, IL 60621

FOR Stephen Villano   Employee Benefit Plan

⑆0710⑈0155 262⑈025592⑈

DAILY JOURNAL

DATE ___October 29, 20-- ___ **SHEET NO.** ___108___

RECEIPT NUMBER	DATE	DESCRIPTION CODE	CHARGE	PAYMENT	ADJUSTMENTS	BALANCE	PREVIOUS BALANCE	NAME
1								
2								
3								
4								
5								
6								
7								
32								
33								
34								
TOTALS			Column A	Column B	Column C	Column D	Column E	

◄ ALL RECEIPTS MUST BE IN NUMERICAL ORDER

Proof of Posting

Column E Total $ ___
Plus Column A Total $ ___
Subtotal $ ___
Minus Column B Total $ ___
Equals Column D Total $ ___

Accounts Receivable Control

Previous Balance $ ___
Plus Column A $ ___
Subtotal $ ___
Minus Column B Total $ ___
Present Acc'ts Rec. Balance $ ___

Daily Cash

Opening Cash on Hand
at Beginning of Day $ ___
Cash Received During Day $ ___
Total $ ___